Health Education for Women

A Guide for Nurses and
Other Health Professionals

Health Education for Women

A Guide for Nurses and Other Health Professionals

Edited by
Vivian M. Littlefield, Ph.D., R.N.
Dean and Professor
University of Wisconsin–Madison
School of Nursing
Madison, Wisconsin
Formerly Chairperson and Clinical Chief of OB/GYN Nursing
University of Rochester
Strong Memorial Hospital
Rochester, New York

APPLETON-CENTURY-CROFTS/Norwalk, Connecticut

0-8385-3669-7

86 87 88 89 90 / 10 9 8 7 6 5 4 3 2 1

Prentice-Hall of Australia, Pty. Ltd., Sydney
Prentice-Hall Canada, Inc.
Prentice-Hall Hispanoamericana, S.A., Mexico
Prentice-Hall of India Private Limited, New Delhi
Prentice-Hall International (UK) Limited, London
Prentice-Hall of Japan, Inc., Tokyo
Prentice-Hall of Southeast Asia (Pte.) Ltd., Singapore
Whitehall Books Ltd., Wellington, New Zealand
Editora Prentice-Hall do Brasil Ltda., Rio de Janeiro

Library of Congress Cataloging-in-Publication Data
Main entry under title:
Health Education for Women: A Guide for Nurses
& Other Health Professionals

   Includes index.
   1. Health education of women.   2. Women—Health
and hygiene—Study and teaching.   3. Obstetrics—
Study and teaching.   4. Gynecology—Study and
teaching.   I. Littlefield, Vivian M.   [DNLM: 1. Gynecology.   2. Health Education.   3. Obstetrics.
WP 100 E24]
RA440.5.E38   1986   613'.0424'071   85-32062
ISBN 0-8385-3669-7

Design: M. Chandler Martylewski

PRINTED IN THE UNITED STATES OF AMERICA

Contributors

Barbara N. Adams, M.S., R.N.,C.
Associate Professor of Nursing (Women's Health Care)
Interim Chairman of Women's Health Care Program
University of Rochester, School of Nursing
Clinician II, Strong Memorial Hospital
Rochester, New York

Jane Ahrens, M.S.
Certified Childbirth Instructor
Childbirth Education Association
Rochester, New York

Patricia M. Allen, B.S.N., R.N.
Nursing Coordinator of High Risk Obstetric Clinic
University of Rochester, School of Nursing
Level III Staff Nurse, Strong Memorial Hospital
Rochester, New York

Carole A. Anderson, Ph.D., R.N.
Associate Professor of Nursing and of Psychiatry
Associate Dean for Graduate Studies
University of Rochester, School of Nursing
Rochester, New York

Margret Banton, M.S.
Formerly Assistant Professor
University of Rochester, School of Nursing
Rochester, New York

Theresa A. Caffery, M.S., R.N.,C.
Instructor in Nursing (Women's Health Care)
University of Rochester, School of Nursing
Clinician II, Strong Memorial Hospital
Rochester, New York

Terry L. Campney Callison, M.Ed., M.S.
Graduate Assistant and Instructor
Department of Psychology
Syracuse University
Syracuse, New York

Patricia Camillo, M.S., R.N.,C.
Full-time faculty
State University of New York at New Paltz
RN/BS Program
OB/GYN Nurse Practitioner at Planned Parenthood of New Paltz
Private Practice: Health Education and Counseling for Women
New Paltz, New York

Patricia Clancy, B.S.N.
Clinical Nurse III
Memorial Sloan-Kettering Cancer Center
New York, New York

Phyllis Collier, M.S.P.H., R.N.
Assistant Professor in Nursing (Women's Health Care)
University of Rochester, School of Nursing
Clinician II, Strong Memorial Hospital
Rochester, New York

Ann Marie Dozier, M.S., R.N.
Senior Associate in Nursing (Women's Health Care)
University of Rochester, School of Nursing
Clinician II
Associate Clinical Chief for OB/GYN Nursing
Strong Memorial Hospital
Rochester, New York

Laurence B. Guttmacher, M.D.
Assistant Professor of Psychiatry
University of Rochester
Rochester, New York

Colleen Keenan, M.S., R.N.,C.
Formerly Assistant Professor
University of Rochester, School of Nursing
Clinician II, Strong Memorial Hospital
Rochester, New York

Dona J. Lethbridge, M.A., R.N.
Assistant Professor
Nursing Department
School of Health Studies
University of New Hampshire
Durham, New Hampshire

Vivian M. Littlefield, Ph.D., R.N.
Dean and Professor
University of Wisconsin–Madison
School of Nursing
Madison, Wisconsin
Formerly Chairperson and Clinical Chief of OB/GYN Nursing
University of Rochester
Strong Memorial Hospital
Rochester, New York

Geri LoBiondo-Wood, Ph.D., R.N.
Associate Professor
University of Nebraska
College of Nursing
Omaha, Nebraska

Barbara Lum, M.S., R.N.
Clinician II (Women's Health Care)
Strong Memorial Hospital
Rochester, New York

Phyllis Sale, B.S.N., R.N.
Clinician I, OB/GYN Outpatient Department
Strong Memorial Hospital
Rochester, New York

Leslie Skillman, M.S., R.N.,C.
Assistant Professor of Nursing (Women's Health Care)
University of Rochester, School of Nursing
Clinician II, Strong Memorial Hospital
Rochester, New York

Mary Sprik, M.S., R.N.,C.
Senior Associate in Nursing
University of Rochester, School of Nursing
Coordinator, Rochester Adolescent Maternity Program
Clinician II, Strong Memorial Hospital
Rochester, New York

Diony Young, B.A.
Public Policy Liaison and Consultant
International Childbirth Education Association
Geneseo, New York

Contents

Preface

This text is designed to provide both process and content for educating women about their health and illness. It is a guide for practicing nurses (including nurse midwives and practitioners), physicians, social workers, health educators, and others to teach women what they need to know to prevent illness, enhance well-being, recover from illness, and have a positive reproductive experience. The text is written with the assumption that the reader has a basic knowledge in obstetrics and gynecology. If the reader's knowledge and experience is limited, then the text must be used as a companion to other clinical texts in women's health care or obstetrics and gynecology.

The uniqueness of the text is that it includes both educational theory and specific content related to women's health and illness. The editor combines a background in education and psychology with long years of clinical experience in women's health. All contributing authors are clinicians, primarily nurses, who currently apply the content of the chapters they write to direct clinical practice. These clinicians and the editor are also involved in health education for women and teach advanced nurse clinicians/practitioners the content presented.

The text is divided into five parts. Part I addresses the questions of why, how, and what related to educating women in health and illness. Part I draws heavily on the literature in education and psychology and condenses the educational process into one chapter of critical content. Selected theories and processes are described to assist women clients to experience involvement in learning and to achieve participation in their own care. What content is needed for women is identified from a life-cycle developmental perspective.

Part II describes content for general and reproductive health promotion. This section describes processes and methodologies for discovering womanhood and sexual self-awareness, making contraceptive decisions, and preparing for stresses of life. In addition, health promotion for women in selected developmental periods and during reproduction is included. The health needs of women who are disabled or homosexual are discussed to assist health providers to focus on the health promotion and well-being of these clients.

Part III describes education when there are special reproductive needs such as adolescent pregnancy, unintended pregnancy, cesarean births, and when pregnancy is at risk. Part IV focuses on gynecological problems. Minor (i.e., vaginal infection) and major (i.e., cancer) problems are described as is education for women undergoing breast surgery for cancer.

Part V describes psychosocial problems that have special relevance for women and for which women frequently seek help from clinicians in obstetrics and gynecology. The authors in this section are a physician and psychiatric nurses who have additional preparation in either obstetrics and gynecology or women's health.

The appendices are designed as tools to use in the clinical setting for a number of care providers who teach women during the reproductive experience. These have been used in clinical settings, for which the editor was the nurse administrator.

Special appreciation is given to the authors who not only wrote chapters in this text, but concurrently created unique health care clinics for women, designed graduate education in women's health care, and conducted research. These authors also cared about each other, their students, colleagues, and the editor. Also, special thanks is given to those typists (Kathy Start, Mike Sprik, and, especially, Sandy Webster) who continued to revise yet another draft. To our committed graduate assistant, Gloria Escalona, is given special praise. Without her, the work would not be a reality.

Vivian M. Littlefield, Ph.D., R.N.

Education for Women's Health: Why? How? What?

Part I addresses the questions of why, how, and what related to educating women for health and in illness. Rationale for why education is especially important to women's health is given in Chapter 1. The educational process for the clinician is described in Chapter 2. Variables influencing learning, theories of teaching–learning, and evaluation of learning are summarized. Literature from education and psychology is cited and applied to women's learning health behaviors as well as their learning in relation to illness and medical intervention. Chapter 3 elaborates on adult learning and decision-making theories. These theories are described because they propose to assist individuals to become actively involved in learning and to achieve participation in health care. Chapter 4 is an organizing framework for the remainder of the book. A developmental framework is proposed to guide the teacher in identifying what content should be taught for women in each age group. Two examples of health teaching (menstrual education and breast self-exam) are given to demonstrate the use of a developmental framework to identify needs of teaching women throughout the life cycle.

Health Education for Women: Why?

1

Vivian M. Littlefield

Introduction. Health education aimed at prevention will be one of *the* most critical components of future health care. There is a growing trend to focus on prevention and alternative approaches to expensive hospitalization. For example, minor surgeries, birth, evaluation of health status, and treatment of chronic and age-related disabilities are being performed outside of traditional health care facilities by a wider variety of health professionals. These alternatives require a major emphasis on education as well as involvement by health care consumers.

Women's health needs, unique because they relate to life experiences versus illness, lend themselves to educational strategies. Illnesses unique to women or for which women are at higher risk are frequently viewed with negative connotations, surrounded with myths, or seen as defeminizing. Education is needed to counter negative attitudes and demystify women's health problems. Education becomes a necessity versus a frill in these circumstances.

Women's changing life-styles and recent socialization encourage new expectations for involvement and participation with health care professionals in preventive as well as illness care. Today's women are expecting accurate; complete information concerning their health, bodies, and development. Women want to be involved in decisions about medical interventions for themselves and their families. This involvement requires well-informed consumers and thrusts on all health professionals (nurses, physicians, social workers, psychologists, and health educators) a major responsibility to provide information.

This text has been written to assist health care professionals to provide education for women in health and illness. It is designed especially for those professionals who are specialists in obstetrics and gynecology with a commitment to provide general health information to the women they serve. Nurses, nurse practitioners, and nurse midwives will find the text useful because a primary focus of their practice is on education. Physicians who are general practitioners, family physicians, or obstetrician–gynecologists will find the text useful if a major thrust of their intervention is educational. Social workers, psychologists, and health educators will also find the information and strategies useful to their practice.

First, the question of *why* a special emphasis on educating women for health and illness care is addressed (Chapter 1). Then the questions of *how* to provide education are described (Chapters 2 and 3). Special approaches and techniques for enhancing women's self-esteem and ability to effectively participate in health promotion and illness care are

3

described. This content is developed from literature and research in adult education and psychology. Finally, the question of *what* content is needed for women in health and illness is addressed (Chapter 4). Topics for education have been selected because they are unique to women, have special relevance or meaning for women, or are health problems for which women are at high risk (Chapters 5 through 26). These topics reflect health–illness needs throughout the life cycle and include, but are not limited to, reproductive health.

WOMEN AND HEALTH: A GOAL

Special emphasis on health education for women is needed because women actually consider health a significant dimension of life (Knutson, 1965) and pursue health as a goal more often then men (Moore, 1980; Rosenstock, 1969). Also, women, more so than men, tend to be considered responsible for the health of others—their spouse, their children, and significant others who are sick (Sandelowski, 1981). Therefore, assisting women to understand healthy life-styles and how to minimize the impact of illness on themselves and their significant others can improve health for the general population.

Because the majority of illnesses today are the result of life-style and behavior, providing health information has the potential to influence health positively. If health can be improved through education, then the cost of health care for society will decrease.

Health Variants Unique to Women

Physical Health. Women's unique biology places them at differential risk for health and illness, and frequently requires specialized health care. For instance, contraceptive choices are complex, and women's unique childbearing functions serve as a major potential for health risks. These risks can result from the biological demands of childbearing, as well as the potential hazards from iatrogenic effects of medical intervention (Corea, 1977).

Examining morbidity and mortality statistics shows that from birth to death, women have lesser mortality rates (with the exception of diabetes) and live longer than men (Tables 1–1 and 1–2). However, women report more physical and mental morbidity and use health services more often than men. Medically, women may have a greater resistance to infections (Waldron, 1976), become less incapacitated with chronic disease, and have cancers that are easier to detect and treat (Pomerleau, 1976; Sandelowski, 1981). Yet, women undergo surgery more frequently, use health services more frequently, even as children (Lewis & Lewis, 1977; Nathanson, 1975), and occupy more nursing home beds than men. Women report their health as less good and more often restricting in their daily activities than do men (Nathanson, 1975).

This presents a paradox (Woods, 1981). Are women as a group more physically healthy than men? This paradox may have its resolution through improved health education of women because one interpretation of the increased treatment of women is that health care professionals, believing myths and stereotypes of women's inadequate health, treat them unnecessarily. Informed and involved women consumers may be able to influence unnecessary medical intervention.

Psychological Health. In the area of psychological health, statistics make women appear less healthy than men. For example, female admissions to outpatient services and inpatient psychiatric private hospitals are higher (Cannon & Redick, 1973; Gove & Tudor, 1973), once admitted they stay longer (Faden & Taube, 1977), and are more often

TABLE 1–1. LIFE EXPECTANCY AT BIRTH AND AT 65 YEARS OF AGE, SELECTED COUNTRIES, SELECTED YEARS, 1969 TO 1976[a]

Country	At Birth		At 65 Years	
	Male	Female	Male	Female
Canada: 1970	69.3	76.2	13.7	17.4
1974	69.6	77.1	13.8	18.0
United States: 1969–1971[b]	67.0	74.6	13.0	16.8
1976	69.0	76.7	13.7	18.0
Sweden: 1970	72.3	77.4	14.4	17.2
1976	72.2	78.1	14.0	17.5
England and Wales: 1970	68.8	75.2	12.0	16.0
1976	69.7	75.8	12.3	16.3
Netherlands: 1970	70.9	76.6	13.6	16.6
1976	71.6	78.1	13.6	17.6
German Democratic Republic: 1970	68.9	74.2	12.9	15.4
1976	68.9	74.5	12.1	14.8
German Federal Republic: 1970	67.3	73.6	11.9	15.0
1975	68.1	74.7	12.2	15.7
France: 1970	69.1	76.7	13.4	17.4
1974	69.5	77.6	13.6	17.8
Switzerland: 1968–1973[b]	70.3	76.2	13.3	16.3
1976	71.7	78.3	14.0	17.7
Italy: 1970	68.5	74.6	13.0	16.1
1974	69.9	76.1	13.6	16.7
Israel[c]: 1970	69.9	73.4	13.5	14.5
1975	71.0	74.7	14.0	15.5
Japan: 1970	69.5	74.9	12.7	15.6
1976	72.3	77.6	14.1	17.0
Australia: 1970	67.4	74.2	11.9	15.7
1975	69.3	76.4	13.1	17.1

Notes: Based on data from World Health Organization: World health statistics, 1970, vol. 1, Geneva 1973, World Health Organization and vol. 1, 1978, United Nations: Demographic yearbook 1976, Pub. No. ST ESA STAT SER R4, New York, 1977, United Nations; National Center for Health Statistics: U.S. Decennial Life Tables for 1969–1971, vol. 1, no. 1, DHEW Pub. No. (HRA) 75-1150, Health Resources Administration, Washington, D.C., May, 1975, U.S. Government Printing Office; Final mortality statistics, 1976, Monthly vital statistics report, vol. 26, no. 12, supp. 2, DHEW Pub. No. (PHS) 78-1120, Public Health Service, Washington D.C., March 30, 1978, U.S. Government Printing Office.
[a]Data are based on reporting countries. Countries are grouped by continent.
[b]Average for the period.
[c]Jewish population only.
(Source: Marieskind, H. I. Women in the health care system: Patients, providers, and programs. St. Louis, Mo.: C. V. Mosby, 1980, by permission.)

prescribed mood-altering drugs (Marieskind, 1980). Some 20 million women become addicted to prescription drugs (Cowan, 1977). Women attempt suicide more often (Williams, 1983) and some 1.2 million women have experienced spouse abuse. Women more frequently report anxiety and stress (Nathanson, 1975). Married women have more ill health than married men or single men or women (Lewis & Lewis, 1977; Nathanson, 1975, p. 60).

However, the reality of psychological health must be evaluated in the social and

TABLE 1–2. LEADING CAUSES OF MORTALITY, UNITED STATES, 1977

Cause	Total	White Female	White Male	Other Female	Other Male
20 to 24 years					
All causes	23,543	5018	16,255	1478	3792
Accidents	12,939	2140	9180	346	1273
Suicide	3694	637	2638	86	333
Homicide	3299	399	1273	328	1299
Malignant neoplasms	1422	434	804	82	102
Heart disease	622	154	260	89	119
Influenzas and pneumonias	272	75	126	29	42
Cerebral vascular disease and stroke	304	98	129	50	27
Congenital anomalies	301	101	152	23	25
Diabetes	103	36	43	15	9
Anemias	83	14	14	23	32
Benign neoplasms	64	28	29	4	3
25 to 44 years					
All causes	101,898	25,646	50,527	8930	16,795
Accidents	22,399	3805	14,536	864	3194
Malignant neoplasms	16,485	7592	6277	1473	1143
Heart disease	14,393	2380	8725	1148	2140
Suicide	8823	2331	5625	219	648
Homicide	8554	829	3317	795	3613
Cirrhosis of liver	5058	1015	2203	681	1153
Cerebral vascular disease and stroke	3737	1315	1236	596	590
Influenzas and pneumonias	2027	561	771	275	420
Diabetes	1477	463	619	188	1207
Congenital anomalies	740	293	342	—[a]	—
45 to 64 years					
All causes	446,096	133,666	242,808	27,411	42,211
Heart disease	158,069	33,791	102,703	8216	13,359
Malignant neoplasms	130,993	52,841	60,593	7305	10,254
Cerebral vascular disease and stroke	24,630	8634	10,200	2800	2996
Accidents	19,000	4647	11,264	758	2331
Cirrhosis of liver	17,821	4938	10,036	983	1864
Suicide	8546	2640	5541	—	—
Influenzas and pneumonias	8010	2311	3974	540	1185
Diabetes	8006	2958	3042	1224	782
Homicide	3837	—	1603	305	1419
65 years and over					
All causes	1,242,342	563,929	565,194	55,137	58,084
Heart disease	548,352	253,601	249,968	23,008	21,775
Malignant neoplasms	232,226	95,373	114,851	8795	13,207
Cerebral vascular disease and stroke	154,623	83,117	55,916	8777	6813
Influenzas and pneumonias	39,871	18,045	18,507	1345	1974
Arteriosclerosis	27,371	15,590	9936	1019	826
Accidents	24,092	10,604	11,189	899	1364
Diabetes	23,599	12,564	7835	2119	1081
Bronchitis, emphysema, and asthma	16,288	4010	11,549	—	550
Cirrhosis of liver	8622	3022	4950	—	406
Nephritis and nephrosis	5834	—	—	589	601
Suicide	4763	—	3567	—	—
Hypertension	4511	—	—	347	—
Hernia and intestinal obstruction	4186	2390	—	—	—
Septicemia	4144	—	—	365	—

Note: Based on data provided by Donald Greenberg, Statistician, Mortality Statistics Branch, Division of Vital Statistics, Washington, D.C., National Center for Health Statistics.
[a]Not a leading cause in this age, color, or sex category.
(Source: Marieskind, H. I. Women in the health care system: Patients, providers, and programs. St. Louis, Mo.: C. V. Mosby, 1980, by permission.)

cultural context in which women live. Women are socialized to express concerns and fears and to seek help when stressed, thus the increased use of health services. This could be viewed positively for prevention and early intervention if health care providers assisted women to use their own resources to restore health and psychological stability when appropriate.

In the area of achievement, women have also not fared well (Horner, 1974; Williams, 1983). A longitudinal study conducted some years ago with gifted children showed only 11 percent of the women versus 50 percent of the men achieved in adulthood even though many of these women were rated more gifted as children (Terman & Oden, 1947, 1959). There are few eminent women in history and less than 2 percent of the Nobel prize winners are women (Kopp, 1979).

Examining the world in which women must achieve sheds light on how difficult this area has been for women. Women have been denied opportunities to develop skills and talents. It is only in recent years that women have been allowed equal schooling, equal opportunities for admission to the major professions, and to compete for major leadership positions. Denying anyone self-fulfillment opportunities is potentially demeaning (Williams, 1983). Conflict occurs because what is expected of women may not fit with what they want and expect of themselves. In the past many women became ill, sought solution in drugs, or attempted suicide. With appropriate education, women can more fully understand themselves and their capacities, choose alternative solutions to missed or unequal opportunities, and begin to contribute their ideas and skills in a way meaningful to their community, their families, and themselves.

Developmentally, one could conclude that women are less mature or adult than men. Women have been described as dependent and seem to accept standards of submissiveness, subjectiveness, and emotionality as female characteristics (Broverman et al., 1970). The expectation for a dependent woman to be a caretaker of children and men brings conflict and confusion. Subjecting one's life to others can result in depression (Williams, 1983). Today's more independent women with multiple roles are indeed a contrast to the dependent women frequently depicted in media, literature, and throughout society. Some women are trying to be primary providers for their families, achieve in a career or a job, and be single parents, good companions, and friends. If women were socialized to be dependent as children, such roles will be difficult to adopt as adults. In addition, being socialized to adopt multiple roles without reasonable limit setting can lead to overload and increased health risks. New skills and knowledge are needed by today's women to prevent inappropriate dependence or assumption of "super women" roles. Health care providers have opportunities to teach these skills.

Reproductive Functions. For centuries women's reproductive functions have been viewed as an illness rather than as a normal process (Williams, 1983). The growing technology for intervention in childbirth (e.g., cesarean sections and forceps), contraception, and menopause attest to the view that women's reproduction must be "medicalized" as opposed to facilitated (Marieskind, 1980). Medical interventions have improved the outcome for some women at high risk for poor pregnancy outcome. Nevertheless, the lack of attention to methodologies that work with rather than interfere in the birth process, perpetuates the belief that women's reproductive system is pathological. Women, too, may share this view unless informed about their bodies and reproductive systems. It is important for women to know about life-style, health habits, and nonmedical approaches to maintaining their reproductive functions in a healthy state. A comprehensive, noninterventionist approach to reproductive health education is essential.

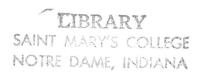

Sexual Health. Women's sexuality has also been inadequately and inappropriately defined. Medical texts continued to perpetuate myths that women's sexuality is less intense than men's and of minor importance (Scully & Bart, 1973), even when new information (Masters & Johnson, 1966, 1970) was readily available about the complexity and intensity of female sexuality.

Newer research findings about female sexual function and capacity have not always been well known and available to health care providers or the lay public. In addition, female sexual function has been compared to young adult men, defining female performance and capacity as inadequate versus different. The richness and variability of female sexuality have thus been ignored and denied, even by professional literature (Fogel & Woods, 1981; Scully & Bart, 1973). Thus female sexual capacity and methodologies for enhancing performance and satisfaction need to be part of health education programs for women. Critical content about female sexuality needs to be taught throughout the life cycle because female socialization has in the past taught women to disregard, misinterpret, or deny their sexuality (see Chapter 6).

Changing Life-styles and Women's Health. It is hypothesized that women's advantage in death rates may change as women change their life-styles, the nature of their work, and become more involved in stress-related situations (Brookes, 1974). This potential, already being demonstrated in some of the leading causes of death (Table 1–2), increases the need for women to have appropriate health education. In addition women's assumption of multiple roles and responsibilities makes more complex their ability and capacity to stay healthy and care for their families.

Health Care Delivery: Inadequate for Women. The health care system has been criticized for its poor and impersonal treatment of women (Sandelowski, 1981). Physicians have been termed "the most powerful purveyors of sexist ideology" (Ehrenreich & English, 1973, p. 5). Women have been unnecessarily treated, operated on (Seaman & Seaman, 1977), and experimented on (Corea, 1977). High costs, withholding of knowledge, failure to respond to convenient time frames for women consumers, and lack of resources for child care have been described as decreasing the quality and quantity of health care for women (Marieskind, 1980) (Tables 1–3, 1–4, and 1–5).

Technology too has significantly impaired women's reproductive health care (Marieskind, 1980) and increased the potential for unnecessary intervention (Banta & Behney, 1978). After reviewing data concerning the increasing technological intervention in such areas as contraception, use of estrogen, obstetrical procedures, mammography, the Pap test, in vitro fertilization, and vaginal surgery, Marieskind (1980, p. 268) concludes that "the impact of the technologies . . . although helpful to some, has not in the masses been positive."

Women have responded to technological interventions and impersonal treatment by complying, withdrawing, protesting, and establishing self-help movements. Sandelowski (1981, p. 154) concludes that the women's health movement was born of the "rape of women's self-determination and control" relative to their own health. Women more so than men have traditionally had few choices concerning how they might pursue health. They have had few opportunities to expand these choices. Women have had to accept medical care they were not satisfied with because there was nothing else. Women have had to submit to a variety of medical and social injustices. Women have not been truly informed consumers of health. Some providers worked to maintain women's ignorance because they believed women were too childlike and capricious to understand the com-

TABLE 1–3. PRINCIPAL REASON FOR VISIT TO PHYSICIAN BY FEMALES AGED 15 AND OVER, UNITED STATES, 1977

Reason	Percent
General, special, and administrative examinations (e.g., annual examination, psychological testing, prenatal checkups, breast and pelvic examinations, school, employment and extracurricular activity examinations)	16.7
Symptoms referable to and diseases of musculoskeletal system and connective tissue (e.g., neck, back, and knee pain or weakness, bone pain, arthritis, bursitis, tenosynovitis, lupus erythematosus)	10.1
Symptoms referable to and diseases of the genitourinary system (e.g., abnormalities of urine, kidney trouble, menstrual disorders, menopausal symptoms, cystitis, complications of pregnancy, cervicitis, pelvic inflammatory disease, vaginitis, breast disease [excluding cancer])	8.9
Symptoms referable to and diseases of respiratory system (e.g., nasal congestion, sinus problems, flu, shortness of breath, tonsillitis, bronchitis, emphysema)	8.8
General symptoms (e.g., chills, fever, pain, weight loss, malaise)	6.9
Diagnostic tests, screening and preventive procedures, test results (e.g., allergy test, glucose level determination, blood tests, mammography, EKG, Pap test, vaccinations, cytology findings)	5.9
Symptoms referable to and diseases of skin, nails, hair, and subcutaneous tissue (e.g., acne, skin infection, rash, hair loss, boils, cellulitis, dandruff, psoriasis, allergic skin reaction)	5.5
Preoperative and postoperative care, progress visits, specific types of therapy, therapeutic procedures (e.g., discussion of cosmetic surgery, suture removal, follow-up visits, physical or respiratory therapy, psychotherapy, tub insertion, cauterization)	5.4
Symptoms referable to and diseases of digestive system (e.g., bleeding gums, difficulty in swallowing, nausea, stomach pain, flatulence, worms, peptic ulcer, appendicitis)	5.3
Symptoms referable to and diseases of eyes and ears (e.g., infection, discharge, hearing dysfunctions, conjunctivitis, otitis media)	5.0
Symptoms referable to and diseases of nervous system (excluding sense organs); congenital anomalies (e.g., convulsions, headaches, multiple sclerosis, epilepsy)	4.4
Symptoms referable to psychological and mental disorders and mental diseases (e.g., anxiety, fears, phobias, depression, alcoholism and drug dependence, sleep disorders, psychoses)	3.2
Medications, family planning (e.g., allergy shots, hormones, renew prescriptions, contraceptive counseling, birth control pills)	3.2
Symptoms referable to cardiovascular and lymphatic systems and diseases of circulatory system (e.g., abnormal pulsations, sore glands, rheumatic fever, hypertension, ischemic heart disease)	3.1
Injury, poisoning, adverse drug effects (e.g., fractures, dislocations, lacerations, puncture wounds, foreign body in eye, burns, motor vehicle accidents, dead on arrival, rape, food poisoning, intoxication)	2.5
Endocrine, nutritional, and metabolic diseases (e.g., goiter, hyperthyroidism, hypoglycemia, ovarian dysfunction)	1.3
Medical and special-problem counseling (e.g., counseling in nutrition or marital, parent-child, money, or work problems)	1.3
Neoplasms (e.g., cancer, benign neoplasms)	0.8
Infective and parasitic diseases (e.g., gastroenteritis, cholera, streptococcal, herpes, or fungus infections, hepatitis)	0.3
Diseases of blood and blood-forming organs (e.g., anemias) etc.	0.2
Uncodable reasons	1.2

Note: Based on unpublished data provided by T. Ezzati from the National Ambulatory Medical Care Survey, 1977, Ambulatory Care Statistics Branch, Division of Health Resources Utilization Statistics, National Center for Health Statistics, Washington, D.C.
(Source: Marieskind, H. I. Women in the health care system: Patients, providers, and programs. St. Louis, Mo.: C. V. Mosby, 1980, by permission.)

TABLE 1–4. PERCENT DISTRIBUTION OF FEMALES WHO REPORTED UNMET HEALTH NEEDS, UNITED STATES, 1974

Age	Percent Reporting Unmet Needs	Unknown
All ages	6.4	0.4
Under 20 years	7.4	0.5
20 to 44 years	7.6	0.4
45 to 65 years	8.0	0.4
65 years and over	6.0	0.8

Note: Based on unpublished data provided by T. F. Drury from the 1974 Health Interview Survey, Division of Health Interveiw Statistics, National Center for Health Statistics, Washington, D.C.
(Source: Marieskind, H. I. Women in the health care system: Patients, providers, and programs. *St. Louis, Mo.: C. V. Mosby, 1980, by permission.)*

plexities of drugs, treatments, and health alternatives. Such a view is in conflict with the reality of many of today's women. The women's movement and women's increasing request to be informed and to participate in established care requires health education that is geared to women's current needs and capacities.

Women's Rights and Professional Responsibility for Health Education

It seems clear that women need information concerning their health. What are women's rights for health education? Individuals can no longer be denied certain information concerning health. The Patient's Bill of Rights adopted by the American Hospital Association in 1973 reflects all patients' right to know and choose the type of care received (A Patient's Bill of Rights, 1973). The Pregnant Patient's Bill of Rights (ICEA, 1979) also establishes the rights of women to information about their reproductive experience. A variety of legal cases and their interpretation recognizes that individuals have a "right to know" and to have *explicit instruction in the use of prescribed medication* and *follow-up care*, and information that they have a *condition requiring continual treatment*. Information can be withheld if the disclosure will cause psychosocial or physiological harm to the extent that the effectiveness of the procedure will be impaired, but not to negate the possibility of the individual's refusal of treatment or of making a "wrong" decision (Redman, 1980).

Women in ever-increasing numbers are seeking information and demanding that

TABLE 1–5. PERCENT OF FEMALES WHO REPORTED UNMET HEALTH NEEDS, UNITED STATES, 1974

Reasons for Unmet Health Needs[a]	All Ages	Under 20 Years	20 to 44 Years	45 to 64 Years	65 Years and over
Cost too high	49.5	49.5	48.7	52.9	44.2
Physician spends inadequate time	15.1	7.5	18.7	16.7	16.7
Difficulty getting appointment	14.3	13.6	17.2	10.6	14.1
Difficulties with transportation	9.6	10.3	5.4	9.2	25.1
Office hours inconvenient	6.3	7.8	6.5	6.6	1.5
Other	25.4	21.1	28.8	25.0	23.5
Unknown reason	9.5	14.8	7.3	7.6	10.2

Note: Based on unpublished data provided by T. F. Drury from the 1974 Health Interview Survey, Division of Health Interview Statistics, National Center for Health Statistics, Washington, D.C.
[a]More than one unmet health need possible per woman.
(Source: Marieskind, H. I. Women in the health care system: Patients, providers, and programs. *St. Louis, Mo.: C. V. Mosby, 1980, by permission.)*

health care providers and facilities offer such information in a framework they can understand and use. The amount of information the woman has a right to and can use effectively without jeopardizing her health is part of many debates among various women's groups and all types of health professionals. Clear lines of what is appropriate knowledge have not been delineated. How much any woman should know is a clinical judgment for individual women in particular health–illness states.

If women have a need and a right for education, what is the responsibility of health care professionals to meet this need? The legal base for medicine "has long included" patient education as an area of practice (Redman, 1980). It is not entirely clear what the full *legal responsibility* of the nurse is for patient education. Some nurses practice acts, and the 1973 American Nurses' Association's (ANA) standards of practice as well as the ANA Statements of Functions, Standards, and Qualifications indicate that teaching is a function and responsibility of the nurse (American Nurses' Association, 1963, 1973). Some nurse practice acts have made explicit the inclusion of independent roles in health education in the scope of nursing responsibility (Redman, 1980, p. 5).

The role of the expanded role nurse, termed Triple A Nurse by Bevis, reflects increased aspects of accountability, authority, and autonomy (Bevis, 1976). As nurses assume more autonomy, have more responsibility for health maintenance and management of illness, the provision of health teaching will likely become more of a responsibility for this group of health care providers.

When a hospital adapts the Patient's Bill of Rights as policy, it becomes the basis for legal action. Thus the patients' right to know their diagnosis, treatment, and prognosis becomes a legal right and health care professionals have a responsibility for upholding the hospital's policy. Whether or not each professional is responsible to see that the other complies is not clear (Redman, 1980). The Bill of Rights, however, places major responsibility for informing patients on the physician. Likely, the near future will see a focus on defining the limits of the right to know and the responsibility of whom should provide health education.

The Joint Commission on Accreditation of Hospitals recommends there be *consistent patient teaching plans* and documentation of patient teaching. Patient education is currently being seen as an integral part of patient care (Jones, 1977). Patient care committees and quality assurance studies are being used to determine what is being done in patient education. There is clearly a focus on increasing the adequacy of patient education by hospital staff eager to provide quality care. The concern for the cost of hospital care, however, threatens to remove resources that allow time for patient education. Careful planning is needed to meet cost containment as well as quality of care goals.

This text allows professionals to incorporate health education into day to day care. The goal of health education that is proposed is to enhance women's appreciation of their bodies, its capabilities, and capacity to adjust to numerous stresses. Especially important is an approach to health education that enhances women's self-esteem, sense of adequacy, ability to cope, and ability to define themselves in ways that do not require the acceptance of inappropriate external notions of what it is to be female.

BIBLIOGRAPHY

American Hospital Association. *A patient's bill of rights*. Chicago, Ill.: AHA, 1973.
American Nurses' Association. *Standards of practice: Functions, standards, and qualifications for practice* (Rev. New York, 1963). Kansas City, Mo.: American Nurses' Association, 1973.

Appelbaum, A. L. Patient education seen as an integral part of patient care. *Hospitals*, 1977, *51*(22), 115–118.

Banta, H. D., & Behney, C. *Assessing the efficacy and safety of medical technologies*. Office of Technology Assessment (U. S. Congress Stock No. 052-003-00593-0). Washington, D. C.: U. S. Government Printing Office, 1978.

Bermosk, L., & Porter, S. *Women's health and human wholeness*. New York: Appleton-Century-Crofts, 1979.

Bernard, J. *The female world*. New York: Free Press, Macmillan, 1981.

Bevis, E. Presentation at a faculty workshop. University of Colorado School of Nursing, Fall 1976.

Brookes, P. Increasing death rate among women? *Nursing Times*, 1974, *70*(23), 881.

Broverman, I. K., Broverman, D. M., & Clarkson, F. E. Sex-role stereotypes and clinical judgments of mental health. *Journal of Counsulting and Clinical Psychology*, 1970, *31*(1), 1–7.

Bullough, B., & Bullough, V. Sex discrimination in health care. *Nursing Outlook*, 1975, *23*(1), 40–48.

Cannon, M. S., & Redick, R. W. Differential utilization of psychiatric facilities by men and women: United States 1970 (Statistical Note No. 81, DHEW Publication No. (HSM)73-9005), National Institute of Mental Health. Washington, D. C.: U. S. Government Printing Office, June 1973.

Carlton, B., & Carlton, M. A. Defining a role for the health educator in the primary care setting. *Health Education*, 1978, *9*(2), 22–23.

Chester, P. Patient and patriarch: Women in the psychotherapeutic relationship. In S. Cox (Ed.), *Female psychology: The emerging self*, pp. 318–334. New York: St. Martin's Press, 1976.

Chodorow, N. *The reproduction of mothering: Psychoanalysis and the sociology of gender*. Berkeley, Calif.: Univ. of Calif. Press, 1978.

Collier, P. Health behaviors of women. *Nursing Clinics of North America*, 1982, *17*(1), 121–126.

Condry, J., & Dyer, S. Fear of success: Attribution of cause to the victim. *Journal of Social Issues*, 1976, *32*(3), 63–68.

Corea, G. *The hidden malpractice: How American medicine treats women as patients and professionals*. New York: Morrow, 1977.

Cowan, B. *Women's health care: Resource, writings and bibliographies*. Ann Arbor, Mich.: Anshen Publishing, 1977.

Cox, S. (Ed.). *Female psychology: The emerging self* (2nd ed.). New York: St. Martin's Press, 1981.

Degler, C. *At odds: Women and the family in America, from the revolution to the present*. New York: Oxford Univ. Press, 1980.

Dorley, S. A. Big-time careers for the little woman: A dual role dilemma. *Journal of Social Issues*, 1976, *32*(3), 85–98.

Dreifus, C. (Ed.). Seizing our bodies: The politics of women's health. New York: Vintage Books, 1978.

Ehrenreich, B., & English, D. *Complaints and disorders: The sexual politics of sickness*. Old Westbury, N.Y.: Feminist Press, 1973.

Ehrenreich, B., & English, D. *For her own good*. New York: Feminist Press, 1978.

Erikson, E. H. The inner and the outer space: Reflections on womanhood. *Daedalus*, 1964, *93*, 582–606.

Erikson, E. H. Once more the inner space. In E. H. Erikson (Ed.), *Life history and the historical moment* (1st ed.). New York: Norton, 1975.

Faden, V. B., & Taube, C. A. Length of stay and discharges from non-federal general hospital psychiatric inpatient units, United States 1975. (Mental Health Statistical Note No. 133) National Institute of Mental Health. Washington, D. C.: U. S. Government Printing Office, May 1977, 1–28.

Fogel, C. I., & Woods, N. F. *Health care of women: A nursing perspective*. St. Louis, Mo.: C. V. Mosby, 1981.

Gordon, L. *Woman's body, woman's right: Birth control in America*. New York: Penguin, 1977.

Gove, W. R., & Tudor, J. F. Adult sex roles and mental illness. *American Journal of Sociology*, 1973, *78*(4), 812–835.

Haller, J., & Haller, R. *The physician and sexuality in Victorian America*. New York: W. W. Norton, 1977.

Horner, M. S. Toward an understanding of achievement-related conflicts in women. In J. Stacy, S. Gerlaud, & J. Daniels (Eds.), *And Jill came tumbling after: Sexism in American education*. New York: Dell, 1974.

International Childbirth Education Association, Inc. (ICEA). *The pregnant patient's bill of rights*. New York: ICEA Publication Distribution Center, 1979.

Jones, P. Patient education—yes—no. *Supervisor Nurse*, 1977, 8(5), 35–43.

Kopp, C. *Becoming female: Perspectives on development*. New York: Plenum Press, 1979.

Knutson, A. L. *The individual, society, and health behavior*. New York: Russell Sage Foundation, 1965.

Lewis, C. E., & Lewis, M. A. The potential impact of sexual equality on health. *New England Journal of Medicine*, 1977, 297(16), 863–869.

Levin, L., & Idler, E. *The hidden health care system: Mediating structures and medicine*. Cambridge, Mass.: Ballinger, 1982.

Marieskind, H. I. *Women in the health care system: Patients, providers, and programs*. St. Louis, Mo.: C. V. Mosby, 1980.

Masters, W. H., & Johnson, V. E. *Human sexual response*. Boston: Little, Brown, 1966.

Masters, W. H., & Johnson, V. E. *Human sexual inadequacy*. Boston: Little, Brown, 1970.

Mechanic, D. Sex, illness behavior, and the use of health services. *Journal of Human Stress*, 1976, 2(4), 29–41.

Montagu, A. *The natural superiority of women*. New York: Collier Books, 1974.

Moore, E. C. Women and health: United States, 1980. *Public Health Reports* (Suppl), 1980, 95(5), 84.

Nathanson, C. A. Illness and the feminine role: A theoretical review. *Social Science and Medicine*, 1975, 9(2), 57–62.

Pomerleau, C. S. Cardiovascular disease as a women's health problem. *Women and Health*, 1976, 1(6), 12–15.

Redman, B. K. *Patient teaching in nursing*. St. Louis, Mo.: C. V. Mosby, 1980.

Rosenstock, I. Prevention of illness and maintenance of health. In J. Kosa, A. Antonoosky, & I. K. Zola (Eds.), *Poverty and health: A sociological analysis*, pp. 168–190. Cambridge, Mass.: Harvard University Press, 1969.

Sandelowski, M. *Women, health, and choice*. Englewood Cliffs, N.J.: Prentice-Hall, 1981.

Scarf, M. *Unfinished business: Pressure points in the lives of women*. New York: Doubleday, 1980.

Scully, D., & Bart, P. A funny thing happened on the way to the orifice: Women in gynecology textbooks. *American Journal of Sociology*, 1973, 78(4), 1045–1050.

Seaman, B., & Seaman, G. *Women and the crisis in sex hormones*. New York: Rawson Associates, 1977.

Sontag, S. *Illness as metaphor*. New York: Farrar, Straus & Giroux, 1978.

Terman, L. M., & Oden, M. H. *Genetic studies of genius*. Stanford, Calif.: Stanford University Press, 1947.

Terman, L. M., & Oden, M. H. *Genetic studies of genius*. Stanford, Calif.: Stanford University Press, 1959.

Tilly, L., & Scott, J. *Women, work and family*. New York: Holt, Rinehart & Winston, 1978.

U.S. Department of Health, Education, and Welfare. *Health-United States, 1978*. (DHEW publication No. (PHS) 78-1232). Washington, D. C.: U. S. Government Printing Office, 1978.

Verbrugge, L. M. Female illness rates and illness behavior: Testing hypotheses about sex differences in health. *Women and Health*, 1979, 4(1), 61–70.

Waldron, I. Why do women live longer than men? *Social Science and Medicine*, 1976, 10(7/8), 349–362.

Williams, J. H. *Psychology of women: Behavior in a biosocial context*. New York: W. W. Norton, 1983.

Woods, N. F. Women and their health. In C. I. Fogel & N. F. Woods (Eds.), *Health care of women: A nursing perspective*, pp. 3–26. St. Louis, Mo.: C. V. Mosby, 1981.

The Educational Process: How?

2

Vivian M. Littlefield

Health Education Viewed as a Therapeutic Tool. The idea that health education is a "therapeutic tool" for health care and promotion is fertile with symbolism. First, a specific therapy is selected after an appropriate needs assessment is made. Second, the *correct* "dosage" is prescribed based on the client's/patient's age, physiological characteristics, special life circumstances, and severity of symptoms. Third, no therapy is ordered without recognizing that inappropriate side effects may occur. Health care professionals monitor these side effects and inform clients/patients and their families to report them. Finally, at key points, reevaluation of the effects of the therapy occurs so that decisions can be made to determine the need for an increase or decrease in dosage, or when therapy is no longer needed.

The term *therapeutic* may seem incongruent with *health* education. Why would a well individual need therapy? If wellness can be viewed on a continuum, then what is therapeutic for well persons would be education that gives them information to assist in maintaining and enhancing their well-being. If the health continuum includes mental health as well as physical health, it would be hard to imagine a completely healthy person every day of her life. Thus, there is a need for "therapeutic intervention" in the form of health education for well women so they can understand developmental and physiological changes that occur with maturing and aging. In addition women need information about potential health risks that women with their specific genetic background and age may encounter. Changing life-styles, balancing multiple roles also impact women in today's complex world. Health education, therefore, becomes an essential "therapy" for optimum health. Figure 2–1 depicts the concept of health education as a therapeutic tool for health promotion and maintenance, illness care and recovery.

Health education can be an appropriate and effective therapeutic tool if used in the above context, and should be based on the same level of knowledge and skill the administration of any therapy would demand. To use this "tool" *therapeutically*, it cannot be applied to everyone in the same manner. Health education needs to be individually applied and evaluated.

This chapter discusses the educational *process* focusing on *how* data are collected to assess learning needs, planning for teaching activities, and evaluating the outcome of health education. Variables that influence learning are also discussed. Chapter 3 expands on teaching–learning theory and introduces decision-making theory. The remaining

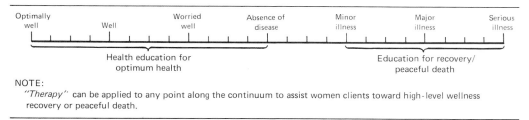

Figure 2–1. Health education as a therapeutic tool.

chapters discuss adaptation of specific methodologies for women in various states of health and illness who seek information from a wide variety of clinical facilities (e.g., outpatient clinics, hospitals, community agencies).

THE PROCESS OF HEALTH EDUCATION

Definitions of Health Teaching

Redman, in her text, *The Process of Patient Teaching in Nursing* (1980), refers to several definitions of teaching. The first, *"activities by which the teacher helps the student to learn"* and a second, *"any interpersonal influence aimed at changing the way in which other persons can or will behave."* These definitions focus the control of what is learned on the teacher. A third definition of teaching is *"communication specially structured and sequenced to produce learning."* This definition does not place control on the teacher (Redman, 1980, pp. 9–10). Redman (1980), however, indicates that the most useful method of viewing health education is to view all interaction with patients or clients as contributing to the broad processes and objectives of teaching–learning. This interaction includes verbal and nonverbal behavior as well as providing information, clarifying thinking, reflecting feelings, teaching a skill, or modeling by example (Redman, 1980).

Process of Health Education

The process used for health education is the same as the problem-solving process used by nurses and physicians. This problem-solving process in nursing has been described by Yura and Walsh (1983) and in medicine by Weed (1971). This process is as critical to teaching as it is to clinical diagnosis in medicine and identification of patient care needs in nursing.

The *first step* in health education is one of *assessment*. Here the woman's needs are assessed prior to deciding what and how much is to be taught by whom. A 14-year-old adolescent making decisions about her own family planning measures would likely need different information than a female physician making the same decision. Frequently, however, the same information is given to all individuals. Different kinds of information are needed by different women because of a different knowledge base, a different emotional response, as well as varying ability to make decisions concerning health. If assessment is omitted, this results in "telling" versus teaching.

The *second* step in health education is that of *planning*. This requires the teacher to consider specific methodological approaches, theories, and content that reflect the individuality of the learner as well as the teacher. Goals for what is to be learned, how it is to be learned, and in what time frame are essential for both the learner and the teacher. This step is often omitted in an attempt to "get all the information across" in a short time. Omitting the planning phase may result in inappropriate "dosage" and inadequate client compliance.

Once the assessment and the planning have been done, the important *third step of implementation* takes place. Once any aspect of the teaching plan has been implemented, *evaluation* begins. This evaluation serves to determine what has been learned and what else needs to be learned. Figure 2–2 demonstrates that the process is continuous with ongoing feedback between the learner and the teacher at each point of contact.

ASSESSMENT

The process of assessment for health education is similar to the assessment of any other health need or problem. The type of data collected in health education varies. Data collection can be ordered around subjective and objective information as in the problem-oriented approach to diagnosis or assessment. What the patient says she needs to learn, what she perceives she knows or has access to finding out from her individual and family support system is subjective information. Objective observations include the woman's

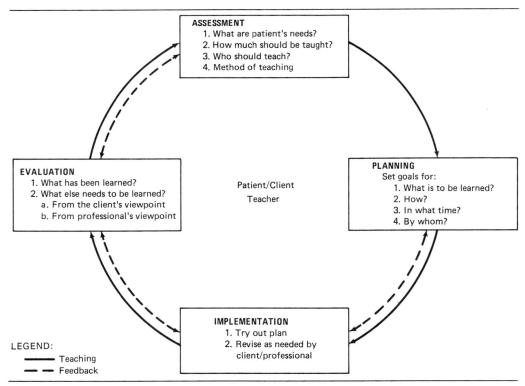

Figure 2–2. The process of patient education.

behavior, age, culture, demonstrated knowledge, and particular stage of health or illness. These data allow an assessment of learning needs.

There are several important variables that may influence learning. Knowledge of how these variables influence learning can assist the health care provider to more effectively plan a given individual's learning experience. A discussion of these variables follows.

Variables Affecting Learning

Age

Adults. The woman's age is an important factor in learning. It seems obvious that children might learn differently than adults, however, health education frequently incorporates learning techniques that have been promoted for children or for more dependent, less experienced learners. The adult education literature suggests that adult learners have certain characteristics that are important to consider in planning learning experiences. These assumptions, identified by Malcom S. Knowles (1970), are:

1. Adults are self-directing human beings
2. Adults use their life experiences as a learning resource
3. Adults' learning is oriented to developmental tasks of their role
4. Adults' time perspective in learning is related to immediacy of application
5. Adults' orientation for learning is problem-centered
6. Adults see themselves as doers
7. Adults resist learning under conditions that are incongruent with their self-concept

These ideas about the adult as a learner have several implications for health education. One of these is that the adult learner should have some control over what is learned. In addition, what is learned will depend on how such learning can be incorporated into important roles. Relevance for the present life circumstance will also be considered by most adults. Because the adult has learned to solve problems and prefers to be actively involved in the learning process, resistance to methodological approaches that exclude active participation may be rejected. Also, learning in an environment that makes learners feel inadequate, or less knowledgeable than they are, is not a positive experience. Under the circumstances the learner might reject what is taught, or avoid the learning situation. Women expressed some of these reasons for not attending mother–baby classes, such as "That nurse doesn't think I know anything. I am not going back. They don't teach what I need to know," and so forth. Indeed some mother–baby classes have focused on the minute detail of the bath, making this task excessively difficult while ignoring the complex baby and all the feelings associated with mothering. (See Chapter 3 for additional information concerning the adult learner.)

Adolescents. Adolescents, too, have unique learning needs. Adolescents may reject learning because of how they feel about the process. Adolescents' conflicts with being independent versus dependent may be reflected in their response to the teacher. Resisting authority may be the issue rather than not learning. The adolescents' need for peer acceptance is such that not learning (changing behavior) may reflect their need to be "in" rather than not knowing what healthy behaviors are.

An important developmental change for adolescents is cognitive development. According to Piaget, adolescents are just beginning to accomplish "formal operations" (Piaget, 1975, pp. 108–117). This means that they have a capacity to reason abstractly.

Adolescents can now take the alternative side of the argument and identify the consequences of a certain behavior or decision. They can also go beyond their immediate field of experience, something that children cannot do. Adolescents can now "think about thinking" and are egocentric in their thought processes. This egocentricity causes adolescents to think they are unique and special. They believe no one else has thought or felt as they do. This is important to remember, because adolescents who have fears or lack adequate information may not ask for information because they cannot imagine others having the same needs. Thus they hypothesize *they* are lacking as individuals because they do not know something. They also may believe that everyone else "thinks as they do." Thus, others' thoughts have the same focus as theirs, i.e., the adolescent (Elkind, 1975). This results in the all too familiar feeling by adolescents that everyone is looking at them.

Because adolescents are so strongly searching for identity, any experience, including a learning experience, must consider the parameters of that identity and allow adolescents to maintain their identity. Asking adolescents to do something that is incongruent with their developing identity may cause them to resist this request. Adolescents are not unwilling or unable to learn, but unable to tolerate threats to their identity. This need for maintaining an identity established with peers is demonstrated in adolescent girls who ask for birth control methods, even when they would prefer not to be sexually active. (See Chapter 15 for specific approaches for educating pregnant adolescents.)

Elderly. The impact aging has on learning ability has been questioned and researched. Many of the findings about differences and declining ability to learn have been challenged. Studies demonstrating a declining ability to learn were conducted by asking elderly individuals to learn meaningless terms. Also impediments to learning such as visual and hearing acuity were not accounted for. It is now thought that, given adequate physiological functioning, the elderly can learn as effectively as younger individuals. Memory is affected by age, but ability to learn new information is not lost. In fact, learning is sometimes enhanced because of increased and widened perspective. Obviously elderly individuals vary greatly in their capacity to learn and need to be assessed individually.

The elderly individual returns to an egocentric attitude, may have difficulty changing lifelong behaviors even with new learning, and may resist a young, inexperienced (life) teacher. Elderly persons are especially sensitive to any situation that may cause them to loose self-respect and decreased status. The physical barriers to learning (sight, hearing, mobility) may be distressing and the reason for nonlearning, especially if elderly individuals are uncomfortable admitting they cannot hear, see, or manipulate objects (Chapter 15 has additional details concerning the elderly learner.)

Being Female. Various authors hypothesize that the uniqueness of being female may have an impact on health behaviors and learning in health education situations. Although evidence for sex differences is neither conclusive nor evidenced by all women, recognizing the potential for differences will assist health professionals in assessing the woman's perspective.

In American culture, women engage in less risk-taking behavior and take more preventative measures than men (Martin, 1978). Thus women seem to be more responsive to health education aimed at prevention. Compared to men, women have been described as being more parochial, rather than scientific, in their health orientation (Suchman, 1965). A parochial orientation includes close relationships with one's ethnic group and friends as well as a family pattern of tradition and authority. Individuals who hold a parochial orientation rely on members of their own group for help and support during illness. Parochial orientations incorporate concern for others, thus learning and observing positive health behaviors may be adopted out of concern and care taking activities for family, friends, and support persons. Women were likely to be better informed about disease and less skeptical of medical care than men (Suchman, 1965). Redman (1980, p. 37) suggests that as modern medicine becomes more "scientific, formal, specialized, complex, impersonal" and focuses on the disease instead of the person, the more likely individuals with a parochial orientation will seek care elsewhere. This may explain the women's self-help movement.

The effort to define feminine cognitive style has been undertaken by several researchers and theorists. Field-independent and field-dependent behaviors have been described with the conclusion that female cognitive style is essentially field-dependent (Witkin et al., 1977). Field-dependent people have a "with people" orientation. These individuals:

1. Are more attentive to and make use of prevailing social frames of reference
2. Attend better and more often to faces of others
3. Tend to manage within the social context they are given
4. Take better account of external social referents in defining their attitudes and feelings
5. Are more in touch with their emotionality and sexuality
6. Suppress rage more often for fear of rejection

These behaviors are contrasted with field-independent cognitive styles that analyze and break down the component parts of a wide variety of fields, see an item as distinct from the background and impose structure on the field. In other words, field-independent persons tend to be analytical. These individuals also problem solve in an objective manner (Witkin et al., 1977). Sherman (1967) argues that these differences in cognitive style do not exist due to genetics or female hormones. She concludes that the differences result because of socialization and emphasis in school. For example, boys were encouraged to be analytical; girls were not. In research with children, field-dependent females were more popular with peers. Girls in today's society are rewarded for concern and attention to other's needs. How could girls not develop cognitive styles accepted, rewarded, and perhaps useful in our society? Recognizing the cognitive style of the potential learner may be helpful. People with field-dependent cognitive styles may respond to the attitudes and feelings of the teacher and learning environment. Thus, the emotional environment surrounding learning will be important for these individuals. A negative attitude on the part of the teacher or failure to recognize how changing the behavior of the woman impacts significant others may prevent learning. Not recognizing how women feel about information provided may also negatively affect the learning situation.

Culture and Values. In addition to age and sex, culture influences how and what one learns. This results because individuals from various cultural orientations hold different values. It is hypothesized that these values influence one's choices about health care and life-style (Kluckhohn & Strodbeck, 1961). Kluckhohn and Strodbeck (1961) conceptualized these differences on six continua. These continua assist the health care professional to recognize that individuals from different cultures may hold different values. Rather than define what values one culture holds, versus another (Italian versus Jewish versus white Anglo-Saxon versus Protestant), Kluckhohn and Strodbeck (1961) define various differences that exist between and within cultural groups (Fig. 2–3). The health care pro-

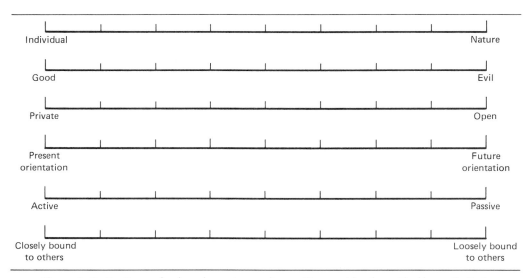

Figure 2–3. Continua of values for various cultures. *(Source: Idea from Kluckhorn, R. R. & Strodbeck, F. L. Variations in value orientations. Evanston, Il: Row, Peterson, 1961.)*

vider can then do an individual assessment in each of the components as opposed to making assumptions about a particular culture. Individuals may not accept teaching because of a different value orientation, not inability to learn or motivation. It is helpful to include in the learning assessment an individual's value orientation as depicted by Kluckhohn and Strodbeck's continua. This allows the teacher to plan the learning experience from the individual's framework.

Individual—Nature Continuum. The individual who would be placed on the individual end of the continuum would view individuals in control of their destiny and accept that they could do things that would make life better, healthier, and so on. The individuals on the far end of the nature continuum would accept the idea that whatever happens, happens and there is little that an individual can do to change the situation. These individuals have difficulty accepting that a change in their own behavior would in fact change the circumstances in which they find themselves. A clinical example of a nature value orientation is the individual who says, "I am not going to get that Pap smear. If I am going to get cancer, I get it. There is nothing I can do." Individuals holding values nearer the nature end of this continuum will take less responsibility for their own health care and accept preventive techniques for futuristic health with less commitment, if at all.

This continuum is reflective of the concept of locus of control (Rotter, 1966). Rotter described the difference in internally versus externally controlled individuals. The internally controlled individual in the end will take a more active stance in seeking information and make an independent decision. The externally controlled person will be more amenable to guidance and suggestion and will look to chance, luck, or powerful others as responsible for providing information and changing life circumstances. Wallston and Wallston (1976) have taken Rotter's concepts and devised a Health Locus of Control instrument for determining whether an individual relies on self, luck, or powerful others in relation to health. They view the concept from a multidimensional perspective. This instrument was designed for behavioral research but may prove useful in clinical assessment situations. It takes 5 to 10 minutes to complete and could be used as an assessment tool. Even using one or two questions from this scale might provide valuable information. For example, the following questions provide information about an individual's reliance on powerful others, self, or chance.

- *Powerful others:*
  Do you usually depend on the doctor to tell you what to do to stay healthy?
- *Chance:*
  Do you think people get sick accidentally?
- *Self:*
  Do you think illness results because of something you have or have not done?

Good–Evil Orientation. Another continuum is termed the good–evil orientation. In this instance, individuals holding a good orientation see men and women as basically good and, therefore, what happens to them is a matter of chance. Individuals holding the evil orientation see men and women as basically bad and the many things that happen in life, such as illness, deformity, or death, as punishment. With this evil orientation, acceptance of illness becomes a matter of accepting punishment as one's due in life. This orientation was seen in the Indian family who refused medical treatment for their child, believing this child's illness to be a punishment for the family's misdeeds. When the Medicine Man was included in the plan of care to assist the family to cope with the evil–punishment issues, medical care was accepted and the child recovered. No amount of teaching would have been accepted by this family if their values and orientation to illness had not been respected.

Private–Open Continuum. Private–open is another continuum described by Kluckhohn and Strodbeck (1961). Individuals on the extreme private end of the continuum are reluctant to share details of their life with others outside of close friends or family. Their willingness to share with health care providers is limited and, therefore, information to make adequate assessments of learning needs or to evaluate the results of teaching are not always available. Those individuals on the open end of this continuum are willing to share, even with strangers, intimate details of their lives. These individuals can share with health care providers without reservation. The health care provider confronting individuals from these different orientations will surely find frustration with the individual who is reluctant to share private details that are necessary to an adequate health assessment. Recognizing that this reluctance to share is not related to adequate assessment techniques will assist the health care provider in appreciating the individual's preferred degree of privacy.

Present–Future Time Orientation. Differences in time orientation are frequently the result of misunderstanding and miscommunication among health care professionals and women who hold present orientations. The health care professional frequently is a futuristically oriented person, believing in "good health practices" for future health, whereas some clients are focused on the immediate present. The time involved in preventive health care for some future year is such that individuals who hold a present orientation have difficulty complying with what seems to be complex requirements, especially when their current life is filled with crises that need attention.

Active–Passive Continuum. Active–passive roles for individuals is another dimension that frequently differs between health care professionals and clients. Becoming actively involved in health care is accepted as a responsibility by health care professionals and individuals who hold active role orientations. On the other hand, others who hold more passive role orientations do not see that they have a responsibility for changing the course of things. This orientational difference can cause severe conflicts. A 14-year-old, pregnant adolescent not responding to dietary restrictions, or the need for rest, or other suggestions to retard her developing symptoms of toxemia, wanted the health professional team to give her "something" to stop the development of edema and her rising blood pressure. It was, in her opinion, the responsibility of the physician to stop the disease. Nothing that "I can do will make it better." She felt that the physicians did not care about her "sickness" when they would not prescribe a "pill," but instead expected her to take responsibility for behavior that would decrease the symptoms.

Relational Orientation. The sixth continuum, defined by Kluckhohn and Strodbeck, is relational orientation or how tightly an individual or family is "bound to others." This also makes a difference in how individuals respond to health teaching. For example, those who are tightly bound to family members frequently cancel their appointments or "fail to show" because "grandmother is sick," or some other family member "needed the car." This commitment to respond to others within the family frequently interferes with some women's ability to follow appropriate health care commitments and practices. An example of an individual tightly bound to others was a pregnant woman considering her family rather than herself. This woman would not eat an appropriate diet during her pregnancy so that her teenage daughter's nutritional needs could be met. This mother felt that the health of her teenage daughter was of primary importance. The teenager was developing rapidly and her future health might depend on adequate nutrition. The pregnant woman denied herself adequate food even though she had severe anemia. Ways needed to be found so that both mother and daughter could maintain an adequate diet on a low income. *No* amount of knowledge of what was adequate nutrition for pregnant women would have helped this woman comply.

Health–Illness Values. A major area of conflict between health care professionals and clients is in the value placed on health. Some clients visualize themselves as ill only when this illness changes their life-style or they cannot function in their work. Other individuals believe in taking "pills" or in going to a health care provider for "every ache and pain." Individuals who hold this latter opinion believe it is the responsibility of health care professionals to solve their problems and that they should not have to do anything to improve their own status. This dilemma is seen clinically in individuals who, when pregnant, cannot accept the fact that although they do not feel ill the initial symptoms for toxemia are important and changes in dietary and rest patterns are necessary. Frequently, regular prenatal visits are also not seen as important because women "feel alright." Another clinical dilemma occurs with women who want medication for the discomforts of stress or menstrual changes. A critical look at the behavior of health care professionals should be taken. It is possible that attitudes of providing medical intervention versus self-help strategies for any symptom has encouraged an illness orientation toward women's health and reproduction. In the past, the discomforts of pregnancy, changes in the menstrual cycle, and menopause have been handled from a medical orientation. Prescriptions have been ordered as opposed to assisting women to cope by adjusting their activities and altering their life-style.

Income Levels and Learning. There are some data indicating that individuals from different income levels learn best by different strategies. This difference, however, may reflect differences in educational levels. The differences mentioned in the literature are worth exploring and will assist in the assessment of individual's preferences for how they learn.

Riessman, Cohen, and Pearl (1964) state that low income individuals prefer physical and visual learning opportunities, content-centered and problem-centered learning, as well as externally oriented experiences. Other preferences of low income individuals are that learning be inductive, related to current situations, and oriented toward one track thinking. These individuals appreciate words that describe action. Middle income individuals, on the other hand, preferred aural learning opportunities, introspective and deductive learning, future oriented situations, and could comprehend a variety of reasons for illness and disease. These individuals had a "word bound" orientation. For example, words had a specific meaning to them, so that clarification was needed between learner and teacher.

A difference between lower class and upper class individuals has been demonstrated to be related to psychosocial deviation. Lower class individuals could tolerate more deviant behavior than individuals in the upper class. Upper class individuals feel they should be self-reliant and did not always seek help when needed. These individuals had a "powerful" sense of personal responsibility toward health maintenance, at least in the psychosocial areas (Blackwell, 1964).

These data should be considered when assessing what an individual needs to learn, as well as how to present it. Never, of course, should individuals be placed in a category because they are "a low income learner." Knowing that there are potential differences, however, allows collection of information about what an individual or a group of individuals might prefer.

Anxiety. Another important variable to consider in assessing and planning learning is the current state or degree of anxiety. Learning is frequently influenced by anxiety. This means normal capacity or readiness for learning may not be completely functional when a state of anxiety exists. Everyone with a moderate or severe level of anxiety has a narrowed perceptual field, more selected inattention, and assimilates less information. In a panic state, detail is magnified.

The influence of anxiety is demonstrated by patients during labor and delivery. Women in labor need repeated, simple explanations for what is happening and what they should do during the later stages of labor. Frequently, activities and discussions that take place around the woman, but are not about the woman, are heard by the woman as relating to her. This occurs because of selected inattention and focused perception. Frequently, ward conversation, related to or intended for another woman, is "learned" and related mistakenly to the woman herself. This is an example of an inappropriate side effect of learning. A humorous incident that makes the point here was when a patient refused to talk to her physician because he had called her an "old bag." The patient had overheard the physician discussing her gallbladder (the "old bag") with the interns. Questions arise about other "side effects" that occur when patients learn inappropriate information. Clinical situations involving crises include the labor and delivery experience, an abortion experience, a patient hospitalized for diagnosis of cancer, and the loss situation when an infant dies. Assessments of patient learning needs in these situations need to take into consideration the impact of anxiety on the patient's perception of what is being said. Also, an appropriate time plan for teaching should be considered. Extensive teaching may need to be delayed until the anxiety is lessened.

Health–Illness States. Another variable influencing the patient's readiness and capacity to learn is an individual's adaptation to illness. A number of theorists have identified stages of adaptation to illness. These stages describe common responses of individuals trying to incorporate a particular illness into their self-concept. Crate's stages (1965) are descriptive and serve as one model for visualizing an individual's response to illness and how this might influence learning (Table 2–1).

The first stage in adaptation to illness, according to Crate, is termed *disbelief*. In this stage, individuals deny that they have an illness and attempt to behave as if they are well. Avoidance, by forgetting or refusing to do things required of them, is a way to deny illness. Individuals may also attempt to control treatment or divert attention to other issues through not learning. Obviously, there is a need to assess an individual's adjustment to illness states prior to proceeding with education that assists them in coping with their illness.

This disbelief stage is seen in pregnant women who deny they have serious complications with their pregnancy that necessitates a change in life-style. A pregnant diabetic, denying that the pregnancy was making her diabetes more difficult to control, found it difficult to "learn" the new dietary restrictions and insulin dosages necessary. A thorough assessment of the patient's problems revealed a need to focus on the impact that pregnancy had on diabetes as well as her emotional response to being "different" from other pregnant women in her group.

The second stage in Crate's adaptation to illness is termed *developing awareness*. Here individuals become less able to maintain denial and more aware of what has happened and its implications. Dependence on others frequently causes conflicts resulting in anger. At first this anger can be diffused. Later it can be more specifically focused upon being sick. Anger can be expressed openly, projected, or directed toward one's self in depression. It is important to recognize the need to express anger at being ill. Attempting to teach anyone to cope with illness may be difficult in this stage. Other family members may need to be taught so that critical information related to safety and survival can be shared.

Reorganization is the third stage in Crate's stages. Here individuals accept the increased dependence that illness demands. Frequently there is some reorganization of roles between family members during this period.

Resolution and *identity change* occur when illness is accepted. Individuals at this stage can now live better with their illness or condition. This is a good time to teach because individuals may be more open to information about their illness and adaptation to illness. A need for support and for an "identity" with others who have the same condition was seen in a group for diabetic pregnant women. There was an identity as a "pregnant diabetic" that meant certain restrictions and limitations on the individuals' life-style and activities. Women in this group expressed the fact that being identified with others like themselves for whom pregnancy was not always easy, helped them accept the strict medical regime that allowed diabetes to have a minimum effect on the outcome of the pregnancy (Littlefield, 1979).

Suchman (1965) identified a fifth stage in adapting to illness called the *recovery* or *rehabilitation* stage. In this stage the person relinquishes the sick role. This stage requires individuals to reestablish relationships and roles that were previously part of their life. This may be difficult for family members. Frequently patients are reluctant to

TABLE 2–1. RELATIONSHIP OF HEALTH–ILLNESS STATES TO HEALTH EDUCATION

| Stage | Characteristics | Readiness | |
		State	Goals

I. Disbelief	Denies illness
	Behaves as if well
	Attempts to control
	  treatment
	Diverts attention
	  from illness
		Resists learning	To increase
			  self-awareness
			  of illness state
			  and its impact on
			  current and future
			  life-style

II. Developing
  awareness
	Denies illness
	Increases dependence
	  on others
	Is angry
	Is depressed
		Resists learning	To recognize conflicts
			To express and resolve
			  anger

III. Reorganization	Accepts fact of
	  illness state
	Accepts increased
	  dependence
	Accepts life change
	Accepts new "identity"
		Is ready to learn	Can now focus on
			  actual health care
			  program

IV. Dependent role	Resists "well" role
	Family members may
	  resist "well" role
		Resists learning	To increase self-
			  awareness and recognition
			  of new wellness
			  state and its potential
			  for return to
			  independence

V. Recovery	Relinquishes
	  dependency and
	  patient role
	Reaccepts independent
	  self
	Reestablishes
	  independent life-style
	  and relationships
		Open to more indepth
		  understanding of
		  illness
			To return to maximum
			  functioning and
			  wellness

(Source: *Developed using Crate (1965), Suchman (1965), and Redman (1980).*)

become "well" again. At times this reluctance relates to lack of knowledge about what is possible; at other times, it relates to an emotional readiness to assume the well role. Learning how to cope with wellness or an improved illness state may be influenced by the individual's family's adaptation and is an important area to assess prior to planning learning experiences.

Assessing Readiness

In addition to collecting data concerning the previously identified variables, the health care professional needs to determine the woman's general state of readiness for health teaching. Two important principles of motivation should be considered while assessing the patient's readiness for learning. These are:

1. Internal motivation is longer lasting and more self-directive than is external motivation, which must be repeatedly reinforced by praise or concrete rewards.
2. Learning is most effective when an individual is ready to learn, that is, when the individual feels a need to know something (Klausmeier & Ripple, 1971).

Observation of the patient's behavior, questions and comments when visiting the clinic, or when nurses interact with her or her family are important ways to collect data about readiness. Direct questioning about specific situations, procedures, or feelings also will allow the health care professional to assess the individual's area of interest, curiosity, or concern. Using "ubiquitous questions" when there is no readily observed behavior or when the woman does not ask questions is sometimes helpful. These questions are phrased so that the woman is given information about what many other women facing the same situation ask. Therefore, permission to have concerns and questions is given by asking ubiquitous questions. For example, for a woman facing the decision concerning an unwanted pregnancy, an ubiquitous question might be, "Many women making a decision like you are, wonder about . . . I was wondering if you had such questions too?"

Summary

The health care professional needs to assess many variables to plan learning experiences. In addition, some assessment of the family and the community resources available to women are needed prior to planning the teaching–learning interaction. It may be that other sources are appropriate and available for teaching individual women. As can be seen, assessment of learning needs and a diagnosis of the learning style and capacity are extremely complex and will take time and skill.

PLANNING THE LEARNING EXPERIENCE

After identifying the client's individual learning needs, plans for learning experiences should include: (1) selection of an appropriate role for the teacher; (2) selection of the best teaching–learning activities; (3) a decision as to the type of learning theory that matches the specific circumstance; and (4) identifying a mechanism for communicating goals, process, and evaluation of learning. This section discusses this planning process and makes suggestions on how to accomplish each of these aspects of planning.

The Teacher's Role

Individuals who teach need to assess their own capabilities, preferences, and knowledge. This allows teachers to select the teaching role most congruent with their own style, abilities, and comfort. Assuming that the health care provider is the only resource for the woman to learn from is a mistake and costly in terms of time. What the woman knows, what the family members know, and what community resources have to offer should also be identified and used when possible and appropriate. For example, in a community where education for childbirth is readily available and adequate, the labor and delivery nurse may assume less of this responsibility and concentrate on evaluating what her individual patients have learned and provide feedback to the teachers of the preparation for childbirth classes as to what has been learned and what additional teaching is needed. Where such resources are not available, then the labor and delivery nurse may herself start a course, or organize a plan for individualized instruction.

Teachers can choose an equalitarian or authority subordinate role. This actual selection of role could be based on the teacher's preference, but instead should depend on the status and circumstances of the learner. For example, women who expect to be directed by health professionals, those who are in a crisis or ill may need a more directive, authoritative teacher. Those who are recovering from illness or seeking to become more independent and self-reliant may prefer a teacher who views them more as equals.

Caplan (1959) believes that the nurse has a special opportunity to establish an equalitarian role because of the perceived "sociological closeness" to the patient. Caplan states that the nurse and other professionals, like social workers and health educators (as opposed to physicians), can function in a "Wise-Sister" (Wise-Brother) role. This role allows clients to feel more comfortable asking questions, sharing information, and being honest about actual health practices. Caplan proposes that this sociological closeness facilitates an open, interactive interchange (Caplan, 1959). It is also possible that some women who value authority and expect to be subordinate to health care professionals will value less the content taught by an individual perceived as equal.

Teaching during labor and delivery demonstrates a need for changing the role of the teacher for individual women as labor progresses. As labor progresses, the woman moves from a more independent (first phase, first stage, 0–4 cm dilated) to a dependent role (transition or 8–10 cm). She is less able to direct her own learning as she approaches the second stage of labor. During the early phases of labor, the woman can identify learning needs and participate actively in the learning process. She is able to make choices and decide on a variety of comfort techniques. In the latter phases of labor, the woman may need direct, firm explanations and specific suggestions for how to behave and what to do.

This need for changing the teacher role can be seen in several other clinical situations. Some of the most illustrative are the new mothers moving through the postpartum experience, adolescents in various states of crises, and women facing a catastrophic illness. These various teacher roles with selected clients are discussed in future chapters. (Chapter 3 provides more detail regarding the advantages and disadvantages of selected roles.)

Selecting Teaching–Learning Activities. Depending on what is to be learned, different types of teaching activities are appropriate. The type of behavior change required of the learner influences the type of instruction and what should be taught (Table 2–2).

For example temporary behavior changes usually require a lesser "dosage" of education than long-term, permanent changes. An increasing number and variety of teaching methodologies are needed as the behavior change becomes more permanent and more critical to the client's health. The importance of the interpersonal relationship with the teacher also increases as more permanent change is required. Additional persons (family, friends, support persons) need to learn the content to facilitate learning and compliance. Table 2–3 demonstrates how these principles can be related to a cessation of smoking instructional program. The "potency" for the instruction program is increased with each individual who does not learn from the previous level of instruction. Readers might identify patients from their own clinical experience for whom different potency levels might be appropriate. Some examples include the individual who has more than one unwanted pregnancy and still does not use contraceptives, the diabetic pregnant woman who can readily discuss the appropriate medical regime for her diabetic and pregnant condition, but does not comply with this regime, the obese individual who does not comply with a weight reduction plan, and the individual who is highly anxious over labor and delivery, parenting, or menopause, even after the usual educational preparation.

Using Learning Principles. Using appropriate learning principles is also important in planning learning experiences. What learning theory should be used requires the teacher to exercise professional judgment (Ausubel, 1965). That is, in applying any learning principle to a particular situation the teacher (1) weighs the claim of one pertinent principle against another by considering relevant aspects, (2) evaluates the momentary

TABLE 2–2. BEHAVIOR CHANGE AND TEACHING ACTIVITIES

Learning Tasks of Patient	Teaching Activities
Temporary and noncritical behavior change *Example:* Activity change during normal pregnancy	Written and oral instruction
Temporary and critical behavior change *Example:* Low salt diet with symptoms of toxemia	Written and oral instruction + Teach client plus another person from patient's support system
Short-term noncritical behavior change *Example:* Practicing LaMaze breathing regularly	Written and oral instruction + Teach client plus another person from patient's support system + Relationship with teacher
Multiple basic behavior change *Example:* Incorporation of new infant into family	Written and oral instruction + Teach client plus another person from patient's support system + Relationship with teacher + Involvement of environment (whole family)

(Source: Redman, B. Personal Communication (1982), by permission.)

situation with the learner's personality and preparation, including state of readiness, fatigue, and current understanding, and (3) considers the appropriateness and the adequacy of the ongoing communication between teacher and learner (Ausubel, 1965).

Another facet of decision making related to selection of appropriate learning principles has to do with the kind and amount of research evidence available for that particular theory. Although empirical evidence is available from animal learning and in controlled laboratory situations, research is needed to determine which principles are appropriate for learning health behaviors. Learning related to health behaviors is different in that learners in this content area are not responsible to the school setting and are in real life circumstances that change the priority and motivational base of learning.

The following principles (Mort & Vincent, 1954) are accepted as having relevance for teaching in a variety of settings. It is logical that they are equally applicable in health education settings.

1. No one learns without feeling some urge to learn.
2. What individuals learn is influenced directly by their surroundings. If an individual is expected to learn something, making this "something" a part of the learner's environment so that the learner may see it, live with it, and be influenced by it increases learning.
3. Persons learn most quickly and lastingly what has meaning to them. A behavior takes on meaning to the learner from its outcome—what that act produces. To produce a thing that a learner wants to learn, assist the person to see the value of this act or behavior from her own perspective or experience and the person is more likely to master the skill necessary to accomplish the task of learning. Thus, the patient's interest is a source of power in motivating learning.

TABLE 2–3. POTENCY OF INSTRUCTION

Example	Goals	Instructional Techniques	Patient Achievement
Woman who is a smoker becomes pregnant and is advised to stop smoking	1. Make patient aware that problem is important and that the goals of the health program are valuable	*Level I:* Provide message and basic information. Verbally: nurse and physician; printed handouts; public education; radio and TV spots	If patient continues behavior (smoking), rate this as failure and move to next level of instructional intensity
	2. Help patient to master and utilize, on her own, a step-by-step medical or health program	*Level II:* Continue with previous level for reinforcement; add programmed instruction; audiovisual instruction; personalized daily or weekly schedule	If patient stops behavior (smoking), rate this as success, but return to last level of instruction for maintenance. If patient continues behavior; increase level of instructional intensity
	3. Continue previous goals, but emphasize that patient must practice for mastery	*Level III:* Continue previous levels as appropriate; add support system; therapist, or group therapy with others having similar problem. Systematic desensitization of emotional or physical resistance to health care program	If patient stops behavior (smoking), maintain at this level, or return to level I for maintenance. If patient who succeeded at level II relapses to former habit, bring up to level III. If patient continues behavior (smoking), increase level of instructional intensity
	4. Same as 3	*Level IV:* Continue previous levels where appropriate: add more direct intervention: more frequent office visits. Reevaluation of individual learning behavior needs	Success at this level requires judgment as to what level is needed for maintenance

4. Readiness to learn is important and can influence learning.
5. Individuals learn in different ways.
6. Security and success are the soil and the climate for growth. Positive reinforcement assists individuals to succeed in learning. What gives satisfaction tends to be repeated; what is annoying tends to be avoided.
7. Learning occurs through attempts to satisfy needs.
8. Emotional tension decreases efficiency in learning. Some degree of emotional tension increases an individual's motivation to learn, but too much emotional tension decreases learning.
9. Some physical defects lower efficiency in learning. Recognition of the influence of physical health on learning should be considered because health education is of necessity frequently delivered to ill individuals.
10. Learning is more efficient and longer lasting when the conditions for it are real

and lifelike. Attitudes, habits, skills for life are best learned when the activities of learning are like those of life. Methods of teaching should be as much as possible similar to those used in actual living.

11. Piecemeal learning is not efficient. Facts and skills are best taught when they are learned, in a pattern and in relation to their use, not as isolated bits of subject matter.

12. Active participation in learning increases learning. The learner gains insight as she learns to organize what she does, practices the desired behavior to be learned, and participates in the learning process from identification of learning needs, to selection of learning activities, to evaluating what she has learned.

13. General behavior is controlled by the emotions as well as the intellect and learning. To be effective, the teacher needs to consider both aspects.

14. Individuals start to learn based on their knowledge base instead of from some artificial knowledge point determined by the learning situation. Growth in terms of learning is a steady, continuous process and different individuals learn at different rates.

15. Learning one thing at a time is impossible. The learner responds to her setting as a whole and takes in many things besides what the learning is focused on.

16. Learning is reinforced when two or more senses are used at the same time. Offering multisensory learning opportunities enhances learning.

17. The average learner is a myth. The individual achievement of a group of learners scatters over a wide range and only a few will be at the "average" point.

Chapter 3 presents more complete information on teaching–learning theory. The expanded discussion in Chapter 3 allows the reader to more easily visualize a variety of approaches that can be selected in numerous clinical settings with women in various stages of health and illness. This brief review has been presented to summarize the educational process.

Writing Objectives. Writing objectives is an important part of planning the learning experience. The importance of clearly stated objectives is reflected in the need to identify what is expected of the learner. Objectives allow evaluation of when learning has taken place. Behavioral objectives are most often recommended. These objectives describe behaviors that learners will exhibit after learning has taken place.

A taxonomy of educational objectives has been developed by a group of psychologists and educators, and is available in Bloom's *Taxonomy of Educational Objectives: The Classification of Educational Goals Handbook I and II* (Bloom, 1956; Krathwohl, Masia, & Bloom, 1964) and in Simpson's work *In the Psychomotor Domain* (1972). These authors divide behaviors into three domains:

1. The cognitive, dealing with intellectual ability
2. The affective, including expression of feelings, interest, attitudes, values, and appreciation
3. The psychomotor, dealing with skills commonly known as motor skills

In each domain, behaviors are ordered into complex behaviors at the upper end of the taxonomy (numbers 5.0 and 6.0) and simple behaviors at the lower end of the scale (number 1.0). Table 2–4 demonstrates these domains, hierarchical differences, and provides a sample objective to demonstrate the three types of objectives.

Obviously different learning activities are needed for cognitive, affective, and psychomotor learning. Thus, the specific objective and its type need to be identified prior to implementing the learning experience so that the appropriate learning experience can be planned. Also, recognition of the different types and hierarchies of objectives will assist the teacher in recognizing the holistic approach needed to learning. Teaching facts and figures is not complete. Values, attitudes, interests, and ability to apply their learning to actual life situations are also needed.

If the reader needs additional assistance to formulate objectives, a programmed approach to learning to write these objectives is available in the September–October 1977 issue of the *Nurse Educator* (Jones & Oertel, 1977). Also Mager's text, *Preparing Instructional Objectives* (1962), is helpful in this area. One idea to limit the difficulty and time involved in writing objectives is to have an "objective bank." That is, an individual or a group of individuals, skilled in writing objectives as well as having knowledge in the specific learning needs of women in a given clinical unit, would write all the possible objectives that could be needed by a particular client. After an appropriate assessment of learning needs, those objectives that are relevant could be selected to be included in an individual woman's plan of care. Appendix A contains an example of behavioral objectives that have been written to cover the entire perinatal experience (see Chapter 12 and Appendix A). A bank of objectives allows the teacher to know the expectations of women in the perinatal experience and avoids the need to create objectives in each individual circumstance.

Use of Contracting for Patient Education

The idea of contracting with a woman for learning should be considered when the learning goals are longterm and involved. "The contract is a mutual understanding of the reason for the education and the problem or areas that will be discussed during the visits" (Redman, 1980, p. 84). The elements to be included in the contract are as follows (Redman, 1980):

1. What is the goal?
2. What does the client have to offer?
3. What does the client expect of the health care provider?
4. What does the health care provider expect of the client?
5. What does the health care provider have to offer?
6. How do client and health care provider plan to work together?
7. When and under what circumstances is the contract to be renegotiated?

Note the inclusion of all the elements reflects a clear goal, mutuality of goals, utilization of both the resources of the health care provider and the woman, the process to be used, and when the evaluation will occur and be renegotiated for a new plan. Signing the contract allows a formal commitment by both provider and client. A study by Stekel and Swain (1977) demonstrated increased effectiveness of learning and compliance when contracting was used in addition to an educational seminar and counseling. Routine care without any of these aspects was not effective in producing learning.

The following are examples of clinical situations where contracting may be appropriate: (1) high-risk pregnant women, such as diabetics; (2) the adolescent who is pregnant or making a choice about abortion; (3) the mother with a preterm infant; (4) the woman with repeated abortions; (5) women with chronic illnesses; and (6) complicated surgical recovery periods.

TABLE 2–4. SAMPLE OBJECTIVES

Taxonomy	Sample Objective
Cognitive Domain	
1. *Knowledge* Knowledge as defined here, involves recall or remembering of information[a]	1. The patient will describe the reasons for practicing breathing exercises prior to labor. 2. The patient will state how the prenatal diet influences fetal development.
2. *Comprehension* Represents the lowest level of understanding. It refers to a type of understanding such that the individual knows what is being communicated and can make use of the material or idea being communicated without necessarily relating it to other material or seeing its fullest implications[a]	1. When bottle feeding the baby, the mother will recognize when the baby is satisfied. 2. The patient will translate the instructions on the birth control pills into appropriate action.
3. *Application* The use of abstractions in particular and concrete situations. The abstractions can be in the form of general ideas, rules of procedures, or generalized methods	1. The patient will apply principles of asepsis when cleaning the baby's cord. 2. Given the general knowledge of the principles of supply and demand in breast feeding, the patient will plan feeding schedules so as to increase her milk supply.
4. *Analysis* The breakdown of a communication into its constituent elements or parts such that the relative hierarchy of ideas is made clear or the relations between the ideas expressed are made explicit or both[a]	1. The patient will identify factors that cause a decrease in breast milk. 2. The patient will distinguish how preparation and no preparation for labor differ.
5. *Synthesis* The putting together of elements and parts to form a whole. This involves the process of working with pieces, parts, elements, and so forth and arranging and combining them in such a way so as to constitute a pattern or structure not clearly present before	1. Upon discharge, the patient will plan daily activities that meet her needs for rest and her new baby's needs for interaction, feeding and rest. 2. The patient will interpret to her husband the feelings she experiences postpartally.
6. *Evaluation* Judgments about the value of material and methods for given purposes	1. The patient will assess the completeness of the care she received in labor and her satisfaction with it. 2. The patient will assess her performance in labor, determining factors in herself and the environment that contributed to her unique performance.
Affective Domain	
1. *Receiving* Awareness. The individual will take into account a situation, fact or event, stage of affairs	1. The patient will be aware that the nurse is available to help during the abortion procedure. 2. The patient will tolerate activity restrictions necessary because of her potential for miscarriage.
2. *Responding* The learner makes a response to a given situation. This response can be at the level of not fully accepting the necessity for responding; and responding on her own; of feeling satisfaction, or pleasure in responding	1. The patient will cooperate with the insertion of the internal fetal monitor. 2. The patient will feel some satisfaction breast feeding her baby.
3. *Valuing* The individual accepts a value, is willing to be identified with that value. From this first level of valuing, the individual can have a preference for the value; more intense valuing involves a commitment to act out the behavior	1. The patient will accept the limitations placed on dietary intake during pregnancy due to the advancing signs of toxemia. 2. The patient will desire to participate actively in the care of her baby.

TABLE 2–4. (cont.)

Taxonomy	Sample Objective
4. *Organization* Putting together the conceptualization of values to form the organization of a value system[a]	1. The patient will regularly choose those alternatives of action that are consistent with good parenting.[b]
5. *Characterization* Here are found those objectives that concern the individual's view of the universe, her philosophy of life, a value system having as its object the whole of what is known or knowable[a]	1. The patient will regulate her life-style during pregnancy in a manner consistent with respect for a healthy outcome of pregnancy for herself and her baby.
Psychomotor Domain	
1. *Perception* The process of becoming aware of objects, qualities, or relations by way of the sense organs[b]	1. The patient will recognize the "feel" of holding a baby with good balance.[a]
2. *Set* A preparatory adjustment of readiness for a particular kind of action or experience	1. The patient will demonstrate panting and pushing behavior needed for the second stage of labor.
3. *Guided Response* The overt behavioral act of an individual under the guidance of the instructor. Prerequisite to preformance of the act are readiness to respond and selection of the appropriate response[b]	1. The patient will discover the most efficent method of diapering a baby through trial of various procedures.[c]
4. *Mechanism* Learned response has become habitual. The learner has achieved a certain confidence and degree of skill. The act is a part of her repertoire of possible responses to stimuli and to the demands of situation where the response is an appropriate one.[b]	1. The patient will use the hand breast pump in removing breast milk.
5. *Complex Overt Response* Performance of a motor act that is considered complex because of the movement pattern required. A high degree of skill has been attained, and the act can be carried out with minimum expenditure of time and energy[b]	1. The patient will skillfully feed her infant who has a cleft lip and palate.
6. *Adaptation* Altering motor activities to meet the demands of new problematic situation requiring a physical response[b]	1. The patient will design her own activity for caring for twins in the home environment.
7. *Origination* Creating new motor acts or ways of manipulating materials out of understandings, abilities, and skills developed in the psychomotor area[b]	Rarely used in patient education.[c]

Note: Objectives not footnoted are those of the author.
[a]Based on Redman (1980) and her adaptation of Krathwohl, D. R., Bloom, B. S., & Masia, B. B. *Taxonomy of educational objectives: The classification of educational goals: Handbook II: Affective domain.* New York: David McKay, 1963, pp. 76–85.
[b]Based on Redman (1980) and her adaptation of Simpson, E. J. *The classification of educational objectives in the psychomotor domain.* In *Contributions of behavioral science to instructional technology: The psychomotor domain.* Mt. Rainer, Md.: Gryphon Press, 1972.
[c]Objective was from Redman's text (Redman, 1980, pp. 81–82).

Use of Written Material for Health Education

Written material is an invaluable resource in health education. Numerous commercial pamphlets are available. Before using these materials, however, the health care provider should screen them according to some criteria that makes their use appropriate, gets at the goals of education for a specific woman or group of women, and does not produce any inappropriate side effects. Table 2–5 lists suggested questions to explore prior to use of any written material for patient education.

In order to identify the grade level of written material, the Dale Chall readability formula is helpful (Fry, 1968) (Fig. 2–4). It allows assessment of the educational level of written material. The material can then be matched to the general educational level of the women the facility serves. It should be remembered, however, that not all individuals read at the educational level obtained; some read above this level, some below. The Dale Chall formula does give an idea of what material would be at a very high level. For example, a study that reviewed the effectiveness of educational material for diabetics found that the material as prepared was comprehensible to only 22 percent of the patients who used it (Mohammed, 1964). Care should be taken not to duplicate this experience. When preparing new materials it is necessary to prepare them so that the information is immediately practicable.

Use of Audiovisual Material for Patient Education

Most people today expect some visual display of what they are to learn. Because some of the concepts that need explaining, such as uterine contractions, are difficult to understand, there is a need to provide visual representation of what we teach. This might include hospital tours, discussions with people who have experienced what the learner is anticipating, as well as films, pictures, and models. Audiovisual resources also need to be screened for appropriateness as well as inappropriate side effects. The criteria identified for written material are relevant to screening audiovisual materials. Additional specific questions, however, need to be asked in making decisions about the appropriateness of audiovisual materials. These appear in Table 2–6.

An example of a film with an emotional impact that was distracting and had negative side effects for some learners was the film, "The Sexually Mature Adult." This film, excellent in its content and ability to teach about sexual response when shown to appropriate audiences, was shown to college-age students in a formal classroom. Because these learners had not chosen to learn about sexual response, the impact of seeing sexual

---

TABLE 2–5. CRITERIA FOR SELECTION OF WRITTEN MATERIAL

1. Is the information critical or relevant to the general content area?
2. Is the information correct?
3. Is the material at the appropriate educational level for the patient population?
4. Do the format and style point out important information, or is the format confusing and the content in a detail not needed by most patients?
5. Does the material meet the objectives for learning set for an individual patient?
6. Do the pictures and drawings create interest and reflect a patient population that your patients can identify with; for example, do pictures and drawings include minority patients or patients from a variety of economic classes?
7. Is the organization of the content appropriate? Is it centered on a single concept? Does it relate content to a condition or a situation the patient might experience? Is it sequenced from implications to appropriate actions?

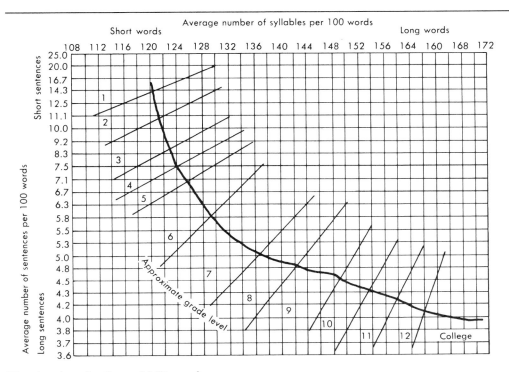

Average number of syllables per 100 words

Short words   Long words

Directions for using the readability graph

1. Select three one-hundred-word passages from near the beginning, middle and end of the book. Skip all proper nouns.
2. Count the total number of sentences in each hundred-word passage (estimating to nearest tenth of a sentence). Average these three numbers.
3. Count the total number of syllables in each hundred-word sample. There is a syllable for each vowel sound; for example: cat(1), blackbird(2), continental(4). Don't be fooled by word size; for example: polio(3), through(1). Endings such as -y, -ed, -el, or -le usually make a syllable, for example: ready(2), bottle(2). I find it convenient to count every syllable over one in each word and add 100. Average the total number of syllables for the three samples.
4. Plot on the graph the average number of sentences per hundred words and the average number of syllables per hundred words. Most plot points fall near the heavy curved line. Perpendicular lines mark off approximate grade level areas.

Example:

	Sentences per 100 words	Syllables per 100 words
100-word sample page 5	9.1	122
100-word sample page 89	8.5	140
100-word sample page 160	7.0	129
	3) 24.6	3) 391
Average	8.2	130

Plotting these averages on the graph, we find they fall in the 5th grade area; hence the book is about 5th grade difficulty level. If great variability is encountered either in sentence length or in the syllable count for the three selections, then randomly select several more passages and average them in before plotting.

Figure 2—4. Graph for estimating readability. *(Source: Fry, E. A readability formula that saves time. Journal of Reading, 11, 514, 1968.)*

TABLE 2-6. ADDITIONAL CRITERIA FOR USE OF AUDIOVISUAL MATERIAL

1. Is the emotional impact of the material conducive to learning, meeting the objectives in the affective realm, or is the emotional impact distracting, overwhelming, or productive of inappropriate side effects?
2. Is the material appropriate to the age level?
3. Are the mode of dress and life-style so obsolete that they detract from the message?
4. Are there so many concepts presented that learning cannot be focused?

intercourse on film was overwhelming to many who were struggling with their own sexuality. Although this film is educational, it is not appropriate for all audiences. Prior preparation for the emotional impact that a film has is essential.

An example of an inappropriate age level film is one on sexuality that has a "grass-hopper telling the story of sex." Adolescent response to this film was negative, and the content covered was lost. The problems of outdated dress and life-style in visual presentations are sometimes distracting and should be considered when older films are used. Some introduction to this fact is needed prior to using the film. Younger audiences have difficulty in believing that the concepts in the film are current or real when the people seem unreal and outdated.

Too many concepts, too much information, as well as emotional issues can be difficult to comprehend in one film. The full impact of the presentation could thus be lost. An example of this last problem is the film "I Am Seventeen and Pregnant." Although this film is excellent in many ways and is a valuable teaching tool for adolescents and their parents, it covers several emotional topics and a wide variety of factual information (pregnancy, contraception, abortion, adoption). It is better shown in segments with discussion taking place at key points. Focusing the learners' attention on key points in the film that meet a specific learning objective is a way to narrow the learning for any session when films cover numerous concepts.

Because individuals respond differently to educational materials, whether written or oral, having a representative sample of women view a film, pamphlet, or chart is a way of assessing its appropriateness for a particular group. Such a review panel can provide information regarding emotional impact, what is unclear, and what type of focusing by the teacher needs to be done when the actual learning experience is offered.

Written and audiovisual materials are readily available from commercial and government sources. Teaching aids are also available from the American Dairy Council, Planned Parenthood, Childbirth Education Association, Maternity Center Association, and local mental health chapters. *Nursing Outlook*, the *American Journal of Nursing*, and *Nurse Educator* are journals that contain descriptions of written and audiovisual materials. State health departments are also an appropriate source for identifying materials. Some communities and medical center libraries have special areas for lay information about health and health practices. The Kaiser Health Education Resource Center in Oakland, California, includes a patient health library as well as health exhibits. There are also resources for instructors and counselors in the various educational and content areas provided by Kaiser (Collen & Soghikian, 1974). Also, companies that produce medical products may advertise instructional materials more or less specific to their products. Several authors have compiled lists of instructional materials (Lenahan, 1968; Wood, 1974, pp. 43–50, 60–66). A special need for a list of materials prepared for Spanish-speaking audiences has been met by Isquith (1974). A list of local teaching materials would be helpful in clinical facilities, libraries, and private organizations concerned with health (see bibliography at the end of this chapter for complete references).

IMPLEMENTATION

Implementing the health education process is difficult to describe in a chapter of this nature. Observation of the teaching–learning behaviors of colleagues is a method by which the reader can visualize this activity. Trying out various activities and roles clinically, and discussing their effectiveness with peers will also assist health care professionals to develop their individual style and determine which of these are effective in a variety of situations. Implementation of a well-thought-out plan may need to be changed when it is not working. Hopefully, when implementation does not work, the instructor will reassess all the factors previously identified to determine the base for the ineffectiveness. Making plans for detailed, systematic feedback about the effectiveness of a teaching method for an individual clinical situation or for overall performance in a clinical setting where several health care professionals function assists in making better decisions about what is effective. Unfortunately, no set pattern is effective with everyone. Flexibility and variety in approach need to be constantly used.

Documentation. Because the planning process and outcome of patient education need to be recorded for the teacher's reference as well as to document what was done, a number of individuals have developed forms to record information about learners, learning needs, progress toward learning, and behavior change related to learning. Resource A provides samples of alternate forms developed for special units and selected learning needs.

Appendixes A and B in this text demonstrate another method for documentation. Individual creativity should allow development of forms that are helpful in a particular clinical setting. The forms in Figures 2–5 through 2–8 are shared to generate ideas about ways to record information. When possible, brevity is helpful in documentation. The more information included, however, the more complete and consistent the teaching is documented. Assessment of learning, plans for teaching, and methods to evaluate learning can also be documented as part of the SOAP (subjective, objective, assessment, plan) format in the problem-oriented record. Each patient problem could have a plan for education or a separate problem related to lack of information identified.

Whatever documentation method is used, the importance of documentation should be noted. In legal terms, only what is documented was provided. It is possible to have clients deny education that was critical to their recovery or health maintenance. Complete documentation clarifies the activity of the teacher and the learner.

EVALUATION

Evaluation in health education can be defined as the process of determining if the educational goals set with an individual or a group of individuals have been met. Figure 2–5 depicts this process. Steele and Brack (1973), adult educators, describe seven essential activities in evaluation. They are: understanding, specifying, describing, comparing, judging, valuing, and influencing.

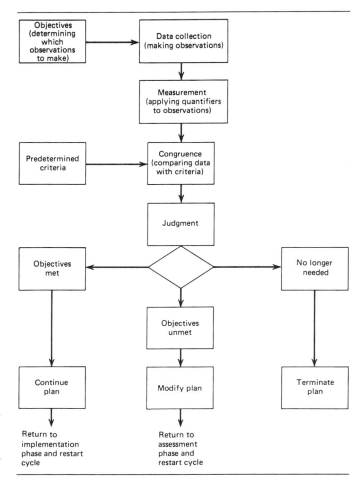

Figure 2–5. The process of evaluation in health education. (Source: Sasmor, J. L. Childbirth education: A nursing perspective. *New York: John Wiley & Sons, 1979, p. 122, by permission.)*

Essential Evaluation Activities

Understanding. For the understanding activity, the evaluator needs to identify the purpose of evaluation. One needs to know who is to use the results, and for what purpose will the information be used (Steele & Brack, 1973). In health education, evaluation data are primarily used so that the teacher can determine if specific learning goals have been met by an individual client. At times evaluation data are used to help the learners have an idea of how their own learning objectives have been met. Frequently, data are needed by administrators to determine effectiveness of an educational program. These data can be used to evaluate staffing patterns, type of educational approach, cost effectiveness, and so forth. Data may be needed by different individuals to justify expenditures on patient education or support for increased expenditures when the outcomes are less than desired. Thus what data are collected for evaluation depend on the purpose to which they are put.

Specifying. The objectives and goals of the teaching plan or program serve as a guide in the activity of specifying. When these are clearly stated, they are more easily evaluated. In evaluating outcomes of health education, goal-free and goal-directed outcomes can be used. For example, behavioral objectives, if used, allow goal-directed evaluation to be conducted to determine if a patient has learned. It is also important to identify other outcomes not in these objectives. For example, a woman's attitude toward health care might be improved as a result of the teaching experience. Failure to examine other outcomes besides the specific goals might cause one to miss both good and bad side effects of the teaching–learning situation.

Specifying includes setting standards for attainment. How many objectives at what level need to be met for an individual to have learned? For evaluation of groups, how many individuals need to meet the objectives? Table 2–7 defines various types of standards. The teacher should be clear about the standard against which the teaching session will be evaluated.

Describing. In the process of describing, the information collected needs to be accurate, bias-free, replicable, germane to the objective, communicable, well-timed, and credible to those who must use it (Steele & Brack, 1973). In health education, the instructor usually does not have experimental type data, but must collect data that demonstrate the effects of teaching in the real-life situation of a busy clinical setting. The most common way of collecting these data clinically is to have patients describe their behavior, or to observe their behavior when they visit the health care facility or are seen in the home by a community health nurse. Being able to phrase questions to obtain data that are descriptive enough to determine if learning is applied in the woman's life situation is indeed a skill and takes time.

Comparing. Description of the teaching–learning situation can be process- or outcome-oriented. In outcome evaluation, encouraged in this chapter, the behavior change observed in the learner is the measure of effectiveness of the teaching. Outcome evaluation is encouraged and used as one criterion in determining if an educational program can receive

TABLE 2–7. STANDARD FOR EVALUATING EDUCATION

1. *Historical standards:* Comparison at different points in time for the individual, the population, the problem, the program, or the technique.[a]
2. *Normative standards:* Comparison with outcomes from another program often in the same region. The ideal comparison group is the true control group in an experimental design.[a]
3. *Absolute standards:* Set by policy makers as, perhaps, a 100 percent solution, even though that may be unrealistic.[a]
4. *Theoretical standards:* Based on what theory and previous research would predict should happen.[a]
5. *Negotiated standards:* Usually somewhere between the theoretical standard and the absolute standard, the compromise made through negotiation.[a]
6. *Arbitrary standards:* Usually based on no information.[a]
7. *Clinical safety standard:* Set by professional nursing groups, hospital accrediting bodies, and individual practice groups.

Note: The standard not footnoted is that of the author.
[a]Adapted from Green, L. W. Toward cost-benefit evaluations of health education: Some concepts, methods and examples. *Health Education Mongraphs,* 1974, 2(Suppl), 36–64.

federal funding or be reimbursed by third party payers in several states (Rinaldi & Kelly, 1977). Outcomes of teaching–learning can be defined at the descriptive level, change in the behavior level, or at the impact on the health level. Recognizing which type of outcome is being used is important at the descriptive level. For example, the teacher can evaluate the patient's ability to describe various contraceptives, their effectiveness, and the client's attitudes toward the use of contraception. *Or* the teacher may prefer to observe how a client inserts a diaphragm, describes taking the pill, or gives an example of declining sex until adequate contraception is obtained. This data collection is an example of change in behavior. At the most rigorous level of outcome, information would be collected concerning frequency of unplanned pregnancies over a lifetime. The process type of evaluation is more frequently done and focuses on what was done by the teacher. The fact that the teacher discussed information is adequate for in-process evaluation.

Patient care audits frequently collect data that health education has been conducted. No attempt is made to determine outcome of teaching. This is becoming less acceptable in patient care today.

Paper and pencil tests can be used to determine outcome. This is possible, but the questions need to be about critical information rather than about "school type" knowledge and facts. Many individuals are threatened or turned off with tests.

Judging. Once data are collected, *judgments* are made as to the worth of the teaching plan. This judgment needs to be based on a realistic idea of what is possible, considering all the other factors that influence learning. If clear standards have been set for what is acceptable, making a judgment as to the effectiveness of a teaching plan is easier. Judgments can be made comparing one health educator's effectiveness to another's or one program to another.

This comparison can also be done formally and be experimentally controlled. For example, women receiving instruction on family planning from two providers or two clinics and a private office can be compared. If one group or individuals within each group are different, such as in pregnancy rates, then an exploration of the teaching process used could be done. Feedback can then be given to those instructors who are less effective in teaching methodologies.

Valuing. Valuing or the process of "interfacing judgments with relevant values and beliefs" (Steele & Brack, 1973) and assigning worth to that which is done, actually asks the teacher to determine the worth of completing the objectives for the learner. An overall indication of patient satisfaction and the ability to handle health problems or developmental crises appropriately, indicate some degree of worth. Some agencies and employers relate value to cost effectiveness. If a particular education approach is very costly, it may not be valued even though patients are satisfied.

Influencing. The process of evaluation and all the previously described activities are considered of little importance unless they are used to *influence* decisions (Steele & Brack, 1973) about the education plan or program for the future. Initially in this chapter when the process of education was described, the reader was encouraged to think of evaluation as ongoing. Feedback is needed whenever any aspect of the teaching plan is implemented. This type of evaluation, termed formative evaluation, allows changes in the teaching plan to occur at any point prior to completing the whole process. A change in any aspect of the teaching–learning plan may need to be done and should be considered when any aspect of the plan is not working.

Methodology Issues in Evaluation. Figure 2–6 depicts a continuum for the methodology used in evaluating patient education. Usually in a busy clinic or hospital setting the health care provider "eyeballs" the outcome and changes strategies and dosage based on her own experience. At the other end of the continuum, the health care provider conducts formal studies to determine the effects of a specific educational approach on learning. Jean Johnson's well-known research (1972) is an example of the latter approach. Obviously, conducting research into effective health education strategies is critical if health care professionals hope to influence future health behaviors. Not all health care providers are prepared to conduct research but could provide important information and raise interesting questions for future research. Most health care providers participate in midlevel approaches that collect outcome data. Outcomes before and after the educational intervention are then compared. These approaches are more often viewed as quality assurance studies. These studies are valuable and contribute to better clinical judgments concerning appropriate approaches for a variety of clients.

Figure 2–7 describes more formal research evaluation designs that can be used in evaluating a program of client education. This approach clearly requires time and expertise. Additional information on various research designs can be found in the bibliography (Fitz-Gibbon & Morris, 1978).

Summary. Table 2–8 summarizes questions to ask if learning is not taking place and Table 2–9 lists questions for teachers to ask concerning attitudes they may convey to learners. These summaries are helpful reminders of many of the points made in this chapter concerning the teaching–learning process.

PROBLEMS FOR LEARNERS AND TEACHERS

A statement of caution needs to be introduced lest the health care provider fall into what could be termed the savior syndrome. With idealistic goals to teach all patients, at all times, all things, in the most appropriate manner so as to change behavior for the better, the health care provider needs to remember that women (and men) at times choose not to learn and fail to take responsibility for their own health care regardless of the teaching. A strong commitment to provide health education does not mean taking full responsibility for the client's health behaviors. An example of a health care provider playing the savior occurred while working with a woman who failed to take birth control pills and repeatedly became pregnant. The nurse went daily to the woman's house to give the patient her contraceptive pill with the rationale that the woman "could not learn to take them." Reasonable efforts based on the best knowledge about what is effective and a genuine concern and caring for women is what is needed and expected. Doing the woman's part or not placing responsibility on the woman is inappropriate. More

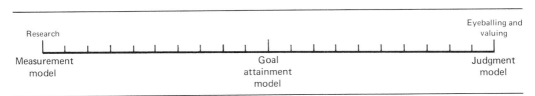

Figure 2–6. A continuum in evaluating education: Methodology issues.

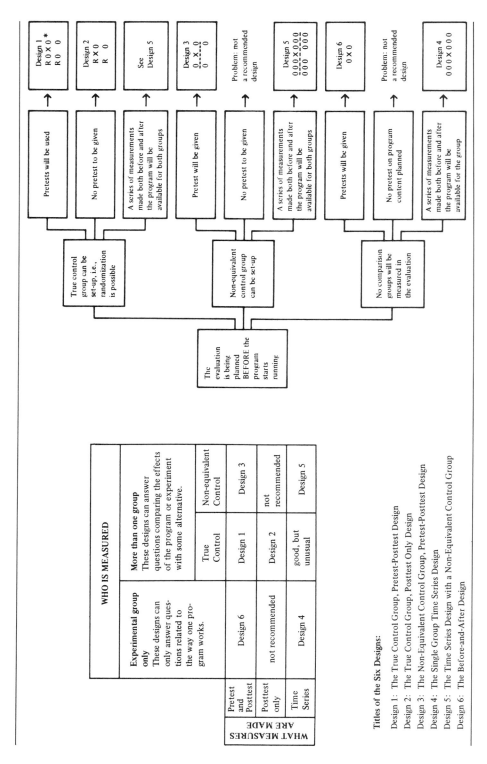

Figure 2–7. Research evaluation designs. (Source: *Fitz-Gibbon, C. T. & Morris, L. L. How to design a program evaluation. Beverly Hills, Ca.: Sage Publications, 1978, by permission.*)

Titles of the Six Designs:

Design 1: The True Control Group, Pretest-Posttest Design
Design 2: The True Control Group, Posttest Only Design
Design 3: The Non-Equivalent Control Group, Pretest-Posttest Design
Design 4: The Single Group Time Series Design
Design 5: The Time Series Design with a Non-Equivalent Control Group
Design 6: The Before-and-After Design

TABLE 2–8. POSSIBLE ERRORS IN TEACHING–LEARNING PROCESS IF GOALS ARE NOT BEING MET

Readiness goals
1. Did the learner ever accept the goals, or were you teaching about what only you believed to be important?
2. What evidence do you have that the goals were appropriate?
3. Were the goals clearly written and understood by teacher and learner?
4. Were goals broken into sufficient intermediate steps to provide guidance?

Teaching–learning
1. Had teaching materials previously been tried with persons of ability similar to your patient and found successful?
2. If previous experience with the materials was not available, in what ways did their characteristics match the patient's readiness?
3. Were the evaluative data gathered often during teaching, to give evidence of areas of success and lack of success?
4. Was teaching continued for sufficient time for learning to be thorough?
5. Were the data gathered for evaluation sufficiently valid and reliable to form an adequate basis for the evaluative decision?
6. Were baseline data obtained for measuring change? People rarely start with no knowledge.

(Source: *Redman, B. The process of patient teaching in nursing (5th ed.). St. Louis, Mo.: C. V. Mosby, 1980, p. 218, by permission.*)

knowledge and skill in getting at the basis for not learning, including motivation to change behavior, is what is needed. This takes understanding of individual differences and values and an appreciation for what changing behavior means to the client.

A review of the medical literature revealed a lack of compliance with the medical regimen in 19 to 72 percent of the cases reported. One study demonstrated a 50 percent noncompliance rate was average (Hayes-Bautista, 1976; Rosenstock, 1975). Although it is not known what techniques or approaches to health education were taken in these medical literature reports, the fact that such a large number of individuals did not comply with the medical care they sought raises questions as to why this occurs. What dosage of instruction would increase compliance?

Another study demonstrated lack of compliance in preventive aspects of health care. Of 1500 individuals surveyed, only 3.5 percent had Pap tests for cancer on a regular basis. Seventy percent of these 1500 individuals had had no tests for cancer in the last 10 years (Public Health Reports, 1965, pp. 130–131). This situation existed even when "large doses" of education concerning the need for such tests were readily available. Why, then, have so few people complied? The Health Belief Model theory hypothesizes that individuals fail to take health actions for the following reasons (Rosenstock, 1960):

1. Individuals do not feel they are susceptible to the disease. These individuals feel that others are susceptible, "but not me." This is one reason some adolescents become pregnant when they know about birth control methods.
2. Individuals feel that the disease, if contracted, would not have serious effects on life. Probably, for this reason only 15 to 20 percent of individuals surveyed follow good dental health practices.
3. Individuals do not know what action to take to avoid the disease or problem. Health education may indicate how you contract something but not what you can do to avoid that "something."
4. The threat of taking action is greater than the disease. An example is seen in

TABLE 2–9. EVALUATION OF TEACHER INFLUENCE

Questions to Ask

I. *Attitudes conveyed*

    1. Am I projecting an image that tells the client that I am here to build, rather than destroy, him/her as a person?

    2. Do I let the client know that I am aware and interested in him/her as a unique individual?

    3. Do I convey my expectations and confidence that the client can accomplish work, can learn, and is competent?

    4. Do I take every opportunity to establish a high degree of private or semi-private communication with my clients?

II. *Freedom and challenge*

    1. Do I allow clients to have a voice in planning and do I permit them to help make the "rules" they follow?

    2. Do I permit clients to challenge my opinions?

    3. Do I teach in as exciting and interesting a manner as possible?

    4. Do I distinguish between clients' learning deficiencies and their personal failure?

III. *Respect and warmth*

    1. Do I learn the name of my client(s) as soon as possible and do I use that name often?

    2. Do I share my feelings with my clients?

    3. Do I practice courtesy with my clients?

    4. Do I notice and comment favorably on what things are important to my client(s)?

IV. *Control*

    1. Do I remember to see small problems as understandable and not as personal insults?

    2. When working with groups do I avoid having "favorites" and "problem clients"?

    3. Within my limits, is there room for clients to be active and natural?

    4. Do I make sure that I am adequately prepared for each teaching session?

V. *Success*

    1. Do I convey to my clients that mistakes are part of the learning process?

    2. Do I provide genuine experiences for success for my clients?

    3. Do I use opportunities to praise (positively reinforce) clients for their success?

    4. Do I set expectations which are, and which are perceived by my clients to be within his/her abilities?

(Source: *Perkey, W. W. The self concept and school achievement. Englewood Cliffs, N.J.: Prentice-Hall, 1970, by permission.*)

individuals who fear the pelvic examination and the consequences of that experience more than the information they would receive from such a screening device.

    5. An additional reason includes the fact that many individuals are not motivated to be healthy. These individuals accept disease and illness as a part of life and choose not to reduce the problem.

As can be seen, individuals do not always learn, either because they have no opportunity to learn or because other reasons make learning, at least at the level of changing behavior, not possible or acceptable. The challenge to the health educator is to discover the "why" behind the nonlearning. For example, a family with a 10-year-old child recently diagnosed as diabetic was assessed to be "unable to learn" the day to day care of their child. This family had had extensive "education" by competent, knowledgeable nurses, physicians, dietitians, and special diabetic educators in individual and group settings. Still, neither the mother nor the daughter could administer insulin. Upon further assessment by the author, it was discovered that this family felt that the diagnosis was wrong and that the child did not have diabetes. Therefore, they did not need to "learn" any of the techniques or change their behavior. Their failure to learn was related to their readiness, rather than inappropriate techniques of teaching or inability to learn what was being taught.

In this example, inadequate assessment was made prior to the initiation of therapy (i.e., patient education) and was, therefore, incomplete. The goals of learning had not been set *with* the patient, but *for* her and her family. The learning need in this case was for an understanding about how diabetes manifested itself and how the decisions were made as to the child's diagnosis. Also, allowing time and assistance to learn effective aspects of incorporating the disease into the parent's concept of the child was important. This example depicts an appropriate "therapy" at the wrong stage in the "illness" without identifying why the therapy was not woking before "increasing the dosage."

RESOURCE A

The following are samples of forms for documentation of teaching–learning. They are presented to encourage individual development of forms for efficient, complete documentation. Appendix A and B in this text demonstrate another approach to documentation (see Chapters 12 and 19).

UNITED HOSPITALS
ST. Paul, Minnesota 55102   990151

PATIENT EDUCATION BARRIERS

PRE-EDUCATION QUESTIONNAIRE SUMMARY	POST EDUCATION QUESTIONNAIRE SUMMARY

PATIENT OBJECTIVE	METHODOLOGY (Circle if used)	EVALUATION (Please sign & date note)
CCU 1. Adjust to Coronary Care Unit environment through an understanding of the purpose of: _____ IV _____ Activity Restriction _____ Oxygen Therapy _____ Diagnostic tests _____ Policies Start date_____	one to one verbal instruction CCU pamphlet	
ANATOMY & PHYSIOLOGY 2. Describe the structure and function of the heart Describe his/her problem _____ (list problem) Start date_____	Group class slide/tape program Heart Model Diagrams Flipchart **Heart-Angina** **Heart-Attack** Heart Attack - whats ahead Heart Attack - what now Patient Manual Chapter one and two	
DIAGNOSTIC STUDIES 3. Explain purpose _____ _____ (list studies) Start date_____	Videotape "Cardiac Catheterization" UHI teaching pamphlets	
RISK FACTORS 4. Describe how to modify _____ _____ _____ _____ (list patient's) Start date_____	Group class slide/tape program Flipchart **Heart-Angina** **Heart-Attack** Heart Attack - whats ahead Heart Attack - what now Patient Manual Chapter three AHA pamphlets	

CARDIAC EDUCATION/REHABILITATION FLOWSHEET MEDICAL

(continued)

PATIENT OBJECTIVE	METHODOLOGY (Circle if used)	EVALUATION (Please sign & date note)

MEDICATIONS
 	
5. Describe name, purpose, dosage, schedule, side effects and contraindications
 	
SAP yes_____ no_____
Anticipated discharge meds
_____
_____
_____
_____
_____
(list patient's)
 	
Start date_____
	Group class
	
	Individual instruction with pharmacist
	
	Date_____
	
	UHI Medication Pamphlets
	
	Patient Manual Chapter six
		TAKE HOME PRESCRIPTIONS
		a. Filled at UHI
		
		   Discharge counseling
		   _____
		
		b. Filled outside UHI

EXERCISE 6. Tolerate 2-3 mets of activity Start date_____	Graded Exercise Progression (calisthenics, walk, bike, stairs)	See discharge note dated_____in patient care section
HOME ACTIVITY 7. Utilize principles of work simplification and adjust activity according to signs and symptoms Start date_____	Graded walking and/or biking schedule Home activity guidelines (instruction and handout) Patient Manual — Chapter Four	

DIET
 	
if appropriate
8. a. state principles of dietary control of hyperlipidemia and obesity
   b. state principles of sodium, potassium and fluid balance
   c. comply with diabetic diet
 	
DIET ORDER_____
 	
Start date_____
	Group class
	
	Individual instruction with nutrition services
	
	Date_____
	
	Patient Manual Chapter five	

PSYCH-SOCIAL-SPIRITUAL 9. Identify stress reducation techniques Recognize and cope with emotional changes Identify community resources Referral to_____ _____ Start date_____	Group support session a. patient b. family Individual consultation Patient Manual Chapters seven and nine	
DISCHARGE INSTRUCTIONS 10. List general care and physician follow up List signs and symptoms which requires a physicians attention immediately; within 24 hours; at next visit.	Discharge Information sheet Patient Manual Chapter eight	
ADDITIONAL OBJECTIVES (i.e., wound care, heart failure, pacemaker, diabetic review) List those appropriate _____ _____ _____		

(Source: United Hospitals, Inc., St. Paul, MN, by permission.)

PRENATAL TEACHING RECORD

Primary Nurse _____ EDC _____ Age _____ G _____ P _____ Education _____
Presented to Clinic at _____ Weeks.   Employment _____
Psych. Social, Economic Comments:_____

	Date	Initial
Danger Signs: (1st Clinic Visit and PRN) Discussed with patient and literature given		
Description of Clinic Routine: (Lab work, B/P, Wt., Urine, Protocols, Making appts, etc.) 1st Trimester 2nd Trimester 3rd Trimester		
Medications: (1st Clinic Visit and PRN) Discussed with patient		
Exercise: (1st Clinic Visit and PRN) Discussed with patient and literature given		
Diet: (PRN and 1st Clinic Visit) Discussed with patient and literature given Comments _____		
Prenatal Classes: (1st Visit and/or before 20 weeks) Discussed with patient and literature given		
Anatomy and Physiology/Growth and Development of Baby Discussed with patient in the 1st trimester Discussed with patient in the 2nd trimester Discussed with patient in the 3rd trimester		
Admission Procedures: (1st Clinic Visit and PRN) Discussed with patient		
Relaxation and Breathing Techniques (30–40 wk) Discussed with patient and literature given		
Anesthesia/Analgesia: (Begin PRN but complete 36–38 wk) Discussed with patient and literature given Choice _____		
Labor and Delivery: (PRN but complete 36–38 wk) Discussed with patient and literature given Tour of labor and delivery		
Type of Feeding: (Start by 32 wk) Discussed with patient and literature given Choice _____		
Contraceptive Method: Discussed with patient and literature given Choice _____		
Child Care: Discussed with patient and literature given Choice _____		

Referrals Made: PRN _____ SS _____ Nutritionist _____ Other __

Special Points of Interest: _____

Initial	Signature	Initial	Signature	Initial	Signature	Initial	Signature

(continued)

SMH **629**

UNIVERSITY OF ROCHESTER
STRONG MEMORIAL HOSPITAL
NEWBORN KARDEX

DELIVERY ROOM ASSESSMENT

Gest Age: by Dates _____ wks.   PR ☐   Coding   SGA ☐
          by Exam _____ wks.   F ☐   AGA ☐
                                      PO ☐   LGA ☐

Resuscitation Yes   Problems with del: _____
               No

Breast Fed: Delivery Room ☐   Did Well ☐
              Labor Room ☐   Did Poorly ☐

Mother's Problems:

This pregnancy _____

Previous pregnancies _____

Pertinent Social History _____

Primary Visitor _____

Interaction with parents:

Time spent together in labor room _____

                                          Positive eye contact ☐
Smiles at baby ☐   Doesn't look at baby ☐
Hugs, touches baby ☐   Doesn't talk about baby ☐
Father held baby ☐
Skin to skin ☐

Comments: _____

Behavior of Baby:

Crying: none ☐   periodic ☐   almost continuous ☐

Affect: difficult to arouse ☐   dozes ☐   eyes open, alert ☐

Color: pink ☐   acrocyanosis ☐   dusky ☐

Void: Yes ☐   Stool: Yes ☐   Jittery: Yes ☐
       No ☐   No ☐   No ☐

Dextrostix: Yes ☐   Temp. _____
             No ☐

Cord Blood: to NBN ☐   to Blood Bank ☐
              to Chemistry ☐   none obtained ☐

Nurse's Signature _____

To Newborn Nursery at _____ a.m.   by _____
                              p.m.

DISCHARGE SUMMARY

                                                    Nurse's
Baby's Condition   **Teaching Needs**   Initials
Activity _____   Bath Demo _____ |
Cry _____   Bath Return _____ |
Color _____   Formula Prep. _____ |
Color _____ |
Feeding _____   Breast Fdg. _____ |
                              Instruct. _____ |
Circ _____   Temp. Taking _____ |
(condition at D/C) |
                              Circ. Care _____ |
                              Metabolic Urine Screen _____ |
                              Received packet _____ |
                              Mother understands instruct. _____ |
Family Interaction Comments: _____

Siblings: _____

Follow-up Lab _____

Discharge Formula Pack: Yes   Type _____
                         No

Discharge Date _____   Time _____ a.m.
                                      p.m.

Nurse's Signature _____

Cradle Picture - Date _____   by _____

Public Health Referral: Yes   No

Reason for Referral: _____

Done By: _____

ADMISSION ASSESSMENT

Admitted at: _____ a.m. / p.m. Date: _____ By: _____

Weight: _____

Aquamephton _____ lmgm at _____ a.m. / p.m.

Signature: _____

Cord Care: _____

Coding: Calculated gest. age by LMP _____ wks.

Clinical est. of gest. age – _____ wks.

Cincinnati Dubowitz Screen
Done   Yes   No

PR □   SGA▪
F □   AGA▪
PO□   LGA□

Nurse's Signature _____

Warming Measures:

None required □
Infra-red □

Isolette # _____   IN _____ a.m. / p.m.

OUT _____ a.m. / p.m.

VITAL SIGN RECORD

Time	Temp	Isolette Temp	Resp	Pulse	Nurse's Initials

ADMISSION BATH & PHYSICAL ASSESSMENT

Time: _____ a.m. / p.m.   Date: _____

Parameters	Normal	Description Abnormal Problems
Heart		
Respiration		
Temp.		
Color		
Cry		
Activity		
Head		
Face		
Neck		
Extrem.		
Chest		
Abdomen		
Genitalia		
Anus		
Skin		
Reflex		
Tone		

Nurse's Signature: _____

Information Packet to Mother & Metabolic Urine Screen Envelope

Nurse's Signature: _____

Transfer to Nursery _____ at _____ a.m.

Nurse's Signature: _____

ISOLATION

Yes   Observation   #1 _____
No   Nursery   #2 _____

Reason: _____

Ordered by Dr. _____

Medications   Yes □   No □

Date IN _____ at _____

Date OUT _____ at _____

CULTURES:

Spec	Date	Time	Initial of Nurse	Result	Date	Time

LAB WORK:

Date	Time	Spec	Result	Initials of Nurse

(continued)

Comments and Signature

Totals

Date	Weight	Temp	Time	Amt. Fed	Void	Stool	Initial

11-7

7-3

3-11

11-7

7-3

3-11

11-7

7-3

3-11

11-7

7-3

3-11

Mother's First Name

Age	EDC	Para	Grav	Mother's Unit #	Baby's Unit #	Type and RH	Baby's Type RH & Coombs	Type Delivery	Date & Time of Birth	Birth Weight	Mother's RM #

Name

Obstetrician | Pediatrician | Apgars | Circ - Date - Time - By | Void p̄ Circ | Nursery

Notif | In | Exam by | Type Feeding

(Source: University of Rochester/Strong Memorial Hospital, Rochester, NY, by permission.)

UNIVERSITY OF COLORADO MEDICAL CENTER

Colorado General Hospital

Colorado Psychiatric Hospital

CASE RECORD

Date
Ward
Name
Hosp. No.

Address

Teaching	Date	Comments
Anesthesia/Analgesia		
1. Pt. is unaware of various options for pain relief.		
2. Pt. has read anesthesia sheet but has not discussed the options.		
3. Pt. can verbalize the pros and cons of each type of pain relief.		
4. Pt. has make choice of pain relief she would like and can give rationale for choice.		
Admission		
1. Pt. can verbalize when to come to the hospital.		
2. Pt. can verbalize where to go depending upon what time of day she arrives.		
3. Pt. is aware of the importance of bringing her clinic card when she comes to the hospital.		
4. Pt. can verbalize entire admission procedure including when to come in, where to go and what to bring.		
Contraceptive Methods		
1. Pt. is unaware of the method of birth control she would like to use following delivery.		
2. Pt. does not desire to use birth control.		
3. Pt. has read literature given her but has not discussed options for contraception.		
4. Pt. has discussed options with partner and team nurses but has not decided on a method.		
5. Pt. has decided on the contraceptive method she and her partner prefer and can give rationale for choice.		

PRENATAL CLASSES ATTENDED

Class	Date	Partner Also
1. Growth and Development		
2. Labor, Delivery, and Anesthesia		
3. Relaxation and Breathing		
4. Film and Tour of L. and D.		
5. Postpartum and Newborn Care		
6. Breastfeeding and Birth Control		

(Source: University of Colorado Health Sciences Center, Denver, CO, by permission.)

BIBLIOGRAPHY

Auerbach, A. B. *Parents learn through discussion*. New York: John Wiley & Sons, 1968.

Ausubel, D. P. Stages of intellectual development and their implications for early childhood education. In P. B. Newhauser (Ed.), *Concepts of development in early childhood education* (Sp. 111). Springfield, Ill.: Charles C. Thomas, 1965.

Blackwell, B. Anticipated pre-medical care activities of upper middle-class adults and their implications for health education practice. *Health Education Monographs*, 1964, *17*, 17–36.

Bloom, B. S. (Ed.). *Taxonomy of educational objectives: The classification of educational goals Handbook I: Cognitive domain*. New York: David McKay, 1956.

Brown, A. J. Evaluation: Role in patient education. *Health Educator*, 1977, *8*, 6.

Caplan, G. *Concepts of mental health consultations, their application in public health social work*. (Children's Bureau). Washington, D.C.: U. S. Government Printing Office, 1959, 264–265.

Carlton, B., & Carlton, M. A. Defining a role for the health educator in the primary care setting. *Health Education*, 1978, *9*(2), 22–23.

Collen, F. B., & Soghikian, K. A health education library for patients. *Health Service Report*, 1974, *89*, 236–243.

Crate, M. A. Nursing functions in adaptation to chronic illness. *American Journal of Nursing*, 1965, *65*, 72–76.

Deets, C., & Schmidt, A. Outcome criteria based on standards: Part 3. *American Operating Room Nurses' Journal*, 1978, *27*, 220–226.

Elkind, D. Egocentrism in adolescence. In J. J. Conger (Ed.), *Contemporary issues in adolescent development*. New York: Harper & Row, 1975, pp. 44–52.

Fabish, M. Will the real health educator please stand up. *Hospital Forum*, 1977, *20*(3), 12–13.

Fitz-Gibbon, C. T., & Morris, L. L. *How to design a program evaluation*. Beverly Hills, Calif.: Sage, 1978.

Fry, E. A readability formulation that saves time. *Journal of Reading*, 1968, *11*, 513–516, 576–578.

Godlove, B. W. (Ed.). Three views of patient education: Finding patient education media: Part I. *Health Care*, 1977, *6*, 21–23.

Green, L. W., & Figa-Talamanca, I. Suggested designs for evaluation of patient education programs. *Health Education Monographs*, 1974, *2*, 54–71.

Hadley, H. *Development of an instrument to determine adult educators' orientation: Andragogical–pedagogical*. Unpublished Ph.D. dissertation, Boston University, 1975.

Hayes-Bautista, D. E. Modifying treatment: Patient compliance, patient control and medical care. *Social Science and Medicine*, 1976, *10*, 233–238.

Improving patient compliance [Editorial]. *Nursing 1978*, 1978, *8*, 40–47.

Isquith, R. N. Health related audiovisual aids for Spanish-speaking audiences. *Health Science Reports*, 1974, *89*, 188–202.

Johnson, J. The effects of structuring patients' expectations and their reaction to threatening events. *Nursing Research*, 1972, *21*, 499–504.

Jones, P. Patient education—yes—no. *Supervisor Nurse*, 1977, *8*(5), 35–43.

Jones, P., & Oertel, W. Developing patient teaching objectives and techniques: A self instructional program. *Nurse Educator*, 1977, *2*, 3–18.

Krathwohl, D. R., Masia, B. B., & Bloom, B. S. *Taxonomy of educational objectives: The classification of educational goals. Handbook II: Affective domain*. New York: David McKay, 1964.

Klausmeier, H. J., & Ripple, R. *Learning and human abilities: Educational psychology* (3rd ed.). New York: Harper & Row, 1971.

Kluckhohn, R. R., & Strodbeck, F. L. *Variations in value orientations*. Evanston, Ill.: Row, Peterson, 1961.

Knowles, M. S. *The modern practice of adult education: Andragogy versus pedagogy*. New York: Association Press, 1970, 39–49.

Lenahan, M. J. Looking for teaching aids? *Nursing Outlook*, 1968, *15*, 48–49.

Lewis, H. L. Nurse practitioner in preventive health education. *Hospital Progress*, 1978, *59*, 80–83.

Littlefield, V. *Andragogical–pedagogical learning orientation in professional continuing education: Impact on learner's use of course content postcourse*. Unpublished Ph.D. dissertation, University of Denver, 1979.

Mager, R. E. *Preparing instructional objectives*. Palo Alto, Calif.: Feoron Publishers, 1962.

Marram, G. D. *The group approach in nursing practice*. St. Louis, Mo.: C. V. Mosby, 1973.

Martin, L. L. *Health care of women*. New York: J. B. Lippincott, 1978.

Mohammed, M. F. B. Patients' understanding of written health information. *Nursing Research*, 1964, *13*, 100–108.

Mort, P. R., & Vincent, W. *Introduction to American education*. New York: McGraw-Hill, 1954, 303–308.

Open medical record: An educational tool. *Journal of Psychiatric Nursing*, 1977, *15*, 25–30.

Patient education through program care needs (Editorial). *Health Educator*, 1978, *9*, 42–45.

Piaget, J. Intellectual evaluation from adolescence to adulthood. In C. J. Guarado (Ed.), *The adolescent as individual: Issues and insights*. New York: Harper & Row, 1975, p. 108–117.

Popham, W. J. *Evaluating instruction*. Englewood Cliffs, N.J.: Prentice-Hall, 1973.

Redman, B. *The process of patient teaching in nursing*. St. Louis, Mo.: C. V. Mosby, 1980.

Redman, B. P. Personal communication in continuing education course for nurses. University of Colorado School of Nursing, 1977.

Riessman, F., Cohen, J., & Pearl, A. *Mental health of the poor*. New York: Macmillan, 1964.

Rinaldi, L. A., & Kelly, B. What to do after the audit is done: Part I. *American Journal of Nursing*, 1977, *77*, 268–269.

Rogers, C. R. *Freedom to learn*. Columbus, Ohio: Charles E. Merrill, 1969, 106.

Rosenstock, I. M. Patients' compliance with health regimens. *Journal of American Medical Association*, 1975, *234*(4), 402–403.

Rosenstock, I. M. What research in motivation suggests for public health. *American Journal of Public Health*, 1960, *50*, 295–302.

Rotter, J. B. Generalized expectancies for internal versus external control of reinforcement. *Psychological Monographs*, 1966, *80*, 1–28.

Sherman, J. Problems of sex differences in space perceptions and aspects of intellectual functioning. *Psychological Review*, 1967, *74*, 290–299.

Simpson, E. M. The classification of educational objectives in the psychomotor domain. In D. P. Ely (Ed.), *Contributions of behavioral science to instruction technology: The psychomotor domain*. (Vol. 3). Mt. Rainier, Md.: Gryphon Press, 1972.

Steele, S. M., & Brack, R. E. Evaluating the attainment of objectives in adult education: Process, properties, problems, prospects. *Publications in Continuing Education*, 1973.

Stekel, S. B., & Swain, M. A. Contracting with patients to improve compliance. *Journal of American Hospitals Association*, 1977, *51*(23), 81–88.

Sturdevan, B. Why don't adult patients learn? *Supervisor Nurse*, 1977, *8*, 44.

Suchman, M. A. Stages of illness and medical care. *Journal of Human Behavior*, 1965, *6*, 114–128.

Wallston, B., & Wallston, K. Development and validation of the health locus of control (HCC) Scale. *Journal of Counseling and Clinical Psychology*. 1976, *44*(4), 580–585.

Weed, L. L. *Medical records, medical education and patient care: The problem oriented record as a basic tool*. Cleveland, Ohio: Press of Case Western Reserve University, 1971.

Weiss, C. H. *Evaluating action programs: Readings in social action and education*. Boston: Allyn & Bacon, 1972.

Wesenberg, C. Consumer health education steps in planning and developing a hospital based program. *Journal Continuing Education in Nursing*, 1977, *8*, 32–34.

Witkin, H. A., Moore, C. A., & Oltman, P. K. Field-dependent and field-independent cognitive styles and their educational implications. *Review of Educational Research*, 1977, *69*(3), 197–211.

Wittrock, M. C., & Wiley, D. *Evaluation of instruction: Issues and problems*. New York: Holt, Rinehart & Winston, 1970.

Wood, M. 300 valuable booklets to give to patients and their families: A source guide (Part I). *Nursing 74*, 1974, *4*, 43–50.

Wood, M. 300 valuable booklets to give patients and their families: A source guide (Part II). *Nursing 74*, 1974, *4*, 60–66.

Wortham, B. R., & Sanders, J. R. *Educational evaluation: Theory and practice*. Worhington, Ohio: Charles A. Jones Publishing, 1973.

Wortman, P. (Ed.). *Methods for evaluating health services*. Beverly Hills, Calif.: Sage Publications, 1981.

You can be too optimistic about your health (Editorial). *Public Health Reports*, 1965, *80*, 130–131.

Yura, H., & Walsh, M. B. *The nursing process: Assessing, planning, implementing, evaluating* (4th ed.). Norwalk, Conn.: Appleton-Century-Crofts, 1983.

Selected Theories and Processes: Special Relevance for Women's Health Education

3

Vivian M. Littlefield, Dona J. Lethbridge, and Barbara N. Adams

Selected philosophical and methodological approaches to women's health education may be indicated because of women's past socialization and current changing roles. As women seek more independence and participation *with* their health care providers, the process of *how* they are informed about health may have an impact on the use of new information and on the woman's self-concept. Adult learning strategies proposed by Malcolm Knowles (1970) have a potential to allow learners to feel in control and confident, that they have the knowledge, abilities, and experiences to effectively manage their future. It is hypothesized that *how* one learns may be equally as important as *what* one learns.

Now that women are seeking to become involved in decisions about their health care, strategies that allow development of decision-making skills are needed to allow more positive and effective decision making. Some women may need assistance in enhancing their ability to make decisions *before* being asked to make complex decisions about their health.

This chapter describes adult learning and decision-making theories. In addition, the use of group process for the health education needs of women is described. This discussion facilitates the recognition that choices of approach to teaching–learning and decision making can be made based on "where the client is." For example, if the client is in a state of crisis, seeking to be more independent in recovering from illness or wanting to have a more equalitarian role in deciding alternatives for her reproductive experience, the approach to learning and decision making should be matched to the woman's needs and current abilities. When the goal is for the woman to be more independent, then the educational process consists of strategies that facilitate independence. When circumstances or preferences require a more dependent role, then the teacher's strategies can be more directive. Group or individual sessions can be selected depending on preference, goals, and time available.

ADULT LEARNING VERSUS TRADITIONAL LEARNING

Malcolm Knowles (1970) has described and promoted adult or andragogical learning theory. Knowles states that adults learn differently than children and that learning opportunities for adults should use selected principles and methodologies.

Briefly, adult learning is defined as an educational process wherein the basis of learning is a free choice of alternative goals for learning and interdependent decision making between student and educator. The teachers perceive their relationship to students as that of helper, resource, consultant, and co-learner. Learning is enhanced by encouraging situations that increase cooperative interaction among learners and their participation in and direction of learning (Hadley, 1975). Knowles (1970) termed this orientation andragogical learning.

The more traditional learning orientation emphasizes acquiring knowledge and skills the educator judges true and effective (Knowles, 1970). The educator's judgment is based on tradition, accepted views and practice, and current knowledge of the physical and social universe. The educator's role is primarily one of authority, a technical expert, director of learning, and judge of achievement. To enhance effectiveness of learning, the educator stresses "techniques to transmit ideas efficiently, development of presentations of subject matter which are logically organized, and motivation of learning by encouraging competitive individual achievement" (p. iv). The educator also maintains control of content to be learned (Hadley, 1975).

The term Knowles (1970) used for this latter approach was pedagogical learning orientation. *Paidos* comes from a Greek word referring to child, thus emphasizing the dependency of the learner on the teacher for knowledge and direction. Table 3–1 describes the major differences in these approaches and focuses on the *extremes* of these orientations so as to depict the meaning of a purely andragogical or pedagogical orientation. The continua can also be viewed as having varying degrees of andragogical or pedagogical focus.

It was a doctoral student (Hershal Hadley) of Dr. Knowles that elaborated on these differences. This student actually developed an instrument to measure degrees of androgogical–pedagogical orientation that a teacher prefers (Hadley, 1975). Thus the following discussion summarizes these difference as reported by Dr. Hadley. The reader is encouraged to review Dr. Knowles's publications and theories (see Bibliography).

The differentiation described by Dr. Hadley is helpful to health professionals not versed in various educational theories. Such a conceptualization allows the recognition that selection of various "degrees" of an orientation can be made for various clinical situations. What degree of andragogical versus pedagogical approach is adequate is a matter of judgment at this point in the development of the theory. The clinician will recognize the parallel between making a clinical judgment about the type and kind of psychological support needed versus an educational decision concerning the type, kind, and degree of educational orientation needed. The scales (Table 3–1) could be used as an assessment tool to determine the educational process present in a particular learning situation. The authors in the remaining chapters of this text lend their opinion as to appropriate orientation. Someday, research may assist in knowing what is appropriate. Currently, much of the research concerning teaching–learning has come from formal educational settings, laboratory, and simulated settings. Obviously the theory should be tested with clients seeking health education. Some of the research (Houle, 1971; Tough, 1977) on learning was done with adults in everyday, nonformal learning situations. These studies are likely to be applicable to well women seeking learning due to life change, preventive health behaviors, and incorporation of chronic, long-term illnesses into their self-concept. The research from formal educational settings and simulated settings is likely applicable to women receiving health–illness education by means of formal groups and via classroom instruction. Most of the literature on patient education does not describe the process used or the educational orientation used. Because of this significant

TABLE 3–1. LEARNING ORIENTATION

Andragogical or Adult Learning						Pedagogical or Traditional Learning
Role of teacher Helper, resource, facilitator.						*Role of teacher* Expert, authority, director.
Relationship of *teacher and students* Informal, warm, accepting, trusting, supportive.						*Relationships of* *teachers and students* Formal, reserved, critically challenging, cautious.
Class climate Cooperative, friendly, sharing, mutuality.						*Class climate* Competitive, rivalrous, intellectually rigorous, judgmental.
Teaching Relaxed, spontaneous, imaginative, flexible.						*Teaching* Systematic, methodical, businesslike, efficient.
Learning activities Group projects, independent study, chosen by students.						*Learning activities* Lectures, chosen by teacher, required by all students.
Evaluation By students & teacher, based on amount & direction of growth toward individual goals, uses various criteria as relevant to student.						*Evaluation* By teacher only, based on formal examinations, based on common standards (norms) of achievement.

Note: These scales were developed by Hershel Hadley under the direction of Malcolm Knowles. They were developed to depict differences in adult and more traditional teaching/learning activites. They demonstrate subdimension continua of the entire teaching–learning experience. Examining a patient's learning experience on each of these subdimension continua will allow the teacher to determine whether adult or more traditional learning orientations should be used.
(Source: *Hadley, H.* Development of an instrument to determine adult educators' orientation: Andragogical–pedagogical. *Unpublished Ph.D. dissertation, Boston University, 1975, by permission.*)

lack of completeness in the health education literature, this author has found it useful to use theories and research from the field of education and psychology and apply these to clinical learning situations. Thus the material presented in the following pages is from education and psychology.

Purposes of Education. One of the primary differences between andragogical and pedagogical orientations is the purpose of learning. The andragogical orientation focuses on growth of the learner as opposed to learning "prescribed subject matter" (Hadley, 1975, pp. 27–35). The philosophies of idealism, realism, perennialism, and essentialism are pedagogical in the purpose of education. In contrast, progressivism and existentialism are cited as andragogical (Hadley, 1975, p. 27). From the literature on philosophy of education, major theorists have advocated one or the other approach. In pedagogical orientations, purposes for learning are given and express "abstract, ideal goals" that are for the good of all learners. These purposes lead to educational programs or teaching situations intended to assure that all learners "achieve identical goals." Andragogical purposes develop from the learners' needs at a particular time and in a specific context. Learning goals are thus continuously created and reconstructed. More importantly, learners participate in this creation and reconstruction of their learning goals (Hadley, 1975).

Carl Rogers sees the different orientation toward purposes of education as the "nub of the question." Rogers states:

> Teaching and the imparting of knowledge make sense in an unchanging environment. That is why it has been an unquestioned function of centuries. But if there is one truth about modern man, it is that he lives in an environment which is continually changing. . . .
>
> We are, in my view, faced with an entirely new situation in education where the goal of education, if we are to survive, is the facilitation of change and learning. The only man who is educated is the man who has learned how to learn; the man who has realized that no knowledge is secure, for security. Changingness, a reliance on process rather than upon static knowledge, is the only thing that makes any sense as a goal for education in the modern world. (1969, p. 104)

The research evidence as to whether emphasizing either purpose leads to more effective learning and use of what is learned is not clear. Guthrie's research (1967) demonstrated that the discovery learning method, more oriented to development of the learner, appears to facilitate transfer of learning, but not retention of knowledge. Expository instruction (more oriented to assimilation of content) facilitates retention but impedes transfer. Gagné (1970) found that learning activities that allow problem solving and actual experiences in transfer of learning actually change the learner. For instance, once a learner uses problem-solving skills, the capacity to use these skills is enhanced in the future. Gagné's research supports a focus on the development of the learner to enhance future abilities.

The literature from adult learning also suggests that adult learners naturally seek learning opportunities for their own development and increased competence. Knox, discussing adult learning in his text, *Adult Development and Learning*, stated that,

> In most instances in which adults purposefully engage in systematic and sustained learning activities, their intent is to modify performance. Their reasons for engaging in the learning activity and their anticipated uses of the new learnings typically relate to a coherent area of activity of performance. (1977, p. 406)

A study concerning adult learning conducted in the United States, Canada, Ghana, Jamaica, and New Zealand found that 90 percent of adult learners stated their motivation for learning was that they anticipated using the knowledge or skill they were learning. Only 20 percent of these adults indicated their motivation for learning was related to curiosity, puzzlement, or wanting to possess knowledge. Thus, the adult most frequently seeks learning that meets his or her own needs and development rather than for the purpose of gaining knowledge per se (Tough, 1971).

Some research also documents adults' pragmatic approach to learning. According to Cross, adult learning is motivated primarily by the desire to solve immediate and practical problems. Adults are interested "not so much in storing knowledge for use at some future time" as they are in applying knowledge to important life goals. Unless earning a degree, adults do not seek traditional academic subjects. This rejection of traditional academic subjects seems to be less a matter of rejecting intellectual challenges than one of evaluating the usefulness of the subject matter (Cross & Zusman, 1977).

Nature of Learners

Internal Versus External Motivation. A major question posed by andragogical–pedagogical learning orientations is whether the learner is dependent and needs to be motivated to learn, or whether learners are independent, self-directed, and intrinsically motivated. In andragogical learning orientations, the individual is seen as self-directing, in control of the learning experience, and motivated to learn without external controls and motivation (Hadley, 1975).

Pedagogical orientations view learners as "empty organisms," dependent on external motivation and direction. This debate about the nature of learners can be identified in the differences of opinion expressed by the behavioral and cognitive theorists in psychology. The behaviorists focus on reinforcement of the behavior of the human organism to promote learning (Skinner, 1974), whereas the cognitive psychologists assume that human beings have built-in "covert mental processes" and that they are the key to facilitating and motivating learning (Davis, 1976, pp. 39–40). The clinical literature also demonstrates this difference of opinion in various approaches to teaching–learning. The use of the words "patient education" versus health education demonstrates a focus on a dependent person who must be given reinforcement versus a person who comes with a desire to learn, consume, and so forth.

The research literature reveals some evidence in support of the andragogical end of the andragogical–pedagogical continuum relative to the learner or individual's internal motivation. Penland (1977) found the two most popular reasons given by adults for undertaking self-planned learning versus enrolling in formal classes were the desire to set their own learning pace and to use their own style of learning, supporting the andragogical concept that adults wish to share in decisions about what and how they learn.

The research by Tough (1977) also supports the intrinsic motivation of most adults to learn without external control or motivation in that a large percent of adults undertake on their own at least one and some undertake as many as five separate learning projects during a 12-month period.

Research has also demonstrated that intrinsic motivation is more effective in producing learning than is extrinsic motivation (Trent & Cohen, 1973). Again, the andragogical principle that adults prefer to learn what they themselves have identified as important is demonstrated (Knowles, 1970). Reflecting on clinical experiences emphasizes how easily women learn what they feel they need to know, only to "forget" simple information about what health care providers thought was critical.

An in-depth analysis of adults who participate in continuous formal educational opportunities was conducted and reported by Houle (1971). From interviews using a structured guide, Houle identified three categories of adult learners. These categories were termed the goal-directed, the activity-oriented, and the learning-oriented. Houle's conclusion as a result of his research was that, although there were no pure types of adult learners, learners could be categorized according to these three types. All of these types allow for self-direction and the students' desire to set their own goals and purposes in learning. Therefore, Houle concluded that adult education could not be fitted into a single pattern. Complexity of focus and purpose of learning opportunities for adults is Houle's recommendation, because adult learners seek learning for a variety of reasons and individual motivations. No doubt Houle's conclusions can also apply to opportunities in health education. Some women seek learning about their health to meet some self-determined goal, others seek such learning for the activity and socialization afforded, others seek understanding and self-insight. All of these reasons are self-motivated and may be unknown to the teacher whose goals are on an entirely different level.

Influence of Learner's Characteristics on Learning. There are certain characteristics of the learner that influence whether learning occurs as well as the degree of learning taking place. Characteristics such as experience, preference of methodology, age, self-concept, ability to problem-solve, and amount of formal education have been demonstrated to influence learning. A selected review of some of these studies follows to demonstrate how the nature of the learner influences what is learned.

Previous Experience and Educational Attainment. Previous experience related to the content and educational attainment may influence the amount of learning. Buckland (1969) demonstrated that the less experienced course participants had difficulty retaining all they learned in a two-day period. Although participants in this course changed their behavior postcourse attendance significantly, this change tended not to reach the level made possible by the course.

Birch and Robinowitz (1951) found that past experiences cause problems in new learning if the learner is "chained to the past." The results of the study by Birch and Robinowitz indicate that what is important in problem-solving behavior is not that an individual is dependent on past experience per se, but rather different kinds of experiences are differentially effective in influencing problem-solving behavior. How and what an individual learned was determined by the amount of positive transfer effect that occurred in subsequential learning. The kind of previous experience functioned to limit the number of the properties of the object that could be perceived by the individual in problem-solving situations.

Preference of Methodology. Sovie (1972) found that participation in continuing education activities was related to a life-style that included time for a wide variety of learning experiences. This life-style of having participated in learning activities was as important as the level of formal education. Cross (1978a), a proponent of andragogical orientations, however, determined that the best single predictor of future educational efforts in an adult was the level of prior educational attainment. Education is, thus, additive. Each year of formal education obtained adds to the probability that the individual will become an active lifelong learner.

Age. Although differences exist as age increases, especially in short-term memory, Lumsden and Sheron (1975) indicated that *rigidity or motivation to learn is as important as ability to learn*. In fact, more recent work on learning with the elderly demonstrates an increased ability to learn in many instances (see Chapter 14).

Self-concept. Weatherby (1978) found that adults who are making major life changes and redirection seek formal educational experiences to legitimize these changes. Meinke (1972) found that individuals with more positive self-concepts attain abstract concepts more effectively than those individuals with less positive self-concepts.

Characteristics of the Learning Experience. A major question concerning the appropriate or most effective learning environment has to do with the "source and direction of control" and the amount of active participation in learning. In a pedagogical approach to learning, learning is thought to be inspired, directed, and controlled by forces external to the learner. In the pedagogical environment, the responsibility of learning rests with the teacher. In an andragogical environment, the learner is an active participant in the learning, and the responsibility for what is learned is placed with the learner. Another question concerns the amount of competitive versus cooperative relationships that could be created in the learning situation. A pedagogical learning experience focuses on meeting established standards or predetermined content. In an andragogical environment, learners are encouraged to feel free to risk, learn from experience, and to measure learning progress by their own standards and learning needs (Hadley, 1975).

Research from the field of psychology supports the effectiveness of active participation in learning (Fincher, 1976) especially in learning problem-solving (Bloom & Broder, 1961). In order to transfer learning from one learning situation to another or to life experiences, the learner's active involvement in learning makes a difference (Gagne, 1965). Knox (1977, p. 425), reviewing the empirical evidence upon which knowledge of adult learning is based, stated

> Both persistence in a learning activity and actual learning achievement can be greatly affected by the educational climate and procedures that enable the identification of congruent expectations and objectives. For example, in some educational programs for adults, time is spent on exploring and agreeing on learning topics and activities that are very prevalent to the participants. This involvement contributes to interest, achievement, and application.

The studies of professionals in formal learning experiences seem to suggest that along with active participation must come a nonthreatening learning environment. Knowles's studies (1970) of adult learners emphasize the need for minimal threat, an opportunity to appear knowledgeable, and to maintain their adult status and social role. The clinical experience of the author and some data from the clinical literature support that individuals seeking health care and adults seeking learning for various reasons are concerned with feeling inadequate in their learning role.

Management of the Learning Experience. Major dilemmas exist for the adult educator concerning methodologies to use in individual and group education experiences. Several authors have suggested various methodologies. Knowles's suggestions appear in Table 3–2. Specific questions arise as to lecture versus discussion, use of audiovisual materials, the teacher and group versus an individual approach. Experience with learners in both academic and patient education classes demonstrate that most people learn in spite of type and quality of methodology. Yet, there is a need to examine various approaches and what each can accomplish. It is also important to develop guidelines for the selection of a methodology based on expected outcomes, type of learning, and characteristics of learner and teacher. Table 3–3 summarizes the advantages and disadvantages of various methodologies. As can be seen, some of these are andragogical and some pedagogical.

A number of studies have in the past focused on specific teaching activities, such as use of media, use of the lecture method, or use of discussion groups. Reviews of these studies have been conducted by a number of scholars. McKeachie reviewed studies and published these results in 1963 and 1970. A 1972 publication by Miton as well as a systematic review by Dubin and Taveggia in 1968 complete these reviews.

Research data are not conclusive and are conficting as to effectiveness of specific methods. Several reasons exist for this fact. Methodologies were evaluated in simulated

TABLE 3–2. SUPERIOR CONDITIONS OF LEARNING AND PRINCIPLES OF TEACHING

Conditions of Learning	Principles of Teaching
The learners feel a need to learn.	1. The teacher exposes students to new possibilities for self-fulfillment.
	2. The teacher helps each student clarify his or her own aspirations for improved behavior.
	3. The teacher helps each student diagnose the gap between his or her aspiration and his or her present level of performance
	4. The teacher helps the students identify the life problems they experience because of the gaps in their personal equipment.
The learning environment is characterized by physical comfort, mutual trust and respect, mutual helpfulness, freedom of expression, and acceptance of differences.	5. The teacher provides physical conditions that are comfortable (as to seating, smoking, temperature, ventilation, lighting, decoration) and conducive to interaction (preferably, no person behind another person).
	6. The teacher accepts each student as a person of worth and respects his feelings and ideas.
	7. The teacher seeks to build relationships of mutual trust and helpfulness among the students by encouraging cooperative activities and refraining from inducing competitiveness and judgment.
	8. The teacher exposes his or her own feelings and contributes his or her resources as a co-learner in the spirit of mutual inquiry.
The learners perceive the goals of a learning experience to be their goals.	9. The teacher involves the students in the process of formulating learning objectives in which the needs of the students, of the institution, of the teacher, of the subject matter, and of the society are taken into account.
The learners accept a share of the responsibility for planning and operating a learning experience and therefore have a feeling of commitment	10. The teacher shares his or her thinking about options available in the designing of learning experiences and the selection of materials and methods and involves the students in deciding among these options jointly.
The learners participate actively in the learning process.	11. The teacher helps the students to organize themselves (project groups, learning–teaching teams, independent study, etc.) to share responsibility in the process of mutual inquiry.
The learning process is related to and makes use of the experience of the learners.	12. The teacher helps the students exploit their own experiences as resources for learning through the use of such techniques as discussion, role playing, case method, etc.
	13. The teacher gears the presentation of his or her own resources to the levels of experience of particular students.
	14. The teacher helps the students to apply new learning to their experience, and thus to make the learning more meaningful and integrated.
The learners have a sense of progress toward their goals.	15. The teacher involves the students in developing mutually acceptable criteria and methods for measuring progress toward the learning objectives.
	16. The teacher helps the students develop and apply procedures for self-evaluation according to these criteria.

(Source: *Knowles, M. S. The modern practice of adult education. New York: Association Press, 1970, p. 52–53, by permission.*)

TABLE 3–3. PROS AND CONS OF TEACHING METHODOLOGIES

Method	Advantages	Disadvantages
Simulation and games	Facilitate transfer of learning Represent real life processes Engage student in activity Cost less than real life situation Permit failure without real life consequence	Give incomplete view of reality May be too simplistic Lack student accountability May not be effective at higher levels of learning
Mastery learning	Assigns major responsibility of learning to student Provides teacher with an evaluation on how well students learn Forces student to work harder Reduces duplication in curriculum Provides structure for low-ability students Results in more competent graduates	May be costly, i.e., initial preparation time Results in high attrition rate May be difficult for anxious students Requires new roles for teachers
Experiential learning	Increases student retention Relates action and concrete events Provides opportunities for relating theory to practice Provides more relevant education	Is time consuming Requires different faculty roles
Lecture	Is inexpensive Requires less preparation time Covers more content Can be changed easily Is effective	Is uni-directional Encourages intellectual passivity Fails to encourage creativity Has low retention rate
Personalized systems of instruction (PSI)	Are viewed positively by students Increase learning Individualize instruction Personalize instruction Reflect higher student achievement	Average higher student Require large amount of time to plan Are not to be used for courses where level of mastery cannot be specified
Discussion	Is responsive to student needs Involves student in learning process Provides wider variety of perspectives Can be effective in changing attitudes Can be effective in learning difficult tasks	Is unreliable in terms of outcomes Is not very effective in conveying content Takes time to develop groups
Audio-tutorial (sic)	Activates several student senses Provides more durable student learning Focuses on student learning not teaching Promotes higher student achievement Is cost effective	Requires large initial investment of time and resources Is not completely self-paced Requires extensive student orientation

Note: Developed by Dr. Albert Smith for the first Regional Conference of the Faculty Development in Nursing Education Project Southern Regional Education Board, Atlanta Georgia, October 16–18, 1977.
(Source: *Sasmor, J.L.* Childbirth education: A nursing perspective. *New York: John Wiley & Sons, 1979, p. 99, by permission.*)

learning situations where the preference of the learner was not considered or controlled for, the learning goals of the learner not identified, and the methodologies not evaluated in relation to application of learning versus recall of content.

The studies reported and experiences in education seem to conclude that the strategy depends on (1) type of learning expected, (2) teacher style, (3) nature of the subject matter, (4) learner style and preference, (5) psychological climate, and (6) interaction of all of these factors.

Type of Learning: Influence on Selection of Teaching Strategies. A study at the University of Michigan using college students found that "instruction that emphasizes meanings of concepts lead to knowledge that is more easily applied in new contexts and is the basis for more flexible and interpretive use by the subject" (Mayer et al., 1975). When preinstructional experiences involved learning without acquiring meaning, it was demonstrated that the subjects' background experiences can seriously affect their perceptions of what new instruction is about and, therefore, affect the organization of the new material (Mayer et al., 1975).

Wittrock (1963) found that when retention and transfer to similar examples are the criteria for measuring learning, giving rules is more effective than not giving rules. The amount of direction influenced the amount of retention and transfer. A maximum amount of direction produced the greatest initial learning; an intermediate amount produced the greatest retention and transfer. Practice and reinforcement were found to affect retention and transfer under certain conditions.

Huckabay, Cooper, and Neal (1977) found that any method, traditional lecture, lecture–discussion, filmstrip, filmstrip–discussion, or a combination of methods was effective when content knowledge was the criterion used to evaluate success. When transfer of learning was the criterion, however, use of audiovisual aids and discussion was preferable. Both studies by Wittrock and Huckabay and colleagues evaluated transfer of learning in simulated situations. In real-life situations, the type of methodology needed to provide transfer learning may be different.

Barnett (1973), in comparing the effectiveness of three instructional formats for physicians in community hospitals, also found that a structured presentation with interactive group discussion led by a moderator seemed to produce the greatest results in applicative use of content learned. However, content test scores had the highest results when a combination of mediated and discussion formats were used. Subjective participant evaluation of the mediated treatment was highest, but this was not statistically significant.

Studies (Baskins, 1967; Beach, 1970) focusing on independent study have also demonstrated improved transfer of learning. Independent study, however, did not show any advantage for retention of knowledge.

The Teacher: Influence on Learning. The influence of the teacher on learning has been shown to lie in the teacher's personality or relationship to discipline. For example, Sherman and Blackburn (1975) demonstrated that personality characteristics were related to teaching effectiveness. The personal characteristics of pragmatism, amicability, intellectual competency, and personal potency were highly correlated with performance. Morstain and Smart (1976) found that faculty with different personalities prefer different teaching–learning techniques. They caution that the preliminary findings from the study concerning the relationship of personality to selection of teaching–learning techniques should be interpreted with caution because the study sample was limited. The study also found that teachers who were categorized as "social" on Holland's personality scale preferred independent study more often than faculty termed realistic, investigative, and enterprising. "Social" teachers were more supportive of the concept that students do their best work when they are on their own. These teachers also placed a greater value on learner freedom and independence in the learning process and preferred courses that were more informal, unstructured, and in which learners set their own goals and standards as well as pursued their own interests. These teachers were more comfortable sharing the educational decision making with learners and tended to prefer the more individually designed teaching–learning arrangements. The orientation of "social" faculty seemed to be closely associated with the andragogical orientation.

In comparison, "realistic," "investigative" teachers tended to have greater preference for more structured, lecture-type teaching–learning arrangements and placed higher value on the importance of formal evaluations of learners. These faculty also had a view of learning that emphasized the acquisition of useful knowledge and skills deemed important for learners' future roles. Learners' development was viewed as proceeding in a structured, systematic manner with periodic formalized evaluative methods. Personality characteristics of "realistic" individuals were postulated as enjoying activities that require explicit, ordered, and systematic behavior. These individuals tend to value concrete and utilitarian items. These individuals are apt to be traditional, materialistic, and pragmatically oriented in their behavior.

Teachers categorized in the "artistic" group by Holland's personality scale had lower scores on "achievement," "assignment learning," and "assessment." These individuals are characterized by their tendency to be impulsive, independent, and nonconforming and might, therefore, express less preference for a more structured and formal learning environment and educational process.

Teacher directiveness–indirectiveness was found to have a linear relationship to students' attitudes toward the subject being taught (Markell & Mayer, 1975).

Learner Style and Preference. The differences in personality and preferences for teaching–learning activities have also been demonstrated in learners. The same researcher, Morstain (1975), reported divergent educational attitudes and orientations in different inter- and intrainstitutional environments and for learners with different personality characteristics and academic aptitudes. It has been proposed that these preferences influence what is effective with individual learners.

Psychological Climate: Influence on Learning. Two studies demonstrated that the psychological experience of students influences their response to the learning situation. Holzemer (1975) found that learners are influenced by the psychological press of the classroom environment. Haines and McKeachie (1967) found that in competitive environments there was poorer achievement and less satisfaction among learners than in a cooperative climate.

Interaction of Method and Learning Style of Learner. Trent and Cohen (1973) suggested, in their review of numerous studies on teaching–learning in higher education, that the interaction of the method and the learning style of the learner was important in learning. Although other studies have failed to demonstrate the existence of interaction, Lewis (1975) concluded that the interaction of the learner's style and preference with the type of instruction seemed to be the important factor in the effectiveness of learning.

Holmes (1974), investigating college students' responses to nontraditional study, found that students' thoughts about the experience depended on "the congruence or lack of congruence between expectations and the reality of the experience." Little emphasis on interaction of method and learner style has been undertaken in health education, but this possibility should be considered.

Evaluation of Student Learning. Another major difference between andragogical–pedagogical learning orientations is the type of evaluation used. In andragogical orientations, the focus is on judging learning by the learners' diagnosis and rediagnosis of their progress and additional needs for learning. Pedagogical evaluation is done by adherence to standards set by the teacher, the educational or professional authorities, or the nature of what is to be learned (Hadley, 1975). Evaluation of learning by health educators, according to external standards, is not done in its strictest sense, but is applied frequently. For example, lists of critical content and necessary information are identified for women undergoing various treatments, surgeries, and childbirth. All content is taught and evaluation is based on increased content knowledge the woman can demonstrate. Increased class hours or reinforcement is used to improve women's ability to cite content taught. Objective "test" series in writing or given orally are designed to determine what has been retained. Behavior is observed for changes in the desired direction. Rarely is there an effort to ask the woman her opinion about her accomplishments in learning or ability to apply the learning to her life situation. Evaluations are sometimes a threat to the learner. Thus, andragogical evaluation strategies may be more appropriate in health education and may allow health professionals to gain a better appreciation of women's self-confidence in using what was taught.

Summary

This review of the major differences in andragogical and pedagogical learning orientations attempted to highlight the many complex decisions to be made about the learning process. Conscious selection of approach and style need to be made and data collected as to the effectiveness. When patients are not learning, an alteration in orientation may help. A major goal of andragogical approaches is to facilitate a sense of confidence and independence in the learner and allow more application of learning to future health and illness situations. Obviously an ideal research focus would be to determine the degree of andragogical–pedagogical orientation needed by various women under the threat of illness, during illness, and for health maintenance. It is highly likely that andragogical approaches are most effective in noncrisis situations. During acute illness or when major life changes occur a more pedagogical approach may be needed. If women and health professionals want women to participate with their care providers, increasing the degree of andragogical orientation for teaching health care could allow the clients to develop increased independence and self-reliance. This is the view of the authors in this text and is reflected in the philosophy of health care promoted by Bermosk and Porter (1979), Sandelowski (1981), the Boston Women's Health Book Collective (1973), and others.

The literature on value orientation, educational level and preference for learning, and states of health or illness (see Chapter 2) also seem to suggest that degrees of andragogical–pedagogical orientation may depend on ethnic background, educational level, and past experience with learning styles as well as state of health.

A study by the author examining the influence of an andragogical versus a pedagogical orientation on learner perception of outcomes found that andragogical–pedagogical orientation was important only when considered with other variables such as congruence of learners' and course goals, learner satisfaction, and learner preference for andragogical or pedagogical orientations (Derby, 1981; Littlefield, 1979). This study was conducted with some 262 professional learners (men and women) and, thus, may not be generalized to patients and health education, but serves to place caution in using one orientation or counting on one approach to learning as the answer to assisting the patient in changing behavior. Another interesting finding of the study with professional learners was that preferences for learning orientation seem to be profession-specific. It was not clear if the preferences existed for women or men. Women preferred both andragogical and pedagogical orientations, and depending on profession, preferred one or the other. Men individually varied in preferring andragogical or pedagogical orientations, but as a group most prefer pedagogical approaches. This difference could not be generalized to health education, but does raise interesting questions about whether men and women have preferences for learning orientation.

Example of Application of Andragogical–Pedagogical Orientations

Annie is a black female, age 32 who has been a class B diabetic for 8 years. She is pregnant with her eighth child. She is highly religious, believing in God's care in influence on her health and that of her baby. She believes that if she maintains her faith all will go well. She enters the high-risk outpatient clinic late in pregnancy (26 weeks' gestation). She is convinced that her many hospitalizations with her last pregnancy 1.5 years ago were due to medical interventions and taking insulin. She delivered a healthy baby girl who is active and developing well. She states that she stopped taking insulin early in this pregnancy because it made her fall and she "feels badly." She will not make regular clinic visits, will not test her blood sugar regularly, take insulin, or completely alter her diet as directed. She states God will care for her. Her religion has influenced her to change her excessive eating, drinking of alcohol and pop, and has influenced her family to have positive relationships and become supportive. Her husband has stopped drinking and is helpful at home as a result of his new religious orientation. She is relieved about this and feels her life is significantly better.

In terms of knowledge about pregnancy and her diabetic condition, testing blood sugar levels, and reason for clinic visits, she will respond with accurate knowledge, then at other times partial, inaccurate knowledge and performance (i.e., testing blood sugar). She will sometimes tell one health team member she has never been told how to do something that another team member has taught her.

An Andragogical Approach. In assessing Annie's learning needs, the andragogical health educator would determine what she perceives as her needs, preferences, and problems prior to an assessment of *what* is known about pregnancy and diabetes. This would allow beginning "where the client is" or stating what her needs for learning are. The social status and role this woman plays within her family and religion would be accepted and used in motivating Annie to care for her own health. For instance, her strong commitment to the caretaker role would be accepted, and efforts to decrease the number and type of hospitalizations and clinic visits would be considered. Annie's experience and knowledge of coping with a complex life circumstance would be recognized and appreciated. Annie would be considered "expert" in this area. Thus, Annie's ideas about how best to incorporate necessary changes in her life would be honored and accepted. The teacher would maintain an equalitarian informal, caring, trusting, and supportive attitude. The teaching methodologies selected would allow active participation and be selected with the patient's input and direction (Table 3–2). Evaluation of Annie's progress in learning would be based on the amount and degree of diabetic control from Annie's perspective, that is, the realistic amount of control possible based on Annie's assessment of what she can accomplish under her complex life circumstances.

A Pedagogical Approach. The teacher would question Annie about her knowledge and begin to cover all topics not completely known. Standards for knowledge and understanding would be set for all pregnant diabetics. Plans would be made to have Annie return for instruction until acceptable knowledge is demonstrated. Pre- and posttests would be created to assure complete and accurate knowledge. Return demonstrations of insulin injections and diet selection would be planned. Methodologies would be selected that allowed systematic and efficient presentation of material and that had been previously tested on pregnant diabetic women. The teacher would make an effort to demonstrate her more extensive knowledge. The pedagogical teacher would direct what was to be learned at each visit. Evaluation of learning would be done by the teacher alone. Learning would be achieved when Annie is able to apply all content taught to life circumstances and maintain complete diabetic control as outlined in the medical protocol.

The author was the teacher for Annie. The pedagogical approach did not work. Annie needed and wanted control and decided *she* would determine what was acceptable performance and knowledge. When a pedagogical orientation was used or attempted, the learner (Annie) withdrew and resisted coming for care. When an androgogical approach was tried, Annie seemed to be more responsive. The outcome of the pregnancy was positive and diabetic control better for Annie than in the past. Obviously other life circumstances facilitated Annie's better performance, but this author feels a comfortable, positive learning circumstance existed. Annie evaluated the experience more positively than the past experience.

THE DECISION-MAKING PROCESS

Ineffective contraceptive behavior, lack of sexual well-being, and chronic stress, among other health problems, demand self-awareness and decision-making skills for successful resolution. The health care provider involved in women's health care must be able to help women develop and enhance these skills. This section describes decision-making theories and suggests their relevance for women's choice of appropriate health behaviors.

Socrates said that competent individuals are "those who manage well the circumstances which they encounter daily and who possess a judgment which is accurate in meeting occasions as they arise and rarely miss the expedient course of action" (D'Zurilla & Goldfried, 1971). Socrates is describing skillful decision- making. Decision making may involve cognitive matters, interpersonal matters, or take place in all aspects of life. One important arena for skillful decision-making ability is that of women's health care. For example, decisions must be made about birth control, childbearing, life changes, and preventive health behaviors.

Steps in Decision Making
A myriad of literature exists about decision making and about problem solving. These terms tend to be used interchangeably. Throughout this discussion, literature describing decision making and problem solving is cited.

It may be said that decisions are made within the context of solving problems. Steps in the decision-making process have been described earlier in the discussions of the educational process. Rephrased in a problem resolution framework, these steps include:

Problem Solving	Education/Assessment Process
1. Identification of a need or a problem	Assessment
2. Collection of relevant information	
3. Production of action alternatives	Planning
4. Choice of a course of action	Implementation
5. Evaluation of the consequences	Evaluation

Identification of a Need or a Problem. Health care providers who understand their own problem-solving process for clinical educational approaches can assist clients to understand the process in relation to deciding their own health care. Identification of the problem in need of a resolution is often considered the most difficult step. This initial step can be viewed negatively or as an opportunity. D'Zurilla and Goldfried (1971) suggest that the initial emotional reaction to a felt need is important and could be viewed as a cue to shift attention to the problem situation.

Janis and Mann (1977) have developed a conflict-theory model of decision making that describes points in the development of the decision-situation. According to their model, unconflicted adherence to the usual course of action for problem resolution results if the individual does not perceive serious risks in adhering to the usual course of action. Additionally, if an individual does not hope to find a better solution to a problem, defensive avoidance of the decision-situation may be the outcome.

Other factors may affect recognition of the decision-situation. D'Zurilla and Goldfried (1973) suggest that the individual needs to inhibit tendencies either to respond on the first impulse or to do nothing. Bloom and Broder (1961), in their classic study of problem-solving strategies, found that less successful subjects tended to be impulsive and quick to give up.

In addition, successful problem solvers compared to nonsuccessful problem solvers

1. Understood the nature of the problem.
2. Understood the ideas contained in the problem (successful problem solvers did not have more knowledge than nonsuccessful problem solvers, but the successful learners could bring relevant knowledge they possessed to bear on the problems presented).
3. Could relate readings and lecture notes to the problem at hand.
4. Could fit knowledge possessed into many uses as opposed to only one use.
5. Substituted a vague concept with an illustrative example.
6. Were actively involved, thought about the problem.
7. Were able to break the problem into "bits and pieces" or simpler terms.
8. Were systematic in their thinking about the problem.
9. Had the ability to follow through on the process of reasoning.
10. Had a self-confident and objective attitude toward the solution of problems.

The classic research on problem solving by Bloom and Broder (1961) seems to indicate that certain learners have characteristics they bring to a learning situation that influence their ability to apply learning to real or problem situations.

Once the decision-situation is recognized, it should be defined. The problem to be solved should be clearly and concisely stated. It may be necessary to redefine the problem into segments and then to deal with the segments separately. This should be done in such a way that when all segments are dealt with, the needs of the total situation are met. Similarly, if the decision pertains to an opportunity or life change, the woman's goal must be identified and defined so that she can assess when her goal has been met.

One example of failure to identify a problem situation in women's health sometimes occurs when a woman becomes repeatedly unintentionally pregnant. She may refuse to admit the pregnancy, deny that she must deal with her condition, or fantasize that she will have the baby and continue with her life course. These women, because of their failure to identify their problem situations, often must undergo second-trimester abortions or accept an unwanted pregnancy after their situation has become obvious to and dealt with by others.

Collection of Relevant Information. If a problem, need, or opportunity has been perceived, information gathering may be necessary, both to better define the problem situation and to prepare formulation of alternative courses of action. In the domain of health, information gathering may involve reading, talking to others, or seeking aid from the health care practitioner.

The information-gathering stage is, for example, essential in deciding a birthing alternative. The expectant couple must learn of the birthing options available to them and then study their own needs and preferences and each birthing option in depth so that later they will be able to choose the appropriate option.

Production of Action Alternatives. The literature on decision making and problem solving suggests that, as alternatives are formulated, judgment should be deferred to encourage the production of creative ideas. A variety of ideas should be sought; the individual should attempt to roam from one logical solution to another during this process (Guilford, 1967). However, the individual's readiness to take risks could affect the formulation of possible choices. More far reaching and out of the ordinary alternatives are possible if the decision-maker tends to be less conservative (Kogen & Wallach, 1967).

On the other hand, an individual who is unable to tolerate periods of indecision or is unduly anxious may be unable to produce alternative choices to action (D'Zurilla & Goldfried, 1973). Janis and Mann (1977) have found that in those situations where there is insufficient time to search for alternatives and to deliberate a state of hypervigilance and states of high anxiety result. In this situation, the formulation of alternatives would be inefficient and incomplete.

In most circumstances it is often suggested that the individuals attempt to formulate as many alternatives as possible. However, Simon (1957) has suggested that because human beings have limited cognitive ability, decision making, rather than being a purely rational process, is one of "bound rationality." Human beings will normally search for alternatives until a good enough versus optimal option is found.

An illustration of the production of alternatives is seen in the situation of the elderly woman who had to choose between giving up her home and moving to an institution for the elderly or staying in her house, which is dangerous during the cold, snowy winter. After much reflection and investigation, she formulated the alternative course of sharing an apartment in a complex for the elderly. When the apartment tenant went to Florida for the winter, the elderly woman moved into the apartment. During the summer, the woman moved back to her home when the apartment tenant returned.

Choice of Course of Action. In this stage, the decision-maker considers the consequences of all alternatives. Each option is evaluated in terms of its costs and benefits, deficiencies, strengths, and weaknesses. Positive and negative values are attached to each of the consequences. Probability ratings are assigned according to the likelihood of occurrence. Theoretically, a numerical score is obtained for each alternative so that the best may be selected.

One study (Scodel, Philburn, & Minas, 1959) looked at betting decisions and the influence of risk. They found that those subjects who selected the alternative with a high probability of winning but a low pay-off were those with a greater fear of failure, higher need for achievement, more other-directed, more socially assimilated, and more oriented to middle class values. Being sophisticated about probabilities and expected values made no difference in choice selection.

The contraceptive literature bears this out. Vigilant contraceptors, i.e., those women who have decided on a course of birth control use and have been successful, have been found to be women with educational and professional aspirations (Jekel, Klerman, & Bancroft, 1973; Shah, Zelnik, & Kantner, 1975). These women seemed to accord the possibility of pregnancy a high negative value and desired a low probability of occurrence.

Simon (1957) suggests that human beings may foresee the positive and negative consequences of an option, but seldom attach numerical probabilities. More likely, individual consequences are examined in totality: Will they occur or will they not? Will a particular solution meet the need without undue negative consequences?

Evaluation of the Consequences. Once a course of action is selected, it must be implemented and evaluated as to outcome. D'Zurilla and Goldfried (1971) state that the individual may need help to act on the decision, to move from thought to action. Furthermore, in some situations the individual may not be capable of carrying out the selected course of action. There may be behavioral deficits such as a lack of assertiveness or lack of social skills, emotional inhibitions such as fear of rejection or performance anxiety, or there may be environmental obstacles. These obstacles must be overcome to allow selected choices that require skills the decision-maker does not have.

If the decision is acted upon with unforeseen or disappointing consequences, the process must be repeated. The problem situation must be reexamined. Perhaps more information is needed or a different alternative should be tried.

An example of disappointing consequences, possibly unforeseen, would be if a couple who investigated alternative modes for childbearing chose a birthing center for their delivery experience and the woman failed to progress with her labor because of fetal distress. The woman would need to consider moving to a hospital for a possible cesarean section.

Increasing Decision-making Ability

In aiding a client to improve decision-making ability, emphasis should be placed on the skill of making decisions rather than the specific instance for which the client is being treated. The ability to make optimum decisions should be transferable from one domain to another. For example, the same rational process would go into deciding on a job change as in choosing a contraceptive method as in buying a new winter coat. This frequently needs to be pointed out to clients confronted with health care decisions.

It is important that the client be encouraged to engage in the decision-making process independently, perhaps using the health care practitioner as a resource. Aldous (1976, p. 274) suggests that if a person has taken on a problem through her own volition, she tends to respond with greater effort at task solution. It is likely that if a client has not identified a problem on her own, vigilant decision making will not ensue at the health care practitioner's suggestion.

D'Zurilla and Goldfried (1973) suggest that the client needs to develop a set or attitude to recognize and accept problematic situations when they occur. Problematic situations are, in a real-life context, the normal state of affairs.

The decision-making process can be taught. Many studies have been done looking at methods of enhancing this ability (see, for example, the comprehensive article by Urbain & Kendall, 1980). Methods included group work in which situations were presented and the participants were helped to formulate alternatives and to evaluate possible consequences.

Coche and Flick (1975) describe their training sessions in detail: The group leader introduces a situation and assists the group in clarification. The group suggests alternative solutions and discusses the feasibility of each. Three to four problems are handled during a session. These authors found that as the groups progressed, there was an increase in relevant alternatives and a decrease in irrelevant ones. These writers specified that they began with cognitive skill training before dealing with more complex personal situations.

Other training groups used role modeling and employed video to set up the decision situation. In encouraging the formulation of wide-ranging alternatives, relaxation and imagery were taught by one therapist to school children.

In working with more than one individual, such as with families or couples, the teaching of communication skills would be an important component, as would negotiation skills. In working with a couple, for instance, both individuals should agree on their assessment of the problem. During information-gathering, the results should be shared rather than withheld or given only in the form of instructions or intentions. The couple should be actively formulating possible alternative courses of action and should come to a consensus on the evaluation of each option. If after assessment of the results, further work is necessary, the couple should also decide on this jointly.

A knowledge base is necessary to identify the decision-situation, otherwise it will not be possible to recognize a problem or an opportunity. In teaching decision-making skills within a women's health context, therefore, basic teaching about women's anatomy and physiology, gynecology and sexuality, and the health care system should take place. Anticipatory guidance about potential life changes would also help the woman to identify decision-situations.

Self-knowledge is another component of the women's health domain of knowledge. Decision-making situations may be identified if the woman is aware of her own needs, motives, and goals. Similarly, self-knowledge gives a basis for the evaluation of alternatives.

Self-awareness, or the process of paying attention to oneself, enables the development of self-insight or knowledge about the self. Self-insight has been studied within a construct termed objective self-awareness (Duval & Wicklund, 1972). This model purports that attention at any given moment is directed either wholly toward the self or wholly toward external events. Stimuli that remind a person of objective status increase self-awareness whereas all other stimuli draw attention outward. The other underlying assumption of this theory is that self-awareness always leads to a self-critical evaluation process in which the person compares herself to some standard on whatever behavioral dimension is salient. This type of comparison is usually aversive in that behavior is generally worse than the standard of comparison. According to Wicklund and Duval (1971), then, the key to objective self-awareness is self-esteem. Real–ideal discrepancies are heightened in the self-aware state.

Causal self-attribution and the feeling of responsibility has been found to increase with an increase in self-focus (Arkin & Duval, 1975; Buss & Scheier, 1976; Duval & Wicklund, 1973). Wicklund and Ickes (1972) found that information seeking increased before decision making, when self-awareness was increased through subjects listening to a tape recording of their own voice.

In 1975, Feingstein, Scheier, and Buss developed the concept of self-consciousness, which they defined as the consistent tendency of persons to direct attention either inward or outward. They suggested that self-consciousness is a state, and that being in such a state is due either to some transient situational variable or to a chronic disposition, or both. They designed the self-consciousness scale of which one subscale, private self-consciousness, measures the tendency to attend to one's inner thoughts and feelings. Studies on objective self-awareness have been replicated using the self-consciousness scale and have obtained similar findings. Other studies (Turner, 1977, 1978a, 1978b) found that self-conscious individuals gave the most lengthy and valid self-descriptions, in other words, demonstrated an increased level of self-knowledge.

Self-knowlege may be developed through increased self-awareness. Self-awareness may be entered into on a transitory basis and is common in the presence of a camera, mirror, or audience. Without these props, however, for the woman not habitually self-conscious, self-awareness must be consciously sought. She will need to practice self-

TABLE 3–4. PRIVATE SELF-CONSCIOUSNESS SUBSCALE

Item	Strongly Agree	Moderately Agree	Agree	Moderately Disagree	Strongly Disagree
1. I'm always trying to figure myself out	1	2	3	4	5
2. Generally, I'm not very aware of myself	5	4	3	2	1
3. I reflect about myself a lot	1	2	3	4	5
4. I'm often the subject of my own fantasies	1	2	3	4	5
5. I never scrutinize myself	5	4	3	2	1
6. I'm generally attentive to my inner feelings	1	2	3	4	5
7. I'm constantly examining my motives	1	2	3	4	5
8. I sometimes have the feeling that I'm off somewhere watching myself	1	2	3	4	5
9. I'm alert to changes in my mood	1	2	3	4	5
10. I'm aware of the way my mind works when I work through a problem	1	2	3	4	5

Instructions: Read each statement carefully. Then, indicate to what extent you agree that the statement describes you.
Scoring: Items 2 and 5 are negatively scored. Scores range from 10 to 50.
(Source: Feingstein, A., Scheier, M. F., & Buss, A. H. Public and private self-consciousness: Assessment and theory. Journal of Consulting and Clinical Psychology, 1975, 7, 256–260, by permission. Copyright 1975 by the American Psychological Association.)

awareness, i.e., establish a self-awareness program. On a routine basis, she would consciously observe herself, asking such questions as "What am I feeling?," "What are my motives?," "How would I describe my mood?," and "How did I come to this conclusion or thought?" A habitually unself-conscious woman may need reminders or a schedule in order to establish a self-aware pattern.

She will also need to know that self-awareness may be difficult. She may have feelings of low self-esteem as she starts to observe her thought processes and actions. Being forewarned of this is helpful and enables understanding of the mechanism underlying feelings of lowered self-worth.

The habitually self-conscious woman may be identified using the private self-consciousness subscale (Table 3–4). The woman with a higher score (closer to 50) would be assumed to have more knowledge about herself. This scale could be used as a quick self-administered scale for women in a number of clinical situations. Having identified the degree of the woman's self-awareness, a specific program could be set up to assist her in increasing her self-awareness.

Summary

This section has described the decision-making process and the value of self-insight or consciousness. The ability to know oneself, one's feelings and needs, is indeed essential for women in a complex society that perpetuates the stereotypes of how women ought to be. Helping a woman understand herself, indeed encouraging her to pay attention to herself, may be essential before women can adequately deal with the challenge of a mutilating surgery or the difficulty of an unintentional pregnancy. Selecting alternatives of treatment, for example radiation or surgery, self-help versus traditional medical care, will require self-insight and knowledge about preferences and comfort with various types of individuals. This self-insight is particularly important in dealing with life choices, (Chapter 7), sexual self-awareness (Chapter 6), and discovering what it means to be a woman in today's world (Chapter 5).

Throughout the discussion on the educational process (Chapters 2 and 3), suggestions have been made to use the group approach for learning. Groups have been used widely and effectively for women, families, and couples. Groups are especially productive for teaching women's health topics because they facilitate support as well as allow presentation of content. Group strategies have a potential to assist women in making decisions, gaining self-confidence, and learning more about themselves in relation to others. The final section of this chapter discusses the application of the teaching–learning process to groups. The reader will note that groups facilitate an andragogical learning orientation *and* have the ability to assist women to develop decision-making skills and self-insights. For more complete information on the group process, additional texts are required (see G. D. Marram's *The Group Approach in Nursing Practice* [1978] or M. E. Loomis's *Group Process for Nurses* [1979]). The following section highlights critical content.

Use of Groups in Women's Health Education

When groups of expectant parents, women facing abortion, couples considering family planning methods, or women preparing for their middle years are organized, the individuals in these groups can be used to support and teach each other. The advantage of the group can be very important, especially for learning affective aspects of health behaviors and for reinforcing women's change in health behavior that is more conducive to health than past behavior.

The group method of learning and the role of the leader have been summarized by Littlefield and Siebert (1978). They are reprinted here (Table 3–5) to provide the reader with a framework and quick summary for organizing and leading groups.

Another facet of group work, group process, refers to an illusive variable that is concerned with the mechanism of change that occurs in groups. It has been described in terms of leadership, membership, interactions, interpersonal learning, and insight depending on whether the group was one of support, task, or psychotherapy. All health care groups would be expected to have a therapeutic objective regardless of the structure and, thus, it would seem appropriate to consider group process goals here in terms described in group treatment literature as curative factors (Loomis, 1979). Yalom (1975) has discussed these human experiences or curative factors that both leaders and members have been able to identify in their groups.

1. *Instillation of hope:* provides a belief that there is an answer to one's problem
2. *Universality:* dispels feelings of being alone resulting in a powerful sense of relief
3. *Imparting of information:* transfers knowledge that is reality based
4. *Altruism:* gives individuals a self-esteem boosting experience through their offers of support, reassurance, and sharing with others
5. *Corrective recapitulation of the primary family group:* fosters change in family behaviors and responses

TABLE 3–5. THE GROUP PROCESS FOR LEARNING

The group method of learning to cope with situational or developmental crises has been employed with great success in many areas of life. The process makes use of the concepts first developed by such self-help groups as Alcoholics Anonymous, where those who have experienced the crises under discussion provide information and support derived from their own experience to others who are anticipating or undergoing such crises.

In planning for or implementing group education, the traditional "school" model with a teacher/lecturer is avoided; instead the group members are encouraged to share their thoughts and experiences with each other. Most learning results from this interaction.

In most groups, the patients themselves set the goals, provide answers, and then apply the answers to their own situation. The role of the group leaders is to focus on assisting the individual group members to find their own answers and to develop their own coping mechanisms. Gwen Marram[a] and Aline Auerbach[b] point out that nurses serving as leaders for such groups can function best by assuming a "wise sister" (or "wise brother") role. This leads to maximum participation by group members who gain self-esteem when they realize they are able to find their own answers to questions and problems.

The following nine basic principles identified by Ms. Auerbach provide valuable information that can be used as guidelines for organizing and leading a group:

1. Learning that takes place during a developmental crisis can facilitate an increased ability to cope with the same condition in the future because it allows new insight into past feelings and behavior.

2. Group members want to learn—that is why they join the group—but many factors influence behavior. The group as a whole can assist in identifying the reasons why a particular member finds it hard to comply with restrictions.

3. People learn best what they are interested in learning. The group leader will do well to ask the members what their concerns and interests are and begin there. If necessary the discussion can always be shifted later by the leader to include critical content.

4. Learning is most significant when the subject is closely related to the individual's own immediate experiences. The leader can apply this principle by taking an example from a member—i.e., the manner in which she handles breast-feeding problems—and using it to illustrate the way the law of "supply and demand" functions.

5. Individuals learn best when they are free to create their own response to a situation. Group leaders can encourage the members to respond freely and creatively by actively listening to every participant's ideas, and by recognizing that different solutions can be valid for different people.

6. Group education is as much an emotional experience as it is an intellectual one. Most group members can be expected to respond emotionally to some problems they encounter; the way this response is received will influence the individual's ability to accept new ideas. For this reason it is extremely important that the group leader accept such responses with skill and empathy.

7. Individuals can learn from one another and frequently do not need an "authority" to supply the answers. The group member who provides an acceptable answer to someone else's problem gains as much from the experience as the individual whose problem she has helped solve.

8. Group education provides a foundation which is useful later for remodeling one's behavior based on one's own experience. This principle was demonstrated in the diabetic mothers group when patients who returned to the group to describe their labor and delivery experiences analyzed them and made plans for changes that would improve any future childbearing experience.

9. Each individual learns in her own way. An important function of the leader is to evaluate continuously each group member's knowledge and understanding of the material presented. Some members may need additional information, follow-up, or assistance with problems that cannot be handled in the group. Each group, as well as each individual within a group, must move at its own pace. This means that the leader needs to be aware of the fact that not only may ideas and content have to be repeated several times, but support must be given to the group as a whole and the individual members on an ongoing basis.

The role of the leader is a key variable in the group learning experience. It can be critical in determining the success of the group as measured by the educational gains made by the members.

Ms. Marram outlines the leader's role as follows:

• To facilitate the benefits of group membership by assisting the members to feel secure and to maintain a sense of belonging and companionship.
• To maintain a viable group atmosphere that enables members to express their real needs and concerns and to be unafraid to risk experimentation.
• To oversee the group's growth by identifying group goals and learning needs.

TABLE 3–5. (cont.)

• To regulate group dynamics, which may mean at times encouraging the active participation of some members and discouraging others from monopolizing the group's time.

In addition, leadership intervention may be employed for the following purposes: to outline and interpret group objectives; to reduce anxiety; and to summarize the group's progress periodically as it approaches its goals. Finally, introducing content into the group's discussions is also a necessary intervention, but one that is performed only after the members are given a chance to share their knowledge about the topic with each other. Because this type of intervention requires in-depth knowledge of a particular subject, leaders often find it useful to call upon other specialists for assistance.

[a] Marram, G. D. *The group approach in nursing practice.* St. Louis, Mo.: C. V. Mosby Co., 1973.
[b] Auerbach, A. B. *Parents learn through discussion.* New York: John Wiley & Sons, 1968.
(Source: *Littlefield, V., & Seibert, G. The group approach to problem solving for pregnant diabetic women.* American Journal of Maternal Child Nursing, *1978, 3(5), 274–280, by permission.)*

6. *Development of socializing techniques:* occurs as a benefit of relating directly and honestly with other group members
7. *Imitative behavior:* allows experimentation with new behavior after observing others
8. *Interpersonal learning:* occurs as individuals become aware of their strengths and limitations and risk new types of expression and behavior
9. *Group cohesiveness:* refers to the attraction of the individual for her group and to other members and their mutual acceptance of one another
10. *Catharsis:* enhances group cohesion and mutual bonds through an open expression of feelings
11. *Existential factors:* represents a cluster of factors including responsibility, basic isolation, contingency, recognition of one's own mortality; those elements of the group that help the members deal with the meaning of their own existence

These group process variables are important to consider when assessing groups and in developing an understanding of how people change through groups. Specific intervention strategies can be used to promote these therapeutic goals within the group.

The therapeutic process or change takes place within the phases or developmental stages of a group. Marram (1978) described these in psychotherapeutic terminology as the introductory or beginning phase, the working-through or middle phase, and the termination phase.

Phase I. The Introductory Phase: Securing a Psychosocial Environment. Initially, groups enter a stage of orientation in which members are searching for norms, structure, and goals. At first they usually depend a great deal on the leader as they look for a role for themselves within the group for which they will be well liked and respected. As they begin to see similarities among members and trust is developed between leaders and members, self-disclosure begins and the basis for group cohesion is found. It is the leader's role in this early stage to help members learn who people are, their strengths, the task of the group, and how it will be managed. She must convey acceptance, understanding, and encouragement to members in order to establish that the group is a safe place for disclosure.

Conflict can emerge when members have fears about sharing, becoming close to others, or being in a group with others who seem to have problems or insecurities. Yalom (1975) sees this occur as members vie with one another and with the leader for dominance and control. Resentment expressed against the leader would be expected because group members usually come to the group with unrealistically high expectations of the leader. The leader is expected to provide all the answers and solve all the problems of the group. No matter how competent the leader is, the group members feel disappointment. With knowledge of this normal phase of group development, the leader does not feel personal assault, but rather continues to redirect the group to explore its own resources.

Phase II. The Working Phase: Locating Responsibility in Members for Change. It is in this stage of group development, as described by Marram (1978), in which members begin to focus on specific problems and take responsibility for their behaviors. They begin to accept feedback from others, initiate verbal exchanges with one another, and assume some of the leadership functions of the group. Feelings, attitudes, and behaviors are explored more openly. Problem solving can take place as the group is able to offer support for changing ideas and activities. The leader maintains an important role within the group by reinforcing an individual's attempts to change a behavior, encouraging the new activity outside the group, and helping the group to acknowledge the change that they see in an individual member.

Phase III. Terminating the Group: Arriving at a Perspective on Self and Others Through Change. The tasks of this stage of group development are to

1. Summarize the experience
2. Establish perspective
3. Bring closure to the group (Marram, 1978)

It is the leader's role to restate the group's objectives that were established early on and to review the progress made with each. Problem areas still needing work should be identified. It will not be disappointing to the group to not have accomplished everything if learning and sharing can be considered a lifelong process. Of equal importance is the recognition that the termination of a group, as with a one-to-one relationship, arouses feelings of anxiety and loss. Time must be allotted for expression of these feelings by the members and the leader. In fact, the leader can promote such a discussion by first revealing her own feelings about the meaning of the group to her and the significance of its ending.

This basic overview of group work is meant to give the reader a beginning step in the establishment and leadership of groups in women's health. Excellent resources on group work are available that provide more extensive theory, practice principles, and the specifics of the role of the health care professional in a variety of types of groups. These are listed in this chapter's bibliography and a resource list at the end of Chapter 15. If the reader has minimal preparation for leading groups, additional reading is necessary.

Summary. This chapter has discussed three approaches to women's health education that have a potential to enhance independence and participation with health care providers. These approaches are also useful to men, but women at this point in time need extra efforts to enhance their self-concept, ability to make complex decisions, and confidence in confronting and challenging health care providers and institutions. This need originates from women's past socialization as well as health care professionals' past insistence on inappropriate medical interventions for women's health–illness care. Using processes for learning that allow women to learn to participate as competent partners in their own care has a potential to change both women's and health care professionals' view of female capacity and abilities.

BIBLIOGRAPHY

Arkin, R. M., & Duval, S. Focus of attention and causal attributions of actors and observers. *Journal of Experimental Social Psychology*, 1975, *11*, 427–438.

Barnett, E. *Comparative effectiveness of three instructional formats in small-goup continuing education for physicians in community hospitals*. Unpublished Ph.D. dissertation, University of Southern California, 1973.

Baskins, S. Experiment in independent study: 1956–60. *Antioch College Reports*, II 1961, 1–4; R. H. Hamilton, An experiment with independent study in freshman history. *Liberal Education*, 1967, *52*, 271–278.

Beach, L. R. Learning and student interaction in small self-directed college groups. Fiscal Report (ED 026 027). Washington, D.C.: U.S. Department of Health, Education & Welfare, 1970.

Bermosk, L., & Porter, S. *Women's health and human wholeness*. New York: Appleton-Century-Crofts, 1979.

Bigelow, G. S., & Egbert, R. L. Personality factors and independent study. *Journal of Educational Research*, 1968, *62*(1); 37–39.

Birch, H.S., & Robinowitz, H. S. The negative effect of previous experience of productive thinking. *Journal of Experimental Psychology*, 1951, *41*, 121–125.

Bloom, B. S., & Broder, L. J. Problem-solving process of college students. In T. L. Harris & W. S. Schwahn (Eds.), *Selected readings in the learning process*. New York: Oxford University Press, 1961.

Boston Women's Health Book Collective. *Our bodies, ourselves: A book by and for women*. New York: Simon & Schuster, 1973.

Buckland, J. K. *An institute as an educational experience in the continuing education of a selected population of nurses*. Unpublished Master's Thesis. Vancouver: British Columbia University, 1969.

Buss, D. M., & Scheier, M. F. Self-consciousness, self-awareness, and self-attribution. *Journal of Research in Personality*, 1976, *10*, 463–468.

Cameron, F. *What research says about learning*. Athens, Ga.: Institute of Higher Education, 1976.

Coche, E., & Flick, A. Problem-solving training groups for hospitalized psychiatric patients. *Journal of Psychology*, 1975, *91*, 19–29.

Cohen, R. E. The functions of experimental participatory experiences in the learning-teaching process. *American Journal of Psychiatry*, 1978, *135*(1), 103–106.

Cross, K. P. Adult learners: A data-based description. In R. E. Peterson, K. P. Cross, S. Powell, T. W. Hartel, & M. A. Rutner, (Eds.), *Toward lifelong learning in America: A sourcebook for planners*. Berkeley, Calif.: Educational Testing Service, 1978a.

Cross, K. P. The adult learner. Address presented at the 1978 National Conference on Higher Education, American Association for Higher Education, Chicago, Illinois, March 20, 1978b.

Cross, K. P., & Zusman, A. *The needs of non-traditional learners and the responses of non-traditional programs*. Berkeley, Calif.: Center for Research and Development in Higher Education, University of California, 1977.

Darby, D. W. The dentist and continuing education—Attitudes and motivations. *Journal of the American College of Dentists*, 1969, *36*(3), 165–170.

Davis, J. R. *Teaching strategies for the college classroom*. Boulder, Colo.: Westview Press, 1976.

Derby, V. L. Learner's and course goal congruence. Impact on learning outcomes. *Journal of Continuing Education*, 1981, *13*(4), 16–24.

Doty, B. A. Teaching method effectiveness in relation to certain student characteristics. *Journal of Educational Research*, 1967, *60*, 363–365.

Dubin, R., & Taveggia, T. G. *The teaching–learning paradox: A comparative analysis of college teaching methods*. Eugene, Ore.: Center for the Advanced Study of Educational Administration, 1968.

Duval, S., & Wicklund, R. A. *A theory of objective self-awareness*. New York: Academic Press, 1972.

Duval, S., & Wicklund, R. A. Effects of objective self-awareness on attribution of causality. *Journal of Experimental Social Psychology*, 1973, 9, 17–31.

D'Zurilla, T. J., & Goldfried, M. R. Cognitive processes, problem solving, and effective behavior. In M. R. Goldfried & M. Merbaum (Eds.), *Behavioral change through self-control*. New York: Holt, Rinehart & Winston, 1973.

D'Zurilla, T. J., & Goldfried, M. R. Problem solving and behavior modification. *Journal of Abnormal Psychology*, 1971, 78(1), 107–126.

Feingstein, A., Scheier, M. F., & Buss, A. H. Public and private self-consciousness: Assessment and theory. *Journal of Consulting and Clinical Psychology*, 1975, 7, 256–260.

Fincher, C. *What research says about learning*. Athens, Ga.: Institute of Higher Education, 1976.

Fogel, C., & Woods, N. *Health care of women: A nursing perspective*. St. Louis, Mo.: C. V. Mosby, 1981.

Gagne R. M. *The conditions of learning*. New York: Holt, Rinehart & Winston, 1965.

Gagne R. M. *The conditions of learning*. New York: Holt, Rinehart & Winston, 1970.

Guilford, J. P. *The nature of human intelligence*. New York: McGraw-Hill, 1967.

Guthrie, J. T. Expository instruction versus a discovery method. *Journal of Educational Psychology*, 1967, 58(1), 45–49.

Hadley, H. N. *Development of an instrument to determine adult educators' orientation: Andragogical or pedagogical*. Unpublished Ed.D. dissertation, University of Boston, 1975.

Haines, D. B., & McKeachie, W. J. Cooperative vs. competitive discussion methods in teaching introductory psychology. *Journal of Educational Psychology*, 1967, 58, 386–390.

Holmes, D. *A comparative study of student learning style in non-traditional and traditional education*. Unpublished Ph.D. dissertation, University of Denver, 1974.

Holzemer, W. *Student ratings of instructional effectiveness and their relationships to the college classroom environment*. Unpublished Ph.D. dissertation, Syracuse University, 1975.

Hongladarom, G., McCorkle, R., & Fugate Woods, N. *The complete book of women's health*. Englewood Cliffs, N.J.; Prentice-Hall, 1982.

Horner, M. Femininity and successful achievements: A basic inconsistency. In J. Bardwick, Douvan, E., Horner, M., & Gutmann, D. (Eds.), *Feminine personality and conflict*. Belmont, Calif.: Brooks/Cole, 1970.

Houle, C. O. *The inquiring mind. A study of the adult who continues to learn*. Madison, Wis.: The University of Wisconsin Press, 1971.

Hovey, D. E., Gruber. H. E., & Terrell, G. Effects of self-directed study on course achievement, retention, and curiosity. *Journal of Educational Research*, 1963, 56, 346–351.

Huckabay, L. M., Cooper, P. G., & Neal, M. C. Effect of specific teaching techniques on cognitive learning, transfer of learning, and affective behavior of nurses in an in-service education setting. *Nursing Research*, 1977, 26(5) 380–385.

Janis, I. L., & Mann, L. *Decision making*. New York: The Free Press, 1977.

Jekel, J. F., Klerman, L. V., & Bancroft, D. R. E. Factors associated with rapid subsequent pregnancies among school age mothers. *American Journal of Public Health*, 1973, 63, 769–773.

Keller, S. The female role: Constants and change. In V. Franks & V. Burtle (Eds.), *Women in therapy: New psychotherapies for a changing society*. New York: Brunner Mazel, 1974.

Klein, S. S. Student influence on teacher behavior. *American Educational Research Journal*, 1971, 8, 403–421.

Knowles, M. S. *The modern practice of adult education: Andragogy versus pedagogy*. New York: Association Press, 1970.

Knox, A. B. *Adult development and learning*. San Francisco: Jossey-Bass, 1977.

Kogen, N., & Wallach, M. A. Risky-shift phenomenon in small decision-making groups: A test of the information exchange hypothesis. *Journal of Experimental Social Psychology*, 1967, 3, 75–84.

Korda, M. *Power: How to get it, how to use it*. New York: Ballantine, 1975.

Lewis, E. Assessment of computer assisted instruction as a tool for advancing adult learning. (ED 140 073). Needham Heights, Mass.: GTE Sylvania, Human Factors Engineering, 1975.

Littlefield, V. M. *Andragogical–pedagogical learning environments in university health professional continuing education courses and their relationship to learner's intent to use course content in patient care*. Unpublished Ph.D. dissertation, University of Denver, 1979.

Littlefield, V., & Siebert, G. The group approach to problem solving for pregnant diabetic women. *American Journal of Maternal Child Nursing*, 1978, 3(5), 278.

Loomis, M. E. *Group process for nurses*. St. Louis, Mo.: C. V. Mosby, 1979.

Lumsden, D. B., & Sheron, R. H. *Experimental studies in adult learning and memory*. Washington, D.C.: Hemisphere Publishing, 1975.

Marieskind, H. *Women in the health system: Patients, providers and programs*. St. Louis, Mo.: C. V. Mosby, 1980.

Markell, C., & Mayer, V. An investigation to empirically determine which instructional procedures produce optimum student growth (ED 129 560). Paper presented at the 48th Annual Meeting of the National Association for Research in Science Teaching, Los Angeles, California, March 17–20, 1975.

Marram, G. D. *The group approach in nursing practice* (2nd ed.). St. Louis, Mo.: C. V. Mosby, 1978.

Marshall, R. E. Measuring the medical school learning environment. *Journal of Medical Education*, 1978, 53(2), 98–104.

Mayer, R. E., Stiehl, C. C., & Greeno, J. G. Acquisition of understanding and skill in relation to subjects preparation and meaningfulness of instruction. *Journal of Educational Psychology*, 1975, 67(3), 331–350.

McKeachie, W. J. Research on teaching at the college and university level. In N. L. Gage (Ed.), *Handbook of research on teaching*. Chicago, Ill.: Rand McNally, 1963 and 1970.

Meinke, D. L. Conceptual learning and the self-concept (ED 132–461). Paper presented at the Annual Meeting of the American Educational Research Association, Chicago, Illinois, April, 1972.

Miton, O. *Alternatives to the traditional*. San Francisco: Jossey-Bass, 1972.

Morstain, B. The relationship between students' personality characteristics and educational attitudes. *Measurement and Evaluation in Guidance*, 1975, 7, 251–258.

Morstain B. R., & Smart, J. C. Educational orientations of faculty: Assessing a personality model of the academic professions. *Psychological Reports*, 1976 (Pt.2), 39(3), 1199–1211.

Penland, P. R. *Individual self-planned learning in America*. Washington, D. C.: U. S. Department of Health, Education & Welfare, Office of Education, 1977.

Redman, B. K. *The process of patient teaching in nursing*. St. Louis, Mo.: C. V. Mosby, 1980.

Rogers, C. R. *Freedom to learn: A view of what education might become*. Columbus, Ohio: Charles E. Merrill, 1969.

Sandelowski, M. *Women, health and choice*. Englewood Cliffs, N.J.: Prentice-Hall, 1981.

Scodel, A., Philburn, R., & Minas, J. S. Some personality correlates of decision making under conditions of risk. *Behavioral Sciences*, 1959, 4, 19–28.

Shah, F. K., Zelnik, M., & Kantner, J. F. Unprotected intercourse among unwed teenagers. *Family Planning Perspectives*, 1975, 6, 39–44.

Sherman, B. R., & Blackburn, R. T. Personal characteristics of and teaching effectiveness of college faculty. *Journal of Educational Psychology*, 1975, 67(1), 124–131.

Simon, H. A. A behavioral model of rational choice. In H. A. Simon (Ed.), *Models of man*. New York: John Wiley & Sons, 1957.

Skinner, B. F. *About behaviorism*. New York: Alfred A. Knopf, 1974.

Sovie, M. D. *The relationships of learning orientation, nursing activity and continuing education*. Unpublished Ph.D. dissertation, Syracuse University, 1972.

Spivack, G., Platt, J. J., & Shure, M. B. *The problem solving approach to adjustment*. San Francisco: Jossey-Bass, 1976.

Tallmadge, G. K., & Shearer, J. W. Relationships among learning styles, instructional methods and the nature of learning experiences. *Journal of Educational Psychology*, 1969, *60*, 222–230.

Tough, A. *Major learning efforts: Recent research and further directions*. Toronto: Ontario Institute for Studies in Education, 1977.

Tough, A. *The adult's learning projects*. Toronto, Canada: Ontario Institute for Studies in Education, 1971.

Travers, R. M. (Ed.) *Second handbook of research on teaching*. Chicago: Rand McNally, 1973.

Trent, J.W., & Cohen, A. M. Research on teaching in higher education. In N. L. Gage (Ed.), *Handbook of research on teaching*. Chicago: Rand McNally, 1973.

Trent, J., & Cohen, A. M. Research on teaching in higher education. In R. Travers (Ed.), *Second handbook of research on teaching*. Chicago: Rand McNally, 1973.

Turner, R. G. Self-consciousness and anticipatory belief change. *Personality and Social Psychology Bulletin*, 1977, *3*, 438–441.

Turner, R. G. Consistency, self-consciousness, and the predictive validity of typical and maximal personality measures. *Journal of Research in Personality*, 1978a, *12*, 117–132.

Turner, R. G. Effects of differential request procedures and self-consciousness on trait attributions. *Journal of Research in Personality*, 1978b, *12*, 431–438.

Urbain, E. S., & Kendall, P. C. Review of social-cognitive problem-solving interventions with children. *Psychological Bulletin*, 1980, *88*, 109–143.

Weatherby, R. Life stages and learning interests. Paper presented at the 1978 American Association of Higher Education National Conference on Higher Education, Chicago, March 20, 1978.

Wicklund, R. A., & Duval, S. Opinion change and performance facilitation as a result of objective self-awareness. *Journal of Experimental Social Psychology*, 1971, *7*(3), 319–342.

Wicklund, R. A., & Ickes, W. J. The effect of objective self-awareness on predecisional exposure to information. *Journal of Experimental Social Psychology*, 1972, *8*, 378–387.

Williams, J. H. *Psychology of women: Behavior in a biosexual context*. New York: W. W. Norton, 1977.

Witkin, H. A., Moore, C. A., & Oltman, P. K. Field-dependent and field independent cognitive styles and their educational implications. *Review of Educational Research*, 1977, *69*(3), 197–211.

Wittrock, M. C. Verbal stimuli in concept formation: Learning by discovery. *Journal of Educational Psychology*, 1963, *54*(4), 183–190.

Yalom, I. D. *The theory and practice of group psychotherapy* (2nd ed.). New York: Basic Books, 1975.

A Developmental Perspective: What?

4

Vivian M. Littlefield

To establish a comprehensive approach to content for health education of women, a life cycle, developmental approach is proposed. If human wholeness and high level wellness are goals, then education for what promotes and maintains health must be a lifelong process. Attitudes and beliefs about what it is to be female are conveyed from the moment of birth. Thus planning for positive attitudes toward female roles and health must begin at birth.

Because of negative stereotyping in selected areas of development, girls require special educational approaches in such areas as female identity, appropriate behavior in competition, nurturing roles, and sexual/reproductive functioning. Specific female health problems/illnesses are also related to age and development. Examining what brings children, adolescents, and women to health care providers assists in anticipating age-related educational needs. Appropriate educational intervention can then be aimed at strengthening women's appropriate use of the health care system while minimizing unnecessary use of the same resources.

This chapter serves as an organizing framework for the remainder of the text. Chapters 5 through 26 provide more detail on developmental and selected female health/ illness educational needs. Tables 4–1 through 4–6 identify age-specific developmental needs that this author concludes have special significance for women's health education. In addition the common and major health concerns and problems of the female child, adolescent, young adult, middle-aged, and elderly are listed. Methodological approaches to individual and group health education are also proposed. Issues concerning what type of facility, and at whose expense a provider/educator should educate women, are raised. The final section of this chapter describes two examples of health education for women using a developmental approach. The examples, breast self-examination and menstruation, are selected because they are unique health education needs for women and the specific needs for learning vary according to age and developmental level. Also, the breasts and menstrual functions of the woman are frequently the focus of negative stereotypes of being female. Using these areas as a specific educational focus can allow incorporation of positive attitudes toward being female as well as specific content related to health prevention.

Comprehensive Health: A Definition

Bermosk and Porter (1979) in *Women's Health and Human Wholeness* have proposed a healthing model for women's health. This model insures that women consumers and providers collaborate in care and in creating a system that is caring about women's health needs beyond a "reproductive and gynecological focus." It proposes modalities that "increase women's knowledge about promotion and maintenance of health . . ." and helps the woman become "more aware of her responsibility in keeping her mind–body–spirit in a balanced state within her environment." This model can also facilitate women and health care professionals to relate in a "complementary–symmetrical" versus a "domination–submission" manner (Bermosk & Porter, 1979, pp. 117–118). The goals of the program are

1. To create in each woman an awareness of her human wholeness.
2. To provide opportunities through which the mind–body–spirit–environment perspective of each woman is expanded to include a variety of pathways available in the healthing process.
3. To develop in each woman a willingness to take responsibility for and to make decisions about her health care.
4. To teach each woman to participate effectively with health care providers and facilitators (Bermosk & Porter, 1979, pp. 118–119).

The services proposed are

1. Integrated and comprehensive health services that will promote, assess, and maintain women's health through all their developmental ages from birth to old age.
2. Oriented to the community and to the women they serve.
3. Based on the principle of shared responsibility between the giver and the receiver of health care.
4. Operated with a team of nurse clinical specialists in collaboration with an extended team of interdisciplinary health providers and facilitators in the community.
5. Operated within an established health care system (Bermosk & Porter, 1979, p. 119).

The following summarization of health education needs of women is written within this philosophy and orientation.

FEMALE DEVELOPMENT AND HEALTH EDUCATIONAL GOALS

Childhood Development Goals

Most psychological theories conclude that life experiences of children influence their self-concept and identity. Therefore, the early years (birth to 11 years) are possibly critical in establishing the child's concept of what it is to be female. What can be accomplished to overcome negative or maladaptive adult roles through education may depend on stereotypes the woman learned as a child. Thus, assisting parents to understand the "female world" (Bernard, 1981) their daughter will experience should be as critical in parent education as details of child care and specific developmental changes.

Because knowledge of what is appropriate parenting for positive mental health in the girl (or boy) is not fully known, education cannot provide "cookbook answers," but must present current knowledge and raise questions about common practices and beliefs that have been demonstrated to be inappropriate for females. Emphasis on the individuality of children with a realistic anticipation of what their future might hold is needed in health education.

An article entitled "X" (Gould, 1980) describes the dilemma of adults when they do not know if a baby is a boy or a girl. The tongue in cheek story of "X" demonstrates the necessity felt in our society to ascribe "sweet and dainty" characteristics to girls and "strong and active" characteristics to boys. The characters in the story of "X" become confused and unable to respond when a boy or girl label is not assigned to a child, X. This child turns out healthy and happy because "it" is "free" from inappropriate stereotypes and can be an individual. Having parents read this story (Gould, 1980) can be a useful device to raise their perception and understanding of children's experience in relation to male and female stereotyping.

Children's literature has perpetuated negative views of females and their roles. Efforts to select bias-free literature that depicts females and their roles in positive ways should be encouraged. Care should also be taken in selecting television shows, movies, and toys. Providing parents with information about the messages presented in these resources may be invaluable.

Table 4–1 identifies developmental tasks that this author concludes are especially important for a healthy girl. The following pages describe these tasks briefly. First, basic differences between boys and girls are summarized.

Basic Differences Between Boys and Girls. Common beliefs hold that girls are naturally more social, more nurturing, more suggestible, and have lower self-esteem than boys. Maccoby and Jacklin (1974) discuss some of these beliefs and present research that supports or refutes these differences (Table 4–2). They conclude that there are few differences that are well established. Documented differences include the greater verbal ability of girls and the greater mathematical and visual–spatial abilities of boys. In addition, sex differences in aggression have been observed in all cultures. Boys are more aggressive verbally and physically (Maccoby & Jacklin, 1974). Whether these differences are entirely biological or sociological is debated. Currently differences between boys and girls are believed to be dependent on the interaction of genetic factors, shaping of behavior by parents and others, and children's spontaneous learning of behavior appropriate for their sex (Maccoby & Jacklin, 1974).

New research (Chodorow, 1978; Gilligan, 1982) concludes that women may construe their world differently than men. This difference has been attributed to women's different modes of thinking about relationships. These differences between boys and girls can be observed in children's play. Boys are more concerned with rules, girls with relationships. Girls will terminate games to maintain relationships. Boys will create rules to resolve conflicts (Gilligan, 1982). Gilligan (1982), author of *In a Different Voice*, found that women in the American culture tend to see the world in terms of connectedness, men in terms of autonomy. Women are thus overthreatened by isolation, men by intimacy. Rather than depreciating either sex's behavior, Gilligan (1982) writes about "differential access of the genders to certain kinds of understanding." She has created new appreciation for a previously unrecognized female sensibility and her work has implications for the future. When world survival may depend on a "sense of connection," humanity may need to "take its cue not from Big Brother, but from sister, mothers, and daughters" (Van Gelder, 1984).

Teaching sessions for parents that present new research and discuss differential abilities of the sexes and that counter myths about females will be insightful. Depending

TABLE 4–1. WOMEN'S HEALTH EDUCATION DEVELOPMENTAL PERSPECTIVE: CHILDHOOD

Age	Critical Content	Educational Goals	Methodology
Childhood Birth–11 yr	*Developmental*		
	Female identity	The child will value femaleness and her own individuality and femininity. The child will define roles for males and females in non-sexist language.	Parental instruction and information about childhood identity within community colleges, mental health, pre-schools, and religious institutions.
	Female socialization	The child will demonstrate situation appropriate (versus sex appropriate) behavior in competition, social interaction, and nurturing.	Play activities supervised by individuals prepared in child development and methods to support individuals versus sex related roles.
	Female competition	The child will demonstrate age appropriate strategies to cope with competition and her own achievement goals.	Parental, pre-school teacher education to discuss methods for increased female ability to compete.
	Examination of sexual apparatus	The child will demonstrate age appropriate understanding of her sexual/reproductive apparatus. The child will describe her sexual apparatus in positive and equalitarian terms.	Parents classes regarding activities that foster positive attitudes toward sex sponsored by mental health and primary care centers.
	Female roles and responsibility	The child will define the responsibilities of various roles without equating these to sex. The child will recognize that being female does not prevent her from being what she wants to be.	Parents classes to discuss roles and alternate life styles and its impact on children. Special focus on how society's view of the female impacts children's concept of being female taught in parent's classes.

Health Promotion

Roles and responsibility for own and others' health

The child will define (and take) age appropriate responsibility for her health.

The child will recognize her rights to participate in decisions regarding her health.

The child will appreciate the role women have played in others' health maintenance and illness care.

Age appropriate responsibility for healthy living done in schools and school health centers.

Include content about females' roles in health in history, civic classes in schools and religious classes.

Health Concerns:
Major Health Problems

Injuries (motor vehicles, poisoning)
Congenital anomalies
Leukemia
Cardiovascular illnesses
Homicide
Sexual abuse

The child will recognize how her life-style and activities affect health.

The child will recognize health and illness vs. good and bad behavior.

The child will demonstrate positive attitudes toward health care providers.

Injuries will be minimized by age appropriate intervention.

Given a major illness, the child will not incorporate a negative self-image for herself or her femaleness.

Efforts to relate cause of illness to activity when appropriate will be incorporated by health care providers.

The child will be protected from birth to adolescence.

Parents classes and support groups will include impact of illness on self-image of the female.

(Source: The critical content was developed using Martin, L. L. Health care of women, New York: J. B. Lippincott, 1978, pp. 1–28; Fogel, C. I., & Woods, N. F. Health care of women, a nursing perspective, St. Louis, C. V. Mosby, 1981, pp. 3–26; Williams, J. Psychology of women: Behavior in a biosocial context, New York: W. W. Norton, 1977. The educational goals and methodology are the authors'.)

TABLE 4–2. DIFFERENCES BETWEEN MALES AND FEMALES (BOYS AND GIRLS) IN THE U.S.A.

	Good Evidence That the Statement is *True*	Good Evidence That the Statement is *False*	Little or Conflicting Evidence on Either Side
1. Girls are more social than boys.		X	
2. Girls are more suggestible than boys.		X	
3. Girls have lower self-esteem than boys.		X	
4. Girls are better at role learning and simple repetitive tasks, boys at tasks that require higher level cognitive processing.		X	
5. Boys are more analytic in their cognitive style.		X	
6. Girls are more affected by heredity, boys by environment.		X	
7. Girls lack achievement motivation.		X	
8. Girls are auditory, boys visual in learning modality.		X	
9. Girls have greater verbal ability than boys.	X		
10. Boys excel in visual–spatial ability in adolescence and adulthood (not childhood).	X		
11. Boys excel in mathematical ability until age 12–13.	X		
12. Boys are more aggressive than girls.	X		
13. Girls have more tactile sensitivity.			X
14. Girls are more fearful, timid, and anxious.			X
15. Boys have higher activity level.			X
16. Boys are more competitive.			X
17. Boys are more dominant.			X
18. Girls are more compliant.			X
19. Girls are more nuturant, "maternal".			X

(Source: *Developed from the discussion "Summary and Commentary" in Maccoby, E. E., & Jacklin, C. N.,* The psychology of sex differences. *Stanford, Calif.: Stanford University Press, 1974, pp. 104–121.*)

on the educational level and/or preferences of parents, the content from Maccoby and Jacklin's article could be read or presented and discussed. A self-administered and self-scored pretest (Table 4–2) could be used to assist parents in identifying their own particular knowledge of male and female differences. Another exercise to use in parent education would be to ask one group to describe a baby after looking at a picture. A second group of parents could describe the same baby informed that the baby was of the opposite sex. Comparisons would likely be enlightening and lead to new insights about how people (including parents) respond to a child depending on sex. After identifying real and perceived differences, then specific developmental tasks that are of special relevance for girls in our society could be discussed.

Sex Role Acquisition in Childhood. Development of sex role identity is a major task of the child. Efforts to understand the factors that influence the acquisition of sex role have been a major task for the behavioral sciences. Numerous unanswered questions exist, but observations of young children confirm that both boys and girls have sex-role preferences by age three. By middle childhood until adulthood, girls demonstrate a widespread preference for the masculine role and ambivalence for clear-cut identification with the feminine role. This is in contrast to boys who show an unequivocal identification with the masculine role (Brown, 1956, 1958; Sherman, 1971). Explanations for these differences are (1) girls perceive the male role as invested with higher status and greater rewards (Brown, 1956, 1958; Williams, 1977), and (2) girls are free to state cross-sex preference and have a greater latitude to engage in a host of male activities (Williams, 1977).

Obviously, early experiences influence this development. Parents need to understand what is involved in the acquisition of sex roles and recognize the influence they have on this development. Many parents fear they will do something wrong. Others have no concept that they influence their children. The degree of parental influence versus other individuals or the child's unique response is open to some debate among theorists, but increasing parents' insights into the child's complex experience will be useful.

Table 4–3 compares male and female acquisition of sex roles and one author's view of the source of influence. Note that teachers, peers, the media, and books are viewed as increasingly important as the child matures. Parents should recognize their influence on the child's environment. (See Chapter 5 for examples of learning strategies in this area.)

Competition. Competition has been viewed as a difficult arena for women. In fact women have been described as noncompetitive and lacking achievement motivation. Horner (1970) found anxiety in women in competition and described this as "fear of success." She concluded that women anticipate negative consequences if they are successful. These negative consequences are a fear of social rejection and loss of femininity (Horner, 1974).

There have been questions raised about whether "fear of success" exists. The data by Horner (1970) seem to conclude that there is something wrong with women that needs to be corrected. However, Sassen (1980) reinterpreted Horner's data and concluded that because Horner found success anxiety only when one person's success was at the expense of another's failure, this was a heightened perception of the "other side" of competitive success. That is, women appreciate the great emotional cost at which success is achieved through competition. They view something "rotten in the system" when only one person can achieve. Women also have a broader view of success and do not see success in only one sphere, i.e., work, corporate success. Women's sensitivity to others' needs and losses could be beneficial, productive, and might be appropriate for a variety of functions and positions in the work world. Women's differences may be a strength as opposed to a limitation.

For women who choose to succeed in male dominated professions (business, corporate structure), there is a need for assistance. Baumrind (1972) suggests the following to assist girls in coping more effectively with competition. It is not that girls need a different kind of preparation for competition than boys, but more conscious attention is required because girls are less likely to be assisted in the acquisition of such skills by prevailing social pressures (Williams, 1977, p. 189).

The following have been identified to encourage competition and the ability of girls to compete:

- A secure emotional base with a warm, nurturant parent who permits exploration, encourages independent action, and is not *too* protective (Hoffman, 1972)
- Encouragement to take risks and extend themselves so as to develop a sense of themselves and their abilities (Hoffman, 1972).

TABLE 4–3. SCHEMATIC REPRESENTATION OF MODEL

Level of Sex Role	Stage	Central Acquisition Tasks		Source of Influence (in order of importance)
		Females	*Males*	
Level I. Learning of appropriate child sex roles	Infancy (0–2 years)	1. Discrimination of males and females 2. Correct categorization of self	1. Same 2. Same	1. Parents 2. Siblings 3. Other adults (e.g., grandparents)
	Preschool (2–6 years)	1. Learning content of sex roles 2. Acquiring gender constancy	1. Same, but more stringent 2. Same	1. Parents and nursery teachers 2. Siblings 3. Peers 4. Media
	Grade school (6–12 years)	1. Elaboration of child sex-role content 2. Development of strong same-sex friendships	1. Same 2. Same	1. Same-sex peers 2. Television 3. Books 4. Teachers 5. Parents
Level II. Preparation for adult sex roles	Early adolescence (12–15 years)	1. Adjusting to menstruation 2. Adjusting to sexual body changes (primary and secondary) 3. Adjusting to sexual feelings 4. Concern with physical attractiveness	1. Adjusting to ability to ejaculate (early maturing) 2. Same for early-maturing boys; less intense 3. Same for early-maturing boys; more intense 4. Less concern	1. Biological factors 2. Same-sex peers 3. Television 4. Books 5. Teachers 6. Parents

Level III. Development of adult sex roles			
Late adolescence (15–19 years)	1. Dating 2. Concern with physical attractiveness 3. Adjusting to sexual behavior 4. Courtship (for some) 5. Decreased academic interest 6. Conflicts about combining vocation with marriage	1. Same 2. Less concern 3. Same 4. Same 5. Increased academic interest 6. Development of vocational interests—no conflict	1. Peers (same- and opposite-sex) 2. Media 3. Parents
Young adulthood (20–35 years)	1. Finding marriage partner 2. Establishing marriage relationship 3. Pursuing occupation (some) 4. Pregnancy 5. Childbirth 6. Breast-feeding (some) 7. Child care (primary responsibility)	1. Same 2. Same 3. Pursuing occupation (all) 4. Fathering 5. — 6. — 7. Child care (secondary responsibility)	1. Peers 2. Spouse 3. Same-sex parent
Middle adulthood (35–50 years)	1. Developing and/or reevaluating marriage relationship 2. Adjusting to children's leaving home (more intense) 3. Adjusting to feelings of loss of youth 4. Developing vocational interests if not done previously	1. Same 2. Same, less intense 3. Same 4. Contemplation of career change	1. Spouse 2. Peers 3. Media
Late adulthood	1. Adjusting to menopause 2. Adjusting to one's own and/or spouse's retirement 3. Adjusting to aging 4. Grandparenting	1. Adjusting to declining sexual potency 2. Adjusting to retirement 3. Same 4. Same	1. Spouse 2. Peers 3. Children 4. Media

(Source: Kopp, C. Becoming female: Perspectives on development. New York: Plenum Press, 1979, pp. 10–11, by permission.)

- Parents who respect the child's personhood and expect competent, autonomous behavior (Baumrind, 1972).
- Opportunities for girls to compete in sports and other contests and win and lose gracefully
- Teaching girls to be assertive in defense of their own persons and rights as individuals
- Socializing girls to assert their individuality and to be independent of pressures either to conform or to rebel

It should be recognized that the skills such as "seeing the other side of competition," viewing success in interpersonal relationships as well as other spheres of life, and attending to others' views and needs are valuable. These skills are more often in the women's domain. Should efforts be made to point up the positiveness of these differing perspectives opposed to saying girls/women cannot deal with competition?

An example of how to teach parents about their child's response to competition follows. A description of boys and girls playing could be shared with parents. These situations would describe conflict and competition. The strengths of approaches to resolving conflict and being competitive could be listed. Questions could be raised as to whether the methods are "female or male" or merely how each sex is socialized and rewarded. Discussion can then be held as to how each sex can be helped to compete in a variety of ways without feeling inadequate or inappropriate.

Sexual Exploration. Children's behavior in examining their sexual anatomy has posed problems for many parents. Explaining reproduction and the role of sex in reproduction has overwhelmed many parents. Yet today parents feel obligated to "handle" this area in ways that promote a healthy attitude toward sex. What are the best ways to approach the topic and allow the child to feel positive about sexual anatomy? A review of several authors on childhood sex education is essential. Several excellent books exist to explain sex and reproduction to children. Parents need help to teach their children in ways that are comfortable for them and their value system. Any teaching session on parenting should include content related to sexual exploration and how to teach about reproduction and intercourse.

Because society still perpetuates negative views about female sexual anatomy and functioning and defines female anatomy as "second class," female children need special emphasis to incorporate positive attitudes toward their reproductive anatomy and sexual functioning. Also, the female internal (versus external) reproductive, sexual structures can foster misunderstanding if special efforts are not made to educate female children about their uniqueness. (See Chapter 6 for a more complete discussion of the special needs regarding female sexuality.)

Responsibility for Own Health. One of the goals proposed for female health is participation with health care providers to maintain and restore health. Ideally, growing up with a sense of responsibility for her own health and taking age-appropriate actions to participate in planning for health at an early age will facilitate a lifelong involvement. For example, the young child could collect data about body functions and parameters of health and assume responsibility for good nutrition and maintaining a healthy life-style. In addition to teaching about what is healthy, health education programs in schools could include responsibility for health and participation with health care providers. Creating experiences with health care providers that are positive would also create a better view of these individuals and may encourage a lifelong commitment to seek the appropriate provider for health promotion or illness care.

Major Health Problems. Major health problems vary according to developmental stages. Thus examining the most common health problems for children will assist the reader to anticipate educational needs for health prevention, promotion, and recovery. This section highlights major health problems of children. Table 4–4 lists these problems more specifically. Accidents, homicide, and sexual abuse are major health problems of children. These problems need educational approaches that allow widespread recognition that these problems exist. Also the resources available to assist parents and children to avoid and/or cope with these problems should be readily known.

An understanding of the child's development is critical in assisting parents to create a safe environment to avoid accidents and decrease violence and abuse. It would be excellent if a massive health education program could be proposed that would allow parents greater understanding of children's needs and the complexities of being parents. There would be many who would question whether education is enough. Others would question whether the cost of such education is worth the potential impact on childhood safety and mental health. It is interesting to speculate on how current financial resources can be redirected and used to assist families to interact in positive ways so as to decrease the need for psychiatric treatment or police protection for family violence.

The remaining health problems of children, e.g., congenital anomalies, leukemia, and cardiovascular illness (Table 4–1), require specific educational effort to assist parents and children to cope with the disease, understand current medical intervention, and avoid negative effects on the child's physical and mental development. A variety of programs and individual teaching sessions are available in increasing numbers across the country. Pediatrics as a medical specialty and nursing have tried to incorporate child development and family needs into illness care and patient education. Such approaches need to be maintained and evaluated for impact and effectiveness. Because illness impacts on self-image, identity, and competence, all of these educational sessions need to consider the impact that illness has on female development. Illness that interferes with selected activities and independence can be especially threatening. Specific recommendations for educational approaches for childhood illness are beyond the scope of this text but are identified for completeness from a developmental perspective. The literature in pediatrics is available for those who work with children or whose female clients request help for their children. Chapter 10 describes special educational needs for handicapped women. It demonstrates the need for education to overcome the negative experience of being handicapped. If preventive intervention and education were available to handicapped or ill children, possibly less intervention would be needed when these children become adults.

Adolescence

Adolescence has been identified as a critical time for special educational approaches related to physical development, sexual response/activity, potential for pregnancy, and assistance with career development. Various approaches to these topics have been tried. Controversy exists as to what is the best educational approach and who (schools, parents, health care providers, parents) should teach adolescents about these topics. These issues are debated elsewhere and should be examined carefully with a complete understanding of adolescent development prior to providing health education to adolescents. Chapter 16 discusses an educational approach for adolescents who are pregnant. The focus of this section is to *highlight critical content* needed for female adolescents.

TABLE 4–4. WOMEN'S HEALTH EDUCATION DEVELOPMENTAL PERSPECTIVE: ADOLESCENCE

Critical Content	Educational Goals	Methodology
Developmental		
Body image/female body changes Secondary sexual characteristics Vaginal changes, secretions Menstrual changes	The adolescent can anticipate changes in the female body. The adolescent views her body changes positively and appreciates her uniqueness without comparing these changes to an unrealistic ideal. Recognizes natural menstrual changes, i.e., cyclic changes in body, emotional response, sexual stimulation and can compare these to her unique response. Defines the need for contraceptives and makes appropriate decisions for self, re: contraceptive use.	Structured separate classes for adolescents and parents regarding changes in body. Well developed library regarding physical in schools and religious institutions (age specific). Audiovisual material available for school and home viewing.
Sexual needs versus need for intimacy	Comprehends the normalcy of the female sexual drive and makes her own age and value appropriate decisions regarding sexual activity. Demonstrates a sense of self-worth and age appropriate decisions regarding sexual activity, avoidance of unwanted pregnancy, veneral disease, etc. Is able to describe the need for intimacy and how it relates to sexual activity. Can define her own goals/needs for intimacy and discuss how these goals/needs do or do not conflict with her own need for identity and achievement.	Formal and informal sex education classes for adolescents by health care agencies, school and religious groups. Classes for parents of adolescents regarding sexuality and current adolescent attitudes and activity, re: sexuality.
Choice of life patterns	Is able to identify various adult roles and responsibilities and realistically describe the activities needed to accomplish these goals. Recognizes the advantages/disadvantages that her own culture places on being female in selecting these roles/responsibilities. Can discuss the "choice" of being a mother from her own, her family's, her culture, and her socioeconomic point of view. Has established tentative life style goals for the immediate (1–5 yr) future that incorporate her individuality, her femaleness, her abilities and the realities of her financial and support structure.	Classes and experitial opportunities to view females in a variety of roles. Community programs for hiring adolescents within their area of interest. Incorporate decision-making regarding realities and when to be a parent in family-life courses in schools, religious and community agencies.

Health Promotion

Assumption of responsibility for own health	Recognizes her responsibility for her current and future health. Initiates health screening and illness care with minimal adult guidance. Can recognize deviations from normal regarding menstrual, breast, and mental outlook changes. Changes life style, health habits, nutritional intake for more positive health when needed. Can identify the major health risks to female adolescents today and her own unique health risks.	Establish adolescent clinics that allow increasing self-responsibility for health. Incorporate criteria for deciding when to seek medical or self-care information in health courses.

Health Concerns for Female Adolescents

Menstrual cycle irregularity/ dysmenorrhea Vaginitis Veneral disease Contraceptive problems Nutritional problems	Can identify illness versus deviations within normal. Appropriately selects need for health care provider versus alteration in health habits and self/parental care. Takes preventive measures when made known by parents/health care providers.	Incorporate these health problems into health education courses in schools, health clinics. Offer parents health-related courses in family practice, HMO's and community colleges.

Major Health Problems

Motor vehicle accidents Suicide Homicide Pregnancy/complications of Substance abuse Neoplasms	Recognizes the health risks for adolescents in her age and ethnic group. Can describe her own risks based on genetic, environmental and life-style circumstances.	Offer classes for adolescents and their parents related to specific health problems based on risk and occurrence.

(Source: The critical content was developed using Martin, L. L. Health care of women, New York: J. B. Lippincott Co., 1978, pp. 1–28; Fogel, C. I. & Woods, N. F. Health care of women, a nursing perspective, St. Louis, Mo.: C. V. Mosby, 1981, pp. 3–26; Williams, J. Psychology of women: Behavior in a biosocial context, New York: W. W. Norton, 1977. The educational goals and methodology are the author's.)

Body Changes, Sexual Activity, and Intimacy. All female adolescents do not have a positive view of their physical development and sexual anatomy. The changing physical characteristics of the female are excellent motivators for learning about the body, body functions, and related health risks and habits. The process by which this content is taught also has a potential to establish positive attitudes regarding female anatomy and physiology. Because most of the female anatomy is internal, efforts to assist female adolescents to understand their vagina, cervix, ovaries, and newly functioning hormonal system are needed. Creating learning experiences that provide both facts and a positive view of female anatomy, sexual response, and reproduction is complex because of the nature of the subject. Thus, special approaches are needed.

Adolescents have stated that they are taught about the "plumbing" but not the emotions and feelings connected with sexual response, hormonal changes, and body image changes. It is continually surprising that many adolescents (as well as adult women) do not understand the mood changes connected with the menstrual cycle or the physical changes associated with sexual stimulation. Incorporating feelings and methods to respond to these feelings in health education is critical. Several authorities on sex education for adolescents conclude that sex education programs that do not effectively deal with sexual morality, tenderness, intimacy, sharing, cooperativeness, personal attachment, and love can make "emotional cripples" of adolescents and encourage "meaningless sex" and sexual promiscuity (Hoyman, 1974; Reiss, 1968). Mary Calderone (Hoyman, 1974) suggests incorporating personal responsibility and allowing adolescents to come to their own conclusions about what is appropriate sexual activity for themselves. Approaching sex education from this perspective seems ideal, but is not easy to accomplish. Adding values and moral discussions, even when allowing for a variety of opinions and views, can lead to misinterpretation by parents and school and community authorities. Thus, preplanning and careful selection of teachers and open communication becomes essential.

Sorenson (1973) found that 52 percent of American adolescents, ages 13 to 19, reported having engaged in sexual intercourse. There were adolescents who were "sexual monogamists" and others who were "sexual adventurers." Most (87 percent) of these adolescents reported having their "heads pretty well together" as far as sex was concerned. These adolescents were more interested in learning about themselves, being independent, and preparing themselves to accomplish useful work, rather than learning about sex per se. These findings support the need to focus sex education on feelings, relationships, responsibility, and the adolescents' value system versus *bits and pieces* regarding sex, pregnancy, and venereal disease.

The need for *intimacy* increases in adolescence (Conger, 1975). Establishing intimate relationships is difficult for the adolescent because self-disclosure is needed for intimacy. The adolescent, fearful of rejection and not fully knowledgeable about herself, may turn away from opportunities of intimacy. Discussing this important need seems critical so that adolescents can recognize a basic human need and constructively learn to establish intimate relationships. In the past (perhaps the present), women have been asked to establish intimate relationships prior to full identity. Some authorities (Sangiuliano, 1980; Scarf, 1980) on female development state that women establish identity sometime in the middle years. In the past, women moved from their parents' home to marriage and, according to Erikson (1965), developed their identity through the men they married. Such a progression forced intimacy prior to identity leaving full development of self-identity to the 40-year-old time period. Many of today's women delay intimacy until identity is more fully developed. Recognizing these competing needs and the complexities of establishing both identity and intimacy is increasingly important for today's adolescent faced with more choices, opportunities, and life-styles.

Choices for Life Patterns. The opportunities for career choices and life-styles currently available to today's female adolescents were not available to many adolescents' mothers. Therefore, discussions regarding careers and their impact on motherhood and marriage are important. The availability of role models who have chosen the career path or family style the adolescent prefers is important. Academic counselors may provide information regarding the demands of a career, but how to incorporate these demands into society's expectation of women is also needed. Also, the adolescent's own values regarding life-style, career, and personal relationships should be considered. "You can be what you want to be," is the goal of education around choice of life patterns. High schools, colleges, and religious and community agencies could incorporate learning opportunities to explore the possibilities and realities of career and life-style choices. The conflicts created for female adolescents with today's multiple choices must be recognized.

Responsibility for Own Health. Opportunities for adolescents to take increasing responsibility for their own health is important to future adult responsibility. Building on childhood experiences and allowing age-appropriate responsibility for health provides challenges to health care institutions and schools. Availability of health services and their responsiveness to adolescent involvement in care may be one of the most critical components in future preventive health care. Speculation regarding what would be comprehensive is complex, but needs to be contemplated and planned. How might current health care facilities be restructured? Should comprehensive health care be available in schools so adolescents can make their own decisions and choices regarding health care? Should special clinics for adolescents be developed in greater numbers? If future female health is to be improved, new innovative approaches need to be developed.

Health Concerns of Adolescents. The health concerns of adolescents (Table 4–4) are centered around gynecological and nutritional problems. If adequate information regarding menstrual changes, vaginitis, venereal disease, and contraception were readily available, focus could be placed on promotion of optimum health. Adolescents need and want information regarding nutrition, how to cope with stress, and establish healthy life-styles.

Health Risks. The major health risks for adolescents, i.e., motor vehicle accidents, suicide, homicide, pregnancy and its complications, and substance abuse (Table 4–2), center around life-style and destructive behaviors. These data support the stance that health education that emphasizes ability to cope with life, the stresses of being an adolescent, and how to handle intimate relationships is needed. Teaching coping strategies may be as important as presenting facts about health risks. Courses, programs, and discussions for parents of today's adolescents are also needed if positive mental, developmental, and physical health are to be maintained. Parents and adolescents alike need opportunities to discuss the complexities of life. Should the schools, religious institutions, community agencies, or parents themselves provide this type of education? All of these resources are needed to provide comprehensive health education for today's adolescents.

Neoplasms constitute the major health hazard for adolescents not imposed by life-style, risk, or psychological stress. Thus, special programs and health care resources for adolescents who must cope with cancer need to be established. Not only must knowledge regarding the disease process and treatment modality be available, but content must be provided relating to coping with the stress of illness and death. The film *Brian's Song,* about a male athlete coping with cancer, is excellent in stimulating discussion regarding family relationships, needs, friendships, male–female interactions, and achievement needs when confronted with a life-threatening illness. Efforts to discuss how differences might have existed if the cancer victim was a woman might be instructive and assist in understanding the complexities of being female. For example, how would the loss of a leg differentially affect the woman? How might the opportunities to achieve through physical feats vary? Would disfigurement caused by illness and drugs be experienced differently?

Young Adulthood

Today, the lengthy preparation for adulthood has established a period of young adulthood. This period is characterized as one in which the youth is "kept in psychological limbo waiting at the door of adulthood" (Allman & Jaffe, 1977, p. 85). This period exists because of changing life-styles, confusion over career choices, instability of the environment, and an inordinate length of time in the educational process for many careers. Also, the freedom to establish intimate or live-in relationships without formal commitment and excessive pressure to become parents can allow more time before full adulthood. The young adult faces questions of commitment, identity, and self-definition.

Identity Versus Intimacy. The major developmental themes begun in adolescence demand more attention and focus for individuals in this age group. The struggle to attain a sense of identity and the development of intimate relationships with people outside the family are crucial and are emphasized by society's expectations for women. Changing values, choices, and opportunities may conflict with past socialization and pose special educational and counseling needs. The desire to achieve in careers and devote some of their life to motherhood poses dilemmas. The close of the safe childbearing period poses a "time crunch" for many women. Young, adult women need information, role models, a clear sense of self, and some "tools" to make appropriate, self-satisfying decisions. Career choices and the resultant achievement orientation conflict with what society has defined as feminine. Critical decisions for life require well developed decision-making skills and knowledge of what the choices mean. Health care providers need to recognize these developmental tasks and how they may impact health educational needs such as contraceptive choices, prenatal care, and gynecological problems.

Preparing for Life Work and Adult Roles. Over 50 percent of today's women over 16 are employed (Marieskind, 1980, p. 162). Females make up 47 percent of the work force (Marieskind, 1980) and thus preparation for work becomes an important focus. Young women and their future partners need accurate information concerning the impact of working mothers on children, male and female relationships, and the woman herself. Good sources for facts and figures include Feinstein (1979), Fogarty, Rapport, and Rapoport (1971), and Solomon (1978). These volumes suggest the diversity and involvement of women in today's work force. (See Chapter 5 for learning exercises related to women and work.)

Table 4-3 depicts the differences and similarities in sex role acquisition for young adult men and women. Note that these tasks parallel except for degree of involvement in child care and the emphasis on career by all men and only some women. Regardless of whether both partners work, child care is the primary responsibility of the woman. At this age, peers and one's spouse become important sources for reinforcement of sex role acquisition. These individuals are important sources to assist in learning and to be educated about possible alternative roles.

Establishing a Family. There have been numerous types of programs, courses, and literature available on childbearing. Incorporating young adult development into these programs would enhance the factual aspects presented relating to pregnancy, childbirth, and parenting. Opportunities to discuss a decision regarding choice of parenting is important as couples choose to be childless, redefine the number of children that is desirable, and lead alternate life-styles that incorporate nonbiological children and homosexual relationships. Education for nontraditional families is needed to assist couples to effectively live the life-style chosen, especially if this counters prevailing norms or past socialization and values. The traditional prenatal education course is limited and now viewed as only a part of the education needed for reproduction and parenting.

Health Concerns. The young adult woman's health concerns center around gynecological problems (Table 4–5). In addition, pregnancy is a major reason this age group seeks health care. This places a responsibility for health education on obstetrical–gynecological specialists. Other health concerns may not get addressed and thus can be overlooked if the focus is only on reproductive health. Questions arise as to whether general health teaching concerning such topics as nutrition, sexual relationships, and depression should be provided by obstetrical–gynecological specialists. Nurses and nurse midwives have insisted on incorporating this teaching into their care. Such teaching increases the time needed with the health care provider, decreasing the income of the individual in many instances. Some opportunity to provide group education is usually a good approach to counter the high costs of individual instruction.

Efforts to enhance the woman's ability to assess her need for professional care versus self-help, support groups, or educational courses is critical. The section on menstruation describes how and what to teach regarding menstruation. This is one health concern where the ability to recognize deviations from normal, use self-help as needed, and go to professional sources at the appropriate time is critical. This information can be passed on to daughters and family members. Future health behaviors can thus be impacted.

Major Health Risks. One major area of health problems for young adult women is complications of pregnancy and abortions (Table 4–5). When a woman's pregnancy is at risk, additional stresses occur and the experience of birth and reproduction can be similar to having an illness. Technological interventions used for high-risk pregnancies can decrease participation and family involvement if efforts are not made to emphasize the human experience. Special educational approaches are therefore needed for the woman whose pregnancy is at risk. For example, educational approaches have been demonstrated to decrease the incidence of preterm labor (Creasy et al., 1980). In a multiple site study it was demonstrated that teaching women to be more in touch with subtle changes in uterine contractions, to monitor their activity and rest patterns, and to come to health providers at the earliest sign of labor allowed intervention and decreased preterm delivery (Creasy et al., 1980). The education needed for diabetic pregnant women and women undergoing ceseren section births are described in Chapters 16 and 18. These chapters demonstrate the large amount of details needed by women whose pregnancies are complicated.

Another area of major health problems for young adult women includes accidents, violence, and suicide. Safety education and education around family violence have not always been part of health care providers' responsibility. However, safety education regarding use of car seats and driving a car posthospitalization and use of medications is now seen as an educational responsibility for nurses discharging patients from hospitals.

TABLE 4–5. WOMEN'S HEALTH EDUCATION DEVELOPMENTAL PERSPECTIVE: YOUNG ADULTHOOD

Critical Content	Educational Goals	Methodology
Development	The Female Young Adult:	
Developing identity versus intimacy	Demonstrates a strong sense of self-identity and estabilishes satisfying mutually supportive intimate sexual and non-sexual relationships.	Assessment of female identity and satisfaction with roles and relationships incorporated into health assessments.
	Recognizes her female identity and how it is consistent/inconsistent with cultural and social norms of her current environment.	Support and self-help groups available for young women in community, higher education, work environment, and health clinics.
Preparing for and/or implementing life work	Chooses life work based on abilities and preferences versus female expectations and/or past/current norms.	Career counseling and support groups for females at the entry level.
	Recognizes the potential for primary, financial, and educational responsibility for self and children.	
	Discusses realistic, data-based information, re: impact of working mothers on children's well-being.	Financial planning and management for women offered.
	Relates this to her own life circumstances, preferences and values.	
	Makes choices, re: career/work versus family, a combination or a family, delayed career/work.	Support groups available to assist in individual decisions about career and/or family.
Establishing family (if desired)	Appropriately selects contraceptives based on individual preference, risks, availability and plans for parenthood.	Prepregnancy classes and individual instruction by health care providers, re: factors involved in decision making.
	Plans children, re: spacing, adequate personal and financial support.	
	Studies the role and responsibility of parenthood, assessing her own and her partner's readiness for the role.	
	Can relate current knowledge, re: what life-style habits result in positive pregnancy outcome.	
	Can identify factors in her own health and her lifestyle that may compromise a healthy outcome for self and baby.	A variety of pregnancy and early pregnancy related classes for choice.
	When pregnant, changes life-style/health habits for benefit of healthy outcome, finds alternative activities/behavior to satisfy own needs/desires.	
	Parents female children according to previous educational goals without sacrificing own needs.	Readily accessible health care providers to answer questions regarding early parenting experiences.
	Assumes or shares responsibility with significant others for appropriate health screening and care of children.	Library holdings regarding parenting, child development, etc.

Health Concerns		
Health Concerns (Young adult women seek health care) Routine exams, screening, pap smears Pregnancy Vaginitis Urinary tract infections Menstrual problems Anemia Nutritional disorders Depression Sexual and relationships difficulties	Assumes responsibility for appropriate individualized risk oriented health screening. Can determine self-care versus medical care needs through self screening (by breast exam, vaginal or cervical changes). Implements self-care and health care interventions for minor health problems. Seeks illness care when appropriate. Seeks learning and/or counseling/therapy when sexual or relationship problems occur. Seeks preferred method (self-study, classes, reading) to obtain critical content in prenatal education when pregnant.	Increase time available for women at health clinics and private physicians' offices for health teaching. Offer general health teaching in OB/GYN services. Establish group education to teach self-screening and appropriate choice of health care resource.
Major Health Risks Motor vehicle accidents Suicide Homicide Neoplasms Complications of pregnancy and abortion Vascular disease of the CNS Pneumonia Chronic diseases Diabetes Cirrhosis Hypertension	Reassesses individual needs and responsibility for contraceptives based on current life circumstances, future plans and new contraceptive technology. Is able to increasingly assess their own mental health status, seeking professional or personal support assistance as appropriate and available. Relates changes in female roles, expectations of females to her own health and sense of worth. If major illness occurs, seeks appropriate care, accepts assistance during illness and takes positive steps to recovery.	Special classes, instruction for high-risk pregnancy needed. Special classes and support groups for individual problems.

(Source: The critical content was developed using Martin, L. L. Health care of women, New York: J. B. Lippincott Co., 1978, pp. 1–28; Fogel, C. I., & Woods, N. F. Health care of women, a nursing perspective, St. Louis, Mo.: C. V. Mosby, 1981, pp. 3–26; Williams, J. Psychology of women: Behavior in a biosocial context, New York: W. W. Norton, 1977. The educational goals and methodology are the author's.)

Perhaps new insights in health professionals' responsibility for accident prevention for the young adult will materialize.

Chapter 26 discusses education to decrease women's tolerance of physical and psychological abuse. Proposals in Chapter 26 for prevention of victimization are intriguing. Incorporating a positive sense of self-worth in women may have the potential to assist women to take steps to improve their circumstances. Early recognition of depression through appropriate education and referral is needed to decrease suicides, a health risk for this age group. The section on depression in Chapter 26 describes how to incorporate this content into health education.

The remaining health risks for young adult women, i.e., neoplasms, vascular disease, pneumonia, and selected chronic disease (Table 4–5), clearly need preventive educational strategies as well as specific education once the disease is manifested. Such educational information is beyond the scope of this text. However, the chapter on life stress and change (Chapter 7) provides ideas and methodologies to assist women to minimize stress.

Middle Years

The health needs of middle-year women are getting much more emphasis. This age group's negative stereotypes are also being challenged and new opportunities and roles are being requested and made available. Chapter 14 identifies major psychosocial needs and health concerns of this age group. This section is therefore brief. Table 4–6 includes critical content, educational goals, and methodologies for women between ages 30 and 50 years.

Developmental Tasks. Important developmental tasks for the middle-year woman are to reevaluate female roles and responsibility and establish goals for the future. These tasks confront men, but are particularly challenging for today's middle-year women because the definition of being female has changed so drastically and is sometimes in conflict with the definition women accepted when they were growing up. Reexamining past roles and becoming aware of new possibilities can consume a large amount of time and can be productive for women's future.

The physical and emotional meaning of menopause is also of primary focus. Myths and stereotypes abound. It is necessary to assist women to recognize the reality of these changes for themselves. The medical profession has at times emphasized the negative. Many women cope with menopause without major problems or negative attitudes. These women's experiences and effective self-help measures need to be shared and used to help other women. Group approaches are especially helpful in these areas. It is clear that educational strategies will have to counter negative attitudes and misinformation to have a "high dosage for the middle-year woman."

Health Concerns and Risks. The health concerns of the middle years center around menstrual problems, thereby bringing women to the gynecological specialist. Other problems, i.e., depression and sexual functioning, are also frequently brought to the gynecological health provider. Thus, education about these conditions needs to be available.

Major causes of death for women between 30 and 50 years of age are summarized in Table 4–6. Some of these conditions are exacerbated because of self-destructive health habits. The educational approach may be to suggest new ways to cope with stress. Once illness has occurred, the woman needs to be helped to incorporate behaviors that will minimize the disease process while allowing quality of life to continue. The chapters on gynecological surgery (Chapter 21) and breast cancer (Chapter 22) describe methods to allow women to cope with the surgical intervention effectively and to minimize impact of the disease on life postsurgery. Many of the suggestions in these chapters are applicable to other surgical interventions this age group may encounter. The sensitive nature of surgery on the breasts and reproductive organs is an added problem for women. Special educational strategies are needed to assist women to confront these sensitivities. Many women who have had help and support describe growth in understanding themselves as women and human beings postbreast or major gynecological surgery.

Late Adulthood and Advancing Years

Developmental Tasks. The developmental tasks that seem to be especially important for women in the 50- to 60-year age group are establishing generativity and living with loss. A reflection on what it has been to be a woman is also instructive. The perspective of a 60-year-old woman can also be instructive to younger women. For the woman beyond 60, maintaining the quality of life while coping with the effects of aging and illness is a major task (Tables 4–7 and 4–8). The health care professional confronts women in circumstances where health is already compromised, thus educational strategies may tend to be focused on the disease, forgetting developmental needs. Recognizing that elderly women are still developing is essential to planning education. Providing opportunities for family and support person involvement is critical. The chapter on education (Chapter 15) for the elderly woman discusses the effects of aging on learning and suggests content and approaches to learning for this age group.

Health Concerns and Risks. The health concerns for women in the 50- to 60-year age group are similar to the middle-year group (Table 4–7). The health concerns of the over 60-year age group (Table 4–8) include loss of hearing, visual acuity, and mental astuteness (Martin, 1978). Other health problems may be increased because of aging and its influence on maintaining self-care activities. The chance of becoming ill with age increases and many women must cope with decreasing independence for long periods of time or for the remainder of their life. The impact such changes have on self-concept and meeting affiliative needs must be considered. Assisting women to incorporate medical intervention without serious compromise of personal needs and goals is a challenge. Counteracting society's negative view of aging and of elderly women is also needed and must be considered when planning teaching sessions. Education for preparation of death is also a right of individuals in this age group.

Summary

We have come full cycle describing a developmental approach to health education for women. Hopefully, this approach has assisted the reader to recognize the comprehensive nature of the educational needs of women. Obviously our current health clinics, hospitals, and community agencies could not offer every woman the total educational package she needs. But, health care professionals can do more than provide information regarding a single complaint. Referral patterns are needed within agencies and clinics for education in each area.

A list of community and educational resources available needs to be offered to women. Cross-specialty consultation and education could be established within hospitals and comprehensive ambulatory clinics. The public educational system could be requested to establish courses, programs, and counseling services around special needs of

TABLE 4–6. WOMEN'S HEALTH EDUCATION DEVELOPMENTAL PERSPECTIVE: MIDDLE YEARS (30 TO 50)

Critical Content	Educational Goals	Methodology
Reevaluation of past female roles and responsibility, establishing goals for the future	The Middle-Year Woman: Can identify satisfaction with past and present roles in light of current development and society's expectation. Takes new/different steps to meet personal and career goals as preferred.	Group and individual sessions for middle years women in community, religious, education and health care settings.
	Establishes appropriate life support systems for changes in life circumstance (loss of children, widowhood, divorce, new career, etc.)	Career counseling and support groups.
Confrontation of physical and emotional meaning of menopause	Discusses normal/frequently experienced menopausal changes.	Groups and individual educational sessions on menopause.
	Reevaluates contraceptive for current circumstances.	Contraceptive materials prepared for the middle-aged woman.
Health Concerns		
Irregularity of menses	Recognizes seriousness of abnormal gyn symptoms and seeks health care.	Individual teaching, re: individual health risks by care provider.
Abnormal bleeding	Institutes life-style/health habit changes based on individual risk/health assessment.	
Physical or emotional symptoms, re: menopause	Incorporates a positive image of the aging female regardless of stereotypes and negative media images.	Health education sessions/courses regarding nutrition, activity, life-style for health and fitness.

Pelvic relaxation Obesity Hypertension Diabetes Anemia Depression Sexual changes, functioning and desires	Uses available health care resources appropriately.	Information available, re: choice of health facility provider.
Major Causes of Death Malignant neoplasms Arteriosclerotic heart disease Suicide Cirrhosis Pneumonia Motor vehicle accidents Hypertensive heart disease	Engages in minimal self-destructive health habits. Given a life-threatening illness for self/significant others, seeks appropriate personal and/or health professional support systems.	Support/educational groups for life crises and illness. Availability of counseling services.

(Source: The critical content was developed using Martin, L. L. Health care of women, New York: J. B. Lippincott Co., 1978, pp. 1–28; Fogel, C. I. & Woods, N. F. Health care of women, a nursing perspective, St. Louis, Mo.: C. V. Mosby, 1981, pp. 3–26; Williams, J. Psychology of women: Behavior in a biosocial context, New York: W. W. Norton, 1977. The educational goals and methodology are the author's.)

TABLE 4–7. WOMEN'S HEALTH EDUCATION DEVELOPMENTAL PERSPECTIVE: LATE ADULTHOOD (50 TO 60)

Critical Content	Educational Goals	Methodology
Developmental		
Establishing generativity given life circumstance	The Woman in Late Adulthood: Finds satisfying social support system for life and health circumstance. Accepts her own responsibility for creating alternatives. Recognizes correct definition of female roles and implements past or current definition depending on "goodness of fit."	Social opportunities available. Discussion groups available for women, re: roles, aging, etc.
Living with loss	Copes with grief and loss in appropriate ways. Accepts changes resulting from aging process without negatively defining self or older females.	Grief support groups.
Health Concerns (seeks care for) Menopausal concerns Menstrual irregularities Estrogen use/nonuse Pelvic relaxation Obesity Hypertension Diabetes Anemia Depression	Maintains previously established responsibility to assess health and seeks appropriate health care interventions where illnesses are minor and require prevention. Assumes mentor, supportive role to females in significant other group related to health maintenance and promotion.	Alternatives for health care available for choice. Opportunities for women to offer help, support to younger women, children, etc.
Major Health Risks Arteriosclerotic heart disease Malignant neoplasms Vascular lesions of the CNS Cirrhosis Hypertensive heart disease Pneumonia Motor vehicle accident	Accepts sick role on temporary basis, moves into rehabilitative phase as appropriate. Complies with medical intervention without compromising personal, independent role functions.	Participatory health care available in all health care settings. Educational opportunities for chronic or long-term illness.

(Source: The critical content was developed using Martin, L. L. Health care of women, New York: J. B. Lippincott Co., 1978, pp. 1–28; Fogel, C. I., & Woods, N. F. Health care of women, a nursing perspective, St. Louis, Mo.: C. V. Mosby, 1981, pp. 3–26; Williams, J. Psychology of women: Behavior in a biosocial context, New York: W. W. Norton, 1977. The educational goals and methodology are the author's.)

TABLE 4–8. WOMEN'S HEALTH EDUCATION DEVELOPMENTAL PERSPECTIVE: ADVANCED YEARS (60 AND BEYOND)

Critical Content	Educational Goals	Methodology
Maintence of the quality of life while coping with aging	Maximizes potential for positive life in spite of aging and negative attitudes toward elderly female.	Individual or group sessions for sharing and learning about aging, potential and real loss.
	Uses past or newly developed strategies for coping with loss, loneliness, potential for death.	
Reevaluation and reflection on what it has been to be female	Can analyze society's and self's definition of femaleness and convey to the younger generation general principles of healthful living.	
	Serves as mentor to younger female family members, friends.	
Health Concerns		
Atrophic vaginitis Pelvic relaxation	Accepts and appropriately uses strategies (life changes and intervention) for coping with age related disabilities, i.e., atrophic vaginitis, osteoporosis, mobility limitation, visual and hearing impairment, etc.	Adequate time in visit to health care provider to teach about changes related to aging and methods to minimize effects.
Osteoporosis Chronic illnesses maligancies cardiovascular	Mobility retention, visual, hearing impairment, etc. Recognizes and/or seeks health care intervention for mental health alterations.	Counseling and support groups in community and elderly group residences.
Aging processes that limit quality of life in: limitations of of activity	Maintains active sexual life based on life circumstances regardless of environmental definition of female sexuality in the elderly female.	Sex education sessions (individual and/or group) available.

(continued)

107

TABLE 4–8 (cont.)

Critical Content	Educational Goals	Methodology
(arthritis, problems of back, spine, and hip) Visual activity Adequate respiratory capacity Ability to hear adequately Mental astuteness Sexual satisfaction		
Loneliness due to loss, grief	Seeks situational support systems for loss, grief.	Education, re: grieving process available.
Depression Reality of death	Prepares for death as is appropriate relevant to health/life circumstance.	
Major Health Risks		
Arterosclerotic heart disease Vascular lesions of CNS Neoplasms Hypertension of the breast Cirrhosis Pneumonia	Accepts intervention for illness care and support including changes in domicile. Responds to the reality of death in positive frame of mind.	Educational and support group sessions for family and elderly female when need residence change and/or illness.

(Source: The critical content was developed using Martin, L. L. Health care of women, New York: J. B. Lippincott Co., 1978, pp. 1–28; Fogel, C. I., & Woods, N. F., Health care of women, a nursing perspective, St. Louis, Mo.: C. V. Mosby, 1981, pp. 3–26; Williams, J. Psychology of women: Behavior in a biosocial context, New York: W. W. Norton, 1977. The educational goals and methodology are the author's.)

women that are not met within health care institutions. A comprehensive approach is needed that allows selection and choice for learning (see Methodologies in Tables 4–1 to 4–8). This will involve community planning and a commitment and a belief in health promotion versus illness care. Certainly, revamping the reimbursement system to pay for health education and reward individuals for staying healthy is necessary before a comprehensive approach can be financed.

The remainder of this chapter describes two areas of unique health education for women as examples of specific health educational needs presented from a developmental approach.

Teaching breast self-examination and menstrual cycle changes are two areas critical to health prevention in women. Because both topics are surrounded with myths and sensitivity, planned strategies to foster positive feelings toward these health strategies are needed. Suggestions concerning how to teach these topics and at what age also serve as an example of recurring topics that should be taught throughout the life cycle. As the woman progresses through the life cycle these topics take on different emphasis and need a different depth of understanding depending on how critical the topic is to a specific woman at a particular age. The specific areas described can be used to incorporate more positive attitudes of being female. These positive approaches can be aimed at the developmental level of the individual, allowing growth and increasing assumption of the responsibility of children, adolescents, and women for their own health.

Breast Self-examination: Improving Behavior

Geri LoBiondo-Wood

Much emphasis is placed on the breasts as a symbol of femininity in American society. Females incorporate these attitudes through lifelong socialization. Mass media uses the ideally proportioned woman to advertise products and sell magazines, movies, and fashions. These types of advertisements reinforce the breasts as a means of asserting one's femininity. The feminist movement has helped to deemphasize some of this publicity. Factors related to self and body image also shape a woman's perception of her breasts. During childhood, attitudes concerning the breasts are formed. During adolescence the woman copes with a number of physical changes in the contours of her breasts and body. During the childbearing years breasts become incorporated into one's body image as a sexual being and as a component of the maternal role. At the time of menopause the breasts, as other body tissues, begin to undergo atrophic changes. Threat of insult from cancer, disease, or surgery at any age potentiate a crisis in a woman's life. Thus, what is taught concerning health prevention needs to be determined by age group as well as the potential for incorporating a positive attitude toward the breasts as a component of being female. First, an overview of the risks women face of breast cancer and the factors that influence women engaging in breast self-examination are discussed. Then critical content and appropriate approaches for each developmental group are discussed.

Risks for Breast Cancer. Breast cancer is the leading cause of cancer death in women between the ages of 15 to 75 years. The best defense against cancer of the breast is early detection. Although statistics relating to other forms of cancer have improved, the statistics for breast cancer have not significantly changed in the past 25 years. Approximately 1 out of every 11 American women will develop breast cancer at some time during her life (Cancer Facts and Figures, 1981).

Risks for developing breast cancer are age-specific. Benign lesions occur primarily in premenopausal women, whereas breast cancer is most frequent in menopausal and post-menopausal women, increasing in incidence throughout the life span (Leis, 1977). Women are at greatest risk over age 50. Other risk factors are a personal or a family history of breast cancer, never having borne children, and first child after age 30. Longer survival rates of treated women have served to stabilize mortality rates over the last 50 years despite the slight increase in incidence of breast cancer.

Breast Self-examination. Breast self-examination (BSE) is one of the best means of early detection and is free and relatively easy to learn. Ninety-five percent of all lumps found in the breast are detected by women themselves (Cancer Facts and Figures, 1981). Breast self-examination is the means by which a woman can learn to recognize normal cyclic changes in her breast and to detect the early warning signs of breast cancer. The warning signs are a lump, thickening, swelling, or dimpling in the breasts; skin irritation, pain or tenderness or distortion of breast tissue; and nipple discharge, retraction, or scaling of the nipple.

A great deal of information is available on BSE and many women know the value of BSE. Yet, many women do not do it at all, do it incorrectly, or do not do it because they feel they cannot judge between abnormal and normal breast tissue (Richards, 1977). Other women hold myths that excessive touching, caressing, or bruising will cause breast cancer.

How a woman views and cares for her breast is a component of her sexual and general health care. Both sexual and general health care habits develop from early and continuing life experience, knowledge of health needs, psychosocial and sexual variables, as well as attitudes and perceptions of one's health needs.

Part of the role of the health care provider is the promotion of health through education and early detection of potential problems. Teaching the value of early detection of breast cancer needs to take a high priority in the health education of women throughout the life cycle. Breast self-examination can also be used to teach age-related and menstrual cycle changes that occur in the breast tissue. This allows the woman to place in perspective her body image and unique developmental pattern. As the normal changes are taught, the health care provider can also assess the client's attitudes toward being female and her comfort with her body and its functions. When problems, negative attitudes, or discomfort are identified, then plans for teaching–learning sessions regarding these areas can be made. Such discussions need to be held when a trust and comfort level has been established between provider and client.

Age-related Needs for Breast Self-examination. The gap between information and use of BSE information is clear. The need to narrow this gap requires strategies that facilitate early detection practices. The performance of BSE should be a lifelong health habit, yet before BSE can be effectively taught, the clients' age-related factors for various breast diseases, developmental issues, motivation, ability to learn, past experiences, and the availability of the appropriate information to adequately learn the skill needs to be assessed.

Although 8 out of 10 breast masses are noncancerous (Questions and Answers About Breast Lumps, 1981) and these benign masses are generally symptomatic of cystic hyperplasia (fibrocystic disease, chronic mastitis), fibroadenomas, interductal papillomas, and mammary duct ectasia, the incidence and type of breast disease are age-specific. Women need to be aware of the most common breast diseases for their age group. For example, cystic hyperplasia is the most common breast disease, occurring between 20 and 25 years of age. It is characterized by multiple, often bilateral firm, mobile and regular shaped lumps. The breasts are frequently tender and painful, especially just prior to the menstrual period. Fibroadenoma is a benign disease occurring between the ages of 15 to 60 years of age, with a median age of 20. It is characterized by a painless, mobile, firm, solid, well-delineated mass. These masses may be multiple and bilateral. Unlike cystic hyperplasia, fibroadenomas do not change with the menses. Interductal papillomas occur most frequently in women between ages 35 and 45 years. Usually there is no palpable tumor or mass. If one is present it is usually soft and poorly delineated from the surrounding breast tissue. The major symptom is a serosanguineous or serous nipple discharge. Mammary duct ectasia generally occurs at or near menopause. There may also be pain, itching, and redness surrounding the nipple. A mass may be soft or firm, palpable, and is usually poorly delineated.

Education regarding breast changes, BSE, and breast cancer should begin during adolescence. This education should be built on health education for the child and her parents and create a sense of responsibility for monitoring the health of her body. Also efforts to encourage positive attitudes toward the breasts as well as other female anatomy should be laid down when the female is a child so that the negative attitudes of touching or manipulating the breasts can be minimized. Then, as the breasts develop in adolescence, there will be a comfort with these changes and an attitude of assuming responsibility for BSE.

Knowledge of breast changes is important in the prepuberty and early puberty period because of the incidence of benign breast disease during adolescence. Breast lumps take on a frightening and threatening meaning at any age. This may be an especially frightening experience to the young girl. Knowledge and experience with BSE gained in earlier years will help an adolescent understand the recent changes in her breasts due to development. Later, the changes due to pregnancy, age, and menopause will be as critical.

Because adolescents are just beginning to learn at the level of abstraction, health education presented in the form of scientific rationales for action rather than imperatives and an opportunity for discussion are desirable and useful approaches (Pidgeon, 1977). Edwards (1980) found that more older women than younger women increased the frequency of BSE after instruction. Thus, special attention to adolescents actually practicing BSE may be needed.

How much a woman feels the need for information or a particular skill affects her readiness to learn. Based on the known risk factors, if a woman or adolescent does not feel that she fits any of the categories, then it may be easier to adopt a "not me" attitude about an issue that may raise anxiety.

Learning may produce a mild degree of anxiety and is a gradual process. Generally, women think that any breast lump is malignant. This may be seen as if the sole intent of BSE, the detection of a health problem rather than a health promoting behavior. Efforts to focus on the health promoting behavior and the fact that most lumps are benign should be emphasized.

Breast self-examination education should be content- as well as process-oriented. Content should stress facts and information regarding breast changes and disease. The process should stress the importance of learning and feeling comfortable knowing the normal appearance and monthly changes in one's breasts.

Sociocultural variables, such as accessibility of health care, a belief about whether or not health care is beneficial, or religious and cultural beliefs that deter one from touching sexual organs, may also affect a woman's motivation to learn. Health providers have a responsibility to assess the needs and the obstacles to BSE in the women they see. Education for BSE does not stop here. Health professionals also need to assess and meet the needs of women in the community so they know the value of BSE.

Assessment. The specific factors that require assessment before beginning a program on BSE teaching are:

1. Age, cultural background, sociocultural background, physical and psychological state of health, and ability to learn.
2. Any past learning or experience with BSE.
3. Knowledge level of breast care, breast disease, and breast cancer.
4. Interest in learning not only the skill of BSE but also interest in learning about age-related and cyclic changes of the breasts.
5. Any previous experience with breast cancer in self, family, or friends.
6. Is the woman at a teaching session by choice, i.e., a woman may join a BSE teaching session at a community center by choice, or an adolescent may be required to be in a health class.

Assessment of knowledge concerning breast cancer and its detection can be done in a variety of clinical settings. Such assessment should be part of all physical health assessments. There is not only a need for information but also a need for discussion time with the women regarding questions and concerns about breast problems and BSE.

When a woman is hospitalized for perinatal care, dilation and curettage, and other medical or surgical problems, it is appropriate to assess needs for BSE teaching. This type of teaching is aimed at preventive and holistic care.

In community settings such as senior citizens groups, women's self-help groups, school and church-related groups, health care professionals could assess and address the needs of larger groups of women. When addressing groups, a variation of the assessment process is necessary. Before the program, the health educator should speak with a contact person from the group to gather information about the group as a whole using the assessment principles. Also, when addressing a group, more time is needed for discussion of fears and questions and for demonstration and teaching of the method. When demonstration is used, a return demonstration to the practitioner is important. It has been found that women who have seen a demonstration and are allowed to return the demonstration to a health practitioner have an increased practice rate than women who just receive an explanation (Fogel & Woods, 1981).

Before beginning any teaching of BSE methods with either individuals or groups, a brief introduction to BSE and a discussion should be allowed. An example of a way to open a discussion is: "We've all heard a great deal about breast lumps and cancer. Certainly any lump found in the body is frightening. But for women breast lumps can be especially frightening. Some ideas we've heard are really myths, such as excessive touching of the breasts causes cancer. What kinds of ideas have you heard or what questions do you think about when considering learning breast self-examination?" A brief early discussion similar to the above can assist the health care provider to more effectively assess points of concern and fear, areas for teaching, and readiness for information.

Goals. The goals for BSE education are that the woman will:

1. List reasons for examining breasts monthly and state that early detection results in an increased cure rate.
2. Identify changes that may occur in breasts both monthly and as they get older.
3. Demonstrate comfort with looking at the contour of her breasts, touching them, and identifying changes.
4. Identify the areas of her breasts that are clinically unimportant (i.e., the infra-mammary ridge).
5. Demonstrate a systematic BSE of the three anatomical sites as outlined by the American Cancer Society (Figure 4–1).
6. Describe BSE as a positive behavior and integrate her information and skill with BSE into her total self-health care.
7. Demonstrate a positive attitude toward being female and a comfort level with her breasts and their functions.

Methods. A great deal of information is available on BSE and breast cancer. Information alone generally does not change behavior. A useful method for teaching BSE is with demonstration and practice. Demonstration includes learning through modeling and discussion of BSE, breast cancer, and breast care. Practice involves the learners' return demonstration of the BSE skill learned. Demonstration and practice combined with didactic information and discussion can aid the acquisition of knowledge and skill. Implementation of this method requires pictures of breasts, a model of a breast with implanted abnormalities, or the use of oneself as a model for visualization.

After the initial assessment and discussion the woman should view the step-by-step procedure of BSE. Included in this procedure should be information regarding time of menstrual cycle when the breasts should be examined. If the woman is postmenopausal, a consistent date, such as the first of the month, should be selected as the appropriate day for BSE. The specific techniques of the breast examination should be in line with the American Cancer Society's Standard Breast Examination (Byrd, 1974). After demonstration of the method, the woman should be allowed to use the breast model or her own breasts to perform the return demonstration. Finally, the woman should be allowed time for questions and concerns. Written information regarding BSE methods and information regarding breast lumps and breast cancer is available through the American Cancer Society. Written information can serve as reinforcement for visual and verbal presentation.

When teaching is achieved with a group, peer support may also be a useful adjunct. Peer support involves pairing a woman with a friend or relative so that they can remind each other to do BSE. Studies done by Edwards (1980) and Israel and Saccone (1979) show that peer support by significant others increases frequencies of health maintenance behaviors. Peer support may be especially useful when teaching in community settings and self-help groups.

Breast cancer is a highly feared disease. Early detection of breast cancer results in higher cure rates and a decreased need for radical surgery. Therefore, education on early detection and the development of positive attitudes toward BSE are an extremely high priority for learning. Once breast cancer is detected, there is another set of teaching and decision-making strategies. Chapter 23 discusses these and the role of health care providers in assisting women to select alternatives in treatment and to take steps for positive recovery. This section has stressed the health promotion component and developmental approach of BSE. The following section describes another unique area of female health

How to examine your breasts

1

In the shower:

Examine your breasts during bath or shower; hands glide easier over wet skin. Fingers flat, move gently over every part of each breast. Use right hand to examine left breast, left hand for right breast. Check for any lump, hard knot or thickening.

2

Before a mirror:

Inspect your breasts with arms at your sides. Next, raise your arms high overhead. Look for any changes in contour of each breast, a swelling, dimpling of skin or changes in the nipple.

Then, rest palms on hips and press down firmly to flex your chest muscles. Left and right breast will not exactly match—few women's breasts do.

Regular inspection shows what is normal for you and will give you confidence in your examination.

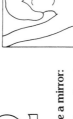

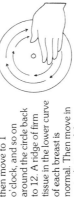

3

Lying down:

To examine your right breast, put a pillow or folded towel under your right shoulder. Place right hand behind your head—this distributes breast tissue more evenly on the chest. With left hand, fingers flat, press gently in small circular motions around an imaginary clock face. Begin at outermost top of your right breast for 12 o'clock, then move to 1 o'clock, and so on around the circle back to 12. A ridge of firm tissue in the lower curve of each breast is normal. Then move in an inch, toward the nipple, keep circling to examine *every part of your breast*, including nipple. This requires at least three more circles. Now slowly repeat procedure on your left breast with a pillow under your left shoulder and left hand behind head. Notice how your breast structure feels.

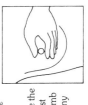

Finally, squeeze the nipple of each breast gently between thumb and index finger. Any discharge, clear or bloody, should be reported to your doctor immediately.

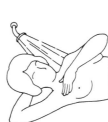

Figure 4–1. A systematic breast self-examination as outlined by the American Cancer Society. *(Source: American Cancer Society. Breast self-examination and the nurse. New York: American Cancer Society, 1976, by permission.)*

education that needs to be approached from a developmental level. Health care professionals located in various care settings can use opportunities to educate women in BSE and to explore through research methods which approaches are most useful in promoting this health prevention measure.

Menstrual Cycle Awareness

Colleen Keenan

Menstruation has many meanings for women in our culture. As a uniquely female experience, menstruation represents an important component of a woman's identity. For nearly 30 years or more of her life, the monthly menstrual event is a reminder of her reproductive potential, or paradoxically, the absence of conception. The cultural meanings of menstruation, with a myriad of symbolic roots such as the life-giving and sustaining qualities of blood as well as the concepts of taboo, contamination, and isolation have been a focal point for the cultural differentiation between men and women.

Events surrounding menstruation also provide developmental markers for critical events in a woman's life. The onset of the first menstrual period, menarche, is an event remembered by virtually every woman. As regular menstrual cycles are established, the pattern is frequently seen as an indicator of healthy functioning. When the pattern is disrupted, concerns regarding illness or the possibility of pregnancy are entertained. Whether the outcome is positive, as in the case of a desired pregnancy, or problematic as in the case of illness or unwanted pregnancy, the interruption of the normal menstrual pattern is a significant occurrence. The cessation of menses in the middle years, menopause, is the final developmental marker related to menstruation and reproductive capacity. With menopause, multiple changes in body image, self-concept role and other factors come into play.

All of these developmental events are experienced in both positive and negative modes. For example, postmenarcheal girls refer to the menses as their "friend." Menstruation has also been commonly known as the "curse." Periods are experienced as bothersome, predictable, familiar, reassuring, and in some instances painful or associated with uncomfortable symptoms. For most women, however, menstruation is a normal fact of life, incorporated into the female identity. Health education can facilitate this process and enhance self-care activities related to menstruation.

Menstrual Cycle Education

Menstrual cycle education is an ongoing process with specific content and methodologies appropriate for the different developmental age groups. From the premenarcheal girl through the woman experiencing menopause, the types of information given, the cognitive level of content, and the learning process are all variable and must be adjusted on an individual basis.

The sources of information available for menstrual cycle awareness and education are used according to the woman's preferred learning style and age appropriateness. For many women, female relatives (mothers, sisters, and in some cases daughters) and peers are an important and often primary source of information. The media (television, newspapers, magazines) can also provide information, particularly about issues related to the menstrual cycle such as the premenstrual syndrome and menopause. Popular literature abounds concerning menstrual health. Schools provide information in the classroom and through written and audiovisual materials concerning menstruation, fertility, and related issues. Self-help and other structured groups are a forum for information sharing, support, and problem solving. And finally, health care providers (nurses, physicians, and others) are a particularly rich and sought after source of information and advice about menstrual cycle matters.

The concept of self-care lends itself well to menstrual cycle awareness and is integrally connected to health education. Self-care "refers to activities that individuals personally initiate and perform on their own behalf in maintaining or enhancing life, health and well-being" (Pender, 1982, p. 150). Specific goals for menstrual cycle health education are to

1. Provide knowledge and a positive attitude about the normal menstrual cycle and its variations from menarche through menopause,
2. Promote positive self-concept and self-esteem by enhancing self-care related to the menstrual cycle, and
3. Facilitate the activation of health seeking behaviors when illness is suspected.

The process used to obtain these goals relies on

1. Assisting the client to obtain information related to her particular needs and knowledge deficits,
2. Promoting the use of information combined with her own experience in order to make decisions concerning the adoption of appropriate self-care measures,
3. Providing reinforcement of appropriate decisions that lead to higher levels of wellness and improved health behaviors, and
4. Maintaining availability of the health care provider on an as-needed basis.

Preparation for Menarche

Menarche is the culmination of several physiological events. Prior to the onset of menses between the ages of 9 and 16, many physical changes are evident. Initially, breast buds develop, followed by pubic and axillary hair. The growth spurt, which accompanies puberty, usually begins about a year before menarche and is usually almost complete by the first menstruation. Secondary sex characteristics are nearly completely developed by this time as well. Tanner (1978) provides a complete discussion of male and female pubertal changes and the reader is referred to that source for more detailed information. The physiological and endocrinal changes underlying the physical changes of puberty are complex and are thoroughly described in other sources, including Mishell and Davajan (1979).

The psychosocial changes encountered during the transition from girlhood to adolescence have been less thoroughly researched and documented in the literature. In recent years, however, several authors (Golub & Catalano, 1983; Grief & Ulman, 1982; Ruble & Brooks-Gunn, 1982; Woods, Dery, & Most, 1983) have examined the psychosocial impact of menarche. Preparation for the onset of menses appears to be a critical variable predicting future menstrual experiences and attitudes (Ruble & Brooks-Gunn, 1982). Regardless of preparation, however, menarche is frequently greeted by the adolescent with mixed feelings of excitement, sadness, fear, and embarrassment. Although preparation for menarche may adequately cover the specifics of the menstrual cycle changes and hygiene (tampons, sanitary pads, etc), other topics such as changing body image and the affective level of experience may not be fully addressed (Golub, 1983). Our culture does not provide for a formal ritualization of menarche and the symbolic rites of passage. Many families do have a quiet celebration or make some gesture marking this important transition, however.

Menstrual cycle education for the premenarcheal girl must be comprehensive, including not only hygiene and basic physiology content but also the affective content so important to paving the way toward viewing the menstrual cycle as a normal, comfortable female experience. Table 4–9 summarizes the critical content and methodologies for this age group.

Assessment. Because preadolescents process information at a concrete cognitive level, the complex topic of menstruation should be handled using basic explanations and terminology. Because of the preadolescent's difficulty in understanding abstract ideas, simple diagrams and representations of female anatomy and of the menstrual cycle calendar are most useful. In assessment of individuals in this age group, however, one must keep in mind that cognitive levels may vary. Assessment should also be based on the expressed learning needs of the individual. Questions posed by the preadolescent can also be useful guides to the most appropriate level of education.

TABLE 4–9. WOMEN'S HEALTH EDUCATION DEVELOPMENTAL PERSPECTIVE: MENARCHE

Critical Content	Objectives	Method

1. Basic anatomy and physiology
  a. Function and location of uterus, ovaries, cervix, and vagina
  b. Ovulation, fertility, contraception
  c. Range of normals for menarche, cycle length, duration, and flow
	1. The adolescent will demonstrate basic knowledge of menstrual cycle and normal reproductive function and structures	1. Parent instruction
		2. Classroom activities
		3. Supportive written materials and audiovisual aids
		4. Concrete language and images

2. Menstrual hygiene
  a. Tampons, pads
  b. Odors
  c. Toxic shock syndrome —prevention
	1. The adolescent will demonstrate comfort with the use of tampons and/or pads and appropriately apply/insert	1. Use of written/verbal instructions
		2. Discussions to alleviate manage hygiene issues

3. Recognition of deviations from normal	1. The adolescent will report suspected deviations to parent or health care provider 2. The adolescent will keep a basic chart of menstrual cycle events	1. Promote ongoing discussions about menstrual cycle with parent(s) and provider 2. Review menstrual charts, reinforcing appropriate documentation
4. Impact of personal and environmental variables (e.g., sports training, stress, nutrition)	1. The adolescent will be aware of potential variables that affect menstrual cycle function and adjusts health behaviors as appropriate	1. Review menstrual cycle charts 2. Reinforce adaptive health seeking behaviors
5. Emotional response to menarche	1. The adolescent will be able to verbalize feelings about her menstrual function 2. The adolescent will express a positive self-image related to normal female reproductive function	1. Parents and health care providers will provide an accepting environment for the adolescent to express her feelings

Learning resources for this age group are primarily parent (usually mother) and family members (older sister, female relative) as well as health education classes. Audiovisual and written materials augment these primary sources.

Goals for Education

1. Set a positive tone for long-term menstrual cycle awareness.
2. Facilitate the pre- and postmenarcheal girl's adjustment to her changing body image.
3. Provide the groundwork for initiating self-care activities related to menstrual cycle health.

Young Adulthood

Contrasted to the ambivalent feelings concerning menstruation prevalent among postmenarcheal girls, the experience of menstruation in young adulthood is generally a familiar, predictable event. The positive and negative aspects tend to be incorporated into the acceptance of feminine identity. Menstruation in this developmental phase is a reminder of fertility, or the failure to conceive. The cyclic pattern of menses is also a reassuring hallmark of health. Conversely, the disruption of the usual menstrual cycle pattern is a cue that a potential health problem may exist. The potential for pregnancy certainly is another consideration for heterosexually active women. In both instances an understanding of the normal menstrual cycle and accurate recording of dates and patterns of flow are critical in order to help identify the potential causes of cycle disruption (Table 4–10).

Age Group. Many factors have an impact on menstrual cycle patterns. The delicate feedback system of the hypothalamic–pituitary–ovarian axis can be easily disturbed by individual and environmental factors leading to menstrual cycle abnormalities. For example, obe-

TABLE 4–10. WOMENS HEALTH EDUCATION DEVELOPMENTAL PERSPECTIVE: YOUNG ADULTHOOD

Critical Content	Educational Goals	Methodology

1. Review of menstrual cycle physiology with increased depth for specific situations
  a. Contraception
  b. Fertility/infertility
	1. The woman will record menstrual data in chart format, identify deviations and seek health care provider consultation when indicated
	2. The woman will monitor, if desired, additional aspects of the menstrual cycle, such as basal temperature and cervical mucus changes
		1. Health care provider instruction
		2. Women's Health Care resources—books and pamphlets
		3. Clarification of misunderstandings
		4. Reinforcement of adaptive health seeking behaviors

2. Menstrual cycle problems
  a. Dysmenorrhea
  b. Menstrual abnormalities: dysfunctional uterine bleeding secondary amenorrhea
  c. Premenstrual Syndrome
	1. The woman will initiate self-care activities where appropriate
	2. The woman will seek health care provider intervention for identified deviations from normal
	3. In the case of the heterosexually active woman, she will consider pregnancy soon after a missed period, to seek health care early in the first trimester
		(1–4 as above)
		5. Alleviate anxiety with thorough explanations and anticipatory guidance to facilitate self-care at appropriate levels

sity, stress, and change in environmental factors can all result in secondary amenorrhea (Gold & Josimovich, 1980). In addition, several medical problems such as endocrine disorders and gynecological dysfunctions such as infection, anovulation, spontaneous pregnancy loss, and neoplasms may be responsible for abnormal bleeding patterns.

Normal Menstrual Cycle Patterns. Menstrual cycle patterns have a broad range of normal variations. The cycle length (calculated from the first day of one period to the first day of the next) is normally about 25 to 36 days. Duration of the menses usually lasts 4 to 7 days. The exact amount of menstrual flow is difficult to correlate with subjective experience. Approximately 30 to 50 cc of menstrual fluid comprise the total flow per menses. Flow is typically heaviest on the first few days and tapers until the end of the menses. It is useful to describe menstrual flow in terms of number of saturated tampons or pads used per day in order to determine abnormally light or heavy flow. The color of menses ranges from bright red to brown with heavier flow usually the brighter red. As blood pools in the vagina with decreased flow, it tends to darken. Clots may also form in the vagina from stasis, although large clots, especially accompanied by cramping, are an indication of dysfunction.

Menstrual characteristics may also vary as a result of contraceptive method. For example, oral contraceptives frequently are responsible for decreased duration and flow during menses. Many of the low estrogen dose pills also are associated with intermenstrual spotting or breakthrough bleeding. The intrauterine device (IUD) commonly causes increased menstrual flow (menorrhagia) and dysmenorrhea because the presence of a foreign body may create a state of chronic inflammation of the endometrium.

Many physical signs of a normally functioning menstrual cycle are evident and can be observed by the woman herself. In addition to the cyclic pattern of bleeding, ovulation at mid-cycle is accompanied by changes in cervical mucus and a slight (1°F) temperature elevation, as measured by daily recorded basal body temperatures (BBT). Many women are aware of a cramping or "pulling" sensation in the lower abdomen at the time of ovulation, and it is not unusual to observe a small amount of spotting mid-cycle. These changes can be used to identify the time of ovulation and are incorporated into the natural family planning method of contraception discussed in Chapter 8.

Common Menstrual Problems. The two most frequently occurring menstrual problems, dysmenorrhea and premenstrual syndrome, are highly amenable to self-care measures, with supportive interventions from the health care provider (see Tables 21–10 and 21–11).

Dysmenorrhea. Dysmenorrhea, the lower abdominal, back, and thigh pain associated with menses, occurs in greater than 50 percent of menstruating women. Usually described as a cramping sensation, dysmenorrhea is a result of uterine contractions mediated by increased levels of prostaglandins that act on the myometrium. Dysmenorrhea usually occurs during the first one to two days of the menses but may precede menstrual flow or continue throughout the period. The severity of pain ranges from barely noticeable to very intense. Associated symptoms such as nausea, light-headedness, and tremulousness are attributable to prostaglandin effects as well.

Self-care measures for dysmenorrhea include heat application to the lower back or abdomen, back and leg massage, rest, and over-the-counter analgesic and antiprostaglandin preparations such as aspirin (see Table 21–10). More severe dysmenorrhea requires consultation with the health care provider. After considering other potential causes of the pain, such as infection, endometriosis, and pregnancy, the health care provider may prescribe a more potent antiprostaglandin medication such as ibuformin (Ponstel), naproxen sodium (Anaprox), or mefamic acid (Motrin).

Premenstrual Syndrome. Premenstrual changes, physical symptoms, and behavior are commonly experienced by women. The premenstrual syndrome (PMS) has been widely discussed in popular literature and in the media. Researchers in the fields of medicine, nursing, and the social sciences have also directed increased attention toward defining PMS, identifying the underlying pathophysiology and treatment. Many different researchers have proposed possible underlying etiologies. For example, estrogen–progesterone imbalance (Dalton, 1977), hyperprolactinemia (Benekek-Jaszmann & Hearne-Sturtevant, 1976), vitamin deficiency (Abraham & Hargrave, 1980), and neurotransmitter mediation (Reid & Yen, 1981), have all been ascribed to cause PMS. It is more likely, however, that PMS is a varying complex of symptoms mediated by sociocultural and psychological variables (Clare, 1983).

The premenstrual syndrome is defined as cyclic variations in affect, and physical symptoms related to the menstrual cycle. Although many women experience symptoms during the 5 to 7 days immediately preceding menstruation, for others, symptoms may last up to 2 weeks before menstruation or more infrequently occur only around ovulation. The somatic symptoms most commonly reported include fluid retention, abdominal bloating, lower back and abdominal cramps, and breast tenderness. Emotional changes include mood swings, irritability, anxiety, and depression. Many women also report cognitive changes, with difficulty in concentrating and inability to complete tasks although this has not been confirmed in controlled studies (Sommer, 1983). Clusters of symptoms usually occur and the types of experiences vary in intensity, duration, and severity from woman to woman. Several authors (Abplanalp, 1983; Abraham, 1980) have stated that PMS is not one syndrome but several. Regardless of the lack of precise understanding about PMS, many women do experience symptoms during the menstrual cycle ranging from barely noticeable to very severe. Although some women easily cope with menstrual cycle changes, others seek help from health care providers. The women suffering from mild to moderate PMS are excellent candidates for self-care regimens that can be facilitated through client education.

Assessment. Perhaps as a result of media attention and increased popular literature women come to health care providers with a broad variety of symptoms related to the menstrual cycle that may or may not be PMS. A thorough health history is mandatory to rule out medical and psychiatric illnesses that may be confused with PMS. Assessment of symptomatology should include type, duration, menstrual cycle and cyclicity, timing, intensity, and previous self-care measures and their effectiveness. In addition, a complete diet history and use or abuse of such agents as caffeine, alcohol, and mood-altering drugs should be assessed.

Once the tentative diagnosis of PMS has been made, further assessment of specific symptom clusters can be undertaken and individualized intervention plans developed. Educational needs should also be assessed on an individual basis. Table 4–11 summarizes the basic self-care regimens for PMS. Medical interventions beyond the basic areas of stress management, dietary modifications, and improved coping strategies are occasionally indicated and are directed at symptomatic relief as well. The use of diuretics, tranquilizers, and other psychoactive medications, bromocriptine (for mastalgia) and antiprostaglandins have all been used with limited success. Natural progesterone vagi-

TABLE 4–11. WOMEN'S HEALTH EDUCATION DEVELOPMENTAL PERSPECTIVE: PREMENSTRUAL SYNDROME

Critical Content	Objectives	Method
1. Definition of premenstrual syndrome	1. The woman will understand the cyclic nature of PMS	1. Individual consultation with the health care provider
2. Charting the menstrual cycle	2. The woman will increase her insight into the specific patterns of her cycle	2. Self-help literature; consultation with health care provider
3. Self-care measures a. Dietary modifications (weight loss, if indicated; reduction or elimination of caffeine, alcohol, refined sugar, salt) b. Enhancement of coping strategies (support network, "time-out", exerting control, participation in self-help groups) c. Vitamin supplementation (Pyridoxine 100–200 mg QD with vitamin B complex) d. Regular exercise	3. The woman will institute self-regulatory behaviors which will increase her sense of control over this health problem 4. The woman will monitor the effectiveness of her self-care measures and make appropriate modifications if necessary	3. Support groups

nal suppositories may also be used and are advocated by those clinicians who hypothesize that PMS is result of a progesterone deficiency (Dalton, 1977; Norris & Sullivan, 1983).

Because the underlying pathophysiology of PMS is poorly understood, and because many psychosocial and physical problems can easily masquerade as PMS, documentation on a daily basis of symptoms experienced over several cycles is mandatory to obtain a diagnosis of PMS. This documentation, or menstrual cycle charting, has additional benefits of providing data recorded at the time of symptoms occurrence, rather than retrospective information that may be incorrect or incomplete. Documentation is also a useful tool to educate women about their unique menstrual cycle changes.

Menstrual Cycle Charting. Menstrual cycle charting has been described in PMS self-care manuals (Harrison, 1982; Sojourner, 1983). Charting is the process of recording menstrual cycle data (menses, other bleeding, amount of menstrual flow, and associated symptoms) in a calendar format. Figure 4–2 is such an example. When several cycles have been recorded, a very accurate picture begins to emerge of the specific menstrual patterns of the particular woman.

The benefits of menstrual cycle charting extend to general menstrual cycle awareness as well. Many women seek health care for menstrual problems and have difficulty providing an adequate history, such as usual cycle length, date of last menstrual period, and the timing of abnormal bleeding or spotting.

In the case of PMS, menstrual charting is one method to facilitate diagnostics. Additionally, women experiencing PMS frequently complain of the sense of being out of control emotionally. Charting can be used as an effective intervention technique to

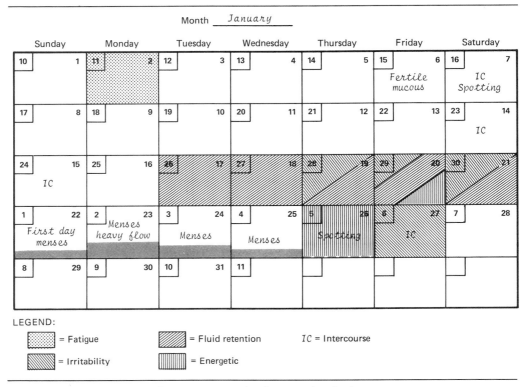

Figure 4–2. Example of menstrual cycle chart.

predict emotional changes before they occur. The woman may then initiate preventive self-care techniques that may decrease the intensity of the symptoms she experiences.

Assessment. Menstrual cycle education for the young adult and adult woman builds on the basic working knowledge she already possesses, provides information applicable to specific situations, and clarifies misconceptions that may impede self-care. Adult women frequently seek out health care providers for specific problems or knowledge deficits. This behavior is typical of adult learners who tend to be self-directed and problem oriented. Many women have specific questions that help the provider gain a clear understanding of the education needed. In addition, sharing of information during the health history also may point to areas of misconceptions that need clarification. A more general focus may be indicated for women seeking knowledge about broader topics such as natural family planning or self-care management of the premenstrual syndrome.

The adult learner is generally able to work with abstract ideas because life experience gives them a wide repertoire upon which to draw. Cognitive level must be assessed individually to insure optimal comprehension of the content.

Learning resources available to the adult woman consist of a wide variety of written materials in the popular literature as well as pamphlets and audiovisual resources prepared specifically for patient education. Peers also provide a rich source of informal knowledge and support through the sharing of common experiences. In a more formal way, self-help and support groups can be very beneficial to women concerning common menstrual cycle problems such as PMS.

Goals for Education. The goals for menstrual cycle awareness education for postmenarcheal young adult women build on the previous goals for the premenarcheal girl and include the same threads of self-care. They are to

1. Enhance self-care activities related to the menstrual cycle through awareness of the normal variations, the appropriate remedies for common problems, and knowledge of the indications for seeking health care provider interventions.
2. Encourage menstrual cycle awareness through charting or record keeping.
3. Increase knowledge of fertility and contraception as it relates to the menstrual cycle.

The Middle Years and the Perimenopausal Period

Table 4–10 describes objectives for education of women in this middle developmental phase. The numerous physiological and psychological transitions of the middle-year women are described in depth in Chapter 14. The underlying physiological processes are clearly reflected in changing menstrual cycle patterns. Cycle length becomes more variable and the amount of flow may increase if uterine fibroids are present. Anovulatory cycles with menorrhagia or metorrhagia are more common. Although many of these changes are the result of normal perimenopausal physiology, they may also indicate dysfunction. This age group is at greater risk for endometrial cancer, which can be associated with abnormal bleeding patterns. Pregnancy may also be suspected when the menses is delayed or missed entirely. These issues may be a source of anxiety as the woman approaches menopause.

Preparation for menopause consists of anticipatory guidance. Many women feel ill-prepared to deal with the changes that occur during menopause. One study (Greene, 1983) found that women preferred health care providers (physicians and nurses) as their primary source of information about menopause. In addition, written information such as pamphlets and group discussions were also cited as preferred sources. In other instances peers and family members may be important "sounding boards" and sources of information.

Assessment. Middle-year women have a rich repository of life experiences upon which to draw. Assessment of these experiences and knowledge is mandatory to develop individualized plans for menstrual cycle education. Areas of knowledge deficit must be identified because myths about menopause still abound. The woman's own goals for self-directed knowledge acquisition must be considered. Opportunities for self-care can then be optimized.

Goals for Education. Midlife women may seek less gynecological health care as they grow older. Because the needs of care during pregnancy and for frequent contraceptive visits decrease, contacts with health care providers may diminish. Important opportunities for on-going education may be missed. Therefore, it is especially necessary to take full advantage of the health visits that do occur in terms of anticipatory guidance for menopause. The goals for menstrual cycle education for the middle-year woman are to

TABLE 4–12. WOMEN'S HEALTH EDUCATION DEVELOPMENTAL PERSPECTIVE: THE PERIMENOPAUSAL PERIOD

Critical Content	Objectives	Method
1. Definition of the menopause (cessation of menses for one year)	1. The woman can state the definition of menopause	1. One-to-one consultation with health care provider
2. Normal menstrual cycle variations and changes (menstrual cycle length, bleeding patterns)	2. The woman will be aware of her of her changing menstrual function	2. Peer, small group discussions
3. Increased risk status for reproductive malignancies (endometrial, breast)	3. The woman will chart her menstrual cycle patterns and report deviations or suspected abnormalities	3. Written and audiovisual resources

1. Provide anticipatory guidance about normal perimenopausal changes, deviations and indications for seeking consultation with the health care provider,
2. Build on previous life experiences and knowledge about the menstrual cycle,
3. Identify knowledge deficits and clarify misconceptions related to the perimenopausal period, and
4. Strengthen adaptive coping skills and self-care activities during this transition period.

Table 4–12 summarizes the critical content and objectives for the perimenopausal woman.

Summary. This section has focused on menstrual cycle awareness as a foundation for self-care and optimal health. Using a developmental perspective, the various stages of menarche, young adulthood, and the perimenopausal period were used to discuss the process of education, promotion of self-care activities, and indications for health care intervention.

CONCLUSION

This chapter has presented an overview of health education for women. The developmental conceptual framework has allowed an organization of the specific needs and health risks of women for health promotion, prevention, and recovery from illness. Women's educational needs were viewed on continua of wellness–illness and self-help professional intervention. Educational approaches to meet these needs were proposed that have appropriate degrees of direct interventions versus facilitation of women's participation in their own health care. Figure 4–3 depicts these three continua. The educational intervention proposed would provide educational "therapy" for those who are ill and "therapy" for the well that maximizes wellness. Special educational approaches for women (versus men) would be available in "larger doses" because women have to overcome negative stereotypes and have a more difficult task to become partners with health care providers due to past socialization. The educational process and educational orientation used has a potential to facilitate participation in health and illness care.

Finally two unique areas of health prevention–promotion were presented as specific examples of how a developmental approach helps identify and plan health education for women.

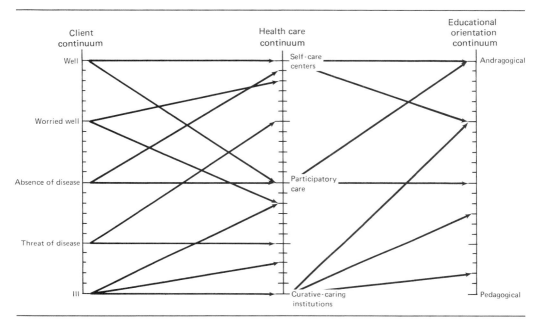

Figure 4–3. Selection of health care facility/educational orientation for women in health and illness.

RESOURCES

For Breast Disease
American Cancer Society, 19 West 56th Street, New York, NY 10019. *(Provides list of cancer centers, information for both public and professional use.)*
Office of Cancer Communications, National Cancer Institute, Bethesda, MD 20205. *(Provides information on cancer-related subjects. Write for nearest office.)*
Women's Breast Cancer Advisory Center, Inc., 1426 Rockville Pike, Suite 406, Rockville, MD 20850. *(Non-profit, consumer-oriented organization. Provides information on all aspects of breast diseases, especially cancer.)*

For Menstruation
Blume, J. *Are you there, God? It's me, Margaret.* Englewood Cliffs, N.J.: Bradbury Press, 1970.
Budoff, P. *No more menstrual cramps and other good news.* New York: Penguin Books, 1981.
Gardner-Loulan, J., Lopez, B., & Quackenbush, M. *Period.* San Francisco: Bolcano Press, 1979.
Harrison, M. *Self-help for premenstrual syndrome.* Cambridge, Ma.: Matrix Press, 1982.
Hongladarom, G., McCorkle, R., & Woods, N. *The compete book of women's health.* Englewood Cliffs, N.J.: Prentice-Hall, 1982.
Reitz, R. *Menopause: A positive approach.* New York: Penguin Books, 1977.
Sojourner, M. *Menstrual cycle changes (PMS): A survivor's guide.* Rochester, N.Y.: Planned Parenthood of Rochester and Monroe County, 1984.
Stewart, F., Guest, F., Stewart, G., & Hatcher, R. *My body, my health: A concerned women's book of gynecology.* Toronto: Bantam Books, 1981.

BIBLIOGRAPHY

Abplanalp, J. Premenstrual syndrome: A selective review. *Women and Health*, 1983, 8(2/3), 107–123.

Abraham, G. The premenstrual tension syndromes. In L. K. McNale (Ed.), *Contemporary obstetric and gynecologic nursing*. New York: C. V. Mosby, 1980.

Abraham, G., & Hargrave, J. Effects of vitamin B₆ on premenstrual symptomatology in women with premenstrual tension syndrome. *Infertility*, 1980, 3, 155.

Allman, L., & Jaffe, D. T. (Eds.) *Readings in adult psychology: Contemporary perspectives*. New York: Harper & Row, 1977.

Angrist, S. S., Mickelson, R., & Penna, A. N. Variations in adolescent's knowledge and attitudes about family life: Implications for curriculum design. *Adolescence*, 1976, *11*(41), 107–126.

Bardwick, J. *Psychology of women: A study of bio-cultural conflicts*. New York: Harper & Row, 1971.

Bardwick, J. *In transition*. New York: Holt, Rinehart & Winston, 1979.

Barry, H., Bacon, M. K., & Child, I. L. A cross-cultural survey of some sex differences in socialization. *Journal of Abnormal and Social Psychology*, 1957, 55, 327–332.

Baumrind, D. From each according to her ability. *School Review*, 1972, *80*, 161–197.

Baxandall, R., Gordon, L., & Reverly, S. *America's working women*. New York: Random House, 1976.

Bem, S. L. The measurement of psychological androgyny. *Journal of Consulting and Clinical Psychology*, 1974, *42*(2), 155–162.

Bem, S. L. Sex role adaptability: One consequence of psychological androgyny. *Journal of Personality and Social Psychology*, 1975, *31*(4), 634–643.

Benekek-Jaszmann, L., & Hearne-Sturtevant, M. Premenstrual tension and functional infertility. *Lancet*, 1976, *1*, 1095.

Bermosk, L. S. & Porter, S. E. *Women's health and human wholeness*. New York: Appleton-Century-Crofts, 1979.

Bernard, J. S. Adolescence and socialization for motherhood. In Dragastine, S. E., & Elder, G. H. (Eds.), *Adolescence in the life cycle*. New York: Wiley, 1975, 227–252.

Bernard, J. S. *The female world*. New York: Free Press, Macmillan, 1981.

Broverman, I. K., Broverman, D. M., & Clarkson, F. E. Sex-role stereotypes and clinical judgments of mental health. *Journal of Consulting and Clinical Psychology*, 1970, *34*(1), 1–7.

Brown, D. G. Sex role preference in young children. *Psychological Monographs: General and Applied*, 1956, *421*.

Brown, D. G. Sex role development in a changing culture. *Psychological Bulletin*, 1958, *55*(4), 232–242.

Buhler, C. Meaningfulness of the biographical approach. In L. Allman & D. T. Jaffe (Eds.), *Readings in adult psychology: Contemporary perspectives*. New York: Harper & Row, 1977.

Bullough, B., & Bullough, V. Sex discrimination in health care. *Nursing Outlook*, 1975, *23*(1), 40–45.

Byrd, B. F. *Standard breast examination*. New York: American Cancer Society, 1974.

Cancer Facts & Figures, 1982. New York: The American Cancer Society, 1981.

Clare, A. The relationship between psychopathology and the menstrual cycle. *Women and Health*, 1983, 8(2/3), 125–136.

Chapman, J. R., & Gates, M. *Women into wives*. Beverly Hills, Ca.: Sage Publications, 1977.

Chapman, J. R., & Gates, M. *The victimization of women*. Beverly Hills, Ca.: Sage Publications, 1978.

Cox, S. *Female psychology: The emerging self*. Chicago: Science Research Associates, 1976.

Condry, J., & Dyer, S. Fear of success: Attribution of cause to the victim. *Journal of Social Issues*, 1976, *32*(3), 63–83.

Chodorow, N. Family structure and feminine personality. In M. Z. Rosaldo & L. Lamphere (Eds.), *Women culture*. Stanford, Ca.: Stanford University Press, 1974.

Chodorow, N. *The reproduction of mothering*. Berkely, Ca.: University of California Press, 1978.

Conger, J. J. *Contemporary issues in adolescent development*, pp. 221–230. New York: Harper & Row, 1975.

Corea, G. *The hidden malpractice*. New York: William Morrow, 1977.

Creasy, R. K., Gummer, B. A., & Liggins, G. C. Systems for predicting spontaneous preterm birth. *Obstetrics Gynecology*, 1980, 55(6), 692–695.

Dalton, K. *The premenstrual syndrome and progesterone therapy*. Philadelphia: W. B. Saunders, 1977.

Darley, S. A. Big-time careers for the little women: A dual role dilemma. *Journal of Social Issues*, 1976, 32(3), 85–98.

Deaux, K., & Taynor, J. Evaluation of male and female ability: Bias works two ways. *Psychological Reports*, 1973, 32(1), 261–262.

Deaux, K., & Emswiller, T. Explanations of successful performance on sex-linked tasks: What is skill for the male is luck for the female. *Journal of Personality and Social Psychology*, 1974, 29(1), 80–85.

Dement, A. L. The college woman as a science major. *Journal of Higher Education*, 1962, 33, 487–490.

Deutch, C., & Culbert, L. A. Sex role stereotypes: Effect on perception of self and others and on personal adjustment. *Journal of Counseling Psychology*, 1976, 23, 373–379.

Diekelman, N. Emotional tasks of the middle adult. *American Journal of Nursing*, 1975, 75, 997–1001.

Edwards, Z. Changing breast self examination behavior. *Nursing Research*, 1980, 29(5), 301–306.

Ehrenreich, B., & English, D. *Complaints and disorders: The sexual politics of sickness* (Glass Mountain Pamphlets No. 2). Old Westbury, N.Y.: The Feminist Press, 1973.

Ehrenreich, B., & English, D. *For her own good: 150 years of the experts advice to women*. New York: Anchor Books, 1979.

Elkind, D. Egocentrism in adolescence. In J. J. Conger (Ed.), *Contemporary issues in adolescent development*. New York: Harper & Row, 1975, 55.

Elkind, D. Erik Erikson's eight ages of man. In L. Allman & D. T. Jaffe (Eds.), *Readings in adult psychology: Contemporary perspectives*, pp. 3–11. New York: Harper & Row, 1977.

Erikson, E. H. Inner and outer space: Reflections on womanhood. In R. J. Lifton (Ed.), *The women in America*. Boston: Houghton Mifflin, 1965.

Feinstein, K. W. *Working women and families*. Beverly Hills, Ca.: Sage Publications, 1979.

Fogarty, M., Rapport, R., & Rapoport, R. *Sex, career and family*. London: George Allen & Univen Ltd., 1971.

Fogel, C., & Woods, N. *Health care of women: A nursing perspective*. St. Louis, Mo.: C. V. Mosby, 1981.

Freeman, J. (Ed.). *Women: A feminist perspective*. Palo Alto, Ca.: Mayfield Publishing, 1975.

Frieze, I. H., Parsons, J. E., Johnson, P. B., Ruble, D. N., & Zellman, G. L. *Women and sex roles: A social psychological perspective*. New York: W. W. Norton, 1978.

Gilligan, C. *In a different voice: Psychological theory and women's development*. Cambridge, Ma.: Harvard University Press, 1982.

Gold, J., & Josimovich, J. (Eds.). *Gynecologic endrocrinology*, (3rd ed.). Hagerstown, Md.: Harper & Row, 1980.

Golub, S., & Catalano, J. Recollections of menarche and women's subsequent experience with menstruation. *Women and Health*, 1983, 8, 49–61.

Golub, S. Menarche: The beginning of menstrual life. *Women and Health*, 1983, 2/3, 17–36.

Gore, W. R., & Tudor, J. F. Adult sex roles and mental illness. *American Journal of Sociology*, 1973, 78(4), 812–835.

Gornick, V., & Moran, B. K. (Eds.). *Women in sexist society*. New York: Mentor Books, 1972.

Gould, L. X, Stories for free children. *Ms*, 1980, 61–64.

Gould, R. L. The phases of adult life. A study in developmental psychology. In L. Allman & D. T. Jaffe (Eds.), *Readings in adult psychology: Contemporary perspectives*, pp. 12–19. New York: Harper & Row, 1977.

Greene, S. *A descriptive study of midlife women's knowledge and sources of information regarding the menopause experience*. Unpublished master's thesis, Rochester, N.Y., 1983.

Grief, E., & Ulman, K. The psychological impact of menarche on early adolescent females: A review of the literature. *Child Development*, 1982, *53*, 1413–1430.

Grieze, I. H., & Ramsey, S. J. Nonverbal maintenance of traditional sex roles. *Journal of Social Issues*, 1976, *32*(3), 133–141.

Hammons, D., & Jablow, A. *Women in cultures of the world*. Menlo Park, Ca.: Cummings, 1976.

Harrison, M. *Self-help for premenstrual syndrome*. Cambridge, Ma.: Matrix Press, 1982.

Hoffman, L. W. Early childhood experiences and women's achievement motives. *Journal of Social Issues*, 1972, *28*, 129–155.

Hoffman, L. W., & Nye, F. I. *Working mothers*. San Francisco: Jossey-Bass, 1974.

Horner, M. Femininity and successful achievement: A basic inconsistency. In J. M. Bardwick, E. Douvan, M. Horner, & D. Gutmann (Eds.), *Feminine personality and conflict*. Monterey, Ca.: Brooks/Cole, 1970.

Horner, M. S. Toward an understanding of achievement-related conflicts in women. *Journal of Social Issues*, 1972, *28*, 157–175.

Horner, M. S. Toward an understanding of achievement-related conflicts in women. In J. Stacey, S. Gereaud, & J. Daniles (Eds.), *And Jill came tumbling after: Sexism in American education*. New York: Dell, 1974.

Hoyman, H. S. Sex education and our core values. *Journal of School Health*, 1974, *44*(2), 62–69.

Hunter, J. E. Images of woman. *Journal of Social Issues*, 1976, *32*(3), 7–17.

Hyde, J., & Rosenberg, B. G. *Half the human experience: The psychology of women*. Lexington, Ma.: D. C. Heath, 1976.

Israel, A. C., & Saccone, A. J. Follow-up of effects of choice of mediator and target or reinforcement on weight loss. *Behavior Therapy*, 1979, *10*(3) 260–265.

Jordon, B. *Birth in four cultures*. Montreal, Canada: Eden Press, Women's Publications, 1980.

Keinston, K. Youth "a new" stage of life. In L. Allman & D. T. Jaffe (Eds.), *Readings in adult psychology: Contemporary perspectives*, pp. 126–144. New York: Harper & Row, 1977.

Kerrins, K. Comparing the self-image of pre-pubescent girls before and after four sessions on body awareness. *Journal of School Health*, 1982, *53*, 1557–1566.

Kjervik, D., & Martinson, I. *Women in stress: A nursing perspective*. New York: Appleton-Century-Crofts, 1979.

Kohlberg, L. Moral development and the education of adolescents. In R. F. Purnell (Ed.), *Adolescence and the American high school*. New York: Holt, Rinehart & Winston, 1970.

Konapka, G. *Young girls: A portrait of adolescence*. Englewood Cliffs, N.J.: Prentice Hall, 1976, 53.

Kopp, C. *Becoming female: Perspectives on development*. New York: Plenum, 1979.

Leis, H. P. The diagnosis of breast cancer. *Cancer Journal for Clinicians*, 1977, *27*(4), 209–232.

Lennane, K. J., & Lennane, R. J. Alleged psychogenic disorders in women—A possible manifestation of sexual prejudice. *New England Journal of Medicine*, 1973, *288*(6), 288–292.

Lerner, R. M. *Concepts and theories of human development*. Reading, Ma.: Addison-Wesley, 1976.

Maccoby, E. E., & Jacklin, C. N. *The psychology of sex differences*. Stanford, Ca.: Stanford University Press, 1974.

MacPherson, K. Menopause as disease: The social construction of a metaphor. *Advances in Nursing Science*, 1981, *3*, 95–113.

Marieskind, H. I. *Women in the health system, patients, providers, and programs*. St. Louis, Mo.: C. V. Mosby, 1980.

Martin, L. *Health care of women*. Philadelphia: J. B. Lippincott, 1978.

Mead, M. *Male and female*. New York: Dell, 1968.

Mechanic, D. Sex, illness, illness behavior and the use of health services. *Journal of Human Stress*, 1976, *4*(2), 29–40.

Miller, J. B. *Toward a new psychology of women*. Boston: Beacon Press, 1976.

Mishell, D., & Davajan, V. *Reproductive endocrinology, infertility and contraception*. Philadelphia: F. A. Davis, 1979.

Mitchell, J. J. Adolescent intimacy. *Adolescence*, 1976, *11*(42), 275–280.

Moore, E. C. Women and health: United States, 1980. *Public Health Reports* (Suppl.), 1980, 95, 9–14.

Muller, C. Women and health statistics: Areas of deficient data collection and integration. *Women and Health*, 1979, *4*(1), 37–59.

Muuss, R. E. Kohlberg cognitive developmental approach to adolescent's morality. *Adolescence*, 1976, *11*(41), 39–59.

Nathanson, C. A. Illness and the feminine role: A theoretical review. *Social Science and Medicine*, 1975, *9*(2), 57–62.

Nathanson, C. Sex, illness, and medical care: A review of data, theory, and method. *Social Science and Medicine*, 1977, *11*(1), 13–25.

Neugarten, B. Adult personality: Toward a psychology of the life cycle. In L. Allman & D. T. Jaffe (Eds.), *Readings in adult psychology: Contemporary perspectives*, pp. 41–48. New York: Harper & Row, 1977.

NIH Publications No. 82-2401. U.S. Department of Health and Human Services. Washington, D.C., November, 1981.

Norris, R. V., & Sullivan, C. *PMS: Premenstrual syndrome*. New York: Rawson Associates, 1983.

Ortmeyer, L. Female's natural advantage? Or the unhealthy environment of males? The status of sex mortality differentials. *Women and Health*, 1979, *4*(2), 121–133.

Pender, N. *Health promotion in nursing practice*, Norwalk, Ct.: Appleton-Century-Crofts, 1982.

Piaget, J. Intellectual evaluation from adolescence to adulthood. In C. J. Guardo (Ed.), *The adolescent as individual: Issues and insights*. New York: Harper & Row, 1975, 108–117.

Pidgeon, V. A. Characteristics of children's thinking and implications for health teaching. *Maternal–Child Nursing Journal*, 1977, *6*(1), 1–8.

Poloma, M. M., & Garland, T. N. The married professional woman: A study in the tolerance of domestication. *Journal of Marriage and the Family*, 1971, *33*(3), 531–540.

Questions and answers about breast lumps (NIH Pub. No. 82-2401, U.S. Dept. of Health and Human Services). Washington, D. C.: U. S. Government Printing Office, 1981.

Redman, B. K. *Patient teaching in nursing* (4th ed.). St. Louis, Mo.: C. V. Mosby, 1980.

Reid, R., & Yen, S. Premenstrual syndrome. *American Journal of Obstetrics and Gynecology*, 1981, *1*(139), 85–104.

Reiss, I. L. Sex education in the public schools: Problem or solution? *Phi Delta Kappan*, 1968, *50*(1), 52–56.

Rich, A. *Of woman born: Motherhood as an experience and institution*. New York: W. W. Norton, 1976.

Richards, J. G. An experiment in public education. In J. Wakofield (Ed.), *Public education about cancer: Recent research & current programs* (UICC Tech, Rep Ser., No 26). Geneva: International Union Against Cancer, 1977.

Richardson, M. S., & Alpert, J. Role perceptions of educated adult women: An exploratory study. *Educational Gerontology*, 1976, *1*, 171–185.

Rollins, B. C., & Canon, K. L. Marital satisfaction over the family life cycle: A reevaluation. *Journal of Marriage and the Family*, 1974, *36*(2), 271–283.

Ruble, D., & Brooks-Gunn, J. The development of menstrual-related beliefs and behaviors during early adolescence. *Child Development*, 1982, 53, 1567–1577.

Ruble, D. N., & Higgins, E. T. Effects of group sex composition on self-presentation and sex-typing. *Journal of Social Issues*, 1976, *32*(3), 125–132.

Russo, N. F. The motherhood role. *Journal of Social Issues*, 1976, *32*(3), 142–153.

Sandelowski, M. *Women, health and choice*. Englewood Cliffs, N.J.: Prentice Hall, 1981.

Sangiuliano, I. *In her time*. New York: Morrow Quill Paperbacks, 1980.

Sassen, G. Success anxiety in women: A contructivist interpretation of its sources and its significance. *Harvard Educational Review*, 1980, *50*, 13–25.

Scarf, M. *Unfinished business: Pressure points in the lives of women*. New York: Doubleday, 1980.

Scully, D., & Bart, P. A funny thing happened on the way to the orifice: Women in gynecology textbooks. *American Journal of Sociology*, 1973, *78*(4), 1045–1050.

Seaman, B., & Seaman, G. *Women and the crisis in sex hormones*. New York: Bantam Books, 1977.

Seiden, A. E. Overview: Research on the psychology of women. I. Differences and sexual reproductive life. *American Journal of Psychiatry*, 1976, *133*, 995–1007.

Seiden, A. E. Overview: Research on the psychology of women. II. Women in family, work and psychotherapy. *The American Journal of Psychiatry*, 1976, *133*, 1111–1123.

Sheehy, G. *Passages: Predictable crises of adult life*. New York: E. P. Dutton, 1974.

Sherman, J. A. *On the psychology of woman: A survey of empirical studies*. Springfield, Il.: Charles Thomas, 1971.

Sojourner, M. *Menstrual cycle changes (PMS): A survivor's guide*. Rochester, N.Y.: Planned Parenthood of Rochester and Monroe County, 1983.

Solomon, B. H. *The experience of the American woman*. New York: Mentor, 1978.

Sommer, B. How does menstruation affect cognitive competence and psychophysiological response? *Women and Health*, 1983, *8*, 53–90.

Sorenson, R. C. *Adolescent sexuality in contemporary America: Personal values and sexual behavior ages 13–19*. New York: Worbel, 1973.

Spots, S. Love: Crisis and consolation for the middlescent woman. *Advances in Nursing Science*, 1981, *3*, 87–94.

Stevenson, J. *Issues and crises during middlescence*. New York: Appleton-Century-Crofts, 1977.

Stage, S. *Female complaints: Lydia Pinkham and the business of women's medicine*. New York: W. W. Norton, 1979.

Tanner, J. *Foetus into man*. Cambridge, Ma.: Harvard University Press, 1978.

Terman, L., & Tyler, L. Psychological sex differences. In L. Carmichael (Ed.), *Manual of child psychology* (2nd ed.). New York: John Wiley & Sons, 1954.

Treiman, D. J., & Terrell, L. Sex and the process of status attainment: A comparison of working women and men. *American Sociological Review*, 1975, *40*, 174–200.

Turner, M. E. Sex role attitudes and fear of success in relation to achievement behavior in women. *International*, 1976, *35*, 2451–2452.

Van Gelder, L. Carol Gilligan: Leader for a different kind of future. *Ms.*, January 1984, 37, 38, 100–101.

Verbrugge, L. M. Female illness rates and illness behavior. *Women and Health*, 1979, *4*(1), 61–79.

Walum, L. *The dynamics of sex and gender: A sociological perspective*. New York: Rand McNally, 1977.

Williams, J. H. *Psychology of women: Behavior in a biosexual context*. New York: W. W. Norton, 1977.

Winick, C. Beige epoch: Depolarization of sex roles in America. In A. E. Winder (Ed.), *Adolescence: Contemporary studies*, pp. 189–197. New York: D. VanNostrand, 1974.

Woods, N. Women and their health. In C. Fogel & N. Woods (Eds.), *Health care of women: A nursing perspective*. St. Louis, Mo.: C. V. Mosby, 1981.

Woods, N., Dery, G., & Most, A. Recollections of menarche, current menstrual attitudes and perimenstrual symptoms. In S. Golub (Ed.), *Menarche*. Lexington, Ma.: Lexington Books, 1983.

Education for Health Promotion

Part II of this text describes content for health promotion in women. Chapters 5, 6, and 7 discuss general health promotion in the area of becoming female, sexual awareness, and coping with life stress. These areas have been clouded with myths and misinformation for women. Therefore, suggestions for content and methodologies to increase women's knowledge and appreciation for their unique biology and experience are proposed. Chapters 14 and 15 focus on health promotion for middle-aged and elderly women. These two age periods have been neglected, and women over forty have been viewed negatively. Such negativism and lack of information has contributed to women's own view of themselves. Educational strategies that assist women to better understand middle years and later developmental changes are therefore essential to positive health. Suggestions for promotion of positive mental and physical health are given.

Reproductive health is considered a life issue versus a medical issue for women. Thus, Chapters 8, 11, 12, and 13 are presented to promote appropriate decision making and participation in reproductive health care by women. The reader who has a basic knowledge of reproduction will find these chapters useful to providing education to women requesting care for contraceptives, birthing, or perinatal care. The reader who is unfamiliar with reproductive health will need an additional reference to supplement content in this area.

Women who have a disability or who are homosexual need general and reproductive health education that considers their perspective and needs. Chapter 9 identifies the special needs of homosexual women and suggests ways to adapt health education to these needs. New emphasis on the rights of the handicapped requires the health care provider to consider the needs of women who have some type of disability. Chapter 10 describes the educational needs of women with physical, hearing, and other disabilities. Several resources for teaching the woman who is handicapped are given.

Discovering Womanhood: An Educational Approach

5

Phyllis Collier

> *Anatomy is destiny.*
> *—Freud*
>
> *No understanding of women will ever be possible until women themselves begin to tell*
> *what they know.*
> *—John Stewart Mill, 1869*

Who am I? Who are we? These questions are often asked by adult women, individually and collectively. Most developmental theorists consider adolescence the "identity stage," when both women and men experience a process through which a more clear and defined sense of self emerges, enabling the individual to move on to other stages and tasks of development. In more recent years, a number of authors and researchers have questioned whether women follow these traditionally defined stages of growth, most of which are based on male norms and experiences. Do women, who have lived by a societally prescribed script for their roles and behavior, experience life in a different way? Are the timing and sequence of their life events, as well as the character of the events themselves, considerably different from those of men? If so, what is known about the uniqueness of the female experience and from where has the information come? This chapter is designed to help women become more aware of the historical and current forces that have influenced their lives as a gender group, as well as to assist them in exploring the significant events and experiences that have composed their individual womanhood.

A popular dictionary defines womanhood as "the state of being a woman; womanly characteristics or qualities; women collectively" (Random House Dictionary, 1967, p. 1641). Biology is probably the most common factor used to identify women—an aggregate of individuals with clear-cut anatomical characteristics (Bernard, 1981). Because of this unique biology, not shared with men, a gender assignment (female) begins at birth. A socialization process accompanies this gender label and continues throughout life. Bernard lists a second factor by which the female world can be conceptualized, that of "place"; the position of women as a group, class, or enclave in the world at large. Although the female world is not closed and independent from the male world, it is a separate entity, the characteristics of which are sometimes difficult to describe.

What does it mean to be a woman? From ancient times, women were rarely seen as simply human beings. Rather, myths were created to explain their differences from men,

133

and describe their perceived mysterious powers and behaviors (Williams, 1977). They were admired for their goodness (mother–nurturer, earth goddess) and feared for their potential for evil (seductress, temptress, sorcerer). These mystery-laden qualities, variations of which continue into the present time, permitted an explanation for events that occurred and limited insights into the true nature of women.

Historically, women's experience has been structured and given its significance by men. There is no known time period or culture in which men have not been the dominant sex (Janeway, 1974). From this environment came the scripts for the female role, that of being a complementary helpmate to men. Women's major sphere was seen as the home, with biological and innate resources for childbearing, mothering, and domestic duties. Desired personal characteristics included being charming, passive, intuitive, adaptable, and submissive to authority. Females were expected to be more emotional, and less logical and rational than men. They were excluded from any kind of major participation or leadership in the public sphere—political, religious, and economic. Likewise, the known educators, authors, and creative artists were men. Wyckoff (1977) describes this as socialization for powerlessness, with the end product being more of a well-developed, intuitive child than an adult woman.

This gender socialization continued throughout the centuries, with some variation as time went by. Individual women or small groups of women made some breakthrough in challenging the system. Eras of change or need—the industrial revolution, world wars— brought about job opportunities for others, particularly the working-class woman. Yet, in spite of gradual progress, the predominant thought was that men's ideas, men's work, and men's lives were more important than those of women.

The social movements of the 1960s and 1970s brought about a profound reevaluation of women's role and position in society. With a newly raised consciousness, women began examining the ideals created for them to live by. With an increased knowledge of each other, they began to see how their experiences repudiated the easy generalizations made about them (Solomon, 1978). Since that time, nearly every cultural script for women has been challenged. This has resulted in changes for women, men, families, and societal traditions and institutions. Some of these changes were accepted with relative ease. Others are still being sorted out.

One outcome of this period of transition was that women began to review the writings and the research literature that described their lives and behaviors. Some conclusions were:

1. There were major gaps in knowledge about women, particularly in the biological and social experiences that were unique to them.
2. Some researchers had found women "theoretically uninteresting" to study (Rosaldo & Lamphere, 1974), whereas others had questioned their ability to be reliable reporters (Williams, 1977).
3. Men were doing much of the research, as well as making decisions on what was important to study and to publish. Little was available from a female perspective.
4. Tools and approaches used to study women were often normed according to male standards and behaviors, with women being labeled different or deviant when they did not measure up to the established criteria (Freize et al., 1978).
5. Bias, based on traditional societal beliefs and stereotypes about women, pervaded much of the literature.

The findings were alarming. In addition to reinforcing traditional expectations for women, these theories and assumptions were frequently used as a basis for diagnosis and treatment, especially in regard to women's reproductive and psychological health care. An era of revisionist literature ensued, with attempts made to correct the gaps and biases, and find new ways to study the female experience. Two important factors were part of this change: an increased number of female professionals designed and conducted research and there was finally a more open climate for women to articulate their experiences from their special vantage point. A goal was to move beyond viewing women as a "variation" from an arbitrary norm, and describe and evaluate the physical characteristics and sociocultural experiences that made parts of their lives unique.

A body of literature that illustrates a transition of approximately 150 years and that was a key part of the reevaluation process is related to human growth and development. Freud (early 1800s) was among the first to publish theories on the psychological development of both men and women, defining psychosexual stages through which they would pass. He believed that both sexes developed similarly until the ages of 4 to 6 years, when female children would discover and be envious that they lacked a penis (Williams, 1977). This critical event had the potential to engender lifelong feelings of inferiority in women, and to place limits on their development (Hyde & Rosenberg, 1976). Although women would never quite be resigned to their "femininity," he believed that childbirth would provide some fulfillment (Freize et al., 1978). A major criticism of Freud is that he did little more than reinforce the cultural stereotypes of his time by focusing on biology, while ignoring social factors that influence roles and behaviors.

Helene Deutsch further developed Freud's theories, particularly beyond the oedipal stages. She also equated femininity with passivity, and viewed motherhood as the most critical feature in a woman's psychological development (Freize et al., 1978).

Karen Horney initially accepted Freud's ideas but later became critical of them. As a counter argument to penis envy, she posed the idea that men may be envious of women's reproductive capacity, and that their striving for achievement was perhaps to compensate for feelings of anatomical inferiority (Freize et al., 1978). Horney also gave recognition to social and cultural influences on development and considered that women might have a psychology of their own.

Erik Erikson reinterpreted the psychoanalytical view of women in a more positive light, seeing women's experience as less negative and pathological than described by Freud and Deutsch. However, he too believed in biological determinism; that the "inner space" of the womb and vagina, and the motherhood role were central to identity formation in women (Williams, 1977). Erikson is also well known for his description of eight life stages, from infancy through old age. The behaviors for each stage are highly male-normed, and current researchers pose the idea that women's life events may occur in a different sequence.

In addition to the biologically focused psychoanalytical models developed by Freud and his followers, several other developmental theories are well known. Social learning theory is frequently used to explain the development of sex differences. Its premise is that children adopt behaviors for which they are rewarded. Thus, if girls are rewarded for traditional feminine behaviors, i.e., being pleasant or nurturing, and are not rewarded for being independent or aggressive, they will make choices about behavior appropriate for them. Imitation, especially of the same-sex parent's behavior and observed learning, behaviors that may be noted and used at a later time, are also tenets of social learning theory. Critics of this theory question whether children are given as strong a sex-typed reinforcement as is proposed; research indicates otherwise. There is also evidence that children do not necessarily imitate the same-sex parent more than one of the opposite sex (Hyde & Rosenberg, 1976).

The cognitive–developmental theory postulates that sex role identity is gained via intellectual steps and is largely self-motivated rather than externally imposed. Children will identify that there are two sexes, adopt a gender identity, and then develop a value for behaviors and attitudes appropriate for their own sex. Culture structures the data that the child uses, however, so a stereotypical sex role may still be present.

Several theorists, previously mentioned, described human development via age-related stages. Most focused on childhood, however, with minimal attention to ongoing adult development. Two more recent authors who describe adult life as a series of predictable, linear, age-specific events are Levinson and Sheehy. Levinson studied only men, and Sheehy's popular book, *Passages,* was heavily based on the male-normed work of Levinson and other stage theorists, even though it describes both sexes. The accuracy of stage theories for women has been questioned for several reasons: Are women being judged according to a male timetable that is inaccurate and inappropriate for quantifying their lives? Are women's lives "predictable?" As an example, do women achieve identity prior to intimacy (using Erikson's stages), or is their sequence in the opposite direction? Sangiuliano (1980) proposes that the sequence and timing of life events may be different for women, and that they are more likely to experience unexpected, critical events that alter their life focus.

A review of developmental theories leaves women with no clear-cut answers regarding what most influences their female identity. Is biology a factor, or are social and cultural influences the major determinant? Are women more naturally passive, dependent, and less achievement-oriented, or are they taught to be so? Is there a more systematic process to help boys/men grow up, whereas women's lives unfold "in great surges of billowing change?" (Sangiuliano, 1980, p. 20). In a world changed by technology, economics, reproductive freedoms, and less clear societal expectations, is it even more difficult to answer these questions?

Bernard (1981) concludes that the female world is:

> . . . still at a stage where broad brush strokes are legitimate. It is not anywhere near the stage . . . where refinement of concepts, perfection of techniques, and elaboration of old ideas are as important as fresh new insights and perspectives. (p. 31)

It is important that the discovery process regarding women's lives be continued, not only for describing the collective female experience, but for looking at the range of individual variations sometimes influenced by age, ethnicity, education, religion, geographical location, and socioeconomic level. Sacks (1982) proposes that there are probably more differences within a gender group than between the sexes. Greater articulation, along with improved research, can help reduce the stereotypes about women and remove some of the limitations that still keep them from full and equal participation in many aspects of society.

This chapter is designed to help women continue to explore and to describe their life events and experiences via an educational experience. The focus is more on awareness and articulation, as opposed to the more specific, cognitive level learning contained in some of the other chapters. Sections of this chapter may be used as an introduction to or in tandem with other chapters.

LEARNING NEEDS

Content Areas. Learning needs could potentially be related to every facet of a woman's life. However, selected content areas that might be most familiar and useful to a variety of women are:

1. History of women
2. Female socialization
3. Life patterns
4. Body knowledge and awareness
5. Health experiences, beliefs, and behaviors
6. Female relationships with others
7. Women's environment
8. Women's work

Assessment. Factors that will help in determining the appropriate educational content and approaches for individuals or groups of women include:

1. Interest in/motivation for self-evaluation.
2. Primary goal(s) for learning—increased knowledge, increased awareness, behavioral change.
3. Specific content areas desired.
4. Preferred educational approach—self-learning, one-to-one, small groups, large groups.
5. Comfort with interaction, self-revelation.
6. Deterrents to self-discovery.
7. Demographic factors—age, socioeconomic level, educational level, ethnic and religious background.

Assessments can be informal or more organized, and education can be conducted in a variety of settings, such as health care facilities, church, neighborhood, and community groups, and women's organizations.

METHODOLOGIES

Three major formats can be used for this type of education: (1) self-learning, (2) individual education, and (3) group work. See Chapters 2 and 3 for a discussion of strengths and weaknesses for each approach; in addition, note content on use of exercises, readings, and audiovisual materials.

Content areas identified earlier are combined with educational methodologies and resources for the remainder of this chapter. Each topic is headed with "Discovering your . . . ," and includes an introduction, educational goals, individual and group learning activities, and background readings.

Discovering Your Heritage

Introduction. Most historical writings contain information about the activities and accomplishments of women. Although the United States had a number of women and minorities who assisted in its founding, it is primarily white men who are celebrated in standard texts (Berkin & Norton, 1979). It was they who explored new worlds, won battles, formed governments, established infrastructural systems, and produced technological inventions—functions traditionally considered to be most significant.

In recent years, historians have begun to examine the experiences and the contributions of women. Through some public records, as well as through diaries, letters, and other less formal methods of documentation, the "hidden" contributions of women to settlement of colonies and territories, to religion, culture, and education have been noted. In addition, topics formerly ignored by scholars, such as childbirth experiences, household technology, and female friendships, have been explored (Berkin & Norton, 1979). More information is available regarding the diversity of women's experiences by socioeconomic levels, rural/urban location, and religious and ethnic background. This "rescue" of women's past provides an awareness that there were many strong and capable female models, and that the work and activities of women were a valuable and worthwhile part of history, also. Future texts and scholarly writings need to reflect both their past and current contributions to society.

It is important that women today recognize the contributions of their foremothers and appreciate their struggles for equality in many areas of life. In an era of rapid change, it is also useful to document and reflect on the customs and activities of today's women, especially in one's own family or cultural group, thus preserving for future generations a personalized view of their heritage.

Educational Goals. To assist women in:

1. Recognition of the historical contributions of women to society.
2. Awareness of female role models in past and current generations.
3. Development of a personal history of their family/cultural group.

Activities
Individual

1. Read historical books on women—general, or those related to a specific time period, socioeconomic or ethnic group, or female cause (voting rights, birth control).
2. Read historical novels. Does the portrayal of women in these books match with the historical description of women's roles and activities during that era?
3. Read autobiographies or biographies of both famous and "ordinary" women.
4. Visit museums. Look for artifacts and materials pertinent to women, i.e, clothing, household items, implements for food preparation, medicines and "cures" for female ailments, craftwork, diaries/writings.
5. Interview your mother, grandmother, or older friends and relatives. Some questions might be:

   • What was it like being a female child in their generation? Were they treated differently from brothers?
   • What were they told regarding do's/don'ts for women?
   • What were they told about menstruation, dating, marriage, sex, childbearing?
   • What was special about the environment in which they grew up, i.e., geography—rural, urban, suburban; ethnic or cultural group; religious orientation; socioeconomic level?
   • What were some of the traditions or rituals carried on by their family? Have they been continued? Why or why not?
   • What choices did they make regarding marriage, having children, work outside the home, career?
   • What do they think about the changes for women in the past 20 years? If they were growing up now, how would their lives be different?

Put the information in writing for future reference.

Group

1. Read historical materials and discuss:

   - Individual women and their contributions. What were their special strengths? What causes did they espouse? What resistance did they receive from society? Examples: Abigail Adams, Marie Curie, Margaret Sanger, Sojourner Truth, Eleanor Roosevelt.
   - Eras of sociopolitical change for women—labor activity of New England mill women; suffragette, Women's Christian Temperance Union, or abolitionist activities.

2. Discuss personal historical female role models during life thus far. Discuss how these women were influential to each participant.
3. Read and discuss selected "historical" classic writings of the 1970s women's movement. Examples:

   - Freidan, *The feminine mystique*
   - Greer, *The female eunuch*
   - Millett, *Sexual politics*
   - Janeway, *Man's world, women's place*
   - Morgan, *Sisterhood is powerful*
   - Chesler, *Women and madness*

   Possible topics of discussion:

   - What earlier historical issues for women did they base their works on?
   - Consider the changes during the 10 to 15 years since these books were written.
   - Compare the theories and ideas in these books with several of the listed authors' current books, i.e., Freidan, *The second stage* and Greer, *Sex and destiny: The politics of fertility*.

Readings:

- Berkin, C., & Norton, M. B. *Women of America: A history*. Boston: Houghton Mifflin, 1979.
- Cott, N. *The bonds of womanhood: 'Women's sphere' in New England, 1780–1835*. New Haven: Yale University Press, 1977.
- Dengler, C. *At odds: Women and the family from the Revolution to the present*. New York: Oxford University Press, 1980.
- Ehrenreich, B., & English, D. *For her own good: 150 years of the experts' advice to women*. New York: Anchor Books, 1979.
- Gurko, M. *The ladies of Seneca Falls*. New York: Schocken Books, 1976.
- Hartman, M., & Banner, L. (Eds.). *Clio's consciousness raised: New perspectives on the history of women*. New York: Harper and Row, 1974.
- Lerner, G. *Black women in white America: A documentary history*. New York: Random House, 1972.
- Rowbotham, S. *Hidden from history*. New York: Vintage Books, 1973.
- Schlissel, L. *Women's diaries of the westward journey*. New York: Schocken Books, 1982.
- Stage, S. *Female complaints: Lydia Pinkham and the business of women's medicine*. New York: W.W. Norton, 1979.

Discovering Your Socialization

Introduction. Most human beings undergo a long and pervasive apprenticeship in maleness or femaleness (sex role socialization) (Katz, 1979). Strong societal and cultural beliefs exist about differences between the sexes, and these are communicated from the moment of birth. After a period of time the child identifies with one sex or another, adopts the behaviors deemed appropriate to the sex, and internalizes the role as part of him- or herself. The socialization process goes on throughout life, with additional expectations potentially related to life stage, marital status, educational level, social position, or changes in societal values.

Stereotypical beliefs about gender attributes and capabilities have served to limit both women and men. However, for women these beliefs have often perpetuated a secondary status in comparison to men, and have inhibited their individuality, discouraged achievement, and restricted autonomy (Fogel, 1981). Numerous authors (Bardwick, 1979; Lasky, 1982; Weitzman, 1982) state that young girls quickly perceive that traditional female characteristics and roles are less valued than those of men, and that these feelings can become deeply internalized.

Theories regarding how individuals arrive at a sex role identity were discussed in this chapter's introduction and in Chapter 4. Regardless of the theory espoused, several forces commonly influence the socialization process in both direct and subtle ways.

Parents are usually the earliest socializers of their children, and it is widely assumed that there is a double standard for raising boys and girls. In many instances this is true. Parents may speak to female and male children in different voice tones, provide sex-typed clothing and toys, and have different expectations for such things as household tasks, dating behaviors, or career choices (Lasky, 1982; Weitzman, 1982). However, Maccoby and Jacklin (1974), after an extensive review of research, concluded that there are surprising similarities in the way parents rear children, with the most notable difference being that boys were handled and played with more roughly and were given more physical punishment as well as more praise and criticism.

Most studies show that parents of higher social class are less rigid about sex distinction, whereas in working and lower class families there is greater concern with "appropriate" masculine or feminine behavior. Birth order may also be an influence, with greater expectations placed on the first born or only child of either sex (Weitzman, 1982).

The media serves as another strong socializing agent. Although progress has been made, women are still quite stereotypically presented in books, television shows, films, and advertisements. Common roles are mother, housewife, nurse, teacher, and secretary. They are more likely to be shown as personally (versus professionally) oriented (Fesbach et al., 1979); they solve problems for children and friends, and are supportive to partners.

Women are shown disproportionately in ads for personal hygiene products and kitchen and bathroom equipment, and rarely as users of mechanical equipment (Fesbach et al., 1979). In an opposite advertising role, women are presented as alluring, charming, and sensual in order to lure consumers to products.

In a variety of ways, schools have conveyed sex-stereotyped messages to students. History and science texts record few achievements by women. Certain types of courses were considered more for one sex or the other. Girls were frequently steered away from math and science, contributing to what some perceive as women's "phobia" in this area. Male athletic programs were given greater priority, and positions of leadership assumed by male students.

At some point in life, usually in adolescence, peers become strong influences in the socialization process. They may reinforce or dispute existing beliefs and behaviors, while adding new ones. A phenomenon noted among young women at this stage is that they begin to equate intelligence with loss of femininity and popularity (Weitzman, 1982).

Given all of the historical and current forces that influence the development of women and men, are they vastly different creatures? On variables commonly measured in this field of study the results are inconclusive, and numerous stereotypes have been disproven (see Table 4–3).

In the everyday world, more tangible evidence of sex-role differences can be noted. Women still bear primary responsibility for household management and child care, even if they are employed outside of the home. Women rarely head corporations or institutions. Few women have won the Nobel prize. In accepting new options open to them, women have been forced to juggle roles and make choices that are not expected of men.

As new worlds opened to women, and family and work relationships became somewhat more egalitarian, several issues ensued. Should women strive to adopt traditional male behaviors in order to "make it," i.e., independence, assertiveness, decisiveness, nonemotionality? Another debate relates to achievement conflicts and dependency needs in women. In spite of many positive gains, breaking free of long-held beliefs has been difficult and many women question whether they have a deep-rooted "fear of success" (Horner, 1972) or a need to be taken care of (Dowling, 1981). Becoming female is a long process of learning, unlearning, and relearning. The changes as well as the things that remain the same can be interesting to explore.

Educational Goals. To assist women in:

1. Developing a definition of femininity.
2. Exploring forces that have influenced their sex role socialization.
3. Developing awareness of sex role stereotypes.
4. Identifying sexist attitudes and behaviors, and ways of responding to them.

Activities
Individual

1. Define "femininity." In what ways do you consider yourself "feminine?" Are there any of your personal characteristics you consider "unfeminine?" Why?
2. What did you learn about the following topics from these people: mother, father, grandmother, school teacher, religious school teacher, your best friend.

   - being feminine
   - success in school
   - dating and marriage
   - your appearance
   - menstruation
   - career
   - having children
   - what men are really like

3. For reflection

   - In what ways has your upbringing as a woman been beneficial to you? In what ways has it hindered you?

Group

1. Discuss: At the present time, how would you define "feminine," "masculine," "androgenous."
2. Respond to the following statements with "agree," "disagree," or "undecided." Discuss the rationale behind your answers.

   - The mother should be awarded child custody when a couple is divorced.
   - Men should not cry.
   - Women should not hold jobs on the night shift.
   - It is important for a man to be "masculine" and a woman "feminine."
   - Wives should make less money than their husbands.
   - A wife and husband should take turns staying home with a sick child.
   - A single man is not capable of caring for an infant.
   - I would vote for a woman for president if she were the best candidate. (Bingham et al., 1983, p. 14–15.)

3. Discuss: How did the following influence what you believe about your role as a woman?

   - Family
   - Racial or ethnic group
   - Socioeconomic status
   - Religion
   - Husband/partner
   - Media

4. Exercise—Have You Ever Met a Woman Truckdriver?
   Discuss:
   a. Is it right for only men to be truck drivers? What is there about the job that makes it unsuitable for women?
   b. Would you like to be a truck driver? Why or why not?
   c. Are the reasons you gave based on what a truck driver actually does? (Bingham et al., 1983, p. 21.)
5. High school stereotypes
   Discuss: What were common beliefs about the following types of women in your high school.

   - Straight-A students
   - Blondes
   - Girls with large breasts
   - Girls who took shop or calculus
   - Cheerleaders

6. Exercise—Sex Role Reversal
   See Chapter 6, Exercise 8
7. List and discuss:

   - Activities/functions that only men can do.
   - Activities/functions that only women can do.

8. Read and discuss current opposing views on female dependency in:

   • Dowling, *The Cinderella complex*
   • Eichenbaum and Orbach, *What do women want: Exploding the myth of dependency*.

9. Define sexism. Discuss personal experiences with it. During the past 10 years, what changes have you noted in the amount and type of sexism that occurs? How do you currently respond to it?

10. Discuss: Would you like to see a truly androgenous society? Why or why not?

Readings

- Bardwick, J. *In transition*. New York: Holt, Rinehart, and Winston, 1979.
- Bingham, M., Edmondson, J., & Stryker, S. *Choices: A teen woman's journal for self-awareness and personal planning*. Santa Barbara, Ca.: Advocacy Press, 1983.
- Brownmiller, S. *Femininity*. New York: Linden Press/Simon & Schuster, 1984.
- Dowling, C. *The Cinderella complex*. New York: Pocket Books, 1981.
- Eichenbaum, L., & Orbach, S. *What do women want: Exploding the myth of dependency*. New York: Coward-McCann, 1983.
- Fogel, C. Issues in the life cycle. In C. Fogel & N. Woods (Eds.), *Health care of women: A nursing perspective*. St. Louis, Mo.: C. V. Mosby, 1981.
- Frieze, I., et al. *Women and sex roles: A social psychological perspective*. New York: W. W. Norton, 1978.
- Gilligan, C. *In a different voice*. Cambridge, Ma.: Harvard University Press, 1982.
- Goffman, E. *Gender advertisements*. New York: Harper and Row, 1979.
- Graham, M., & Birns, B. Where are the women geniuses? Up the down escalator. In C. Kopp (Ed.), *Becoming female: Perspectives on development*. New York: Plenum Press, 1979.
- Halas, C., & Matteson, R. *I've done so well—Why do I feel so bad?* New York: Ballantine Books, 1978.
- Schaef, A. *Womens reality: An emerging female system in the white male society*. Minneapolis, Mn.: Winston Press, 1981.
- Shulman, A. *Memoirs of an ex-prom queen*. New York: Alfred A. Knopf, 1972.

Discovering Your Life Patterns—Past and Future

Introduction. Historically, there was only one life plan for women. They and others assumed that they would become wives and mothers, in that order, with a partner whose financial acumen and achievements would sustain them both. Even in the early 1960s, a group of college women described their dream life as including marriage, a professional husband, three children, a home in the suburbs, a round of daily activities, an income above $20,000, and a station wagon (Sangiuliano, 1980).

At some point, developmental theorists began to identify stages of both childhood and adult development. The adult stages included tasks and events for young adulthood, middle years, and aging. For women, these tasks fitted well with their accepted role—children in their twenties, "empty nest" syndrome in their late forties. Sheehey (1976) gave credence to changing female roles for women when she described them as Caregivers (traditional), Either-or-women (who choose between love and work), or Integraters (who do both). Sheehey, however, still held that life events follow a fairly predictable pattern.

Sangiuliano (1980) is of the opinion that women's lives are more likely to be unpredictable and that they almost always lead a serial life of hibernation and renewal, postponement, and actualization. She states that critical events, which contain an element of the unexpected, often disrupt the status quo and jolt women into taking stock of their lives.

Women may be described as "late bloomers" in planning for and living their own lives. At this stage it is important to gather data on how they perceive their lives unfolding, what motivates them, and what plans they have for the future, as new options become available.

Educational Goals. To assist women in:

1. Assessing their individual life patterns, and comparing them with those of other women.
2. Evaluating the style by which they live their lives.
3. Exploring the process of planning and goal setting for the future.

Activities
Individual and/or Group

1. On a blank sheet of paper, draw a line that represents your life. The line can be straight, slanted, jagged, convoluted. Place a mark and a brief description at significant points in your life. Put a mark at the spot you are at present.
   Discuss with others: What do the shapes of the lines convey? What was considered a significant event? (Sangiuliano, 1980, p. 27)
2. Reflect/Discuss: Are you a person who plans your life, or do events, relationships, jobs just "fall into place?" What are advantages/disadvantages to either style?
3. Respond to the following questions:

   • When do you feel most fully alive?
   • What do you do well?
   • What do you need to learn to do?
   • What wishes should you be turning into plans?
   • What underdeveloped or misused resources do you have?
   • What should you start doing now?
   • What should you stop doing now? (source unknown)

4. Styles—How do you:

   • Ask for something
   • Get something you really want when there may be some resistance
   • Deal with conflict

5. If you could choose a job or career other than your present one, which five would you most likely consider?
6. In each of the following areas, list your most important goals for the next month, the next 6 months, the next 2 years.

   • Your relationship with yourself
   • Your relationship with another

- Work, creativity
- Financial prosperity
- Health and appearance
- Recreation and/or travel
- The world around you (Gawain, 1982, p. 49)

7. Write your own eulogy.

Readings

- Baruch, G., Barnett, R., & Rivers, C. *Life prints: New patterns of love and work for today's women*. New York: A Plume Book, 1983.
- Bingham, M., et al. *Choices: A teen woman's journal for self-awareness and personal planning*. Santa Barbara, Ca.: Advocacy Press, 1983.
- Bradley, B., et al. *Single: Living your own way*. Reading, Mass.: Addison-Wesley, 1977.
- Gawain, S. *The creative visualization workbook*. Mill Valley, Ca.: Whatever Publishing, 1982.
- Goodman, E. *Turning points: How people change, through crisis and commitment*. New York: Doubleday, 1979.
- Sangiuliano, I. *In her time*. New York: Morrow Quill Paperback, 1980.
- Sheehey, G. *Passages*. New York: E.P. Dutton, 1976.

Discovering Your Body

Introduction. Women are generally more attuned to their bodies than are men (Murray, 1972; Sandelowski, 1981). Several reasons are offered for this: (1) women's role is more identified with their body and some of its functions (pregnancy, childbearing), (2) women experience cyclic phenomena (hormonal changes, menstruation), thus having a more constant reminder of the natural working of the body, and (3) women are under cultural pressure to be "beautiful" and thereby pay more attention to their outward appearance. Women may be more likely to equate their self with their body, whereas men's sense of self more commonly comes from work and achievement (Murray, 1972).

Greater attunement to their bodies, however, does not mean that women feel more positive about them. In fact, due to negative socialization, the opposite has often been true. As examples, natural body odors and pubic and limb hair have been labeled offensive, and menstruation called "the curse." Societal and media standards for beauty leave women with an internalized ideal that few can measure up to (Murray, 1972). Female clothing has frequently not been designed for body comfort—from the corsets and bustles of yesteryear to today's high heeled shoes. Women have also lived with the persistent exploitation of their bodies or body parts (especially breasts, legs, and genitalia) for the selling of everything from automobiles to pornographic materials.

These multiple societal influences often contributed to women feeling that their bodies were not their own. A factor that reinforced this feeling was that they frequently did lack knowledge of basic body parts and functions. The need to rely on "experts" for normal physiological events, as well as for care related to true disease processes, helped reduce a sense of self-control.

The women's movement encouraged women to reclaim their bodies—to be knowledgeable and accepting of them without having to conform to unrealistic standards for weight, shape, cosmetic appearance, or dress. A further outcome was that women sought information about their bodies and questioned some of the treatments and procedures routinely performed on them. Self-care routines, such as breast self-examination, enabled many women to assume responsibility for monitoring their own breast tissue; pelvic self-examinations helped others to visualize and identify sexual organs previously labeled "down there."

Greater acceptance of their physical selves, as well as the recent emphasis on preventive health care, especially in regard to nutrition, exercise, and stress reduction, has stimulated many women to focus on their bodies in a more healthful way. Blum (1977) credits women with having greater ability to take health information and allow it to interact with feelings, thus providing insight that will more likely lead to a positive behavioral change. An educational process that combines these factors has the potential to help women become more comfortable with, more knowledgeable of, and more responsible for their bodies. Rather than being a source of dissatisfaction, the female body can be celebrated.

Educational Goals. To assist women in:

1. Recognition of influences on their standards for beauty and the ideal body.
2. Becoming familiar with body parts and their feelings about them.
3. Reflection on the unique responses and capabilities of the female body.
4. Accepting responsibility for their bodies.

Activities
Individual

1. Exercise—The Outer Physical
   See Chapter 6, Exercise 11
2. Place your body in contact with various environmental textures and reflect on the sensations experienced. Examples—a hot shower, cool grass, rain, wind, sand, mud.
3. In writing, list ways your body gives you messages. Examples—cyclic phenomena, symptoms of fatigue, stress.
4. List your common activities or practices that are potentially *helpful* and *harmful* to your body.
5. Ask your health care provider to explain body parts and functions or disease processes as they occur for you.

Group

1. Review and discuss advertisements and commercials that use women's bodies to sell products. What response do you have to them? What messages are conveyed?
2. Exercise—Body Drawings
   See Chapter 6, Exercise 12
3. Exercise—Body Touching
   See Chapter 6, Exercise 13
4. Discuss the issue of women and weight, using either of two books:

   • Orbach, S. *Fat is a feminist issue*.
   • Chernin, K. *The obsession: Reflections on the tyranny of slenderness*.

5. Describe a memorable experience related to your body. Compare experiences with other women. Examples: your first menstrual period, being pregnant/giving birth, losing a body part, receiving a massage.
6. Discuss: What does it mean to "take control" of your body?

Readings

- Ayalah, D., & Weinstock, I. *Breasts*. New York: Summit Books, 1979.
- Boston Women's Health Book Collective. *Our bodies, ourselves* (2nd ed.). New York: Simon and Schuster, 1976.
- Chernin, K. *The obsession: Reflections on the tyranny of slenderness*. New York: Harper Colophon Books, 1982.
- Federation of Feminist Women's Health Centers. *A new view of women's body*. New York: Simon and Schuster, 1981.
- Goffman, E. *Gender advertisements*. New York: Harper and Row, 1979.
- Orbach, S. *Fat is a feminist issue*. New York: Berkley Books, 1978.
- Rush, A. *Getting clear: Body work for women*. New York: Random House, 1973.
- *Women: A journal of liberation*. 1982, 8(2). Entire issue on women and their bodies.
- Woods, N. Woman's body. In C. Fogel & N. Woods (Eds.), *Health care of women: A nursing perspective* (Ch. 5). St. Louis: C. V. Mosby, 1981.

Discovering Your Health

Introduction. Chapter 1 provides an overview of women's health issues, their unique needs and risks, historical and current problems related to provision of care, and a rationale for specialized health education for women.

Fortunately, we have moved beyond the days of viewing women as being societally limited because of their biology, or of being inherently or fashionably sick as a part of their feminine role. Likewise, the biased judgments and labeling of women in regard to their physical and psychological care have lessened, and the quality and quantity of research on women has improved. Women are generally more knowledgeable and participatory in their health care than they were a decade ago.

Health has also assumed a new dimension. No longer considered just the absence of disease or the sum of one's biological, psychological, and social parts, it is viewed as a more complex phenomenon that is dynamic and changing. Health may be experienced on a continuum from wellness to illness (Ardell, 1977; Travis, 1975). It is also subject to personal definition, based on individual beliefs and values, or perhaps on whether or not a person feels well (Sandelowski, 1981).

This multidimensional view of health is especially relevant for women, whose health is frequently considered in terms of their reproductive status and needs. Health for women includes other varied aspects of physical and emotional well-being in the context of the changes and transitions that women have experienced. Sandelowski (1981) states that if health includes achievement of full potential, then women as a group are not yet healthy. She adds that a feminine definition of health includes:

> . . . the ability to change because we choose to . . . knowing ourselves well . . . exploring ourselves, our bodies and minds . . . finding pleasure from our own bodies . . . loving and nurturing the self . . . assuming personal power and responsibility, and the

ability to define how we conform to and how we differ from society's expectation of us . . . most important, it is to refuse to be a victim. (p. 93)

In defining and quantifying the health of women, transitional needs and risk factors need to be considered. What, if any, are the consequences of earlier sexual activity, having fewer children, increased participation in the work force, and living longer (Woods, 1981)? What about increased smoking among women, increased exposure to toxins and environmental hazards, and greater participation in the aggressive/risk-taking professional world? Will women's positive health behaviors—greater concern with health, more familiarity with the system, earlier care-seeking for minor symptoms— provide a balance for the changing risk factors?

Riessman (1983) warns against a new form of medicalization of women's health care during this time of transition. As physicians acknowledge women's experiences, learn more about their physiology, and develop helpful treatments, some common problems can be stripped of their political content and returned to traditional medical management. Riessman cites several examples of this, such as regimens for PMS/dysmenorrhea and weight control, and suggests that women maintain an awareness of the social phenomena that remain a part of these conditions. She proposes that women can retain control of their health care by acquiring a good knowledge base, practicing self-care (preventive health behaviors, use of alternatives to medication and technological treatment) and by working collaboratively with traditional providers in decisions related to medical regimens. An educational process can help women define and set goals for their individual health, as well as maintain ownership of the milieu of women's health in general.

Educational Goals. To assist women in:

1. Developing a personal, holistic definition of health.
2. Recognizing their personal biological and life-style health risks, and planning for reduction of those risks.
3. Maintaining awareness of psychosocial and political issues that remain a part of women's health care.
4. Maintaining an active role in care and decisions related to their health.

Activities
Individual

1. Define "health" and "women's health."
2. Write a personal definition of "good health" for you.
3. Do one of the following:

    • Complete a standard health history which includes a personal and family history.
    • Do a multigenerational "family tree" of health, listing longevity, chronic or serious illnesses, cause of death.

    Evaluate your individual risk based on the information you compile.
4. Complete a life-style assessment that will help evaluate wellness levels and preventive health behaviors.
    Tools:

    • *Wellness–worseness continuum*. In D. Ardell (Ed.), *High level wellness*. Emmaus, Pa.: Rodale Press, 1977.

- *Wellness inventory*, available from John Travis, M.D., Wellness Resource Center, 42 Miller Ave., Mill Valley, CA, 94941.
- These and other assessment tools are also reprinted in P. Flynn, *Holistic health: The act and science of care*. Bowie, Md.: Robert J. Brady Co., 1980, Chapter 6.

5. Do a gynecological family history
   a. Age of menarche, menopause. Occurrence of dysmenorrhea, premenstrual syndrome. Beliefs and behaviors related to menstruation.
   b. Occurrence of gynecological conditions—congenital anomalies, fibrocystic breasts, ovarian cysts, ectopic pregnancies, fertility problems, etc.
   c. Occurrence of cancers—breast, uterine, cervical, ovarian, vulvar.
6. Keep a health diary. It can be related to your general well-being or to a specific item, i.e., menstrual cycle, mood changes, pregnancy, eating habits, responses to exercise, responses to a treatment regimen. Evaluate periodically. Are there patterns of which you were previously not aware? Does day-to-day data disprove anything you perceived was occurring?
7. Set two health goals for yourself, using the following format.
   a. What I want to accomplish in the next _____ months.
   b. How I plan to do this.
   c. How I might block myself.
   d. How I will know that I have accomplished the goal in item a. (Flynn, 1980, p. 131)

Group

1. Share definitions of "health" and "women's health."
2. After individually assessing biological and life-style risk factors, have each member present her risk profile to the group. Discuss preventive or risk-reducing behaviors.
3. Discuss psychosocial or political factors that may be a part of common female conditions. Examples: obesity, anorexia nervosa, depression, dysmenorrhea.
4. Discuss: Why do you think women live longer and are generally healthier than men?
5. Discuss: In what ways are you your own health care provider? How do you decide what you will treat or deal with, and when you will involve a health care provider?
6. Describe/discuss situations where a decision was made regarding your health. Who made the decision? (you, your provider, both) What comprised the decision-making process? Who was "in charge" of the situation? If the situation was problematic, how could it have been changed?

Readings

- Bermosk, L., & Porter, S. *Women's health and human wholeness*. New York: Appleton-Century-Crofts, 1979.
- Boston Women's Health Book Collective. *Our bodies, ourselves* (2nd ed.). New York: Simon & Schuster, 1976.
- Corea, G. *The hidden malpractice*. New York: William Morrow, 1977.
- Ehrenreich, B., & English, D. *Complaints and disorders: The sexual politics of sickness*. Old Westbury, N.Y.: The Feminist Press, 1973.

- Flynn, P. *Holistic health: The art and science of care*. Bowie, Md.: Robert J. Brady, 1980.
- Fogel, C., & Woods, N. *Health care of women: A nursing perspective*. St. Louis, Mo.: C. V. Mosby, 1981.
- Martin, L. *Health care of women*. Philadelphia: J. B. Lippincott, 1978.
- Pelletier, K. *Mind as healer, mind as slayer*. New York: Dell, 1977.
- Riessman, C. Women and medicalization: A new perspective. *Social Policy*, 1983, *14*(1), 3–18.
- Sandelowski, M. *Women, health and choice*. Englewood Cliffs, N.J.: Prentice-Hall, 1981.
- Verbrugge, L. Sex differentials in health. *Public Health Reports*, 1982, 97(5), 417–437.

Discovering Your Relationships

Introduction. Human relationships have undergone changes during the past decade. The changes can be noted in patterns of relating, in duration and continuity of acquaintance, and in the values placed on friendships between different groups of people.

Several factors have influenced this transition. "Communicating" has come to be considered an important attribute, and skills for such have been taught in places as diverse as encounter groups and boardrooms. The mobility of American society has moved people from long-term family and community relationships to a more "revolving-door" sequence of acquaintances. But most of all, the changes that have occurred in and for women have caused the rethinking and reworking of their relationships with their families, with men, and with other women. Traditional as well as revisionist literature speaks of the impact of these changes.

A woman's first close relationship is usually with her mother, beginning at infancy. Mothers hold female children more frequently, are more verbal with them, and spend more time in close proximity than with their sons (Magrab, 1979). Through childhood and adolescence mothers serve as role models, and many of the daughter's sex role behavior patterns are attained from her.

Much is written about the ambivalence of the mother–daughter relationship. Traditional theorists focus on women living through their daughters or seeing them as rivals. Eichenbaum and Orbach (1983) pose that women may be reworking their own mother–daughter relationship at the same time they are parenting daughters, and thus conflicting feelings and behaviors occur. However, not all mother–daughter relationships are conflictual, even at the adult separation stage. Magrab (1979) suggests that when opportunities beyond the wife and mother role are fully available to women, and when husbands and other persons or agencies participate in child care, then the mother–daughter identity bond may be less intense. In a current-day role reversal, daughters sometimes serve as role models for mothers who have aspirations for changing their own lives.

Fathers are sometimes termed the forgotten parent for their daughters. In traditional families, they are usually less involved in child care and consider little girls, especially, the responsibility of their mothers (Lamb, Owen, & Chase-Lansdale, 1979). Yet, fathers exhibit much warmth to their daughters, and often the special feeling of being "daddy's little girl" emerges. Sometimes girls who are socialized to stereotypical feminine behaviors use cuteness and charm to get what they want from their fathers.

From much of the existing literature, the father's major influence on daughters is to reinforce traditional feminine behavior. Studies of women who are successful in careers, however, show that they frequently have close relationships with both parents, and that expressive and achieving behaviors were equally encouraged (Bardwick, 1979; Lamb, Owen, & Chase-Lansdale, 1979). Thus, future fathers who more fully participate in childrearing and who have less stereotypical attitudes of women can provide a positive reinforcement as daughters explore their changing options.

The relationships between adult women and men are also changing. Namely, women are moving from secondary status to a more equal and participatory role as they interact with men. Communication can be more direct; women need not resort to flirtation or other subtle ways to be heard. Women can initiate relationships, and need not give up such things as name and job if they enter into a marriage partnership.

Moving away from sex-stereotyped forms of interacting has provided freedoms for men, too. Yet, the changes have not been without difficulties as the issues of power and responsibility are resolved. Women's socialization has prepared them to relate to others in a more intimate way (Bernard, 1981) and to be more expressive and disclosing (Henley & Freeman, 1976). This is somewhat opposite of male socialization. In several studies, men indicate more often than women that their emotional needs are satisfied in a marriage relationship; women also report seeking support from female friends and relatives (Bernard, 1981; Warren, 1975). It is probably still more difficult for women to have close male friendships outside of marriage, because of the sexual innuendo that accompanies it.

Women's friendships with other women have often been considered secondary to their relationships with men. There is a popular stereotype that women do not like or trust each other. The theoretical rationale stated that little girls are sometimes ostracized from dyadic "best friends" groups during childhood, or are in competition with each other for boys during adolescence, and thus develop feelings of distrust. Boys, on the other hand, can substitute for each other and are more used to group and team play (Bardwick, 1979).

Female friendships have also been devalued because it was considered that women talked about less important things (clothes, children), whereas men talked about ideas, business, and politics.

The women's movement and consciousness-raising helped women recognize the value and uniqueness of female friendships. Women relate in a more supportive, intimate style and female friendships are "richer in spontaneity and confidences exchanged" (Booth, 1972, pp. 186–187). Women have become more aware that female friendships can be a choice and can be given priority, not scheduled around other persons or events (Eichenbaum & Orbach, 1983). Seiden and Bart (1975, p. 208) state that friendships among women must be relegitimatized "so that men and women may take them seriously and recognize that women may well make sacrifices to maintain them."

In intense, supportive female relationships, women are sometimes surprised and ashamed that feelings of jealousy or envy at other's achievements still surface, or that friends will disappoint or anger them. Eichenbaum and Orbach (1983) state that this is inevitable as long as women do not feel good or whole within themselves, and that in the future, some healthy feelings of competition may connote self-awareness and security.

Educational Goals. To assist women in:

1. Evaluating early family relationship patterns.
2. Looking at same-sex and opposite-sex patterns of relating.
3. Appreciating the value of friendships.

Activities
Individual

1. Reflect on childhood relationships with your mother and father. Did they relate to you in a similar or different way? What did each give you in the way of praise, punishment, physical affection, information about what it meant to be a girl, access to their work and activities? If you had a brother, was he treated similarly by each parent? What do you recall as being "special" between you and your mother, and you and your father?
2. List five favorite aunts, uncles, cousins, or grandparents. Consider why you named each one.
3. Trace your relationship with four childhood friends, female or male. When and why did any of them cease? If they still exist, what stages have they gone through?
4. Draw three concentric circles denoting three levels of friendship. Fill in each circle with 3 or 4 names.

   - Inner circle—your closest, most intimate friends who live in close geographic proximity to you.
   - Second circle—intimate friends who live at a distance; good friends just outside your most intimate group.
   - Third circle—good, but perhaps sporadic friendships.

   Over the past 10 years, have the individuals named moved from one circle to another? Why? If you are married, or in a steady relationship, in which circle is your partner?
5. Read books about long-term relationships, or changing relationships. Examples:

   - Marilyn French, *The women's room*.
   - Sara Davison, *Loose change*.
   - DuBois, E. (Ed.). *Elizabeth Cady Stanton, Susan B. Anthony: Correspondence, writings, speeches*. New York: Schocken Books, 1981.

Group

1. Discuss your relationship with your mother. What has been positive; what traumatic? Are you and your mother alike? More alike than you would wish? How similar or dissimilar are your life patterns? Optional: Use Nancy Friday's *My mother, myself*, as a discussion starter.
2. Read and discuss *Men are just desserts*, by Sonya Friedman.
3. Exercise—Intimacy
   See Chapter 6, Exercise 14
4. View a movie that explores female relationships. Discuss. Examples:

   - *The turning point* (Anne Bancroft, Shirley McLaine)
   - *Terms of endearment* (Shirley McLaine, Debra Winger)

5. Discuss: Did you ever cancel plans to go out with a female friend(s) because a man asked you out at the last minute? At what age or life stage did this occur? Why did/do you do it?

6. Individually list the attributes you most seek in a close friend. Do you have any friend who has all of these qualities? Is it possible for one or two friends to meet all your needs? If you are married or in a steady relationship, is it fair to expect a partner to meet most of your needs? Discuss.

The individual activities can also be adapted for group use.

Readings

- Arcana, J. *Our mother's daughters*. Berkeley, Calif.: Shameless Hussy Press, 1979.
- Bardwick, J. *In transition*. New York: Holt, Rinehart & Winston, 1979. Ch. 8, "Women's attitudes toward women."
- Bernard, J. *The female world*. New York: The Free Press, 1981. Ch. 12, "Kinship, network, and friendship groups."
- Caplan, P. *Barriers between women*. New York: SP Medical and Scientific Books, 1981.
- Eichenbaum, L., & Orbach, S. *What do women want: Exploding the myth of dependency*. New York: Coward-McCann, 1983.
- Friedman, S. *Men are just desserts*. New York: Warner Books, 1983.
- Friday, N. *My mother, myself*. New York: Delacorte Press, 1977.
- Goodwin, G. *A mother and two daughters*. New York: Avon Books, 1983.
- Lamb, M., Owen, M., & Chase-Lansdale, L. The father–daughter relationship: Past, present, and future. In C. Kopp (Ed.), *Becoming female: Perspectives on development*. New York: Plenum Press, 1979.
- Seiden, A., & Bart P. Women to women: Is sisterhood powerful? In N. Glazer (Ed.), *Old family/New family*. New York: D VanNostrand, 1975.
- Shain, M. *When lovers are friends*. Philadelphia: J. B. Lippincott, 1978.

Discovering Your Environment

Introduction

ENVIRONMENT—The aggregate of surrounding things, conditions or influences, especially as affecting the existence or development of someone or something.*

This segment does not contain any theoretical background or research studies. Rather, it includes a series of exercises and activities to stimulate women to think about their surroundings. Environment can include stimuli that give pleasure, encourage thought, help you dream and plan, open new horizons, acquaint you with other cultures, or cause you to experience deep feelings. Environment can be moods or feelings, people, places, geographic terrain, weather, colors. It can already exist, or it can be created by an individual or group.

Discovering the Existing Environment

1. Explore different geographic terrains within 100 miles of your home. How do you respond to different areas?

   - a craggy shore
   - summer woods with sun filtering through the trees

---

*The Random House dictionary of the English language, New York, Random House, 1967, p. 477.

- open fields
- a busy city block

2. Explore your town or city by block or area. Who lives there? What aura is created? What kind of women live there? What kind of diversity or homogeneity exists?
3. Treat yourself to a new physical experience, a facial, massage, hot tub bath, vigorous climb.
4. Attend a lecture/program/film on a topic that is totally new to you.
5. If your circle of friends is fairly homogenous, get acquainted with women from other racial or cultural groups. Learn about their customs and beliefs. Group exchange visits can be useful.
6. Read books about women from backgrounds other than your own. Examples:

   - Alice Walker, *The color purple* (black women)
   - Jane Howard, *A different woman* (white women)
   - K. Kahn, *Hillbilly woman*

7. Explore the religious groups represented in your town. What beliefs do they have about women?

Creating Your Own Environment

1. Imagine a room of your own that would be your hideaway. No one else can enter it unless you invite them in.

   - Where would the room be located?
   - How would it be furnished?
   - What colors and textures would be prominent?
   - For what purpose would you use the room?
   - Who else might be permitted to visit?

   Draw a sketch of the room. Actually create the room.

2. For one day, pretend to be another woman you have always wanted to be, either real or imagined. Dress and act the part accordingly.
3. Imagine yourself as the first female ——— (President, conductor of the New York Philharmonic, Orioles baseball player, Pope).

Discovering Your Work

Introduction. Women have always worked, within the sphere of their homes and sometimes outside of them. Yet their reasons for working, their tasks, work status, and salaries have usually differed from those of men. Moreover, what they do in terms of labor for their household or community is not truly considered "work."

Kessler-Harris (1981) describes the agricultural society of colonial days when mother, father, and children worked side by side in a relatively egalitarian manner to produce food, clothing, and other items necessary for survival. With the coming of the industrial revolution large numbers of men and women were employed in mills and factories. The term work gradually came to be associated with production in the public sphere that had a market value, and women who remained in their households became known as "nonworking women" or "nonworking mothers."

From this era through the mid-nineteenth century, several facts were evident. Jobs were classified as distinctly male or female, women received lower pay than men, and were not considered appropriate for management positions. They were not admitted to the apprenticing trades or to most of the unions that were formed (Kessler-Harris, 1981; Woods & Woods, 1981). Many were steered toward acceptable work roles—nursing, elementary school teaching, and secretarial jobs—that were perceived as natural extensions of their helping character.

Beliefs about female employees were that they worked primarily for extra money for the family, would quit to have children, lost more days due to illness, and in some instances, took jobs away from men (Freize et al., 1978; Woods & Woods, 1981).

Why were women not "successful?" Numerous authors pose that women have traditionally seen femininity and work achievement as mutually exclusive. Horner's (1972) research suggesting that women fear success was readily accepted; it gave theorists a rationale for women's ambivalence (Bardwick, 1979). However, at this same time women were beginning to examine their systematic exclusion from the real world of work. Although they made up a large part of the labor force they were not of it (Bernard, 1981). Housewives constituted a major unpaid labor group, pink collar workers were recipients of especially low wages and minimal benefits, and professional women had been excluded from mentorships and the "old boy networks" that helped men move up the career ladder.

Attitudes and behaviors have changed. Freize and colleagues (1978) state that women now work not only for financial reasons but for personal satisfaction. Bardwick (1979) further elaborates that as women recognize their equal right to choose what they will do, they will stop constructing the self in roles of relating and giving, and rather will build it through independent achievement.

Although having greater options in the work force has benefited women at all levels, some problems have occurred also. Men and women have had to learn to relate to each other in a new way as they worked on a more equal status. Women have experienced role proliferation; most who work still have the major responsibility for household management and child care. Work hazards and toxins need to be considered, especially for pregnant women in certain work sites. Stressors associated with new roles are also present.

A major discussion centers around whether women who rise in the professional and corporate world will experience more coronary heart disease, a condition common to men in this field. Haynes and Feinleib (1980) surveyed three groups of women—white collar, clerical, and housewives—and found that it was not the corporate but the clerical women who had the highest rate of coronary heart disease. Associated stressors were little power within the work environment, poor job mobility, an unsympathetic boss, and suppressed hostility.

Although the world of work has been opened to women in a new way, they are not totally "of" it yet. Women need to be aware of both the benefits and the risks of this transitional period.

Educational Goals. To assist women in:

1. Evaluating past and future work patterns, and the reasons for those patterns.
2. Exploring the benefits and the risks of work to their physical and emotional health.
3. Setting goals for future work.

Activities

1. On a large piece of paper draw a grid of your work life outside of your home. Along the left, list your jobs chronologically, from earliest to most recent. At the top of subsequent vertical columns, list headings of job duties, salary and benefits, why I worked, level of job satisfaction, what I learned, why I left. Complete for each job.
   For reflection:

   • How would you describe the pattern of your work life?
   • Were there any significant changes over time, especially in why you worked?
   • If you have a family, how have their needs influenced your work pattern? (full time/part time, moves for husband's/partner's job, children's education, etc.)
   • To what degree has your work pattern been a choice?

2. If you have been primarily a mother and homemaker, complete a similar grid. In the left hand column, use stages of your life, such as prechildren, with small children, with adolescent children; pre- and postdivorce, etc.

3. Consider the issues of "role proliferation" for yourself, that of having many parts of your life that consume attention and energy.

   • List your roles. Examples: secretary, wife, lover, mother, student, volunteer, club president, friend.
   • Which roles seem most easy/difficult to manage?
   • Which role elicits most conflict in you?
     What or who contributes to the situation?
   • How have you worked at resolving the conflict?
   • Did you list "self" as a role?

4. List your work goals and plans for the next 10 years.

Group

1. List five words that you think describe a "job" and five that describe a "career." Compare.
   Discuss:

   • How are they different or similar?
   • Which do you have?
   • Is homemaking or volunteer work a career?

2. After individually completing the work grid described in individual activity 1, compare and discuss.

3. Describe your first day at work outside of your home. If you worked at home for a long period of time and then reentered the outside work force, describe that day.

4. Discuss: What is a mentor?

   • Have you had one in your work life?
   • In what way did this person help you?
   • What were the advantages/disadvantages to having a male/female mentor? Did it make any difference?
   • If you did not have one, how might a mentor have made a difference for you?

5. Describe and compare the ambiance of your current work settings (small/large personnel group, private/open surrounding, regimented/casual, slow paced/hectic, human-oriented/mechanical).

   - Is the work atmosphere conducive to the task?
   - Is the work setting one in which you are comfortable and productive? Why or why not?

6. Discuss sexual harassment on the job.

   - What is it? How is it exhibited?
   - Describe personal experiences.
   - What are some of the difficulties in labeling and resolving it?
   - How can it be stopped?

7. Discuss: Do you work in a "man's world?"

   - Why or why not?
   - Are there differences in the work goals, work styles, communication and decision-making patterns of men and women?
   - What do both sexes need to learn about each other in the work setting?

8. List all the potential health hazards in your work setting (home or elsewhere). Consider lighting, ventilation, temperature, noise level, equipment, product content, management/organization style, interpersonal relationships, position in which most work is completed (sitting, standing, moving), miscellaneous stressors.

   - What are the major risks to your health in your current work setting?
   - What preventive measures have been taken by you or your organization? What else could be done?
   - Is there anything in your work setting that could present problems for women with special needs? (Pregnant, handicapped)

9. Role play conversations or interviews around situations that you think might be difficult for you. Examples: asking for a raise or promotion, entering a new field of work for which you have interest but minimal experience, discussing reorganization of household tasks with your family because you have decided to go back to school.

10. Discuss the work you would like to be doing 10 years from now. What steps will you need to take to reach that goal? What supports and barriers are present that will be influential?

Readings

- Bardwick, J. *In transition*. New York: Holt, Rinehart, and Winston, 1979. Ch. 3, "Work, the need for fulfillment."
- Carr-Ruffino, N. *The promotable woman: Becoming a successful manager*. Belmont, Calif.: Wadsworth, 1982.
- Cassedy, E., & Nussbaum, K. *9 to 5: The working woman's guide to office survival*. New York: Penguin Books, 1983.
- Hennig, M., & Jardim, A. *The managerial women*. New York: Doubleday, 1977.
- Howe, L. *Pink collar workers*. New York: Avon Books, 1977.

- Kanter, R. M. *Women and men of the corporation*. New York: Basic Books, 1977.
- Kessler-Harris, A. *Women have always worked*. Old Westbury, N.Y.: The Feminist Press, 1981.
- Mintor, M., & Block, J. *What is a woman worth?* New York: William Morrow, 1983.
- Norris, G., & Miller, J. *The working mother's complete handbook*. New York: A Sunrise Book/E. P. Dutton, 1979.
- Oakley, A. *Woman's work: The housewife, past and present*. New York: Vintage Books, 1976.
- Rosen, B., Rynes, S., & Mahoney, T. Compensation, jobs, and gender: Should a female nurse make as much as a male truck driver? *Harvard Business Review*, 1983, *61*, 170–190.
- Terkel, S. *Working*. New York: Pantheon Books, 1974.
- Woods, N., & Woods, J. Women and the workplace. In C. Fogel and N. Woods (Eds.), *Health care of women: A nursing perspective*. St. Louis, Mo.: C. V. Mosby, 1981.

BIBLIOGRAPHY

Ardell, D. B. *High level wellness*. Emmaus, Pa.: Rodale Press, 1977.
Bardwick, J. *In transition*. New York: Holt, Rinehart & Winston, 1979.
Berkin, C., & Norton, M. B. *Women of America: A history*. Boston: Houghton Mifflin, 1979.
Bernard, J. *The female world*. New York: The Free Press, 1981.
Bingham, M., Edmondson, J., & Stryker, S. *Choices: A teen woman's journal of self-awareness and personal planning*. Santa Barbara, Calif.: Advocacy Press, 1983.
Blum, L. H. Health information via mass media: A study of the individual's concepts of the body and its parts. *Psychological Reports*, 1977, *40*, 991–999.
Booth, A. Sex and social preparation. *American Sociological Review*, 1972, *37*, 123–192.
Corea, G. *The hidden malpractice*. New York: William Morrow, 1977.
Dowling, C. *The Cinderella complex*. New York: Pocket Books, 1981.
Eichenbaum, L., & Orbach, S. *What do women want: Exploding the myth of dependency*. New York: Coward-McCann, 1983.
Fesbach, N., Dillman, A., & Jordan, T. Portrait of a female on television: Some possible side effects on children. In C. Kopp (Ed.), *Becoming female: Perspectives on development*. New York: Plenum Press, 1979.
Fogel, C. Issues in the life cycle. In C. Fogel & N. Woods (Eds.), *Health care of women: A nursing perspective*. St. Louis, Mo.: C. V. Mosby, 1981.
Freize, I., Parsons, J., Johnson, P., Ruble, D., & Zellman, G. *Women and sex roles: A social psychological perspective*. New York: W. W. Norton, 1978.
Gawain, S. *The creative visualization workbook*. Mill Valley, Calif.: Whatever Publishing, 1982.
Gilligan, C. *In a different voice*. Cambridge, Mass.: Harvard University Press, 1982.
Haynes, S., & Feinleib, M. Women, work, and coronary heart disease. *American Journal of Public Health*, 1980, *70*, 133–141.
Henley, N., & Freeman, J. The sexual politics of interpersonal behavior. In S. Cox (Ed.), *Female psychology: The emerging self*. Chicago: Science Research Associates, 1976.
Horner, M. Toward an understanding of achievement-related conflicts in women. *Journal of Social Issues*, 1972, *28*(2), 157–175.
Hyde, J., & Rosenberg, B. *Half the human experience: The psychology of women*. Lexington, Mass.: D.C. Heath, 1976.
James, M. *Breaking free*. Reading, Mass.: Addison-Wesley, 1981.
Janeway, E. *Between myth and morning: Women's awakening*. New York: William Morrow, 1974.

Katz, P. The development of female identity. In C. Kopp (Ed.), *Becoming female: Perspectives on development*. New York: Plenum Press, 1979.

Kessler-Harris, A. *Women have always worked*. Old Westbury, N.Y.: The Feminist Press, 1981.

Lamb, M., Owen, M., & Chase-Lansdale, L. The father–daughter relationship: Past, present, and future. In C. Kopp (Ed.), *Becoming female: Perspectives on development*. New York: Plenum Press, 1979.

Lasky, E. Self-esteem, achievement, and the female experience. In J. Muff (Ed.), *Socialization, sexism, and sterotyping: Women's issues in nursing*. St. Louis, Mo.: C. V. Mosby, 1982.

Lerner, H. Female dependency in context: Some theoretical and technical considerations. *American Journal of Orthopsychiatry*, 1983, 53(4), 697–705.

Maccoby, E., & Jacklin, C. *The psychology of sex differences* (Vol. 1/Text). Stanford, Calif.: Stanford University Press, 1974.

Magrab, P. Mothers and daughters. In C. Kopp (Ed.), *Becoming female: Perspectives on development*. New York: Plenum Press, 1979.

Muff, J. (Ed.). *Socialization, sexism, and stereotyping: Women's issues in nursing*. St. Louis, Mo.: C. V. Mosby, 1982.

Murray, R. Body image development in adulthood. *Nursing Clinics of North America*. 1972, 7(4), 617–629.

Riessman, C. Women and medicalization: A new perspective. *Social Policy*, 1983, 14(1), 3–18.

Rich, A. *Of woman born: Motherhood as an experience and institution*. New York: Norton, 1976.

Rosaldo, M., & Lamphere, L. (Eds.). *Women, culture, & society*. Stanford, Calif.: Stanford University Press, 1974.

Rush, A. *Getting clear: Body work for women*. New York: Random House, 1973.

Sacks, S. Rethinking gender identity: A continuing process. In J. Muff (Ed.), *Socialization, sexism, and sterotyping: Women's issues in nursing*. St. Louis, Mo.: C.V. Mosby, 1982.

Sandelowski, M. *Women, health, and choice*. Englewood Cliffs, N.J.: Prentice-Hall, 1981.

Sangiuliano, I. *In her time*. New York: Morrow Quill Paperbacks, 1980.

Seiden, A., & Bart, P. Woman to woman: Is sisterhood powerful? In N. Glazer (Ed.), *Old family/new family*. New York: D Van Nostrand, 1975.

Sheehy, G. *Passages*. New York: E.P. Dutton, 1976.

Solomon, B. (Ed.). *The experience of the American woman*. New York: A Mentor Book, 1978.

Stage, S. *Female complaints: Lydia Pinkham and the business of women's medicine*. New York: W. W. Norton, 1979.

Stoll, C. *Female and male: Socialization, social roles, and social structure*. Dubuque, Iowa: William C. Brown, 1974.

Travis, J. W. *Wellness workbook*. Mill Valley, Calif.: Wellness Center, 1975.

Walum, L. *The dynamics of sex and gender: A socialization perspective*. Chicago: Rand McNally College, 1977.

Warren, M. *The work role and problem coping: Sex differences in the use of helping systems in urban communities*. Paper presented at American Sociological Association, San Francisco, 1975.

Weitzman, L. Sex role socialization. In J. Muff (Ed.), *Socialization, sexism, and sterotyping: Women's issues in nursing*. St. Louis, Mo.: C. V. Mosby, 1982.

Williams, J. *Psychology of women: Behavior in a biosocial content*. New York: W.W. Norton, 1977.

Woods, N. Woman's body. In C. Fogel & N. Woods (Eds.), *Health care of women: A nursing perspective*. St. Louis, Mo.: C. V. Mosby, 1981.

Woods, N., & Woods, J. Women and the workplace. In C. Fogel & N. Woods (Eds.), *Health care of women: A nursing perspective*. St. Louis, Mo.: C. V. Mosby, 1981.

Wyckoff, H. *Solving women's problems*. New York: Grove Press, 1977.

Education for
Sexual Self-awareness

6

Phyllis Collier

Much has been written about female sexuality throughout history. However, the content was frequently shrouded in myth and mysticism, was influenced by the social perception of women's role at the time, and was seldom written by women themelves. Fortunately, we live in a different era, where we have begun to view sexuality as more than genital acts and where an increasing amount of research and written information related to female sexuality is available. In addition, women are challenging the myths and the stereotypes of the past, and are exploring and redefining the nature and the expression of their sexuality. Educators, counselors, and providers of women's health care can learn from women as well as help them in this process of growth and self-discovery.

In defining human sexuality, components frequently included are:

1. Biological sex—female/male.
2. Gender identity—one's sense of being female or male; may potentially be different from biological sex.
3. Sex role—an individual's perception of what constitutes appropriate behavior, attitudes, beliefs, and emotions for a woman or a man and how that is practiced or conveyed in relationships with others (Martin, 1978).
4. Sexual orientation—heterosexuality, bisexuality, homosexuality, and practices related to that preference.
5. A range of pleasurable and erotic behaviors experienced by an individual, alone or with other persons.

In a more inclusive definition of this complex phenomenon, Roberts states (1980, p. 241)

> . . . Our sexuality is part of our basic identity. It encompasses our total sense of self as male or female. It involves our attitudes, values, feelings, and beliefs about masculinity and femininity; how we feel about our physical selves—the limits, the joys, and the embarrassments of our bodies. It is the integration of our needs for affiliation and inti-

---

Except when specific credit is given, the exercises in this chapter have been developed by the author or adapted from uncredited materials used in numerous sexuality workshops and seminars. Excellent background sources were books or training manuals by Calnek and Levine (1981), Helmich and Loreen (1979), and Read (1979).

macy, and our expressions of love and affection, as well as our fears, fantasies, and decisions regarding our erotic conduct. Human sexuality is expressed in our full range of interactions with others. It influences and is influenced by our interpersonal relationships, our family roles, and our social life-styles. Thus sexuality is integral to the establishment of self-image, self-understanding, and personal identity and to the formation of human relationships.

Much of our sexuality is learned, rather than being innate. Sexual learning often parallels social learning (Roberts, 1980) and is influenced by family, peers, culture, religion, the media, and societal trends. The accumulation of knowledge, values, and beliefs related to sexuality occurs throughout life, often in a manner that is "chaotic and disorderly . . . never quite completely integrated" (Roberts, 1980, p. 298). Thus, many have difficulty sorting through the conflicting messages, double standards, and life experiences that influence their personal sexual code.

Female sexuality traditionally was seen as a response to male sexuality and intercourse, with minimal acknowledgment of the uniqueness of the female experience (Hite, 1976). "Good" women were considered to be passive partners, with little interest in or need for sex other than for purposes of procreation. Their opposites were the sexual temptresses, the women with uncontrollable erotic appetites.

Over time, a number of myths and barriers have hindered the process of exploring and defining the nature of female sexuality.

1. Sex was considered more important for men than for women.
2. Women were socialized to be sexually dependent on men, as opposed to having autonomous needs and desires (Huerter, 1979).
3. Expression of sexuality was inseparable from female role socialization (Martin, 1978).
4. Behaviors of all kinds were more rigidly defined and regulated for women (Williams, 1977).
5. There was a major lack of factual information regarding female sexuality, and much bias in what was available.
6. Women tended to see their individual experiences and feelings as unique, and had difficulty talking about them with other women (Huerter, 1979).
7. Sex/sexuality was seen as a source of problems, rather than as an essential and important part of one's identity (Roberts, 1980).

Of the theorists and researchers who studied female sexuality, Freud was among the first to give increased credence to its existence and its normalcy. Yet, he was very much a product of the societal beliefs of the late 1800s and his theories reinforced the idea of women's expression of their sexuality through motherhood (anatomy is destiny) and of the sexual superiority of the male (penis envy). In addition, he defined "mature" feminine sexuality as the ability to have vaginal orgasms rather than "immature" clitoral ones (Freize et al., 1978; Williams, 1977).

In the early 1900s, Havelock Ellis published his cross-cultural studies of human sexual behavior. His work disputed the myth that women had little or no sex drive and emphasized the varieties of sexual behaviors practiced by both men and women. He was also an advocate of societal equality for women, and worked for the reform of divorce laws and the public availability of birth control methods.

More scientific research in the field of sexuality took place in the fifties and sixties. Studies by Kinsey and Masters and Johnson were instrumental in opening this field as a valid one for study, as well as for providing contradictory evidence to the prevailing

Freudian views of female sexual functioning. Kinsey found that more women masturbated and had premarital sexual experiences than had been thought, that some women were capable of multiple orgasms, and published his belief that the clitoris, rather than the vagina, was the primary response site for the female (Lewis, 1980). Masters and Johnson (1966) found the sexual response cycle to be similar for both sexes and negated the difference between vaginal and clitoral orgasms. These studies, plus some of the societal changes of the decade that followed, set the stage for revisionist views of female sexuality.

In the 1970s numerous social movements occurred that built upon one another. Several provided impetus for the rethinking of female sexuality: (1) the women's movement, with its emphasis on sexual equality and reproductive freedoms; (2) the "sexual revolution," which engendered more open discussion and questioning of sexual norms; and (3) the human potential movement, which focused on personal growth through the discovery of the self. During this period women openly challenged the systems that had denied them equal status and participation in all realms of society. Concerns related to sexual health focused on gaps in information and research, bias on the part of care providers (particularly among obstetrician–gynecologists and mental health providers), and the lack of opportunity to express what they knew about their sexuality and be taken seriously.

One outcome of this era was that women began to share information and experiences with each other. Through formats such as consciousness-raising groups and health collectives they validated the commonality as well as the diversity of the female experience. Change was effected on many fronts as women became more knowledgeable and assertive; this was especially noticeable in the areas of sexual and reproductive options.

The social and political phenomena that accompany female sexuality throughout history are important to examine. Current information related to female psychosexual development and sexual functioning adds another dimension of knowledge.

Women's psychosexual development includes a biological as well as a psychosocial component. Genetically, the union of X chromosomes from both the mother and the father normally results in a female offspring. A gender assignment (female) begins at birth and the child is socialized according to parental and societal beliefs regarding that sex. The capacity for sexual response is present at birth, and both vaginal lubrication and orgasmic patterns have been noticed in female infants (Kolodny et al., 1979). Beyond infancy, gender identity and gender role begin to develop. Female children identify and adopt behaviors deemed appropriate to their sex, as learned from parents and the culture at large. Theories vary as to how this process takes place (see Chapter 4 and introduction to Chapter 5). Childhood is also a time when natural curiosity about genitalia occurs, and negative messages from parents and others can be internalized.

Puberty pushes adolescent females into a major phase of psychosexual development. Development of secondary sex characteristics brings on a critical reassessment of body image. Menstruation introduces the potential capacity to reproduce. Personal sexual values are being developed and a preference for the gender of a partner is being established (Lion, 1982). Social pressures to be popular or to "be a woman" sometimes force current-day teenagers to become sexually active before their sexual identity and values are formed.

Although adult sexuality is not usually considered in terms of a developmental stage, women may undergo new life experiences, development of more mature heterosexual or homosexual relationships, pregnancy, childbearing, lactation, and parenting. Given the negative sexual socialization in women's past, it may also be a stage of unlearning and reexploration of what their sexuality incurs.

Female sexual anatomy and physiological response has some unique aspects, also. Sexual organs are more contained within the body, resulting in a less visible awareness of what takes place. Both men and women follow the same general phases of the sexual response cycle—excitement, plateau, orgasm, and resolution. However, Masters and Johnson described more variations in the response pattern for women. The most notable difference is that women need not totally complete the resolution phase before restarting a new cycle, thus making them capable of having multiple orgasms.

Approximately 90 percent of women have experienced orgasm at some time; 75 percent experience it on a fairly regular basis (Martin, 1978). However, as few as 30 percent of the women in Hite's (1976) survey reported achieving orgasm from intercourse alone; most needed additional clitoral stimulation. The role of orgasm as a determinant of women's level of sexual satisfaction has elicited varying responses. There is no longer doubt about its importance to women, but Kitzinger (1983) proposes that both society and numerous sex researchers have made it THE measure of sexual success. Although some women may feel that sex without orgasm is unsatisfactory, others may place equal importance on the total experience of lovemaking and the feelings and pleasures engendered.

Studies show that approximately 65 to 80 percent of women masturbate, and many find that it gives them a more intense orgasm (Martin, 1978). In recent years women have practiced it both for a pleasurable individual sexual experience as well as for getting in touch with their bodies and becoming orgasmic.

Female sexuality has many components—biological, psychological, social—as well as its long history of myths and beliefs. It is still in the process of being studied and redefined. In contrast to the past, however, female sexuality:

1. Is an integral part of a woman's life.
2. Is as important to women as it is to men.
3. Is autonomous and not dependent on men or male sexual behaviors.
4. Is influenced by some unique physiology and social experiences.
5. Includes options and choices.
6. Is a cause for celebration and not merely a source of problems.

Sangiuliano (1980) has proposed that many women have "postponed" the development of an autonomous sexual identity; that the restrictions and discomforts of the past, as well as the new unknowns hinder them in exploring this part of themselves. Kerr (1977) states that although women now have permission to be free, many of them are not. The changing rules have opened the door to new attitudes and behaviors for others, but sometimes new myths and expectations accompany them. As an example, whereas orgasms were once considered unimportant to the sexual experience, some women now feel "cheated" if they are unable to attain multiple orgasms.

In spite of many positive gains in the area of female sexuality, not all women fully know and value themselves as sexual beings. Stressors still exist. An educational process that deals with both facts and feelings can assist clients as they choose their individual path toward sexual wholeness.

Providers who assist women in this process need not be "experts" or sex therapists. They do need; however, in-depth factual knowledge and a level of comfort with their own sexuality. In addition, they need skills to assess needs and provide interventions for women who are seeking to understand their sexuality. Methodologies in this chapter are designed for both individual and group education in a variety of settings, such as hospitals, health centers, women's groups, and church and community organizations.

LEARNING NEEDS

Learning needs related to sexual self-awareness fall into three major categories—affective learning, cognitive learning, and specific skills. They cannot all be distinctly separated, i.e., some factual information has an emotional component, also. The learning needs are focused around the characteristics of a sexually healthy person as described by Lion (1982); they have a positive body image; see their sexual organs and bodily functions as normal and natural; have a cognitive knowledge of sexuality that is factual and free from myth; see sex as a function of sexuality, not an object to be gained; are aware of and appreciate their own and others' feelings and attitudes regarding sexuality; and experience harmony in their physiological, psychological, and sociological lives.

Affective Learning Needs
Awareness of:

1. Components of female sexuality and how the parts are interrelated.
2. Past sociocultural influences on present sexual values and behaviors.
3. Comforts/discomforts related to various areas of sexuality.
4. Enhancers/deterrents to personal sexual growth.
5. Individual goals/expectations regarding sexuality.

Cognitive Learning Needs

1. Female growth and development.
2. Female anatomy and physiology.
3. Sexual response cycle.
4. Range of sexual expression and preferences.

Specific Skills

1. Body awareness and pleasuring.
2. Communication—with peers, partners, providers.

Assessment. Assessment of female sexuality and related learning needs can involve knowledge and motivation levels, feelings, concerns, and life experiences. It should include what is communicated verbally as well as the nonverbal clues given, such as comfort versus embarrassment or anxiety related to sexual topics. In talking with women about their sexuality, the following principles should be kept in mind (Hogan, 1980; Lion, 1982; Seimens & Brandzel, 1982).

1. Give "permission" to talk about sexuality by initiating a routine question during a health history or interview or in a group discussion. This establishes the provider as a person who is willing to discuss the subject.
2. Start with topics that are generally less emotionally loaded for the average person. Example: How they learned about sex, as opposed to their sexual practices.
3. Establish a vocabulary common to all involved. Clarify words or descriptive terms that are unclear or unknown.
4. Use open-ended questions or comments when possible, although sometimes directness is useful or appropriate.
5. Use a universal approach, connoting common human experiences. Example:

"Many women find that they enjoy masturbation" or "Some people find it difficult to talk with their partner. . . . Has this been your experience?"

6. Assume a range of sexual values, experiences, and orientations.
7. Be reassuring, empathetic, and nonjudgmental.
8. Provide an unhurried atmosphere; allow time for the woman to express herself.
9. Provide privacy, especially for a one-to-one discussion.
10. Do not force anyone to talk about their sexuality if they are not ready to do so.

The following are some examples of sexual assessment tools that can be used in a variety of settings.

1. *Client check list*
   Designed for use in health care settings. Could also be adapted for assessment of learning needs of a group.

   Listed below are topics about which many patients seek discussion. It will be helpful to your provider if you will check those you would like to talk about on this visit.*

The check list will be returned to you at the end of your visit.

_____ Premarital counseling	_____ Finances
_____ Pregnancy	_____ Sexually transmitted disease
_____ Contraception	_____ Sexual inadequacy of partner
_____ Breast self-examination	_____ Marriage problems
_____ Douching or other feminine hygiene practices	_____ Failure to please partner
_____ Menopause	_____ Sexual practices
_____ Menstruation	_____ Divorce
_____ Parenthood	_____ Being single
_____ Painful intercourse	_____ Widowhood
_____ Inability or difficulty in reaching orgasm	_____ Options in life-style
_____ Homosexual feelings	_____ Pressures from friends
_____ Masturbation	_____ Social pressures
_____ Sterilization	_____ Loneliness
_____ Abortion	_____ Security
_____ Doubts about whether or not you are normal	_____ Effects of medications, drugs, alcohol
_____ Difficulty in responding to partner	_____ Sexual assault, rape
	_____ Other (list)

2. *Introductory assessment statements*
   Designed for use in a health history, or a counseling interview. Selected ones could be used in a group.

---

*From *NAACOG Technical Bulletin*, Number 1, April 1977.

- What questions do you have regarding sex/sexuality?
- How do you feel about the sexual part of your life?
- Have you noticed any changes in your sexual functioning/intimate relationships?
- If you could change something related to your sexuality, what would it be?

3. *Assessment process for a sexual problem/concern**
   May follow a problem identified during the introductory assessment.
   Data to elicit:
   a. Description of problem in client's terms.
   b. Onset, course. Constant versus occasional; relationship to an event, medication, drug/alcohol use; factors that increase or relieve the problem.
   c. Perceptions of why the problem has occurred.
   d. Expectations, goals for treatment.
   e. Who else is involved or knows about the problem, impact on relationships.
   f. Previous professional or other help sought.
      Phrases to expand information:

      - Can you describe it . . . more?
      - How is it different from what it used to be?
      - What else is on your mind about this?
      - How do you feel about . . . ?
      - What has been the most difficult part of this situation for you?

4. *Miscellaneous open-ended assessment questions*
   Designed for individuals or group; can be written or stated verbally, then discussed.
   a. Regarding my sexuality:

      - I feel great about _____
      - I wish I felt better about _____
      - I know a lot about _____
      - I wish I knew more about _____

   b. I feel positive—neutral—negative about:

Being a woman	Foreplay
Being the age I am	Intercourse
Menstruating	Oral-genital sex
My body (generally)	Masturbation
My breasts	Fantasizing
My genitals	Orgasms

   c. Messages I got about sex from:

Mother	Clergy/church
Father	Lovers
Friends	Spouse

---

*Adapted from N. Woods, *Human sexuality in health and illness* (1979).

Teacher   Children
Media

   d. One thing I would like to change about my sexuality is _____
       _____

5. *Assessment of cognitive knowledge*
    This is occasionally done by administering written exams, with questions and/or
    diagrams that need completing. Often used to measure knowledge of sexual
    anatomy and physiology and other factual information. Knowledge levels can also
    be informally assessed through conversations with clients.

EDUCATIONAL METHODOLOGIES

Format. Several formats have been used for sexuality education, the two most common
being the individual and group approaches. Both require a teacher/care provider. A third
type of format is the self-help/self-care approach in which women themselves take full
responsibility for their own learning.

Individual Education. An advantage of one-to-one sexuality education is that it can be
initiated as soon as needs are made known, and can be tailored specifically to the person
and the situation. Some women will ask questions or articulate needs in a private session,
but would not feel comfortable doing so in a group. A disadvantage of individual education is that the client does not have the benefit of hearing directly about other women's
experiences. It is also less time-efficient for the provider, particularly if the educational
process is a lengthy one.

Group Education. Groups are frequently used for sexuality education. Both the commonality and the diversity of individual experiences and beliefs help to stimulate discussion
and self-evaluation within a group. Women frequently learn from each other in this type
of format. A disadvantage is that some women may get "lost" in a group that is attempting to deal with many needs.

Self-help Education. Self-help groups are voluntary groups organized by peers who share
a common need or concern (Kush-Goldberg, 1979). They are sometimes formed because
of dissatisfaction with traditional services related to education or care. During the 1970s,
many women's health groups were formed for this reason, with sexuality being a common
topic for discussion. The inclusion of a professional in this kind of group has the potential
for changing the egalitarian atmosphere; however, many groups use providers as guest
presenters or consultants for their learning needs.

Techniques. A variety of techniques and materials can be used to educate women about
their sexuality.

Books and Other Reading Materials. There are many excellent books and pamphlets
available for women. *Our Bodies, Ourselves*, by the Boston Women's Health Book
Collective, was one of the first to both provide more detailed medical information in
understandable terms and be written from a feminist perspective. Some books are primar-

ily informational; others have a self-help approach (assertiveness, relaxation, body pleasuring). There are materials for various age groups, educational levels, or points of view.

Reading materials are excellent for self-education, and can be used at the client's own pace. They can also be assigned as supplements to other types of sexuality education, such as a lecture or a discussion session. (See list of recommended reading at end of chapter.)

Audiovisual Aids. Films, filmstrips, and tapes can add variety if they are used for a specific purpose. Visual materials can be used to present information (female changes at puberty, sexual response cycle) or a scenario that can be used as a basis for discussion. Explicit sexual films, developed for educational purposes, can also be used. These films introduce participants to behaviors they have generally experienced only in private situations, or perhaps not at all (body massage, masturbation, heterosexual or homosexual lovemaking). The purpose is to increase awareness of the varieties of pleasuring behaviors and to desensitize the participant to discomforts that may be present in relationship to a behavior. The educator should always prepare the individual or group for the films, and a discussion period that helps people get in touch with their response should follow.

Process Exercises. These are structured exercises, usually done in a group, that allow participants to interact around their sexual values, beliefs, and experiences. This design helps women to evaluate and publicly articulate their feelings, and to test their beliefs with those of others. Response to exercises can be written, verbal, or sometimes involve body movement. Some formats that are commonly used for sexuality exercises are:

- *Dyad–Triad Groups*
  In a large group, people are divided into two's and three's for the task or discussion. This enables everyone to more quickly and fully participate. Some participants may also be more comfortable sharing feelings with just a few people, especially when first doing these types of exercises. For some exercises using a triad two people can interact and the third can be an observer/reporter.
- *Fishbowl Technique*
  Several participants get into the center of a group and complete an exercise, while the others observe. Afterward other group members can respond and discuss.
- *Continuum*
  Participants move from one side of the room to the other, placing themselves on a continuum between two extremes, depending on their response to a given issue. "Strongly agree" is one end of the room and "strongly disagree" the other. A variation on this is the forced choice approach, when people must select the "best" of only two answers and move to one side of the room or the other. The continuum model can also be used for written exercises.

Lectures. Lectures are an efficient way of presenting material, but should be used to a limited degree in sexuality education. The greatest drawback is that they generally do not allow for feedback or interaction among attendees. An alternative is a "mini-lecture" of factual material (growth and development, sexual response cycle, anatomy and physiology) coupled with a discussion/application period.

Demonstrations. Demonstrations of several types may add clarity to a content or process area. For example, models of the female body may be used to show how a breast or a pelvic examination is done, or how a diaphragm is inserted. Role plays of an interactional process—talking with a teenager about body changes, asking a care provider a question, relating needs to a partner—provide some how-to's for a client or a group.

Problems in Providing Sexuality Education. For most women, talking about their sexuality engenders some anxiety. Many have been brought up to consider sex a private matter, not to be discussed with others. Other women may experience feelings of embarrassment, guilt, or shame because of the ambivalent sexual messages they have received. There may be concerns related to normalcy and whether or not they are like other women. Any of these factors can interfere with the learning process, on a one-to-one or group basis.

For women with a high level of discomfort with their bodies, the individual exercises related to body pleasuring and masturbation may be problematic. Nevertheless, individuals do have a choice in responding to an educator/provider, or in attending a group learning experience. Many women elect to do so, in spite of their discomforts, in order to become more knowledgeable and aware of their sexual feelings. A supportive atmosphere, a graduated learning approach beginning with less anxiety-producing topics, and a facilitator aware of both verbal and nonverbal clues can enhance the educational process.

Sample Methodologies for Identified Learning Needs

Earlier in this chapter, three major areas of learning needs were identified—affective, cognitive, and specific skills. This segment includes examples of exercises and other educational approaches to the learning needs listed in each category. In addition, a sample format is given for a sexuality series for groups.

Adult learning theory is used as a basis for the educational program in this chapter. The content is based on the expressed needs of the learner and makes use of the knowledge and experience of the learner in a highly participatory way. The teacher serves as a facilitator and evaluation is conducted by both learner and teacher.

Affective Learning Approaches. The affective component of sexuality includes feelings, values, beliefs, and one's level of awareness and understanding of them. Most of the exercises listed can be adapted for individual or group use, depending on the setting or the preferences of the persons involved.

Exercise 1: Definition of Sexuality
On a blackboard, newsprint, or piece of paper list words or phrases that describe what sexuality means to you. Discuss:

- Where did your definition of sexuality come from?
- Did you change your personal definition after doing the exercise? Why?
- Is there a difference between sexuality and sex? Between sexuality and sensuality?

Exercise 2: Definition of Sexuality
On a large blackboard or piece of paper write the word "sexuality" at the top. Draw two lines, one that represents expression of sexuality by a person alone, and one representing behaviors with other persons. Fill in several examples of behaviors (on a continuum, from nongenital to genital) to get the group started. Away from the lines, add miscellaneous words that also describe sexuality or sexual expression (Fig. 6–1). Invite participants to add words or phrases that they would include in a broad definition of sexuality. Encourage creativity in this exercise. Discuss:

- Same questions as in Exercise 1
- Placement of behaviors on the continuum lines.

Exercise 3: Sexual History
Write a history of your sexuality beginning with your earliest childhood memories. Some items to include:

- First feelings of being female
- Socialization of male/female children in your family or cultural group
- Menarche, menstruation experiences
- Age you first recalled having pleasurable body or genital feelings
- How/what you first learned about sex
- Messages about sex from your family, church, school teacher, peers, the media
- Dating
- Touching/pleasuring behaviors alone or with someone else
- Intercourse experiences
- Marriage, singlehood
- Your sexual response
- Feelings about intimate relationships
- Parts of your sexuality you feel comfortable/uncomfortable about
- Ways in which you like to express your sexuality
- Goals for sexual growth

This exercise can be kept private or shared with others.

Exercise 4: Influences on Sexuality
On paper, make two lists:

- Events/persons that made me feel *positive* about my sexuality
- Events/persons that made me feel *negative* about my sexuality

Discuss:

- Events/persons most influential in each life stage—childhood, adolescence, young adulthood, middle years, aging
- Early positive and negative feelings that still affect you.
- Ways in which you have dealt with negative experiences.

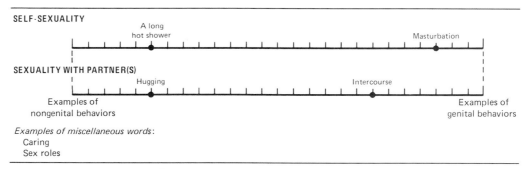

Figure 6–1. Exercise 2: Definition of sexuality.

Exercise 5: Sexual Life Line
On a blank piece of paper, draw your sexual life line, indicating all the important sexual events in your life. Label the events and note the age they occurred. Rate them with a plus or minus, depending on whether they were positive or negative (Sangiuliano, 1980, p. 213).

Exercise 6: Word Game
On a blackboard or sheets of newsprint, list words that might be part of a sexual vocabulary. Write or call out (while someone records) all words you know that mean the same as those listed. Examples:

menstruation	masturbation
pregnant	intercourse
breasts	oral sex
vagina	male/female homosexual
penis	

Discuss:

- Which words do you feel comfortable/uncomfortable using?
- Which words do you use or not use with your mate, friends, mother, child, clients?
- Which words did you use 10 years ago but do not use now, or vice versa. Why?
- What are some ethnic or geographic differences in word usage?

Exercise 7: Sexual Myths
Describe one bit of information, fact, or attitude that was conveyed to you as a child that you now know is a myth. Discuss:

- Who told you the myth and when did you decide it was no longer true?
- Who was your main source of sex education?
- What verbal and nonverbal messages were conveyed in the process of your education?
- Do you wish your sexuality education had been different? If so, in what way?

Exercise 8: Sex Roles
Imagine yourself growing up in your family as a boy rather than a girl. How might your life have been different in areas such as:

- Childhood toys and play
- Relationship to father and mother
- Subjects taken in high school
- Choice and implementation of a career
- Dating patterns
- Marriage relationship
- Responsibilities for home and child care

Exercise 9: Open-ended Sentences
Complete the following sentences. These can be printed on paper and done individually or called out verbally in a group while participants take turns responding (Helmich & Loreen, 1979, pp. 62–63).

- Men are _____
- Women are _____
- Sex is _____
- Sexuality is _____
- Marriage is _____
- Loving someone is _____
- I feel good when someone _____
- I am most hurt when someone _____
- Being normal means _____
- I like to daydream about _____
- Sometimes I like to be alone because _____

Exercise 10: Forced Choice

Choose the "best" answer for each scenario and explain the reason for your choice. Fishbowl technique is good for this exercise.

- The worst thing for me would be a lifetime of:
  - _____ mental retardation
  - _____ no family
  - _____ severe physical disability
- The best birth control method for a 14-year-old girl is:
  - _____ the pill
  - _____ foam and condoms
  - _____ no method
- While cleaning your daughter's room you find a sizeable collection of "beefcake" magazines. You would:
  - _____ totally ignore it
  - _____ throw it in the trash can
  - _____ ask her to share it with you
- A teenage neighbor tells you he is gay. You:
  - _____ recommend counseling
  - _____ suggest he go out with girls more
  - _____ ask him why he thinks he is gay
- Masturbation:
  - _____ should be left to experience
  - _____ should be taught by nurses and doctors
  - _____ should be taught by parents
- Intercourse is primarily for:
  - _____ fun and pleasure
  - _____ honesty and openness
  - _____ physical relief

Exercise 11: The Outer Physical

Use as a homework assignment. Feelings/responses to the exercise can be discussed with a care provider or group.

Take some time to think about your body:

- What about your body are you proud of? How do you stress it?
- What about your body are you embarrassed about? How do you hide it?

- Where do your models for physical attractiveness come from?
- Which parts of your body do you associate with pleasure? With pain?
- Which parts don't you like?
- How much do you feel that people like or dislike you for your body?
- Do you feel that your appearance really expresses who you are?

After thinking about your body, go to a room with a full-length mirror, where it is quiet and you can be alone for at least 15 to 20 minutes. Take off all your clothes and jewelry. Look at yourself in the mirror.

- Are you pleased to see yourself?
- Are you comfortable being nude?
- Do you feel that you have the right to touch and look at yourself?

Now look at your body in detail. Start at the top of your head and work down to your toes. Include your back side, too. Touch each part as you go. Talk out loud; say what you are feeling. Make statements about your body parts and any connected feelings that seem important to you.

Do something pleasant for your body—a long hot bath, a head-to-toe massage, some relaxing yoga exercises (Rush, 1973, pp. 17–18).

Exercise 12: Body Drawings
On a piece of paper, draw your internal and external sexual organs. Share with group members. Discuss:

- Which parts/organs were included? Omitted?
- What variety of parts did participants consider "sexual"?
- Which parts have you actually seen?
- Which organs are a mystery to you?

Exercise 13: Touching
Prepare a handout with front and back view outlines of the female body on either half of the page. Label one side "opposite sex" and the other "same sex." For each drawing, shade in the parts where it is "ok" for you to be touched, by same and opposite sex friends (Calnek & Levine, 1981, p. 44).

Exercise 14: Intimacy
For each behavior listed, fill in the name of a *specific* male and female with whom you could do that activity. If you are married or have a steady partner, what man (or woman) besides your partner could you add to the list? Complete individually and discuss.

With . . . for . . . to whom would you . . .

Male		**Female**
_____	Spend an evening in front of the fire	_____
_____	Eat at an elegant restaurant	_____
_____	Give a facial massage	_____
_____	Spend an out-of-town weekend	_____
_____	Go to a concert	_____
_____	Read poetry to	_____
_____	Spend all day Sunday in bed	_____

_____	Go to an X-rated movie	_____
_____	Ask for a $10 loan	_____
_____	"Cry your eyes out"	_____
_____	Celebrate a raise	_____
_____	Have intercourse	_____
_____	Sleep in a tent	_____
_____	Hug because you felt like hugging someone	_____

Discuss: What was easy/difficult about this exercise?

- What are some societal barriers to intimacy?
- Is it difficult to have friends of the opposite sex after you are in a steady relationship?
- If you could not fill in all the blanks, why not?

Exercise 15: Sexual Freedom*
Complete and discuss:

Two times or places I felt most sexually free:

  1. _____
  2. _____

Two times or places I did not feel sexually free:

  1. _____
  2. _____

Exercise 16: Sexual Possibilities
Complete, using this rating scale:

  1 have tried
  2 would like to try
  3 might like to try
  4 unsure whether I would try
  5 doubt that I would try
  6 would never try

  _____ Taking a nude walk alone in the woods
  _____ Having intercourse with someone of the opposite sex
  _____ Engaging in oral sex
  _____ Making love on a waterbed
  _____ Engaging in extramarital sex
  _____ Posing in the nude for an art class
  _____ Intercourse with a female in the dominant position
  _____ Making love with someone of your same sex
  _____ Masturbating
  _____ Making love outdoors
  _____ Using a vibrator
  _____ Engaging in a sexual relationship with someone much younger

---

*Exercises 15 and 16 are adapted from Read, 1979, pp. 33–34.

‗‗‗‗‗‗ Taking the initiative for starting foreplay
‗‗‗‗‗‗ Having a full body massage
‗‗‗‗‗‗ Watching others engage in sex

Exercise 17: Sexual Orientations
Complete individually; discuss, if desired.

- My sexual orientation is: (heterosexual, bisexual, homosexual)
- I first realized this when ‗‗‗‗‗‗
- Some of the feelings and behaviors that I think are different for me from other life-styles are ‗‗‗‗‗‗
- I am very happy with this orientation because ‗‗‗‗‗‗
- Some negative experiences because of this life-style have been ‗‗‗‗‗‗

Exercise 18: Goals for Personal Sexuality
Complete individually; discuss, if desired.

- Regarding my sexuality:
    I feel very good about ‗‗‗‗‗‗
    I am still not sure about ‗‗‗‗‗‗
    I still feel uncomfortable about ‗‗‗‗‗‗
- During the past 5 years I have ‗‗‗‗‗‗
- During the next 5 years I would like to ‗‗‗‗‗‗

Exercise 19: Sexuality Journal
Keep a journal over time about your experiences as a woman and as a sexual human being. You may want to begin with a sexual history (Exercise 3), then move to current experiences. Record feelings, events, new information or insights received, dreams, fantasies, and so on. Include drawings, pictures, and other illustrative materials.

Cognitive Learning Approaches. Cognitive learning involves knowledge, comprehension, and application of factual material. Sexuality learning that fits in this category includes the knowledge of sexual terminology and content such as female growth and development, anatomy and physiology, the sexual response cycle, the various modes of sexual expression, and the sexual problems and dysfunctions that women may experience.

The following are some suggested approaches for teaching this content. Each topic includes readings for the client from popular sources and additional resources and techniques for the educator, which can be adapted for group or individual use.

Topic: Female Growth and Development

1. Client readings

   - Sheehy, G. *Passages.*
   - Scarf, M. *Unfinished business.*

2. Techniques and resources
   A. Mini-lecture on life stages
      (1) Resources

         - Burnside, I., et al. *Psychosocial caring throughout the life span.* New York: McGraw-Hill, 1979.
         - Fogel and Woods (1981), Ch. 6, "Issues in the Life Cycle."

- Gilligan, C. *In a different voice*. Cambridge, Mass.: Harvard University Press, 1982.
- Lion (1982), Chs. 3, 4, 5, 6. "Sexuality in the life stages."

B. Exercises
  (1) For each life stage you have lived through—childhood, adolescence, young adulthood, middle years, aging—write a paragraph that describes the major events that occurred during that time. What were key factors regarding your socialization as a woman? What were issues/concerns related to sexuality for each stage?
  (2) Draw your life line (Chapter 5, Discovering Your Life Patterns—Past and Future, Activity 1).
  (3) Discussion questions

   - Has your life followed a "traditional" course? Why or why not?
   - Some of the popular literature describes men and women as following the same pattern through all the life stages. How might women's pattern of life be different and why? Is it "unfair" for care providers to judge women according to whether or not they have completed the traditional developmental tasks for each life stage?
   - Does socialization regarding sexuality still differ for men and women? How? Why?

Topic: Female Anatomy and Physiology

1. Client readings

- Boston Women's Health Book Collective. *Our bodies, ourselves*, Ch. 2, "Sexuality."
- Federation of Feminist Women's Health Centers. *A new view of a woman's body*, Chs. 2, 3, 4.

2. Techniques and resources
  A. Mini-lecture
    (1) Resources

     - Fogel and Woods (1981), Ch. 5, "Woman's Body."
     - Siemens and Brandzel (1982), Ch. 2, "Sexual Anatomy."

  B. Audiovisual

     - Federation of Feminist Women's Health Centers. *A new view of a woman's body*. Color photos of female breasts and genitalia.
     - Netter, F. *The Ciba collection of medical illustrations—Reproductive system*. 1970, 2, Rev. Summit, N.J.: Ciba Pharmaceutical. Color drawing of normal pelvic anatomy.
     - Corrine, T. Color slides of variations in female external genitalia. Available from Focus International, 1776 Broadway, New York, NY 10019.

  C. Exercises
    (1) Affective Learning Exercise 12, Body Drawings
    (2) Group exercise (in dyads or triads). With materials such as construction paper, balloons, straws, ping-pong balls, scissors, tape, paste, etc., con-

struct a three-dimensional model of the female reproductive organs. Compare and discuss.

(3) Homework: Affective Learning Exercise 11, The Outer Physical

- With a mirror, examine external genitalia. Some women may also want to do a pelvic self-examination and visualize internal structures. (Technique described in Ch. 2, *A New View of a Woman's Body* by the Federation of Feminist Women's Health Centers.) Alternative: View anatomy while health care provider is doing examination.

(4) Discussion questions:

- What words were you taught as a child for your genitals? Were they general and vague (e.g., "down there")? Specific?
- How did you feel about touching your genitals and examining them closely?
- How closely connected are you to your female organs? Would it make a major difference if you lost one of them or if they did not function normally? Examples: Uterus—infertility, hysterectomy. Breast—mastectomy.

Topic: Sexual Response Cycle

1. Client readings

- Barbach, L. *For yourself: The fulfillment of female sexuality*, Ch. 5.
- Siemens, S., & Brandzel, R. (1982), Handout (Fig. 6–2)

2. Techniques and resources
   A. Mini-lecture on sexual response cycle
      (1) Resources

      - Siemens & Brandzel (1982), Ch. 3, "Physiologic Response to Sexual Arousal." (Fig. 6–2, Tables 6–1 & 6–2)
      - Kolodny, R. et al. (1979), Ch. 2, "Sexual Anatomy and Physiology."
      - Katchadourian, H., & Lunde, D. (1979), "Biological Aspects of Human Sexuality." (2nd ed). New York: Holt, Rinehart, & Winston, 1980.

   B. Audiovisual
      (1) Films

      - *The Sexually Mature Adult*
      - *Physiological Responses of the Sexually Stimulated Female in the Laboratory*

   C. Exercises
      (1) Review Figure 6–2 (female sensual–sexual response). Discuss the variety of activities which can initiate the SR cycle.
      (2) Draw your own sexual response pattern. Describe each step with a few phrases or sentences.

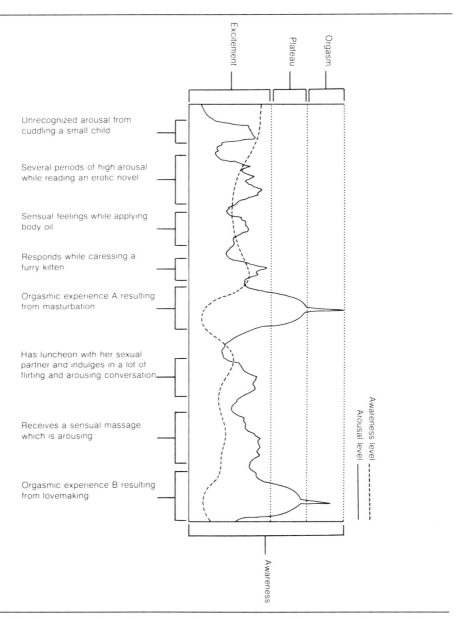

Figure 6–2. Female sensual-sexual response. This figure represents a four-hour span in the life of a hypothetical woman. It represents physiological responses to a variety of erotic stimuli. She becomes aroused a number of times but is not always aware of it. Two typical orgasmic episodes are included. They are complete with excitement, plateau, orgasm, and resolution phases. (Source: *Siemens, S., & Brandzel, R. Sexuality: Nursing assessment and intervention. Philadelphia: J. B. Lippincott, 1982, by permission.*)

TABLE 6–1. PHYSIOLOGICAL CHANGES IN WOMEN DURING THE SEXUAL RESPONSE CYCLE

Body Part Responding	Excitement	Plateau	Orgasm	Resolution
Breasts	Nipples and areola become tumescent	Increases	No change	Return to normal size rapidly
	Venous pattern becomes more defined	Increases	Veins become very evident	Veins return to normal more slowly than nipples
	Whole breast starts to engorge	Increases	No change	Returns to normal size more slowly than nipples
	Nipples become erect	Erection continues	No change	Nipples return rapidly to normal
Skin	A measles-like rash may appear on the epigastrium, breasts, and chest of 75% of women and 25% of men	Color increases in intensity. May extend over body, face, and neck	No change	Disappears rapidly, usually in reverse order of appearance. A fine film of perspiration appears on one-third of all orgasmic persons
Muscles	Long muscles of arms and legs become increasingly tense. Restless, involuntary movements become increasingly rapid	Mouth may be open. Jaws may be clenched. May frown, scowl, or grimace. Arms and legs may move in a clutching motion. Pelvis may thrust involuntarily	All muscles may have involuntary spasms. Voluntary muscle control lost	Muscle-tension largely dissipates within 5 min
Heart	Tachycardia	Heart rate elevates to 100–175 beats/min	Heart rate increases to 110–180 beats/min	
	Hypertension	Blood pressure elevates 20–80 mm Hg systolic and 10–40 mm Hg diastolic over normal	Total blood pressure elevation may reach 30–100 mm Hg systolic and 20–50 mm Hg diastolic over normal	
Lungs	Respiratory rate is variable depending upon degree of excitement	Hyperventilation occurs during high sexual tension just before orgasm	Respiratory rate may elevate to 40/min during a strong orgasm	Respiratory rate returns to normal rapidly

(continued)

179

TABLE 6-1. (cont.)

Body Part Responding	Excitement	Plateau	Orgasm	Resolution
External genitalia				
Clitoris	Corpus cavernosa and corpus spongiosum begin to engorge, increasing the diameter of the shaft and glans. A few shafts elongate	Shaft and glans retract against the pubic bone and disappear under the hood	Shaft and glans remain retracted	Tumescence may last 5–10 min after orgasm. Returns to normal position in 5–10 min after orgasm
Labia majora	In the nullipara, the labia thin and flatten against the perineum	Labia almost disappear against the perineum	No change	If woman is orgasmic, there is a rapid decrease to normal size in 1–2 min
	In the multipara, the labia engorge and may become 2–3 times normal size	The labia become pendulous and separate	No change	If woman is orgasmic, there is a decrease to normal size in 10–15 min
Labia minora	The labia engorge 2–3 times normal size and, because of the swelling, act as an extension of the vagina	Engorgement continues. In the nullipara, color changes from pink to red. In the multipara, labia become bright red. All color changes occur within 3 min of orgasm	Colors remain as in late plateau. The proximal portions contract rhythmically	Intense color fades within 10–15 sec. The remainder fades relatively rapidly
Internal genitalia				
Clitoris	Vestibular bulbs may engorge to 2 or 3 times normal size. Crura increase in size to a lesser degree	Engorgement continues	Vestibular bulbs empty during orgasmic contractions	Bulbs immediately refill from the venous plexi
	Bulbocavernosi and ischiocavernosi muscles develop increasing tension	Muscular tension increases	Bulbocavernosi and ischiocavernosi muscles contract sharply at 0.8 sec intervals. Three to 15 contractions are possible	Probable immediate reduction of myotonia with orgasm and almost immediate return of muscle tension when bulbs refill

	Excitement	Plateau	Orgasm	Resolution
Vagina	Vaginal walls produce clear lubricant within 10–30 sec of sexual arousal. This lubricant is called a transudate Congestion begins in the walls of the lower third of the vagina. There is lengthening and distention of the inner two-thirds of the the vaginal barrel with a ballooning effect at the cervical end Color changes from purple-red to a darker purple	Less lubricant produced The lower third of the vagina becomes grossly engorged, which reduces the lumen. This is called the *orgasmic platform*. There is a further increase in width and length of the vagina A deep purple color develops	No observed change The orgasmic platform is reduced by the spastic contractions of the circumvaginal muscles	Lubrication rarely continues during this phase Orgasmic platform dissipates rapidly Color returns to normal over 10–15 min
Uterus	The uterus and broad ligaments become engorged. The greatest engorgement occurs in the multipara The uterus moves up and back into the false pelvis. This helps create the balooning effect of the upper third of the vagina	Engorgement continues Uterine elevation completes	No change noted No change is evident in position. Uterine contractions similar to the first stage of labor occur	The nullipara loses vasocongestion within 10 min. The multipara needs 10–20 min to lose congestion. If she is not orgasmic, resolution requires 30–60 min Initially the uterus descends rapidly. Full descent is achieved after 5–10 min. If orgasmic, the cervical os opens slightly. It does not close for 20–30 min

(Source: Siemens, S., & Brandzel, R. Sexuality: Nursing assessment and intervention. Philadelphia: J. B. Lippincott, 1982, pp. 53–69, by permission.)

TABLE 6–2. FREQUENTLY ASKED QUESTIONS ABOUT SEXUAL RESPONSE

I have read that a woman's nipples become erect. Why don't mine?

There are always some variations to the standard patterns. Women with asymmetrical breasts or flat or inverted nipples often do not have simultaneous nipple erection. Some women with inverted nipples have no erection.

My nipples seem to get erect twice during sex—once when I get aroused and once more after orgasm. What makes them do that?

Sometimes the engorgement of the areola is so great that it seems to surround the erect nipple and it appears that the nipple erection is lost. Then, if the areola tumescence is lost before the nipple erection, it appears that the nipple has become erect twice.

My partner says that I get all red and blotchy in the face when I'm having sex. Is that normal?

Tell your partner that you are really excited. The intensity of the "sex flush" is determined by the degree of arousal and the intensity of the orgasm.

When I come, my heart is beating so fast it scares me. Is that normal?

A higher heart rate is expected during orgasm. For women, variation in the rate of heart beat is related to intensity of orgasm. The heart beats most rapidly with orgasms from masturbation.

The romantic novels always talk about panting when you are coming, but I don't seem to do that. What's wrong with me?

The research done by Masters and Johnson indicates that men always hyperventilate during orgasm, but that often a woman with very mild sexual tension may not.

I was rubbing my clitoris and when I got really excited, it disappeared. What happened?

The crura, the ischiocavernosus muscle, and a suspensory ligament to the pubic bone retract the clitoris so actively during plateau that there is at least a 50 percent reduction in length as it is pulled under the clitoral hood.

My clitoris doesn't get any bigger or get "erect." Am I undersexed?

Clitoral engorgement may be visible to the naked eye or microscopic. Smaller clitorides tend to have a greater relative size increase than larger ones. Erection, in the sense of penile erection, does not occur with the clitoris.

My partner "rides high" to try to give more stimulation to my clitoris. It doesn't seem to help me have an orgasm. Is anything wrong with me?

The penile shaft rarely touches the clitoris during insertion and thrusting. "Riding high" pushes the penis against the anterior portion of the vagina and the urinary meatus, which may provide some extra stimulation to these areas, but the penis does not usually succeed in making clitoral contact while inserted.

The color has changed in my labia since my pregnancy. It is a darker pink most of the time and when I am excited it gets very dark red. Why is this?

Pregnancy increases the vascularity of all the pelvic structure and this increase in blood supply causes a darker color. Nothing is wrong with this coloration. It is an indication that there is enough vasocongestion to result in orgasm. Very dark colors of red or wine may indicate you developed labial or pelvic varicosities during pregnancy.

I don't lubricate very much. Does that mean I'm not very sexy?

Lubrication starts within seconds and some women develop sufficient lubrication for coitus almost immediately. Sometimes, a woman may be lubricating very adequately but the transudate remains inside the vagina and is not evident at the introitus. Using the finger to move some of this lubrication to the labial and clitoral area may increase arousal and permit easy entrance of the penis. For many women, the immediate appearance of transudate is not an indication that they are ready for coitus. Most women prefer and need extensive loveplay before they feel aroused to the point of desiring penetration.

I get really excited and lubricate well for a while, but then I seem to get dry and sex becomes uncomfortable.

Women who stay at plateau levels of excitement for a period of time or those who have partners who maintain insertion and thrusting for a long period of time may want to plan ahead and use additional lubricant. A water-soluble lubricant such as K-Y Jelly is available at any pharmacy. A longer lasting lubricant with silicone has been developed by a doctor. It is available upon prescription. Oil-based

TABLE 6–2. (cont.)

lubricants such as petroleum jelly (vaseline) or many of the massage oils and hand lotions should be avoided because they may interfere with the normal flora in the vagina.

Sometimes I feel that everything stops just before an orgasm. What is this?

During very high sexual tension, the pelvic muscles may have a spastic contraction lasting 2–4 sec before the regular contractions start. It is important that effective stimulation continue during this time to ensure full orgasmic response.

Is it true that some women ejaculate?

Some women respond with orgasm and "ejaculation" when an area on the anterior vaginal wall is palpated. This area is called the Grafenberg spot in honor of the first person who wrote about it. It is assumed that this "ejaculate" originates in the glands that surround the urethra tissue, which is homologous to the male prostate gland. Much more research needs to be done before clinical applications can be made.

(Source: *Siemens, S., & Brandzel, R. Sexuality: Nursing assessment and intervention. Philadelphia: J. B. Lippincott, 1982, pp. 53–59, by permission.*)

Topic: Varieties of Sexual Expression and Orientations

1. Client readings
   - Adair, N., & Adair, C. *Word is out: Stories of some of our lives*. New York: Delta Special/New Glide Publications, 1978.
   - Barbach, L., & Levine, L. *Shared intimacies*. New York: Anchor Press/Doubleday, 1980.
   - Hite, S. *The Hite report*. New York: Macmillan, 1976.
   - Vida, G. (Ed.). *Our right to love: A lesbian resource book*. Englewood Cliffs, N.J.: Prentice-Hall, 1978.

2. Techniques and resources
   A. Mini-lecture
      (1) Resources
         - Kolodny, et al. (1979), Ch. 14, "Homosexuality and Transsexualism."
         - Ponse, B., In Kirkpatrick (1980), Ch. 10, "Finding Self in the Lesbian Community."
         - Read, (1979)
            Ch. 6, "Masturbation"
            Ch. 7, "Arousal and Response"
            Ch. 8, "Intimate Behavior"
            Ch. 9, "Sexual Life-styling"
            Ch. 10, "Sexual Expression"
         - Schwoyer, C., In Lion (1982), Ch. 7, "Variations in Sexuality."
   B. Audiovisual
      (1) Films
         - "Touching," Psychological Films
         - "Bodies"
         - "Margo" (female masturbation), Multimedia Resource Center
         - "Rich and Judy," "Free" (heterosexual lovemaking), Multimedia Resource Center

- "Holding" (female homosexual lovemaking), Multimedia Resource Center
- "VirAmat" (male homosexual lovemaking), Multimedia Resource Center
- "Like Other People" (handicapped couple discussing affectional and sexual needs), Perennial Education

C. Exercises
(1) List ways in which you express or get in touch with your sexuality, individually and in relationships with others. What additional methods would you like to add to your sexual repertoire? Why?
(2) Affective Exercise 16, Sexual Possibilities
(3) Affective Exercise 17, Sexual Preferences
(4) Sexual Behaviors
Read the following list of sexual behaviors/categories and, using your own information, write a definition of each (Lion, 1982).

Singles	Transexualism
Marrieds	Nymphomania
Celibacy	Sadomasochism
Heterosexuality	Incest
Homosexuality	Fetishism
Bisexuality	Prostitution
Androgeny	

How did you learn this information? Have you known or interacted with persons whose sexual behavior fits any of your definitions? As you interacted, what was your response? Open? Uncomfortable? Interested? Relieved? Scared?

Discuss:

- Variations in group members' response to definitions and reactions.
- How differences were tolerated in the group.

Also see Chapter 9 for content on lesbian sexuality.

Topic: Female Sexual Dysfunctions

1. Client readings

- Barbach, L. *For yourself: The fulfillment of female sexuality*, Chs. 1–5.
- Boston Women's Health Book Collective, *Our bodies, ourselves*, Ch. 2, "Sexuality."

2. Techniques and resources
A. Mini-lecture
(1) Resources

- Fogel & Woods (1981), Ch. 19, "Sexual Dysfunction."
- Lion (1982), Ch. 8, "Sexual Dysfunction and Therapeutic Approaches."
- Siemens & Brandzel (1982), Ch. 12, "Psychogenic Sexual Dysfunction:

Approaches to Treatment"; Ch. 13, "Sexual Dysfunction: Organic Causes"; Ch. 14, "Drugs That Affect Sexual Function."

    B. Exercises
        (1) List/discuss reasons why you think some women have problems and dysfunctions related to their sexuality. What internal/external factors may be influential?
        (2) Discuss: How important is orgasm to sexual satisfaction? To gender identity?
        (3) Discuss: Have you ever had a sexual problem? What? How did it affect you? How did it affect your relationships with others? What did you do about it? If you sought help, what options or services were available?

Specific Skills Learning Approaches. Sometimes sexuality education involves teaching women specific skills to help them enhance their sexual repertoire or overcome a sexual concern or dysfunction. Examples of this include general body pleasuring, relaxation, masturbation, and communication with a partner. This educational approach usually includes some didactic/instructional content, use of audiovisual materials for illustration, and affective level discussion with the individual or the group members. This is followed by homework and individual practice sessions, with periodic feedback to the instructor and group, if appropriate.

Topic: Body Pleasuring
Teaching women body awareness as well as specific techniques for self-pleasuring usually is done through a graduated series of activities. Initial exercises are usually more low-key, less threatening ones, such as general relaxation techniques. At the woman's desired pace, activities can move from nongenital to genital pleasuring. This format is often used for women who want to become orgasmic, but is also appropriate for women without this problem who want to enhance their range of sexual expression.

Moving through a program such as this requires commitment on the part of the client to spending a certain amount of time per day or week in a private, uninterrupted setting for practice of the exercises. Requirements need not be rigid, however, and some women may be interested in only selected activities. Content can include:

1. Basic knowledge and awareness of body parts and functions; related attitudes and feelings. (Suggestions given in affective and cognitive sections.)
2. Relaxation techniques.
3. Nongenital touching/pleasuring.
4. Genital touch/pleasuring.
5. Additional aids—use of fantasy, erotica (films, literature and art), vibrators, oils and lubricants, sensual clothing.

Two popular books that describe this series of activities and give specific exercises are:

- Barbach, L. *For yourself: The fulfillment of female sexuality*. New York: Anchor Press/Doubleday, 1976.
    Ch. 3, "Where Are You Now?"
    Ch. 4, "The First Steps Toward Change"
    Ch. 7, "Why Masturbation?"

Ch. 8, "Exercises"
Ch. 9, "Elaborating on What You've Learned"
• Heiman, J., LoPiccolo, L., & LoPiccolo, J. *Becoming orgasmic: A sexual growth program for women*. Englewood Cliffs, N.J.: Prentice-Hall, 1976.
Ch. 2, "Getting to Know Yourself"
Ch. 3, "Exploring by Touch"
Ch. 4, "Touching for Pleasure: Discovery"
Ch. 5, "Touching for Pleasure: Focusing"
Ch. 6, "Going Further"
Ch. 7, "Using a Vibrator: A Little Help from a Friend"

Additional resources include:

1. Books
   See resource list on Sexuality Self-Help for Women
2. Films
   • "Becoming Orgasmic: A Sexual Growth Program for Women," Focus International. A three-film series based on content in Heimen, et al. (1976). "Discovery" and "Self-Pleasuring" complement material in Chs. 2–7, and can be used for women with or without a partner. The third film, "Sharing," is for women with a partner and follows the content of Chs. 8–10.
   • "Margo" (female pleasuring and masturbation), Multimedia Resource Center.

Topic: Communication About Sexuality
Communicating sexual desires or concerns is often difficult. Both men and women have been socialized to think that sexual expression is "doing what comes naturally," and hence needs little discussion. In addition, some women still see men as being "in charge" of their sexuality, and hesitate to verbalize their own preferences and desires for fear of threatening or hurting their partners.

Poor communication can, in the least, inhibit the fullest actualization of a relationship. It can also lead to false assumptions and expectations that result in frustration, resentments, and feelings of powerlessness on the part of either partner. Turner (1977) states that dysfunctional communication and sexual dysfunction often go hand in hand. An educational process can serve as a catalyst for more effective communication in a relationship.

1. Readings
   • Barbach (1976), Ch. 5, "Letting Your Partner Know."
   • Heiman, et al. (1976), Ch. 8, "Sharing Self-Discovery with a Partner"; Ch. 9, "Pleasuring Each Other."
   • Kerr, C. *Sex for women*. New York: Grove Press, 1977, Ch. 8, "Asking for What You Want."
   • Shandler, M., & Shandler, N. *Ways of being together*. New York: Schocken Books, 1980.
   • Turner, N. Overcoming poor sexual communication patterns. *Medical Aspects of Human Sexuality*, July, 1977.

2. Exercises in an educational setting
   A. Define (preferably in writing) what you would like to discuss with your partner regarding your sexual relationship. Include what you like about sex

with him/her, problem areas, your wants/needs, things you would like to do differently.

B. Rehearse a conversation with a partner. Practice opening statements and ongoing segments of the discussion. Work on refining and becoming comfortable with what you wish to convey. If doing individually, practice in front of a mirror. You may also want to role play potential responses from your partner as part of your monologue. If in a group setting, role play with another person.

C. Practice use of "I-statements" in a conversation with another person. Avoid use of second and third person pronouns such as "you" and "they" and inquisition words such as "why" and "when." Begin sentences with "I" and use words that describe feelings. Begin with a topic not related to sexuality such as your response to a political situation or controversial events. Then move to a dialogue related to sexuality.

Examples:

Indirect Expression	**Direct Expression—"I"-Statements**
You drive like a maniac!	I am scared when the car goes over 65.
You never spend any time with me.	I feel lonely when you are not here.
I think you are selfish when you forget to blow in my ear.	I love having you blow in my ear.
People who don't enjoy X-rated movies are prudes.	I enjoy movies with explicit sex. I really get turned on.
When do you plan to go to bed?	I'd like to give you a body massage.

3. Exercises with partners
   A. Listening
      While one partner shares feelings, the other one listens for an allotted period of time (5–10 minutes). Then roles are reversed. Do daily for one week. This can be used for general as well as sexual communication. (Turner, 1977, p. 100)
   B. Specific feedback
      Practice communicating specific needs and wants related to sexuality.
      (1) Use "I"-statements.
      (2) Follow unclear or unspecific statements with "tell me more about that" or "would you please elaborate on what you mean."
      (3) Try paraphrasing the partner's statement before jumping to conclusions about what was said. "I think I'm hearing you say that . . ."
      (4) Include some suggestions for meeting the expressed need (Turner, 1977, p. 100). Examples:

      • I need more time with you; I would like to take you out to dinner.
      • I would like more variety in our lovemaking; Let's read *The Joy of Sex* and try some new things.
      • I really enjoy being held when I'm feeling down; I'm going to ask you for that more often.

C. Readings
   Read magazines, novels, self-help books, or professional materials related to sexuality. Discuss. (See reference list at end of chapter.)
D. Lists and journals
   Individually make a list of what you would like to give to and receive from your partner in a relationship, generally and sexually. Discuss. Keep personal journals regarding your sexual growth as an individual and as a couple. Share if desired.
E. Outside resources
   Attend lectures, sexual self-awareness seminars, relationship enrichment programs that are designed to increase awareness and communication.

Group Learning Approaches. Affective, cognitive, and special skill learning related to sexuality can be taught individually or in groups. Education with other women has several potential advantages.

1. Experiences, feelings, and concerns common to many women become known. The feeling of being "the only woman in the world," which frequently occurs in regard to sexual matters, is decreased.
2. The stimulus of being in a group—responding to information, contrasting personal beliefs and practices with the varied ones of other participants—can facilitate a more immediate self-awareness and self-evaluation process.
3. A more personalized awareness of the range of ways in which other women express their sexuality can lead to increased tolerance of others' preference.
4. Information, options, and problem-solving techniques can be learned from peers, as well as from the facilitator/educator.

Groups for sexuality education can range from primarily information giving with surface-level discussion to a more intense interaction where women attempt to get at their feelings and may reveal intimate personal experiences. Discussion regarding the approach should take place before the group begins.

The educator should follow general guidelines for leading groups. Some specific suggestions for conducting sexuality groups are:

1. Although your main role is to be a resource person and facilitate group process, do not hesitate to selectively share some of your own feelings and experiences. Your behavior and comfort with the topic can serve as a role model for the group.
2. Participants may need to intellectualize about sexuality at first, before dealing with feelings. This is normal for a sensitive topic.
3. Watch closely for both verbal and nonverbal communication. Silence and body language are common ways of responding.
4. When someone takes a risk in revealing herself, be supportive. Do not leave her hanging.
5. Be flexible; revise content and process according to the response of the group.
6. In dealing with controversy, acknowledge the diversity of viewpoints. It is not necessary to come to a consensus regarding sexual issues.
7. Do not let "experts" (persons who have attended sexuality groups before, professionals who have some expertise in the field of human sexuality) dominate the group.

At the first group meeting, participants should discuss and agree to some guidelines. Items often included in a contract are:

1. Each person is entitled to her own beliefs and opinions and has the right to be heard. There are no "right" or "wrong" responses.
2. Everyone has the right to speak or not. Although participation in group discussion is desirable, it is also voluntary.
3. Information shared within the group may be of a very personal nature and should remain confidential.
4. When possible, I-statements should be used ("I think," "I feel," etc.) rather than generalizing to others ("Some people say . . .").
5. Once a group is established, it should not be interrupted by guests or new participants, unless the group agrees to this. Members should commit themselves to attending all sessions, for the sake of continuity and group building.
6. Although a leader or facilitator is present, group members also share responsibility for the progress of the group, and need to give feedback to the leader and each other periodically.*

Sample Format for Group Education

The following is a 10-session series on female sexuality, each designed to last 1½ to 2 hours.

Session 1

1. Get acquainted
2. Discussion of purpose and goals
3. Assessment of learning needs, desired content and process for the group
4. Contracting—"rules" for the group
5. Definition of sexuality
   A. Definition of sexuality, Exercise 1 or
   B. Definition of sexuality, Exercise 2

Session 2

1. Early and current influences on sexuality. Choose from:
   A. Open-ended assessment, Exercise 4b or 4c
   B. Influences on sexuality, Exercise 4
   C. Sexual life line, Exercise 5
   D. Sexual myths, Exercise 7
   E. Sex roles, Exercise 8
   F. Sexual words—Word game, Exercise 6
2. General values and clarification regarding sexuality
   A. Open-ended sentences, Exercise 9
   B. Forced choice, Exercise 10

---

*Adapted from Calnek and Levine (1981, p. 13).

Session 3

1. Female anatomy and physiology
   A. The outer physical, Exercise 11
   B. Body drawing, Exercise 12
   C. Cognitive section—under Female Anatomy and Physiology
2. Sexual response cycle—Cognitive section, under Sexual Response Cycle

Session 4

1. Intimacy
   A. Touching, Exercise 13
   B. Intimacy, Exercise 14
2. Friendships—female/male, female/female

Session 5

1. Solo sexuality (body pleasuring, masturbation)—Specific Skill section, under Body Pleasuring

Session 6

1. Varieties of sexual expression and orientations
   A. Sexual freedom, Exercise 15
   B. Sexual possibilities, Exercise 16
   C. Cognitive section—under Varieties of Sexual Expression and Orientations

Session 7

1. Female sexual concerns and dysfunctions; types of therapy, Cognitive section—under Female Sexual Dysfunctions

Session 8

1. Communication about sexuality—Specific Skill section, under Communication about Sexuality

Session 9

1. Read *Lady Chatterley's Lover* by D. H. Lawrence.
2. Discuss: Is this a beautiful story of a woman's sexual unfolding or a male author's view of female sexuality?

Session 10

1. Evaluation and feedback
2. Future goals
   A. Goals for personal sexuality, Exercise 18

Special Groups. The content and approaches to sexuality education listed thus far are appropriate for most women. However, events and circumstances can create the need for a more specific approach for some women. Life stage changes, pregnancy, illness, or disability are all factors that have the potential for altering how women feel about themselves and their bodies, and their usual patterns of sexual expression. Educational approaches must be adapted accordingly. For each of the groups, pertinent content is listed and resources for further information are given.

Adolescent Women. Learning needs:

1. Physical and emotional changes of puberty
2. How pregnancy occurs
3. Changing relationships with males and females
4. Options related to sexual behaviors
5. Contraceptive methods

Readings:

- Bell, R. *Changing bodies, changing lives: A book for teens on sex and relationships*. New York: Random House, 1980.
- Carson, D. *Girls are equal too*. An Aladdin Book/Atheneum, 1973.
- Fleming, A. In E. Lion (1982), Ch. 4, "Sexuality in Adolescence."
- Gordon, S. *The sexual adolescent: Communication with teenagers about sex*. North Scituate, Mass.: Duxbury Press, 1973.
- (Also see Chapter 16.)

Middle Years/Aging Women. Learning needs:

1. Role and life stage changes
2. General physiological changes; menopause
3. Normal changes in sexual response cycle

Readings:

- Butler, R., & Lewis, M. *Love and sex after 60*. New York: Perennial Library/Harper & Row, 1976.
- Dresen, S. The middle years: The sexually active middle adult. *AJN*, June 1975, 75:1001–1005.
- Gress, L. Human sexuality and aging. In M. Barnard, et al. (Eds.), *Human sexuality for health professionals*. Philadelphia: W. B. Saunders, 1978.
- Hotchner, B. Menopause and sexuality: Gearing up or down. *Topics in Clinical Nursing*, January 1980, *1*, 45–52.
- Markley, V. In E. Lion (1982), Ch. 5, "Sexuality and Adulthood; Ch. 6, "Sexuality and Aging."
- Moran, J. Sexuality: An ageless quality, a basic need. *Journal of Gerontological Nursing*, September/October 1979, 5, 13–16.
- Solnick, R. (Ed.). *Sexuality and aging*. The University of Southern California Press, 1978.
- (Also see Chapter 14.)

Pregnancy and Childbearing. Learning needs:

1. Role changes
2. Body image changes
3. Sexual activity during pregnancy; alternate positions and methods of pleasuring
4. Birth and lactation as a sexual experience

5. Conflict between sexuality and motherhood
6. Partner relationships during pregnancy

Readings:

- Barbach, L., & Levin, L. (1980), Ch. 7, "Being Pregnant and Being Sexual."
- Bing, E., & Coleman, L. *Making love during pregnancy*. New York: Bantam Book, 1977.
- Cronenwett, L., & Newmark, L. Fathers' response to childbirth. *Nursing Research*, 1974, *23*, 210–127.
- Hollender, M. H., & McGhee, J. B. The wish to be held during pregnancy. *Journal of Psychosomatic Research*, 1974, *18*, 193–197.
- Lion, E. (1982), Chapter 10, "Sexuality during pregnancy, the postpartum period and lactation."
- Newton, M. Meeting sexual and emotional needs during pregnancy. *Family Health*, October 1977, *9*, 15–16.
- Newton, N. Interrelationships between sexual responsiveness, birth, and breast feeding. In J. Zubin & J. Money (Eds.), *Contemporary sexual behavior: Critical issues in the 70s*. Baltimore: Johns Hopkins University Press, 1973.
- Rossi, A. Maternalism, sexuality and the new feminism. In J. Zubin & J. Money (Eds.), *Contemporary sexual behavior: Critical issues in the 70s*. Baltimore: Johns Hopkins University Press, 1973.

Handicapped Women. Learning needs:

1. Body image changes
2. Personal and societal perceptions of the individual as a sexual being
3. Modifications in position and forms of sexual pleasuring specific to handicapping condition.

Readings:

- Bullard, D., & Knight, S. (Eds.). *Sexuality and physical disability: Personal perspectives*. St. Louis, Mo.: C. V. Mosby, 1981.
- Cole, T. M. Sexuality and physical disabilities. *Archives of Sexual Behaviors*, 1975, *4*.
- Egan, J., & Osborne, J. Sexuality and spinal cord injury. In E. Lion (Ed.), *Human sexuality in nursing process*. New York: John Wiley & Sons, 1982.
- Kolodny, R., et al. *Textbook of human sexuality for nurses*, Ch. 11, "Sex and the Handicapped." Boston: Little, Brown, 1979.
- Task Force in Concerns of Physically Disabled Women. *Toward intimacy: Family planning and sexuality concerns of physically disabled women* (2nd ed.). New York: Human Sciences Press, 1978.

BIBLIOGRAPHY

Barbach, L. *For yourself: The fulfillment of female sexuality*. New York: Anchor Press/Doubleday, 1976.
Barbach, L., & Levin, L. *Shared intimacies: Women's sexual experiences*. New York: Anchor Press/Doubleday, 1980.

Bell, A., & Weinberg, M. *Homosexualities: A study of diversity among men and women*. New York: Simon & Schuster, 1978.

Calnek, J., & Levine, S. *Human sexuality: A training manual for job corps centers*. Rochester, N.Y.: Genesee Region Family Planning Program, 315 Alexander Street, 1981.

Freize, I., Parsons, J., Johnson, P., Ruble, D., & Zellman, G. *Women and sex roles*. New York: W.W. Norton, 1978.

Helmich, J., & Loreen J. *Sexuality education and training: Theory, techniques, and resources* (2nd ed.). Planned Parenthood of Seattle/King County, 2211 East Madison, Seattle, Washington, 1979.

Heiman, J., LoPiccolo, L., & LoPiccolo, J. *Becoming orgasmic: A sexual growth program for women*. Englewood Cliffs, N.J.: Prentice-Hall, 1976.

Hite, S. *The Hite report*. New York: Macmillan, 1976.

Hogan, R. *Human sexuality: A nursing perspective*. New York: Appleton-Century-Crofts, 1980.

Huerter, R. Female sexuality. In D. Kjervik & I. Martinson (Eds.), *Women in stress: A nursing perspective*. New York: Appleton-Century-Crofts, 1979.

Katchadourian, H. (Ed.). *Fundamentals of human sexuality* (3rd ed.). New York: Holt, 1980.

Kerr, C. *Sex for women*. New York: Grove Press, 1977.

Kirkpatrick, M. (Ed.). *Women's sexual development*. New York: Plenum Press, 1980.

Kitzinger, S. *Woman's experience of sex*. New York: G. P. Putnam's Sons. 1983.

Kolodny, R., Masters, W., Johnson, V., & Briggs, M. *Textbook of human sexuality for nurses*. Boston: Little, Brown, 1979.

Kush-Goldberg, C. The health self-help group as an alternative source of health care for women. *International Journal of Nursing Studies*, 1979, *16*, 283–294.

Lewis, M. The history of female sexuality in the United States. In M. Kirkpatrick (Ed.), *Women's sexual development*. New York: Plenum Press, 1980.

Lion, E. (Ed.). *Human sexuality in nursing process*. New York: John Wiley & Sons, 1982.

Martin, L. *Health care of women*. Philadelphia: J. B. Lippincott, 1978.

NAACOG Technical Bulletin, Number 1, April 1977.

Read, D. *Healthy sexuality*. New York: Macmillan, 1979.

Roberts, E. Sex education vs. sexual learning. In M. Kirkpatrick (Ed.), *Women's Sexual Development*. New York: Plenum Press, 1980.

Rush, A. K. *Getting clear: Bodywork for women*. New York: Random House, 1973.

Sangiuliano, I. *In her time*. New York: Morrow Quill Paperbacks, 1980.

Sherfey, M. J. *The nature and evolution of female sexuality*. New York: Random House, 1972.

Siemens, S., & Brandzel, R. *Sexuality: Nursing assessment and intervention*. Philadelphia: J. B. Lippincott, 1982.

Turner, N. Overcoming poor sexual communication patterns. *Medical Aspects of Human Sexuality*, July, 1977, *11*, 99–100.

Williams, J. *Psychology of women: Behavior in a biosocial context*. New York: W. W. Norton, 1977.

Woods, N. Woman's body. In C. Fogel & N. Woods (Eds.), *Health care of women: A nursing perspective*. St. Louis, Mo.: C. V. Mosby, 1981.

Woods, N. *Human sexuality in health and illness* (2nd ed.). St. Louis, Mo.: C. V. Mosby, 1979.

RESOURCES

General Readings in Human Sexuality

Bell, A., & Weinberg, M. *Homosexualities: A study of diversity among men and women*. New York: Simon & Schuster, 1978.

Bell, R. *Changing bodies, changing lives: A book for teens on sex & relationships*. New York: Random House, 1980.

Carrera, M. *Sex: The facts, the acts, and your feelings*. New York: Crown, 1981.

Clark, D. *Loving someone gay*. New York: A Signet Book/New American Library, 1977.

Comfort, A. *The joy of sex*. New York: Simon & Schuster, 1974.

Kaplan, H. *The new sex therapy*. New York: Bruner/Mazel, 1974.

Katchadourian, H., & Lunde, D. *Fundamentals of human sexuality* (3rd ed.). New York: Holt, Rinehart & Winston, 1980.

Masters, W., & Johnson, V. *Human sexual response*. Boston: Little, Brown, 1966.

Masters, W., & Johnson, V. *The pleasure bond*. Boston: Little, Brown, 1974.

Mead, M. *Male and female*. New York: New American Library, 1974.

Nelson, J. *Embodiment: An approach to sexuality and Christian theology*. Minneapolis: Augsburg, 1978.

Offit, A. *The sexual self*. New York: Ballantine Books, 1977.

Read, D. *Healthy sexuality*. New York: Macmillan, 1979.

Robinson, P. *The modernization of sex*. New York: Harper & Row, 1976.

Sarrel, L., & Sarrel, P. *Sexual turning points: The seven stages of adult sexuality*. New York: Macmillan, 1984.

Solnik, R. (Ed.). *Sexuality and aging*. Los Angeles: The University of Southern California Press, 1978.

Female Sexuality

Ayalah, D., & Weinstock, I. *Breasts*. New York: Summit Books, 1979.

Baetz, R. *Lesbian crossroads: Personal stories of lesbian struggles and triumphs*. New York: William Morrow, 1980.

Barbach, L. *For yourself: The fulfillment of female sexuality*. New York: Anchor Press/Doubleday, 1976.

Barbach, L., & Levin, L. *Shared intimacies: Women's sexual experiences*. New York: Anchor Press/Doubleday, 1980.

Boston Women's Health Book Collective. *Our bodies, ourselves* (2nd ed.). New York: Simon & Schuster, 1976.

Federation of Feminist Women's Health Centers. *A new view of a woman's body*. New York: Simon & Schuster, 1981.

Freize, I., Parsons, J., Johnson, P., Ruble, D., & Zellman, G. *Women and sex roles*. New York: W. W. Norton, 1978.

Hite, S. *The Hite report*. New York: Macmillan, 1976.

Kerr, C. *Sex for women*. New York: Grove Press, 1977.

Kitzinger, S. *Women's experience of sex*. New York: G. P. Putnam's Sons, 1983.

Ladas, A., Whipple, B., & Perry, J. *The G Spot*. New York: Holt, Rinehart, & Winston, 1982.

Martin, D., & Lyon, P. *Lesbian woman*. New York: Bantam Book, 1972.

Millett, K. *Sexual politics*. New York: Avon Books, 1970.

Sangiuliano, I. *In her time*. New York: Morrow Quill Paperbacks, 1980.

Sherfey, M. J. *The nature and evolution of female sexuality*. New York: Random House, 1972.

Williams, J. *Psychology of women*. New York: W. W. Norton, 1977.

Sexuality Self-help for Women

Barbach, L. *For yourself: The fulfillment of female sexuality*. New York: Anchor Press/Doubleday, 1976.

Blank, J. *My playbook: For women/about sex*. Burlingame, Calif.: Down There Press, 1975.

Blank, J., & Cottrell, H. *I am my lover*. Burlingame, Calif.: Down There Press, 1978.

Dodson, B. *Self love and orgasm*. Betty Dodson, Publisher & distributor, P.O. Box 1933, New York, NY 10156, 1983.

Heyma, J., LoPiccolo, L., & LoPiccolo, J. *Becoming orgasmic: A sexual growth program for women*. Englewood Cliffs, N.J.: Prentice-Hall, 1976.

Ray, S. *I deserve love*. Millbrae, Calif.: Les Femmes, 1976.

Rush, A. *Getting clear: Body work for women*. New York: Random House, 1973.

Sisley, E., & Harris, B. *Lesbian sex*. New York: Simon & Schuster, 1977.

Texts Written for Health Professionals

Barnard, M., Clancy, B., & Krantz, K. *Human sexuality for health professionals*. Philadelphia: W. B. Saunders, 1978.

Green, R. (Ed.). *Human sexuality: A health practitioners text*. Baltimore: Williams & Wilkins, 1975.

Hogan, R. *Human sexuality: A nursing perspective*. New York: Appleton-Century-Crofts, 1980.

Kolodny, R., Masters, W., Johnson, V., & Biggs, M. *Textbook of human sexuality for nurses*. Boston: Little, Brown, 1979.

Lion, E. *Human sexuality in nursing process*. New York: John Wiley & Sons, 1982.

Munjack, D., & Oziel, L. *Sexual medicine and counseling in office practice*. Boston: Little, Brown, 1980.

Siemens, S., & Brandzel, R. *Sexuality: Nursing assessment and intervention*. Philadelphia: J. B. Lippincott, 1982.

Woods, N. *Human sexuality in health and illness* (2nd ed.). St. Louis, Mo.: C. V. Mosby, 1979.

Books/Training Manuals for Sexuality Education

These books contain theory, educational approaches, and additional resources for sexuality education. Both general education as well as specific topical areas are covered. Some books include suggestions for age group adaptation.

Beresford, T. *How to be a trainer*. Baltimore, Md.: Planned Parenthood of Maryland, 1980.

Calderwood, D. *About your sexuality: About the program* (Rev ed.). Boston: Unitarian Universalist Association, 1983.

Calnek, J., & Levin, S. *Human sexuality: A training manual for job corps centers*. Rochester, N.Y.: Genesee Region Family Planning Program, 1981.

Dollar, M. *Trainers' resources, No. 3—Human sexuality*. Regional Training Center for Family Planning. Atlanta, Ga.: Emory University School of Medicine, 1977.

Helmich, J., & Loreen, J. *Sexuality education and training: Theory, techniques and resources* (2nd ed.). Seattle: Planned Parenthood of Seattle/King County, 1979.

Morrison, E., & Price, M. *Values in sexuality: A new approach to sex education*. New York: Hart, 1974.

Schiller, P. *Creative approach to sex education and counseling*. New York: Association Press, 1973.

Audiovisual Resources for Sexuality Education

Center for Marital and Sexual Studies, 5199 E. Pacific Coast Highway, Long Beach, CA 90804

Churchill Films, 622 North Robetson Blvd., Los Angeles, CA 90069

Concept Media Filmstrips, 1500 Adams Avenue, Costa Mesa, CA 92626

Focus International, 1776 Broadway, New York, NY 10019

MultiMedia Resource Center, 1525 Franklin Street, San Francisco, CA 94109

Perennial Education, Inc., 477 Roger Williams, P.O. Box 855, Ravinia, Highland Park, IL 60035

National Organizations

Additional information and materials for sexuality education can be obtained from these organizations.

American Association of Sex Educators, Counselors, and Therapists (AASECT), 3422 N. Street, NW, Washington, D.C. 20007

Institute for Family Research and Education, 760 Ostrom Avenue, Syracuse, NY 13210

Institute for Sex Research, Morrison Hall, Indiana University, Bloomington, IN 47401

National Gay Task Force, 80 5th Avenue, New York, NY 10011

Planned Parenthood Federation of America, 810 Seventh Avenue, New York, NY 10019 (or local affiliates)

Sex Information and Education Council of the U.S. (SIECUS), 122 East 42nd Street, New York, NY 10017

Unitarian Universalist Association, 25 Beacon Street, Boston, MA 02108

Understanding and Managing Stress

7

Terry L. Campney Callison

> *Yet do I hold that mortal foolish who strives against the stress of necessity.*
> —*Euripedes,* Mad Heracles, *l. 281.*

One of the challenging aspects of writing about stress is integrating the burgeoning volume of literature aimed at both professional and popular audiences. The considerable attention given to this topic reflects that stress is a phenomenon that affects virtually everyone at various phases of the life cycle.

Management of stress is particularly relevant to women who, in addition to taking care of themselves, must often assume responsibility for the health and welfare of other family members. Furthermore, women are highly vulnerable to stress as a function of the numerous roles they must assume. With the considerable responsibility and influence that women hold with regard to health care in a family, women should be specifically targeted as recipients of a broad range of health care information. Educational efforts should focus on making women an integral part of the health care team. By acknowledging the woman's vital role as a partner in the health care of herself and her family, the first step will have been taken in enlisting cooperation from the patient.

Health care professionals have the task of identifying symptoms of stress, addressing the issue with women clients, and actively involving them in promoting wellness (Shaw, 1981). An important step in this process is educating the client in techniques designed to reduce the perception of stress. The effects of stress reach well beyond the individual who is experiencing them. In addition to the toll taken on one's body, the individual's stress may well affect family, friends, colleagues, and productivity.

From birth to death, humans are confronted with stress-inducing stimuli. The dependent infant employs crying as a response to unmet needs. In each successive developmental stage, individuals expand their repertoire of responses to cope with frustrations that block their goals, disrupt their lives, and tax their resources. Major demands of childhood include those associated with socialization processes and challenges introduced by schooling. Adolescents, influenced by intense peer pressure, strive for independence and struggle with the development of a personal identity. Young adults face major decisions related to education, career choice, and establishing relationships with potential partners. Couples often struggle financially in establishing a home, and emotionally in deciding whether to have children. Responsible parenting requires long-term commitments of

196

time, energy, and money. When children have left home, partners often find themselves reassessing their relationship in terms of different needs than those upon which the relationship was established. Older adults face major financial and emotional changes upon retirement, and health concerns assume paramount importance as infirmities set in on their aging bodies. Major disruptions, which are particularly stress-inducing, result from such unanticipated events as serious illness, death of a loved one, unemployment, or a sudden loss of income. Relocation to a new community, change of employment, divorce, poverty, and birth or adoption of a child are stressful events that often strain the individual's resources to cope and adapt. In many cases, these events have not been previously experienced, and therefore, require novel responses that are perceived as threatening to the individual.

The link between stress and illness has been well documented in the literature (Ibrahim, 1980); however, the research is frequently criticized because the complexity of stress-related phenomena poses difficult methodological problems that may result in confounding of variables (Janis, 1982). Research on the stress–illness link includes the relationship between life events, stress, and illness (Andrews & Tennant, 1978; Kimball, 1982; Paykel, 1978; Rabkin & Struening, 1976), personality (Cohen, 1980), and life-styles and depression (Stewart & Salt, 1981). Nathanson (1977) reported that women experience more instances of morbidity than men, and Schmale (1972) found that feelings of hopelessness or helplessness preceded symptoms of physical or psychic disease. Fox (1978) elaborated on issues and research related to the development of cancer, Sklar and Anisman (1981) reported stress-induced alterations in the growth of tumors, and Bahnson (1981) suggested that stress induced by loss and depression, combined with personality variables, were factors in increased vulnerability to cervical cancer.

Because illness is a socially approved reason for obtaining at least temporary relief from regularly assumed responsibilities at home or work (Parsons, 1951), increased stress may contribute to the perception of illness, adoption of illness behavior (Mechanic, 1962; Pilowsky, 1969), and subsequent seeking of treatment by a health care professional. Roghmann and Haggerty (1973) found an association between psychosocial stress and increased utilization of health care services among families with dependent children. Because relief from symptoms associated with stress is sought from the health care professional, responsibility for addressing the problem lies with the practitioner. Although the expediency of prescriptive medication may be tempting, the interest of the client is not served well if the source of the problem is neither acknowledged nor dealt with. The practitioner who is truly concerned with the promotion of wellness behavior must enlist the client as a full and responsible partner in treatment. If the client can be taught effective techniques that reduce stress and promote perceptions of control and responsibility for her own health, then prescriptive medication, which engenders feelings of passive dependence, becomes a poor substitute for effective health care.

Whenever a decision is made to implement changes in one's life, four possibilities exist: (1) the individual can attempt to change the situation, (2) change oneself, (3) modify both, or (4) change cognitions about the situation or oneself. High levels of stress may create feelings of helplessness and the client's ability to take action may be impaired. She must be firmly encouraged to take action that will allow her to develop the perception of at least some measure of control. This requires supportive statements from the practitioner, which include the message that dramatic changes are unlikely to occur quickly, but that steps can be implemented to help her gain confidence in her ability to take charge of the troubling aspects of her life.

Stress Research Models

Scientific investigation of stress phenomena began approximately 50 years ago. The foundation for stress research was laid by physiologist Walter B. Cannon (1929), whose observations on somatic manifestations associated with acute emotions have been regarded as classic. Cannon proposed that psychological aspects of stress could lead to physiological changes that might result in disease. Harold Wolff (1953) combined principles of physiology and psychiatry to describe protective adaptive reactions, i.e., coping mechanisms, used as a response to stressful stimuli. Wolff proposed that a particular stimulus might be considered noxious for one person but not for another. Hans Selye (1956) developed the general adaptation syndrome as a comprehensive biological model to describe the physiological stress response that occurs in the body. Selye acknowledged that stress was unavoidable and that a certain amount was necessary to maintain homeostasis. Research on the relationship between stress and life events was aided by Thomas Holmes and Richard Rahe's (1967) social readjustment rating scale. Subsequently known as the schedule of recent events, this scale represented an early attempt to quantify psychosocial aspects of the impact of life changes as a vehicle to predict a stress response. Irving Janis (1958) and Richard Lazarus (1966) made major contributions to the development of a cognitive approach to the field of stress research. An individual's appraisal of an event and the meaning attached to the event are central tenets of the cognitive model.

Thus, attempts to empirically study phenomena associated with stress have produced three major theoretical models: physiological, life events, and cognitive. Each of these three conceptualizations poses different research questions and methodological strategies in addressing the relationship between stress and disease. Problems develop when proponents of a particular stress model limit their definition to include only that which is specified by the model they support. In the physiological model, stress is a term applied to physiological responses that are viewed as adaptations to demands placed upon the body. Psychological variables (e.g., attitudes, values, motivations) are included under the general rubric of "stressors," which may be considered contributing factors in the organism's responses (Selye, 1956). In the life events model, stress is conceptualized as an environmental event that requires unusual responses and puts a strain on the individual's resources. Major disruptions (e.g., fire, tornado, imprisonment, birth of a child, loss of a loved one) are considered stressful events, with the affected individual being regarded as "stressed" (Holroyd, 1979). Finally, proponents of the cognitive model conceptualize stress as a transaction between the system (individual, social, or biological) and the environment, whereby adaptive resources are threatened (Lazarus, 1966). Psychological processes (i.e., appraisal of the perceived threat and coping strategies) that mediate both adaptive demands and the individual's responses to these demands are believed to profoundly influence the organism's physiological state, thereby providing the link to stress-related disorders (Holroyd, 1979).

Acknowledging the value and contribution of each body of literature is essential to developing a healthy eclecticism in effectively working with patients. Recognition, assessment, and management of stress require the practitioner to be equipped with an armamentarium of knoweldge, which can be tailored to the unique needs of each individual.

The scientific community lends credence to research that has been empirically tested by methodologically sound criteria. As scientists, we must adhere to these criteria to be taken seriously by our profession. Our approach to the assessment and the management of stress will, therefore, be based upon established empirical evidence, with the hope that it will enable the practitioner to become a more critical consumer of the literature and will provide a base of empirical evidence upon which sound clinical decisions can be made.

The voluminous literature related to stress is a result of numerous authors addressing stress-related phenomena from diverse perspectives and theoretical orientations. Because they do not uniformly agree on a specific operational definition of stress, it is necessary for the reader to determine precisely what is being represented. As a consumer of the literature, the health care professional must be cognizant of these perspectives to both assess the client's interpretation and assist her in effectively coping with what she perceives as "stress."

Jenkins (1979) has developed a comprehensive model of the interaction between stress and the organism (Table 7–1), in an attempt to integrate various theoretical orientations that reflect the multifaceted phenomena associated with stress. In this model, Jenkins categorizes stress into four clusters, or "levels": biological, psychological, interpersonal, and sociocultural. Each level is defined in terms of adaptive capacity, stressors, alarm reaction, defensive reaction, and pathological end-state. Jenkins's model integrates physiological components of the biological model, sociocultural changes related to the life events model, and perceptual appraisal and coping phenomena associated with the cognitive model. With such diversity, it is no wonder that individuals find it difficult to define "stress" in a manner that satisfies proponents of the various perspectives.

Physiological Model. Hans Selye (1956, 1974, 1979), who conducted much of the early research in the field, defined stress as "the nonspecific response of the body to any demand." Physiological stress involves visceral and neurohumoral reactions to noxious stimuli that disturb or injure tissue structure or function (Lazarus, 1966). Selye (1956) demonstrated that tissue systems defend against noxious stimuli and that the defenses are nonspecific with regard to the type of noxious agent. This nonspecific system of defenses is what Selye refers to as the general adaptation syndrome, which includes three distinct stages: the alarm reaction, the stage of resistance, and the stage of exhaustion. Also known as the biological stress syndrome, the general adaptation syndrome follows a medical model in chronicling manifestations of stress in the body over a period of time.

Life Events Model. In a sociological context, from which the life events model evolved, Smelser (1963) used the term structural strain to refer to the stress stimulus that produces sociocultural disequilibrium and requires adaptation. Holmes and Rahe's (1967) work with the schedule of recent events (SRE) served as a springboard for research on life events. In developing the SRE, the assumption was that all life changes are stressful and require adaptation. Vinokur and Selzer (1975) refined this concept by modifying the SRE to reflect both desirable and undesirable life events in determining a life stress score. Sarason, Johnson, and Siegel (1978) added yet another dimension in their life experiences survey (LES). This instrument, which is also based on the SRE, allows the respondent to identify an event, rate the event in terms of its desirability or undesirability, and finally rate it with regard to personal impact of the experience. Comprehensive and provocative critiques (Dohrenwend & Dohrenwend, 1978; Rabkin & Struening, 1976) of research on life events have focused on methodological weaknesses and may well influence future work on this model.

Makosky (1980) has criticized sexist aspects of the item content in scales used to measure life events. Questions relating to the world of work (e.g., promotions, demotions, firing, or conflicts with supervisor) would be relevant to a larger proportion of men than women, whereas areas of direct stress that might affect women (unplanned pregnancy, abortion, rape, child care difficulties, sex discrimination) are glaringly absent. The content is likely to "produce misleading and inaccurately low life-change and/or stress

TABLE 7–1. A MODEL DEPICTING THE INTERACTION OF STRESS AND THE ORGANISM

	Adaptive Capacity	Stressors	Alarm Reaction	Defensive Reaction	Pathological End State
Biological level	State of physique, nutrition, vigor Natural or acquired immunities	Deprivation of biological needs Excess inputs of physical or biological agents	Arousal—hunger, thirst pain, fatigue Changes in physiological function	General adaptation syndrome Physiological compensation Shifts in metabolism Changes in pain threshold	Deficiency diseases "Exhaustion" Addictions Chronic dysfunction Structural damage
Psychological level	Resourcefulness, problem solving ability Ego strength Flexibility Social skills	Perceptions and interpretations of danger, threat, loss, disappointment, frustration, or sense of failure or hopelessness Loss of self-acceptance Threat to security	Feeling of deprivation—boredom, grief, sadness Feelings of anxiety, pressure, guilt Fear of danger	Ego defenses—denial, repression, projection Defensive neuroses Perceptual defenses—wishes, fantasies, motives Planning Problem solving	Despair, apathy Chronic personality pattern disturbances Psychoses Chronic affective disorders Meaninglessness
Interpersonal level	Primary relationships including family Network of social supports	Social isolation Lack of acceptance Insults, punishments, rejections Changes in social groups, especially losses	Antagonism, conflict, suspicion Feelings of rejection, punishment	Defensive, rigid social relating Avoidance Assuming sick role Aggressiveness "Acting out" Enlisting social supports	Chronic exploitation Becoming an outcast Imprisonment Permanent disruption of interpersonal ties Chronic failure to fulfill roles
Sociocultural level	Values Norms and practices "Therapeutic" social institutions Systems of knowledge and technology	Cultural change Role conflict Status incongruity Value conflicts with important others Forced change in life situation	Communication of concern and alarm Expressive behavior of crowds Mobilization of social structures	Culturally prescribed defenses—scapegoating prejudice Explanatory ideologies Legal and moral system Use of curers and institutions	Alienation, anomie Breakdown of social order Disintegration of the cultural systems of values and norms

(Source: *Adapted from Jenkins, C. D. Psychosocial modifiers of response to stress. Journal of Human Stress, 1979, 5(4), 3–15.*)

scores for women" (p. 118). The degree of stress experienced is another issue, because it is unknown whether women and men respond to similar stressors with the same amount of stress. Reliable scales are needed to measure objective stressors (events and conditions in a woman's life), along with subjective stress (feelings related to these events and conditions) (p. 125).

The stress literature contains an abundance of research that has been conducted on men; nevertheless, a large gap exists in the knowledge about stress in the lives of women and its impact on women's mental health.

Although the health care professional may find it inconvenient to have clients complete an instrument such as the SRE or LES, the theoretical concepts that underpin these instruments may be used to assess the client's level of stress. A broad, open-ended question such as, "What has been going on in your life (since I last saw you)?" can serve as a stimulus for the discussion of major events that have placed some demand on the individual. If the desirability or undesirability of the event is not apparent in the client's response, this dimension, as well as its impact, may be elicited by the question, "What was that like for you?" An empathic response to the client's concerns, e.g., "It sounds like you have had a tough time," is likely to draw further verbalization from the client. Using such counseling techniques as allowing the client to ventilate, eliciting feelings, listening, and conveying empathy, the practitioner establishes a sense of genuineness, which paves the way for strong rapport with the client. Nonverbal cues (e.g., steady eye contact, head nodding) serve to encourage further verbalization.

Any seeming relationship between the client's reported event and her state of wellness or illness should be probed by the practitioner. In addition to creating an awareness of such a relationship, if none exists, this may also serve to confirm the client's suspicions regarding the possibility of a relationship between her state of wellness and stress-inducing demands of her life. When the client's input is solicited, her position as a valued and knowledgeable member of her own health care team is reinforced. Additionally, it provides the practitioner with valuable feedback for further discussion of aspects of the situation that may either exacerbate or reduce perceptions of stress. At this point, the practitioner can educate the client in alternative methods of reducing stress.

Consider the case of 27-year-old Tricia B., who denied specific complaints upon arriving for a routine gynecological and breast examination. During the breast examination she expressed fear that she might have one or more lumps in her breast. Although she believed she had detected lumps during an earlier attempt at self-examination, she was unable to find them at the time of our examination; furthermore, she was somewhat uncertain as to what form a suspicious lump might be expected to take. In determining that her understanding of the breast self-examination was minimal, the practitioner stated that the client was in a better position than anyone else to know the shape and feel of her own breast. Tricia was told to expect changes in her breast to coincide with the various phases of her menstrual cycle. Techniques of breast self-examination were demonstrated, and the client was given the opportunity to practice. Finally, she was instructed to perform the self-examination at the conclusion of each menstrual period, and it was suggested that it could easily be performed in the shower. At a subsequent check-up, the client indicated that she was performing regular breast self-examination and had developed an awareness of changes that occurred in conjunction with phases of the menstrual cycle.

Using the simple, but effective, management techniques, the practitioner was able to both allay fears associated with a perceived threat and enhance the client's sense of control with minimal educational effort. Additionally, the client received acknowledgment of her responsibility as owner of her breast, and she was enabled to assume both responsibility and a sense of control for regular monitoring of her body.

Cognitive Model. Holroyd, Appel, and Andrasik (1983) proposed that psychological stress exists when the individual recognizes an imbalance between either internal or environmental demands and her resources for coping with such demands. In the cognitive model, the stress stimulus is one of perceived threat to important values or goals (Lazarus, 1966). The concept of appraisal of a perceived threat refers to the evaluation of an event in terms of significance to the individual's well-being and her resources or options for responding. Coping involves both intrapsychic and behavioral efforts to tolerate or reduce levels of stress (Holroyd, Appel, & Andrasik, 1983).

As one appraises a situation in terms of its potential threat, Janis's (1958) concept of "the work of worrying" comes into play. This includes mental rehearsal of anticipated losses and development of cognitive reassurances that can serve to reduce fear when the crisis is subsequently confronted. This fits nicely with Bandura's (1977) concept of self-efficacy, which refers to one's confidence in her own ability to cope and do what is necessary to successfully resolve the problem.

The effects of coping on physiological stress responses are still unknown, but current thought is that the way in which an individual copes with stress may be the key variable in predicting a physiological stress response. Effective coping may be more important to the deterrence of illness than an absence of stress (Antonovsky, 1979; Cohen & Lazarus, 1973; Cullen, 1980; Dill & Feld, 1982; Folkman, Schaefer, & Lazarus, 1979; Miller, 1980; Mulder & Mulder, 1980; Roskies & Lazarus, 1980).

Preparatory intervention in the form of information-giving may reduce clients' feelings of helplessness by increasing their personal involvement as active participants in the treatment process (Hamburg & Adams, 1967; Janis, 1983; Miller, 1980). Pranulis, Dabbs, and Johnson (1975) demonstrated that hospitalized patients felt a greater sense of control when given the role of active collaborator with health care professionals. Attention was diverted from their own emotional reactions, as passive recipients, to focus instead on information, in making them active participants in the treatment. Perhaps the crucial factor in ultimately attaining a high level of patient compliance is that of engendering both trust and commitment through acceptance of the patient as a competent partner in her own health care team.

Cognitive Factors

Stress is perceived and experienced subjectively and may be reflected in either physical or psychological symptoms. Regardless of its etiology, the individual is experiencing stress if that is her perception. In this context, stress can be viewed as both a producer and a product of physiological and psychological wear and tear that drains the body of this potential capacity for optimal health.

There is no way to escape the perception of stress in our lives. However, stress can be reduced to a manageable level with effort, accompanied by a commitment to change.

Research on commitment has shown that when a verbal commitment has been made to someone who is esteemed (e.g., a health care professional), the prospect of both social and self-disapproval for reneging serves to bind and stabilize the commitment (Janis & Mann, 1977; Kiesler, 1971; McFall & Hammen, 1971).

The scientific literature is filled with research where stress is either manipulated as an independent variable (i.e., as a causal agent) or measured as the dependent variable (an effect). As interest in the causes and effects of stress has increased, emphasis has focused on the psychosocial perspective, with many current therapies following a cognitive–behavioral approach to the reduction and management of stress (Ellis & Harper, 1977; Epstein & Fenz, 1965; Janis & Rodin, 1979; Meichenbaum & Jaremko, 1980). This modality has firm roots in attribution theory, which involves the individual's perception of an event, and the interpretation, explanation, and meaning attached to that event (Janis & Rodin, 1979; Shaver, 1981; Storms & McCaul, 1976; Veronen & Kilpatrick, 1983).

The evaluation of emotions, internal sensations, health, and illness requires an active process of taking in sensory data, encoding, and organizing it in the brain, appraising it in terms of existing schema, creating tentative hypotheses, and selectively seeking additional information to either confirm or disconfirm the hypotheses. Emotions, feelings, health, and illness are inferred through the perception of sensations. The interpretation of one's bodily state is an ongoing cyclical process triggered by the perception of arousal sensations that, in turn, lead to a search for explanations (Pennebaker, 1980).

The attention paid to cognitive factors in the emotional experience is central to the cognitive labeling theory of Schachter and Singer (1962). In an ingenious experiment, they demonstrated that emotions are the result of a cognitive perceptual process, whereby the individual becomes aware of arousal, seeks an appropriate explanation, and then attaches a meaningful label to the arousal. Information is appraised by combining situational factors from the external environment with sensory data received internally to perceive the state of one's emotions, internal sensations, health, and illness. This perceptual process is uniquely built upon the individual's prior experience and current state of reference. Sensory, encoding, appraisal, and labeling factors are totally unique and subjective for each individual, so that no two people are experiencing an emotion or event in the same way. Building upon this cognitive labeling theory provides a useful model for integrating perception and attribution in understanding their role in emotions, feelings, and health and illness behaviors. This theoretical base is central to developing a full appreciation of the complexities of the stress phenomenon.

The perception of personal control, as an important factor in reducing stress, is supported by a considerable body of literature (Averill, 1973; Ball & Vogler, 1971; Bowers, 1968; Glass, Singer, & Pennebaker, 1977; Houston, 1972; Janis & Rodin, 1979; Johnson & Sarason, 1978; Kanfer & Seider, 1973; Langer, 1983; Lapidus, 1969; Lefcourt, 1981; Pervin, 1963; Pranulis, Dabbs, & Johnson, 1975; Seligman, 1975; Staub, Tursky, & Schwartz, 1971; Suls & Mullen, 1981; Thompson, 1981; Weisenberg, 1977; Weiss, 1970). The meaning attached to both stressful events and their controllability appears to be a central factor in predicting and understanding an individual's reaction in coping with aversive stimuli.

Although the topic of perception has been addressed in the stress literature by cognitive theorists, less attention has been devoted to the perception of illness or wellness and its relationship to specific behaviors. Does the world view of the client who perceives herself as "ill" differ from that of one who views herself as "well?" Are different behaviors associated with each mind set? Expectations of the patient, her family, friends, colleagues, and employer may be affected by the way the individual interprets and acts on perceptions of illness or wellness. It is conceivable that one's perception of wellness could be instrumental in the employment of denial as a defense mechanism to ward off the threat associated with illness and disease. The severity of a perceived threat, combined with a perceived lack of control, may be significant determinants in the client's subjective view of her state of health.

In the case of 38-year-old Sally, a graduate student who professed excellent health, the discovery of a small, but malignant melanoma produced a high level of stress. Unable to work, think, eat, or sleep in accordance with her normal patterns, Sally became hypervigilant about her body and spent much of her waking hours obsessed about her present and future health. Although she had a well-developed support system of family and friends, combined with highly competent medical personnel, fears about her health were paralyzing her efforts to maintain a heavy schedule of responsibilities associated with being a student, instructor, teaching assistant, and wife. Sally reported:

> Before I had even received results from the biopsy, I went to a medical library to read what I could about the disease. The sentence I remember most clearly was, "Melanoma is a highly lethal form of cancer." Even though I knew it was very serious, since the husband of a friend had died with melanoma at the age of 32, I was unable to stop ruminating over the sentence which, like a broken record, kept being repeated in my head. Suddenly, I felt that I was living on borrowed time, and the threat of dying seemed very real. Although my body did not feel any different, I was overwhelmed and sickened by the knowledge that I was harboring what was potentially a highly lethal disease. Even in casual conversation, when people asked, "How are you?" I proceeded to give them a full medical report! My family and friends were so patient and supportive, but I don't know how they tolerated my singular focus. Many mornings I awakened and immediately pulled the covers over my head in a symbolic attempt to withdraw and simply shut out the world. With outpatient surgery scheduled just two days before Christmas, my greatest wish was to simply hide in a corner and be left alone while everyone else enjoyed the holiday festivities. Tears were always close to the surface and they flowed freely, with disconcerting regularity. It is an understatement to say that I was positively miserable.
>
> Although I was well-versed on the literature showing a relationship between positive attitude and successful outcome in cancer patients, I had been unable to internalize this information. The emotional aspect of being terrified precluded my ability to effectively manage the stress. I was used to being in control, and I was simply unprepared to deal with the heretofore unknown feelings of helplessness. Intellectually, I could understand what was happening, but I was emotionally unable to deal with it.
>
> One morning, after months of agonizing and dragging myself through this "blue funk," I decided that I had to actively change my thinking. It was through a process of conscious awareness that I was able to readjust my perceptions. I dealt with facts: my surgeons both said that I was fine and had an excellent prognosis; the pathology report following surgery disclosed no abnormal cells; except for feeling tired, my body was fine—and perhaps the tiredness was due to the fact that following the biopsy, I had discontinued a long-standing regimen of regular exercise. If everything pointed to the fact that I was well, then indeed, I was physically healthy, and all that was left was to straighten my head! At that point, I was able to regain my energy and begin to act like myself once more.
>
> I know that my 'self-talk'—that continuing monologue that goes on in one's own head—was negative, and that I had to force myself to make it positive. When the negative rumination began, I said, sometimes out loud, 'Stop it!' As a conscious process, this was effective. From that point on, I rather quickly regained a sense of well-being and viewed myself as actively taking control, which was a familiar role that provided stability.

It appears that Sally had fairly well-defined ideas about those elements that constituted illness versus wellness behaviors, but unresolved emotional conflicts—primarily involving fear—precluded a swift transition from one to the other. Resolution involved a process of cognitive restructuring. When she determined that objective evidence supported a state of wellness, she was able to modify her subjective evaluation to one of perceived control, which allowed her to regain emotional stability and to adopt behaviors associated with wellness.

Research on alcohol- and drug-related problems in women suffers from the same limitation as research on stress, in that it has primarily been conducted with male subjects, and the results have been improperly generalized to women (Bardwick, 1971; Makosky, 1980; Morrissey & Schuckit, 1978; Sadava, Thistle, & Forsyth, 1978).

Research needs include a further examination of the relationship between premorbid variables and the development of cancer (Fox, 1978), along with studies to strengthen the link between stress and psychic and somatic disease. Janis (1982) suggests prescriptive rules to improve research strategies and obtain meaningful results.

Use of Groups

Physical exercise, yoga, meditation, and psychotherapy are among the stress reduction strategies that may employ groups. Teaching stress management techniques in a group setting is cost effective from the standpoint of reaching a wider audience with fewer professional contact hours than are consumed when working on a one-to-one basis.

Although economic benefits of group work are clear, the research data are less conclusive. The possibility of "evaluation apprehension," i.e., increased arousal or motivation stemming from the perceived threat of judgment by others (Cottrell, 1968, 1972; Henchy & Glass, 1968), may either facilitate or deter the effectiveness of group work. Henchy and Glass (1968) contend that the threat of being evaluated is almost always a factor when tasks are performed in the presence of others. Cottrell (1968, 1972) suggests that the presence of others forces individuals to anticipate both positive and negative outcomes, and that group members may act as an anticipated source of incentives.

Groups also provide an opportunity for social comparison, i.e., comparing oneself to others who are in similar situations, which may be important in assessing the individual's social relations (Pettigrew, 1967). Social comparison processes may affect one's perception of the magnitude or importance of what is believed to be a social deficit.

Stimulation from social sources, and the response to social stimuli, occurs in a dynamic context. Within a group, each individual maintains a sense of preparedness to respond to the unexpected, as part of the process of adaptation to changing demands of the immediate environment (Zajonc, 1980). Latane and Cappell (1972) have demonstrated increased levels of arousal when the subject is in the presence of others.

Research on the role of affiliation (the need to be with others) in human stress has lacked methods of demonstrating a reduction in anxiety as a result of the presence of others. Theories of affiliation proposed by both Schachter (1959) and Bovard (1959), however, assume that the presence of others produces a calming effect for those who are experiencing stress. Perhaps the most critical factor in group work includes the opportunity for members to provide comfort and to reduce the uncertainties of each other (Zajonc, 1980).

Psychosocial and Biological Factors

Emotions and Life Change. Research by Stewart (1982) supports a sequence of emotional orientations through which an individual moves when experiencing life transitions or crises. The initial period of disorientation is manifested by feelings of passivity, helplessness, and loss. This phase is followed by one in which the individual attempts to gain mastery and autonomy. In the final stage, the individual works toward achieving a "complex, accepting, and realistic orientation to the situation" (p. 1103).

Serious Illness. Stress affects the entire family when one of its members faces an acute illness (Linn, 1982). In times of serious illness, family relationships are not likely to improve if they were unstable in times of health (Gaudinski, 1977). In the clinical setting, observation of interactions between client and family will provide an indication of anxiety levels and the type of support that might ameliorate additional stress, caused by feelings of guilt and helplessness on the part of family members.

An alternative approach to care for the terminally ill is the hospice, where patient, family, and friends cope by confronting the reality of impending loss in a supportive atmosphere (Mahar, 1981).

Loneliness. Loneliness is an emotion that can be experienced in solitude or in the midst of a large crowd. It is a gnawing sense of detachment that tends to magnify other stressors in the environment (Silverman, 1981). One of the mediating factors in the experience of loneliness is the ability to exercise personal control over one's relationships to attain a desired level of contact (Perlman & Peplau, 1981). Averill (1973) found evidence supporting the idea that reduced levels of stress and enhanced performance are an outgrowth of feelings of personal control. In a study of college couples who reported feelings of loneliness and depression after the relationship had dissolved, those partners who initiated the breakup and desired an end to the relationship reported feeling less distressed (Hill, Rubin, & Peplau, 1976).

Body Image. The relentless pursuit of youth, beauty, and excitement is a constant source of stress and discontent for many women, regardless of age, size, or physical attributes. In this context, the issue of body image is particularly relevant to women. As depicted in the mass media, the idealized woman is young, thin, glamorous, sexy, exciting, and seemingly happy. Although this image is unrealistic, repeated exposure to this illusion has the effect of reinforcing the stereotype (Zajonc, 1968). Many women experience a sense of frustration, failure, and loss of self-esteem when they perceive themselves as less than this idealized image.

Self-esteem is inherently linked to physical attractiveness, as defined by society (Israel, 1977; Langer, 1983; Nowak, 1977). The idea of women forever maintaining a youthful appearance is deeply rooted in our culture and is reinforced through the encouragement and approval of men. It is paradoxical that many women who attempt to look like an adolescent would shun the idea of acting like one, because the implication is clearly one of immaturity.

Keeping in mind that the concept of attractiveness is culturally defined, the idea of thinness, as a desirable and attractive ideal for women, is peculiar to Western cultures. In this context, it has been estimated that nearly 50 percent of American women are overweight. Every popular magazine geared toward women includes a regular diet column and exhorts either a new diet and exercise plan or a multitude of low calorie recipes. Health spas, exercise clubs, and tanning salons abound with the implied promise of a rejuvenated, slender body to match the glamour and excitement that will accompany it.

Eating Disorders. For the majority of women, the idealized female image is unattainable, and the disillusionment is painful. Compulsive eating disorders are closely tied to body image, along with the issues of power and control. The extremes of both anorexia nervosa and obesity provide signals of fear and unmet needs; both are characterized by feelings of helplessness in changing any part of their lives. Anorexia nervosa is a disorder peculiar to Western cultures, particularly adolescent females (Boskind-Lodahl, 1976; Bruch, 1978). The obsession to be thin, combined with the perception of being fat, wreaks havoc on body organs as the individual slowly starves herself—sometimes to death. Bulimia, a related eating disorder, is equally destructive. Eating binges, accompanied by guilt and shame, are often followed by vomiting and the taking of laxatives to purge the body of food taken in. Because these disorders frequently occur in tandem, the combination of symptoms is referred to as bulimarexia. Psychological referral of both the patient and her family is usually necessary to enable the bulimaretic to understand and manage this over-controlling behavior.

Although obese women claim a desire to be thin, the spectre of possibly becoming a different person, if one should indeed become thin, is frightening enough to serve as an impetus for maintaining excessive weight (Orbach, 1978). As is sometimes the case with seemingly unwanted adolescent problem pregnancies, compulsive eating disorders may represent acting out behaviors. It is as though the individual, because of deep insecurities, is desperately asking a parent, partner, or spouse, "Despite what I do to make myself unhappy or unattractive, do you and will you still love me?" Such testing of a relationship is manifested in many forms and serves as a continuing source of stress to all parties involved. The basis for these insecurities might be most appropriately explored in counseling.

Although obesity knows no gender, the hatred and disgust toward excessive weight in our culture is directed at women. In her provocative exploration of the genesis and treatment of obesity, Orbach (1978) comments on the symbolic meaning of obesity in a feminist context:

> Fat is a response to the many manifestations of a sexist culture. Fat is a way of saying 'no' to powerlessness and self-denial, to a limiting sexual expression which demands that females look and act a certain way, and to an image of womanhood that defines a specific social role. Fat offends Western ideals of female beauty and, as such, every 'overweight' woman creates a crack in the popular culture's ability to make us mere products. Fat also expresses the tension in the mother–daughter relationship, the relationship which has been allocated the feminization of the female. This relationship is bound to be difficult in a patriarchal society because it demands that the already oppressed mothers become the teachers, preparers, and enforcers of the oppression that society will visit on their daughters. (pp. 21–22)

Orbach states that although insight is gained through exploration of the symbolic meanings of fat as rebellion toward oppression, ". . . getting fat remains an unhappy and unsatisfying attempt to resolve these conflicts." Indeed, "obesity is an unsatisfying personal solution and an ineffectual political attack" (Orbach, 1978, p. 23).

In extensive group work described by Orbach, clients focus on building a positive body image and self-concept, bringing hidden fears of being thin to higher levels of awareness, removing judgments about body size, developing self-acceptance, and learning assertion skills.

Revised tables of optimal height and weight ranges for small, medium, and large body frames, longitudinally developed by the Metropolitan Life Insurance Company (1983), have generally been accepted as the standard for a healthy American population. Although the weight for each body type remained stationary for many years, the 1983 revision lowered optimal weight ranges for both women and men in all categories. It should be noted that for the women whose "normal" weight is at the upper end of the range for her height and body frame, dieting may be both ineffective and unnecessary.

Aging. With the process of aging being both natural and inevitable, there is no turning back the clock to restore one's body to what it was in earlier years. It seems that the key to aging gracefully lies in acceptance and enjoyment of each phase of the life cycle. However, stereotyping of the elderly as "worn out and useless" is but one example of contemporary society's devaluation of anything but youth.

A decline in self-esteem may result when aging individuals assume the self-image and behaviors that portray negative stereotypes of the elderly (Snyder & Swann, 1978). Diminished self-esteem has been shown to induce a decreased belief in one's ability to control the environment (Rodin, 1980). Retirement may serve as the catalyst that brings issues of aging into sharp focus where they await resolution (Bradford & Bradford, 1979).

In addition to reviewing updated care practices for the elderly (Hooker, 1976), research has focused on positive aspects of aging (Huyck, 1977) and use of technology to assist the handicapped elderly (Bray & Wright, 1980; Breuer, 1982; Sargent, 1981).

Recently, a client enthusiastically remarked, "I am almost 80, and I'm glad to be old. I have experienced so much during my lifetime, and I always enjoy talking with younger people to keep up with new things that are happening." She showed a keen interest in research being described, asked thoughtful questions, and later wrote a note to convey additional ideas. Although her family has experienced a number of acute personal tragedies, this woman has risen above them. In her words, "I have had to accept the reality of these situations. There was nothing I could do to change them, so I accepted the reality and went on with the business of living." This woman's attitude was so positive and refreshing that I left our encounter feeling rejuvenated. "Old" is something I believe she will never be.

Another example of reinforcing the aging stereotype is a recent game on the market, aimed at an older population, that encourages participants to "remember when." Although reminiscence can be self-affirming in one context, as a game it serves to devalue both present and future, with the implication that good times are only found in reliving the past. At any age, people need to feel useful, and they must be encouraged to set goals toward specific things to which they can look forward.

In the health care setting, older women may have sexual concerns that they are reluctant to mention. Many women experience unsatisfactory marital intercourse in later years (Huyck, 1977). Postmenopausal women may experience discomfort during sexual intercourse when thinning tissues and membranes, along with reduced lubrication from vaginal secretions, are caused by reduced production of estrogen.

Diminished sexual needs and desires of her partner and/or reduced availability of partners, particularly for single older women, constitute legitimate concerns that postmenopausal women may wish to discuss. Loewenstein (1980) suggests that men who tend to experience a decline in energy in their fifties may well be jealous of women "who may be performing at peak capacity in every way at that age, probably because they had a later start" (p. 166). Bardwick (1971) notes that in our sexually repressive society, a woman often needs 15 years of sexual activity to reduce inhibitions and enjoy her sexual capabilities. Women between the ages of 35 and 60 have demonstrated greater sexual interest, responsivity, and orgasmic capacity than younger women (Huyck, 1977; Loewenstein, 1978).

In any routine physical assessment, questions regarding sexual problems should be addressed as matter-of-factly as any other function. Just as the practitioner queries, "Any problems with urination?" the question, "Any sexual problems or concerns?" may open the door for dialogue. Although this might appear trivial, many women have never spoken to a health care professional about sexual concerns because *both* parties have been reluctant to broach the topic! This could be viewed as an indictment of our society's contradictory values, attitudes, and behaviors that cloud the issue of sexuality.

Occupational Stress. Change and adaptation are stressors commonly found in an occupational setting. Change is a source of stress because it requires adaptation to the disruption of behavioral, physiological, and cognitive patterns of functioning. How the change is perceived is particularly important, because adjusting to a change thought to be beneficial is easier than adjusting to change that is judged negative. However, any change can be viewed as stress provoking (Beech, Burns, & Sheffield, 1982; Holmes & Rahe, 1967).

Researchers studying occupational stress (Davidson & Cooper, 1981) have examined blue collar stress (Poulton, 1978), white collar stress (Cooper & Marshall, 1978; Greenwood & Greenwood, 1979), age discrimination toward women (DeGooyer, 1982), exclusion of women from jobs due to occupational health hazards (Stellman, 1977), family stress exacerbated by employment of the wife and/or mother (Asmundsson, 1981), coping with the mental work load (Mulder & Mulder, 1980), and costs of job-related stress (Diamond & Kirmeyer, 1982).

The burnout stress syndrome (Paine, 1982), viewed as a professional hazard (Freudenberger, 1981; Morrow, 1981; Shubin, 1978), is widely prevalent among health care professionals (Gardner & Hall, 1981; Pines & Maslach, 1978; Wilder, 1981). A number of researchers have focused attention on the impact and management of stress in the nursing profession (Appelbaum, 1981; Baer, 1982; Baldwin & Bailey, 1980; Barstow, 1980; Garbin, 1982; Grout, 1980; Hartl, 1982; Scully, 1980).

Nursing, waitressing, and secretarial work—jobs that are primarily filled by women—have been identified as highly stressful occupations. Although the job demands on waitresses are largely physical and demands on secretaries are of a more mental and manual nature, the work of nurses requires high levels of physical, mental, and emotional output.

Changing technology requires many secretaries, among others, to interact with a computer terminal during much of their working time. The advent of the computer has produced, along with its remarkable capabilities, a new set of stressors for those who sit at a computer terminal for lengthy stretches of time. Attention to these problems is in order because of the impact of computer use at home, school, and work. The National Institute of Occupational Safety and Health (NIOSH, 1981) projects that 45 to 50 percent of the working population will work at least part-time on video display terminals by the year 1990.

In addition to frustration, which is not an infrequent by-product of working with computers, other complaints include visual problems (eye fatigue, irritation, and difficulty with focus or accommodation), musculoskeletal difficulties, nervous tension, irritability, and stomach problems (Harvard Medical School Health Letter, 1983; NIOSH, 1981; Springer, 1983).

Visual problems can be reduced by maintaining a visual display with sharp focus (constrast between light and dark areas of at least 8 to 1). If vision is focused primarily at the screen, room lighting should be kept low; if the eyes are trained primarily on paper, room lighting should be relatively bright. Glare can be eliminated by shading windows, positioning the video display screen at right angles to the light source, or by wearing tinted glasses. For every 30 minutes of work with a close focus, workers should spend at least 2 minutes focusing on objects at a minimum distance of 30 feet.

Aches and pains often result from sitting too long in furniture designed for work in a precomputer era. Adjustable height on chairs is a must, and the video screen should be positioned straight ahead, so that the individual is not forced to continually be looking either up or down. A footstool is helpful in raising legs off of the chair seat so that circulation is not impaired, and getting up every 30 minutes for a stretch break is helpful in reducing fatigue. Head, arm, and shoulder movements help relieve tension in the trapezius muscles, which receive the most strain.

Additional factors that add to stressful conditions in this rapidly growing field include insufficient training, monotony of the task, isolation from others, and attempts to keep pace with the speed and efficiency of the machine.

Learning to manage computer-related stress is particularly important because it has the potential to affect individuals with almost no limit on age. The two-year-old whose parent has her matching shapes, colors, and numbers on a video display terminal will never know what life was like before the personal computer. Similarly, the 68-year-old grandmother who spent her summer at a camp for computer instruction does not want to miss the phenomenon (Elmer-DeWitt, 1983).

Another comment on the impact of the computer is in order. The computer is based upon mathematical principles—an understanding of which is necessary for a full appreciation of this tool. In the recent past, women were not encouraged to pursue a strong mathematical background, which has led to the development of impaired mental health in the form of math anxiety in many women (Donady, Kogelman, & Tobias, 1980). Because this has limited potential job opportunities for many women, females of every age must be encouraged with the message that they can do and be whatever in this world that they choose. Encouragement from a health care professional, who is viewed with esteem, can be especially important to an adolescent who has turned her back on others, or the divorcee who is attempting to restructure her life. These insidious sources of stress endanger the individual's health and welfare by dampening enthusiasm, destroying self-confidence, and curtailing potential. The cognitive notion of perception is applied: if a woman appraises a situation as being beyond her reach, the self-fulfilling prophecy usually works to assure that this will be the case.

Managing Stress

With an understanding of the concept of stress, the task at hand is to assist clients to reduce their perceived level of stress. Teaching and learning strategies, based upon principles of adult learning, have been previously covered in Chapters 2 and 3. Using these techniques, a treatment plan may be tailored to the needs of the individual; this is critical to the success of any approach.

In teaching clients to manage stress, which occurs on either a regular or intermittent basis, the focus is on nonprescriptive therapy in a natural setting (Girdano & Everly, 1979; Morse & Furst, 1979; Randolph, 1981; Shaw, 1981). That is, the goal of the practitioner is to teach and guide the client in ways that reduce dependence on the health care system. The idea is to instill the client with a sense of control so that she can independently and successfully cope with stressful events that confront her.

The client must be assured that a certain measure of stress in one's life is both essential and inevitable, and a balance is necessary for optimal health (Selye, 1956). Accepting those things that cannot be changed is essential to the development of strategies to attack those things that can be modified. Harnessing negative energy and using it productively are important steps in appraising the positive and useful aspects of stress. Likewise, developing strategies to confront the challenges of change are essential to effectively manage stress (O'Neill & O'Neill, 1974; Selye, 1974; Sheehy, 1976).

Biofeedback is a noninvasive modality for facilitating relaxation, where the client is actively involved as a participant (Brown, 1977; Cauthen & Prymak, 1977; Morse & Furst, 1979; Randolph, 1981). Electronic instruments attached to the body record physiological responses. Instruments usually include an electromyograph, which measures muscle activity, and a thermistor, which measures skin temperature. The client is trained to interrupt physiological arousal when its presence is indicated by feedback in the form of a tone or light on the instrument. Exercises and other self-regulation modalities

(Beech, Burns, & Sheffield, 1982; Morse & Furst, 1979; Sutterley, 1981), often used in conjunction with biofeedback, include autogenic training (Green, Green, & Walters, 1976; Rosa, 1973), body therapies (Greenwood & Greenwood, 1979), deep breathing (Schwartz, 1978), guided imagery (Pelletier, 1976), meditation (Carrington et al., 1980; McQuade & Aikman, 1974; Woolfolk & Richardson, 1978), progressive relaxation (Jacobson, 1958), self-hypnosis (Sparks, 1962; Woolfolk & Richardson, 1978), systematic desensitization through reciprocal inhibition (Wolpe, 1958), and yoga (Patel, 1973) to attain a deep level of relaxation, termed the relaxation response (Benson, 1975).

Holroyd (1979) suggests that to be effective, treatment strategies must take into consideration those complex cognitive and behavioral interactions with environmental demands that occur in natural settings beyond the confines of the biofeedback laboratory. Meichenbaum (1977) encourages the use of videotaped models to demonstrate desirable coping behaviors, as part of a cognitive–behavioral approach.

Ineffective Coping. In the pursuit to reduce stress in their lives, individuals may develop ineffective and/or destructive responses to stressful stimuli, including denial, complaining, compulsive gambling, and alcohol and drug abuse (Morrissey & Schuckit, 1978; Sadava, Thistle, & Forsyth, 1978). Denial of stressful aspects simply serves to drive the problem inward and delay the prospect of confronting the issue. Complaining to others is ineffective in resolving problems that need to be openly and honestly addressed. Compulsive gambling, excessive consumption of alcohol, and drug abuse have well-established track records as contributors to the escalation of existing difficulties (Applebaum, 1981). The task is to develop appropriate and effective methods to reduce the stress of life.

Proper care of the body is a major feminist value, which assumes greater importance with increasing age (Weg, 1967). Treating one's body with respect throughout the life cycle assumes proper rest, food, and exercise, with moderation or abstinence from cigarettes, alcohol, and other drugs.

Personal Time. One of the more effective techniques in reducing perceived levels of stress is the establishment of regular periods of uninterrupted, personal time for the individual (Goldfein, 1977). This might entail announcing to others that she is unavailable at regular, specified times, when she cloisters herself to be freed from pressures of doing anything at all. This personal time can be used to relax, reduce fatigue, and simply think. When pressures of a fast-paced life-style sometimes force the individual to consider *thinking* a luxury, this private, personal time is ideal for sorting out mental demands and restructuring thought processes.

Rest. As for bodily rest, there is simply no substitute, and the client should be encouraged to make time available for adequate rest to restore herself, both physically and mentally. Unfortunately, individuals often respond to an overload of demands by reducing sleep in order to "catch up." The health care professional is in an ideal position to state, with authority, that the client owes herself the necessity of adequate rest.

Time Management. The perception of being stressed often involves an overwhelming sense of too little time to meet demands that confront the individual. An excellent resource for evaluating commitments and establishing priorities is Lakein's (1973) self-help book on time management, which covers such topics as decision-making, establishing priorities, scheduling, procrastinating, overcoming fear, developing willpower, and making time for oneself. Goldfein (1977) and Woolfolk and Richardon (1978) are also excellent self-help sources.

In many cases, individuals set themselves up as recipients of stress by placing unrealistic expectations on themselves and/or those with whom they come in contact at home, on the job, or in social settings. An example is the attempt to emulate the superwoman myth—an ideal that is well rooted in contemporary culture. A realistic appraisal of the source of these expectations (Ellis & Harper, 1977; Woolfolk & Richardson, 1978) might assist the client in assessing possible rigidity in her own thinking, along with her need for control over others.

Nutrition. Proper care and feeding of the body are essential to maintain feelings of wellness and reduce symptoms of stress. Results of nutrition research suggest detrimental effects on the body from long-term dietary intake of highly processed foods, refined white sugar, salt, caffeine, and chemical additives and preservatives—all of which have been linked to stress (Ballentine, 1978; Burkitt, 1978; Girdano & Everly, 1979; Rosenburg, 1983; Stauth, 1978). Even if the individual is dieting, it is important to maintain the body at optimal levels by eating well-balanced, unhurried meals at regular intervals and with an emphasis on fresh fruits, vegetables, and high fiber grains. Fad diets that exclude fats, carbohydrates, or proteins should be avoided, because these elements are needed by the body (Ballentine, 1978; Burkitt, 1978; Girdano & Everly, 1979; Stauth, 1978). Dieters who find it stressful to adhere to a strict intake regimen might modify feelings of deprivation by allowing themselves one day each weekend to eat foods that have been restricted by the diet.

For information regarding nonmeat sources of protein, Lappé (1975) has compiled a classic resource. The Cooperative Extension, which has an office in each county across the United States, is an excellent resource for current information—most of which is available at no charge to the public—on all aspects of nutrition, dieting, exercise, and healthful living.

Exercise. A program of regular exercise is not only good for the body, but it also provides a sense of doing something positive for oneself. At least some exercise is appropriate for the individual, regardless of age or physical condition. Walking, running, aerobic exercise, swimming, skiing, self-defense arts, tennis, bicycling, golfing, jumping rope, weight-lifting, or working out at an exercise gym are activities that can relieve stress (Girdano & Everly, 1979; McQuade & Aikman, 1974). As little as 10 to 15 minutes of exercise each day can provide evidence of increased muscle tone. The Boston Women's Health Book Collective (1976) offers sound guidelines for choosing an exercise. Once again, the individual must schedule time for exercise and put forth the effort to maintain it on a regular basis.

Relaxation. Relaxation techniques are highly effective in reducing levels of stress. Yoga, meditation, biofeedback, self-hypnosis, and the relaxation response are all used to eliminate external stimuli by focusing on total body relaxation. Use of progressive relaxation techniques has the effect of decreasing the heart rate and breathing, lowering the blood pressure, and slowing the activity of the nervous system.

Diversion. Diversions in one's routine can be employed to reduce stress. Listening to music, reading, writing, taking a different route home, or attending a concert, play, or movie are all ways of diverting attention from routine elements in one's life and focusing on different stimuli.

Cognitive Restructuring. Cognitive restructuring is a coping technique that involves the interpretation of an event from a rational, rather than emotional point of view (Beech, Burns, & Sheffield, 1982; Dill & Feld, 1982; Ellis & Harper, 1977; Folkman, Schaeffer, & Lazarus, 1979; Janis, 1983; Meichenbaum, 1977). A perceived threat may be reconceptualized in nonthreatening terms (Girodo, 1977). The client must first become aware of negative aspects of her internal dialogue or "self-talk," which serves to perpetuate irrational fears associated with a threatening event. A conscious awareness of one's self-talk is necessary before changes can be made to eliminate negative aspects of these cognitions. The health care professional can assist the client by challenging irrational thoughts and guiding toward less self-defeating alternatives (Ellis & Harper, 1977). Most importantly, the practitioner should demonstrate support by encouraging the client in her attempts to successfully meet the demands of anticipated stress, thereby promoting a sense of control (Langer, 1983; Lefcourt, 1981).

Support Systems. Perhaps the most critical factor in reducing stress is a well-developed social support system of family and friends (Cobb, 1976; Epting, 1982; Lieberman & Borman, 1979; Silverman, 1980). This group consists of those who know the individual and her vulnerability, and are in a position to provide strong support in a continuing relationship. Ideally, in an intimate relationship, partners serve as each other's therapist in a mutual support system to soothe the battle scars of daily living.

The development of supportive social networks has been examined by Gottleib (1981) and Maguire (1983), whereas Warren (1981) reported on the use of helping networks as a coping mechanism in urban environments. Frydman (1981) found that the use of supportive social resources reduced the "pathogenic impact" of stress, and Caplan, Killilea, and Abrahams (1976) reported positive results through the use of a multidisciplinary support system.

Reproduction. Stress is often a by-product of issues surrounding the reproductive phase of one's life (Loewenstein, 1978). From puberty to menopause, decisions must be made about birth control and whether—or when—to have children (Luker, 1975; Williams et al., 1975). Unplanned pregnancies are difficult at any age, but are particularly so when they are unwanted (Baldwin, 1973; Boston Women's Health Book Collective, 1976; Yamamoto & Kinney, 1976) or occur in adolescence (Colletta & Gregg, 1981). Unresolved emotional conflicts related to either abortion or relinquishing a child for adoption may haunt the woman for her lifetime. Because of the personal nature and unique factors involved for each client, individual counseling is indicated for women with problem pregnancies.

Loss. Marital disruption (Bloom, Asher, & White, 1978; Chiriboga, 1979), including separation from or loss of a partner or loved one (Bahnson, 1981; Bowlby, 1980; Ramsay & Noorbergen, 1981; Silverman, 1981), is particularly stress provoking, and subsequent adaptation can be a painful, yet an enlightening period of personal growth (O'Neill & O'Neill, 1974). Loss of a loved one through separation, divorce, or death—even if the relationship was less than optimal—seems to trigger feelings associated with other losses that have occurred in earlier years. Use of supportive networks, development of new friendships and activities, combined with "tincture of time," are useful in easing the deep psychological pain and stress that accompanies feelings of loss.

Family Violence. Victims and perpetrators of family violence experience continuing levels of stress that may peak intermittently. Battered women (Petit, 1981) and their children may find temporary refuge in shelters designed to provide an alternative to living with the threat of physical abuse. Child abusers (Collins, 1977) can develop alternative coping strategies in supportive self-help therapy groups such as Parents Anonymous.

Disability. Living with a disabling handicap is a constant source of stress. Although innovative devices to assist the handicapped are available (Bray & Wright, 1980; Breuer, 1982; Hale & Barr, 1979; LaRocca & Turem, 1978), the cost of this technology is frequently prohibitive. A number of agencies may provide financial assistance, but this is woefully inadequate to meet the needs of those who could benefit from assistive devices (see Chapter 10).

Self-help. Self-help resources are widely available to assist individuals in coping with and reducing life stress (Gartner & Riessman, 1977). Individuals may be challenged to think positively (Buscaglia, 1982) and rationally (Ellis & Harper, 1977), examine their problems in relation to predictable life crises (Loewenstein, 1980; Sheehy, 1976), restructure their lives (O'Neill & O'Neill, 1974), evaluate their appearance (Orbach, 1978), and form or join mutual self-help groups (Lieberman & Borman, 1979; Silverman, 1980). Weber and Cohen (1982) have examined beliefs and self-help approaches from a cross-cultural perspective. The popular literature is abundant with resources to help the individual explore specific concerns from a variety of perspectives.

Effecting change is a three-step process: first there must be a desire to change, followed by the behavioral intention as evidenced by a stated commitment to change. Finally, action must be employed to enact the desired change.

There exists a widespread belief that it is easier to change oneself than to change the stress-inducing situation, and this may account for the fact that self-help techniques suggested for both individuals and groups primarily focus on making changes in oneself.

The Health Care Professional as a Resource

Because the health care professional maintains contact with a large and diverse population, and is viewed as a source of information, she has a responsibility to become well acquainted with community resources. It is essential to have a working knowledge of agencies to which clients can be referred for problems relating to individual and family counseling, medical, dental and health care, employment, child care, financial assistance, food cupboards, battered women's and children's shelters, support groups, and recreational programs. Information for quick reference is available through the community's Chamber of Commerce, United Way, Department of Social Services, Cooperative Extension, and Health Department. The practitioner's ability to simply create an awareness of community resources designed to assist clients may serve to reduce the perception of isolation and helplessness.

Stress, Change, and Growth

Change, in and of itself, is a producer of stress. Living in a society that places a high priority on technology requires adaptation, and humans must become more and more complex to keep pace with the tools of technology (von Puttkamer, 1983). Environmental stressors will persist, but individuals must demonstrate creativity and develop tools to turn down the "noise" of stressful stimuli. Only then can we effectively utilize the energy produced by associated arousal.

Because life change is often stressful, but inevitable, we must integrate thinking and reasoning with sensing and feeling to establish priorities that, in turn, will lead us toward greater growth both as individuals and as part of society. As Tielhard de Chardin (1965) observed, "When we learn to live with the uncertainty of growth, it becomes joyous certainty."

AUDIOVISUAL RESOURCES

The following audio cassettes, films, slides, and pamphlets are available in English. There is a serious lack of stress-related patient education material available for use with non-English speaking populations.

Audio Cassettes

Carrington, P. Learning to meditate: Clinically standardized meditation—(CSM) self-regulated course. Pace Educational Systems, P.O. Box 113, Kendall Park, New Jersey 08824, 1979. *(Consists of three 1-hour tapes, plus workbook designed for self-paced instruction in meditation. The workbook contains forms for personal evaluation and follow-up at 3-month intervals.)*

Madden, J. Relaxation/Centering. Human Effectiveness Consultants, 818 State Tower Building, Syracuse, New York 13202. $6.50. *(A two-sided tape that features techniques of deep muscle relaxation and centering, aimed at reducing tension in both body and mind.)*

Films

Managing Stress. CRM/McGraw-Hill, P.O. Box 641, Del Mar, California 92014. *(Available in 16 mm film or 3/4 inch videocassette, color, 33 minutes; purchase $575, rental $95; free preview for purchase consideration. Awarded the Mental Health Association's Best in Show Award for 1979; explores tension generated from within the individual and from within organizations; case study interviews demonstrate techniques of handling stress to increase productivity.)*

Mental Health Association. Learning to cope: How to deal with your tensions. Screenscope, Inc., Suite 2000, 1022 Wilson Boulevard, Arlington, Virginia 22209. 16 mm color, 25 minutes. *(Focuses on management of tensions associated with the inevitable hassles of daily living.)*

Stress. New York State Department of Health, Albany, New York. 16 mm, black and white, 20 minutes. *(Describes stress, its sources, and implications for health; techniques are presented for reducing levels of stress.)*

Slides

Chaisson, G. M. The nature and management of stress. Biomedical Communications, University of Arizona Health Services Center, Tucson, Arizona, 1978. 54 slides, 24-minute audio cassette tape, and guide. *(Depicts symptoms and diseases correlated with stress, and differentiates between coping and adaptation; covers the General Adaptation Syndrome, bodily and intrapsychic responses, and effectiveness of methods of coping with stress.)*

Pamphlets

Stress: Blue Print for Health, 25(1), 1974. Blue Cross Association, 676 North St. Clair, Chicago, Illinois 60611. Health care professionals can obtain up to 100 copies of this pamphlet, at no charge for distribution to patients, by contacting the Public Relations Department of their regional Blue Cross/Blue Shield office. *(An easy to read, 94-page guide to understanding stress throughout the life cycle. Written by authoritative researchers in the field of stress, chapters cover stress associated with childhood, adolescence, middle years, aging, home, occupation, and environment; includes techniques designed to reduce stress. Highly recommended.)*

Public Affairs Pamphlets. Public Affairs Committee, Inc., 381 Park Avenue South, New York, New York 10016. Individual pamphlets may be purchased for $.50, and the 32-page Health Packet costs approximately $12.00. Individual titles can be purchased in low quantity rates. These easy to read, informative, 10- to 28-page patient education pamphlets cover a wide range of health related issues, including nutrition, birth control, chronic diseases, emotional problems, aging, alcoholism, drugs, menopause, obesity, death, social and economic problems, child development and family relations, mental and physical health, and intergroup relations.

- Freese, A. S. *Understanding stress*. Public Affairs Pamphlet No. 538.
- Irwin, T. *How to cope with crises*. Public Affairs Pamphlet No. 464.
- Ogg, E. *Partners in coping: Groups for self and mutual help*. Public Affairs Pamphlet No. 559.

Books

Lakein, A. *How to get control of your time and your life*. New York: New American Library, 1973. *(Written by a leader in the field of time management, a practical approach to the problem is addressed in an easy-to-read text. Topics covered include such stress-inducing areas as decision making, establishing priorities, scheduling time, procrastinating, overcoming fear, developing willpower, and making time for oneself. Highly recommended.)*

REFERENCES

Andrews, J. G., & Tennant, C. Editorial: Life event stress and psychiatric illness. *Psychological Medicine*, 1978, *8*, 545–549.

Antonovsky, A. *Health, stress, and coping*. San Francisco: Jossey-Bass, 1979.

Applebaum, S. H. *Stress management for health care professionals*. Rockville, Md.: Aspen Systems, 1981.

Asmundsson, R. Women at work: Stresses within the family. In C. Getty & W. Humphreys (Eds.), *Understanding the family: Stress and change in American life*. New York: Appleton-Century-Crofts, 1981.

Averill, J. R. Personal control over aversive stimuli and its relationship to stress. *Psychological Bulletin*, 1973, *80*, 186–303.

Baer, C. L. Effective time management. In D. C. Sutterley & G. F. Donnelly (Eds.), *Coping with stress: A nursing perspective*. Rockville, Md.: Aspen Systems Corporation, 1982.

Bahnson, C. B. Stress and cancer: The state of the art, Part 2. *Psychosomatics*, 1981, *22*(3), 207–220.

Baldwin, A., & Bailey, J. T. Work-site interventions for stress reduction. *Journal of Nursing Education*, 1980, *19*(6), 48–53.

Baldwin, B. Problem pregnancy counseling. In R. C. Wilson (Ed.), *Problem pregnancy and abortion counseling*. Saluda, N.C.: Family Life Publications, 1973.

Ball, T. S., & Volger, R. E. Uncertain pain and the pain of uncertainty. *Perceptual Motor Skills*, 1971, *33*, 1195–1203.

Ballentine, R. *Diet and nutrition: A holistic approach*. Honesdale, Pa.: Himalayan International Institute, 1978.

Bandura, A. Self-efficacy: Toward a unified theory of behavioral change. *Psychological Review*, 1977, *89*, 191–215.

Bardwick, J. *Psychology of women*. New York: Harper & Row, 1971.

Barstow, J. Stress variance in hospice nursing. *Nursing Outlook*, 1980, *28*(12), 751–754.

Beech, H. R., Burns, K. E., & Sheffield, B. F. *A behavioral approach to the management of stress*. New York: John Wiley & Sons, 1982.

Benson, H. *The relaxation response*. New York: William Morrow & Co., 1975.

Bloom, B. L., Asher, S. J., & White, W. W. Marital disruption as a stressor: A review and analysis. *Psychological Bulletin*, 1978, *85*(4), 867–894.

Boskind-Lodahl, M. Cinderella's stepsisters: A feminist perspective on anorexia nervosa and bulimia. *Signs 2*, 1976, *2*(2), 342–356.

Boston Women's Health Book Collective. *Our bodies, ourselves: A book by and for women* (2nd ed., rev.). New York: Simon & Schuster, 1976.

Bovard, E. W. The effects of social stimuli on the response to stress. *Psychological Review*, 1959, *66*, 267–277.

Bowers, K. G. Pain, anxiety, and perceived control. *Journal of Consulting and Clinical Psychology*, 1968, *32*, 596–602.

Bowlby, J. *Loss: Sadness and depression. Attachment and Loss, Vol. III*. New York: Basic Books, 1980.

Bradford, L. P., & Bradford, M. I. *Retirement: Coping with emotional upheavals*. Chicago: Nelson-Hall, 1979.

Bray, J., & Wright, S. *The use of technology in the care of the elderly and the disabled: Tolls for living*. Westport, Conn.: Greenwood Press, 1980.

Breuer, J. A. *A handbook of assistive devices for the handicapped elderly: A new help for independent living*. New York: Haworth Press, 1982.

Brown, B. B. *Stress and the art of biofeedback*. New York: Harper & Row, 1977.

Bruch, H. *The golden cage*. Boston: Harvard Press, 1978.

Burkitt, D. The link between low-fiber diet and disease. *Human Nature*, 1978, *1*(12), 34–41.

Buscaglia, L. *Living, loving and learning*. New York: Holt, Rinehart & Winston, 1982.

Cannon, W. B. *Bodily changes in pain, hunger, fear, and rage*. Boston: C.T. Branford, 1929.

Caplan, G., Killilea, M., & Abrahams, R. B. *Support systems and mutual help: Multidisciplinary explorations*. New York: Grune & Stratton, 1976.

Carrington, P., Collings, G. H., Benson, H., Robinson, H., Wood, L. W., Lehrer, P. M., Woolfolk, R. L., & Cole, J. W. The use of meditation–relaxation techniques for the management of stress in a working population. *Journal of Occupational Medicine*, 1980, *22*(4), 221–231.

Cattell, R. B., Eber, H. W., & Tatsuoka, M. M. *Handbook for the sixteen personality factor questionnaire* (16 PF). Champaign, Ill.: Institute for Personality and Ability Testing, 1978.

Cauthen, N. R., & Prymak, C. A. Meditation versus relaxation: An examination of the physiological effects of relaxation training and of different levels of experience with transcendental meditation. *Journal of Consulting and Clinical Psychology*, 1977, *45*(3), 496–497.

Chiriboga, D. A. Marital separation and stress: A life course perspective. *Alternative Lifestyles*, 1979, *2*(4), 461–470.

Cobb, S. Social support as a moderator of life stress. *Psychosomatic Medicine*, 1976, *38*(5), 300–314.

Cohen, F. Personality, stress, and the development of physical illness. In G. C. Stone, F. Cohen, N. E. Adler, & Associates (Eds.), *Health psychology*. San Francisco: Jossey-Bass, 1980.

Cohen, F., & Lazarus, R. Active coping processes, coping dispositions, and recovery from surgery. *Psychosomatic Medicine*, 1973, *35*, 375–389.

Colletta, N. D., & Gregg, C. H. Adolescent mothers' vulnerability to stress. *Journal of Nervous and Mental Disease*, 1981, *169*(1), 50–54.

Collins, M. C. *Child abuser: A study of child abusers in self-help group therapy*. Littleton, Mass.: Public Sciences Group, 1977.

Cooper, C. L., & Marshall, J. Source of managerial and white collar stress. In C. L. Cooper & R. Payne (Eds.), *Stress at work*. New York: John Wiley & Sons, 1978.

Cottrell, N. B. Social facilitation. In C. G. McClintock (Ed.), *Experimental social psychology*. New York: Holt, 1972.

Cottrell, N. B. Performance in the presence of other human beings: Mere presence, audience and affiliation effects. In E. C. Simmel, R. A. Hoppe, & G. A. Milton (Eds.), *Social facilitation and imitative behavior*. Boston: Allyn & Bacon, 1968.

Cullen, J. Coping and health: A clinician's perspective. In S. Levine & H. Ursin (Eds.), *Coping and health*. New York: Plenum Press, 1980.

Davidson, M. J., & Cooper, C. L. A model of occupational stress. *Journal of Occupational Medicine*, 1981, *23*(1), 564–574.

DeGooyer, J. Women, work and age discrimination. *Graduate Women*, 1982, *76*(5), 21–23.

Derogatis, L. R., Rickels, K., & Rock, A. F. The SCL-90 and the MMPI: A step in the validation of a new self-report scale. *British Journal of Psychiatry*, 1976, *128*, 280–290.

Diamond, A., & Kirmeyer, S. L. Stress in the workplace. *Human Ecology Forum*, 1982, *12*(3), 13–15.

Dill, D., & Feld, E. The challenge of coping. In D. Belle (Ed.), *Lives in stress: Women and depression*. Beverly Hills, Calif.: Sage, 1982.

Dohrenwend, B. S., & Dohrenwend, B. P. Some issues in research on stressful life events. *Journal of Nervous and Mental Disease*, 1978, *166*, 7–15.

Donady, B., Kogelman, S., & Tobias, S. Math anxiety and female mental health: Some unexpected links. In C. L. Heckerman (Ed.), *The evolving female: Women in psychosocial context*. New York: Human Sciences Press, 1980.

Ellis, A., & Harper, R. A. *A new guide to rational living*. North Hollywood, Calif.: Wilshire, 1977.

Elmer-DeWitt, P. Mixing suntans with software. *Time*, 1983, *122*(8), 61.

Epstein, S., & Fenz, W. D. Steepness of approach and avoidance gradients in humans as a function of experience. *Journal of Experimental Psychology*, 1965, *70*, 1–2.

Epting, S. P. Coping with stress through peer support. In N. D. C. Sutterley & G. F. Donnelly (Eds.), *Coping with stress: A nursing perspective*. Rockville, Md.: Aspen Systems, 1982.

Folkman, S., Schaefer, C., & Lazarus, R. S. Cognitive processes as mediators of stress and coping. In V. Hamilton & D. Warburaton (Eds.), *Human stress and cognition*. New York: John Wiley & Sons, 1979.

Fox, B. H. Premorbid psychological factors as related to cancer incidence. *Journal of Behavioral Medicine*, 1978, *1*(1), 45–133.

Freudenberger, H. The burned out professional: What kind of help? *Proceedings of the First National Conference on Burnout*. Philadelphia, Pennsylvania, 1981.

Frydman, M. I. Social support, life events, and psychiatric symptoms: A study of direct, conditional and interaction effects. *Social Psychiatry*, 1981, *16*, 69–78.

Garbin, M. Stress research in clinical settings. In D. C. Sutterley & G. F. Donnelly (Eds.), *Coping with stress: A nursing perspective*. Rockville, Md.: Aspen Systems, 1982.

Gardner, E. R., & Hall, R. C. W. The professional stress syndrome. *Psychosomatics*, 1981, *22*(8), 672–680.

Gartner, A., & Riessman, F. *Self-help in the human services*. San Francisco: Jossey-Bass, 1977.

Gaudinski, M. S. Psychological considerations with patients on respirators. *Aviation, Space, and Environmental Medicine*, 1977, *48*, 71–73.

Girdano, D., & Everly, G. *Controlling stress and tension: A holistic approach*. Englewood Cliffs, N.J.: Prentice-Hall, 1979.

Girodo, M. Self-talk: Mechanisms in anxiety and stress management. In C. D. Spielberger & E. G. Sarason (Eds.), *Stress and anxiety* (Vol. 4). New York: Wiley, 1977.

Glass, D. C., Singer, J. E., & Pennebaker, J. W. Behavioral and physiological effects of uncontrollable environmental events. In D. Stokols (Ed.), *Perspectives on environment and behavior*. New York: Plenum Press, 1977.

Goldfein, D. *Every woman's guide to time management*. Millbrae, Calif.: Les Femmes, 1977.

Gottleib, B. H. *Social networks and social support*. Beverly Hills, Calif.: Sage, 1981.

Green, E. E., Green, A. M., & Walters, E. D. *Outline of verbal procedure used in developing voluntary control of internal states in autogenic feedback training*. Topeka, Kan.: The Menninger Foundation, 1977.

Green, E., Green, A. M., & Walters, E. D. Biofeedback training for anxiety tension and reduction. In J. White & J. Fadiman (Eds.), *Relax: How you feel better, reduce stress and overcome tension*. New York: Dell, 1976.

Greenwood, J. W., III, & Greenwood, J. W., Jr. *Managing executive stress: A systems approach*. New York: John Wiley & Sons, 1979.

Grout, J. W. Stress and the nurse: A selected bibliography. *Journal of Nursing Education*, 1980, *19*(6), 58–62.

Hale, G., & Barr, P. *The source book for the disabled: An illustrated guide to easier and more independent living for physically disabled people, their families, and friends*. New York: Paddington Press, Distributed by Grosset & Dunlap, 1979.

Hamburg, D., & Adams, J. A perspective on coping behavior: Seeking and utilizing information in major transitions. *Archives of General Psychiatry*, 1967, *17*, 277–284.

Hartl, D. E. Stress management and the nurse. In D. C. Sutterley & G. F. Donnelly (Eds.), *Coping with stress: A nursing perspective*. Rockville, Md.: Aspen Systems, 1982.

Harvard Medical School Health Letter. The DDT's: The new social disease. *Harvard Medical School Health Letter,* 1983, *8*(5), 1–2, 5.

Henchy, T., & Glass, D. C. Evaluation apprehension and the social facilitation of dominant and subordinate responses. *Journal of Personality and Social Psychology,* 1968, *10,* 446–454.

Hill, C. T., Rubin, Z., & Peplau, L. A. Break-ups before marriage: The end of 103 affairs. *Journal of Social Issues,* 1976, *32,* 147–168.

Holmes, T. H., & Rahe, R. H. The social readjustment rating scale. *Journal of Psychosomatic Research,* 1967, *11,* 213–218.

Holroyd, K. A. Stress, coping, and the treatment of stress related illnesses. In J. R. McNamara (Ed.), *Behavioral approaches in medicine: Application and analysis.* New York: Plenum Press, 1979.

Holroyd, K. A., Appel, M. A., & Andrasik, F. A cognitive–behavioral approach to psychophysiological disorders. In D. Meichenbaum & M. E. Jaremko (Eds.), *Stress prevention and reduction.* New York: Plenum Press, 1983.

Hooker, S. *Caring for elderly people: Understanding and practical help.* London: Routledge & K. Paul, 1976.

Houston, B. K. Control over stress, locus of control, and response to stress. *Journal of Personality and Social Psychology,* 1972, *21,* 249–255.

Huyck, M. Aging: The ultimate experience. *Vassar Quarterly,* 1977, *73,* 3–7.

Ibrahim, M. A. Editorial: The changing health state of women. *American Journal of Public Health,* 1980, *70*(2), 120–121.

Israel, J. Confessions of a 45-year-old feminist. In L. Troll, J. Israel, & K. Israel (Eds.), *Looking ahead.* Englewood Cliffs, N.J.: Prentice-Hall, 1977.

Jacobson, E. *Progressive relaxation.* Chicago: University of Chicago Press, 1958.

Janis, I. L. Stress inoculation in health care. In D. Meichenbaum & M. E. Jaremko (Eds.), *Stress reduction and prevention.* New York: Plenum Press, 1983.

Janis, I. L. Postscript: Improving research strategies (1982). In I. L. Janis (Ed.), *Stress, attitudes, and decisions: Selected papers.* New York: Praeger Publications, 1982.

Janis, I. L. *Psychological stress.* New York: John Wiley & Sons, 1958.

Janis, I. L., & Mann, L. *Decision making: A psychological analysis of conflict, choice, and commitment.* New York: Free Press, 1977.

Janis, I. L., & Rodin, J. Attribution control and decision-making: Social psychology in health care. In G. C. Stone, F. Cohen, & N. E. Adler (Eds.), *Health psychology.* San Francisco: Jossey-Bass, 1979.

Jenkins, C. C. Psychosocial modifiers of response to stress. *Journal of Human Stress,* 1979, *5*(4), 3–15.

Johnson, J. H., & Sarason, I. G. Life stress, depression and anxiety: Internal–external control as a moderator variable. *Journal of Psychosomatic Research,* 1978, *22,* 205–208.

Kanfer, F. & Seider, M. L. Self-control: Factors enhancing tolerance of noxious stimulation. *Journal of Personality and Social Psychology,* 1973, *25,* 381–398.

Kiesler, C. A. (Ed.). *The psychology of commitment.* New York: Academic Press, 1971.

Kimball, C. P. Stress and psychosomatic illness. *Psychosomatic Research,* 1982, *26*(1), 63–71.

Lakein, A. *How to get control of your time and your life.* New York: New American Library, 1973.

Langer, E. J. *The psychology of control.* Beverly Hills, Calif.: Sage, 1983.

Lapidus, L. B. Cognitive control and reaction to stress: Conditions for mastery in the anticipatory phase. Proceedings of the 77th convention of the American Psychological Association, 1969.

Lappé, F. M. *Diet for a small planet* (Rev. ed.). New York: Ballantine Books, 1975.

LaRocca, J., & Turem, J. S. *The application of technological developments to physically disabled people.* Washington, D. C.: Urban Institute, 1978.

Latane, B., & Cappell, H. The effects of togetherness on heart rate in rats. *Psychonomic Science,* 1972, *29,* 177–179.

Lazarus, R. S. *Psychological stress and the coping process.* New York: McGraw-Hill, 1966.

Lefcourt, H. M. Locus of control and stressful life events. In B. S. Dohrenwend & B. P. Dohrenwend (Eds.), *Stressful life events and their contexts.* New York: Prodist, 1981.

Lieberman, M. A., & Borman, L. D. *Self-help groups for coping with crisis: Origins, members, processes, and impact*. San Francisco: Jossey-Bass, 1979.

Linn, L. J. Psychosocial needs of patients with acute respiratory failure. In D. C. Sutterley & C. L. Donnelly (Eds.), *Coping with stress: A nursing perspective*. Rockville, Md.: Aspen Systems, 1982.

Loewenstein, S. F. Toward choice and differentiation in the midlife crises of women. In C. L. Heckerman (Ed.), *The evolving female: Women in psychosocial context*. New York: Human Sciences Press, 1980.

Loewenstein, S. F. An overview of some aspects of female sexuality. *Social Casework*, 1978, 59(2), 106–115.

Luker, K. *Taking chances: Abortion and the decision not to contracept*. Berkeley, Calif.: University of California Press, 1975.

Maguire, L. *Understanding social networks*. Beverly Hills, Calif.: Sage, 1983.

Mahar, I. The hospice concept: An alternative approach to terminal care. In C. Getty & W. Humphreys (Eds.), *Understanding the family: Stress and change in American family life*. New York: Appleton-Century-Crofts, 1981.

Makosky, V. P. Stress and the mental health of women: A discussion of research and issues. In M. Guttentag, S. Salasin, & D. Belle (Eds.), *The mental health of women*. New York: Academic Press, 1980.

McFall, R. M., & Hammen, L. Motivation, structure, and self-monitoring: Role of nonspecific factors in smoking reduction. *Journal of Consulting and Clinical Psychology*, 1971, 37, 80–86.

McQuade, W., & Aikman, A. *Stress: What it is, what it can do to your health, how to fight back*. New York: E. P. Dutton, 1974.

Mechanic, D. The concept of illness behavior. *Journal of Chronic Disease*, 1962, 15, 189–194.

Meichenbaum, D. *Cognitive–behavioral modification: An integrative approach*. New York: Plenum Press, 1977.

Meichenbaum, D., & Jaremko, M. *Stress prevention and management: A cognitive–behavioral approach*. New York: Plenum Press, 1980.

Metropolitan Life Insurance Company. *Metropolitan height and weight tables*. New York: Metropolitan Life Insurance Company, March 1983.

Miller, N. E. A perspective on the effects of stress and coping on disease and health. In S. Levine & H. Ursin (Eds.), *Coping and health*. New York: Plenum Press, 1980.

Miller, S. When is a little information a dangerous thing? Coping with stressful events by monitoring vs. blunting. In S. Levine & H. Ursin (Eds.), *Coping and health*. New York: Plenum Press, 1980.

Morrissey, E. R., & Schuckit, M. A. Stressful life events and alcohol problems among women seen at a detoxification center. *Journal of Studies on Alcohol*, 1978, 39(9), 1559–1576.

Morrow, L. The burnout of almost everyone. *Time*, September 21, 1981, 84.

Morse, D. R., & Furst, M. L. *Stress for success: A holistic approach to stress and its management*. New York: Van Nostrand Reinhold, 1979.

Mulder, G., & Mulder, L. J. M. Coping with mental work load. In S. Levine & H. Ursin (Eds.), *Coping and health*. New York: Plenum Press, 1980.

Nathanson, C. A. Sex, illness, and medical care: A review of data, theory, and method. *Social Science and Medicine*, 1977, 11, 13–25.

National Institute of Occupational Safety and Health (NIOSH). Potential health hazards of video display terminals. Washington, D. C.: U.S. Government Printing Office, June 1981.

Nowak, C. A. Does youthfulness equal attractiveness? In L. Troll, J. Israel, & K. Israel (Eds.), *Looking ahead*. Englewood Cliffs, N.J.: Prentice-Hall, 1977.

O'Neill, N., & O'Neill, G. *Shifting gears: Finding security in a changing world*. New York: M. Evans, 1974.

Orbach, S. *Fat is a feminist issue*. New York: Berkley, 1978.

Paine, W. S. An ecological perspective on the burnout stress syndrome. *Human Ecology Forum*, 1982, 12(3), 15–19.

Parsons, T. *The social system*. Glencoe, N.Y.: The Free Press, 1951.

Patel, C. H. Yoga and biofeedback in the management of hypertension. *Lancet*, 1973, *11*, 1053.

Paykel, E. S. Contribution of life events to causation of psychiatric illness. *Psychological Medicine*, 1978, *8*, 245–253.

Pelletier, K. *Mind as healer, mind as slayer*. New York: Dell, 1976.

Pennebaker, J. W. Self-perception of emotion and internal sensation. In D. M. Wegner & R. R. Vallacher (Eds.), *The self in social psychology*. New York: Oxford University Press, 1980.

Perlman, D., & Peplau, L. A. Social psychology of loneliness. In S. Duck & R. Gilmour (Eds.), *Personal relationships (3): Personal relationships in disorder*. New York: Academic Press, 1981.

Pervin, L. A. The need to predict and control under conditions of threat. *Journal of Personality*, 1963, *34*, 570–587.

Petit, M. Battered women: A (nearly) hidden social problem. In C. Getty & W. Humphreys (Eds.), *Understanding the family: Stress and change in American family life*. New York: Appleton-Century-Crofts, 1981.

Pettigrew, T. F. Social evolution theory: Convergences and applications. In D. Levine (Ed.), *Nebraska Symposium on Motivation*. Lincoln, Neb.: University of Nebraska Press, 1967.

Pilowsky, I. Abnormal illness behavior. *British Journal of Medical Psychology*, 1969, *42*, 347–351.

Pines, A., Maslach, C. Characteristics of staff burnout in mental health settings. *Hospital and Community Psychiatry*, 1978, *29*(4), 233–237.

Poulton, C. E. Blue collar stressors. In C. L. Cooper & R. Payne (Eds.), *Stress at work*. New York: John Wiley & Sons, 1978.

Pranulis, M., Dabbs, J., & Johnson, J. General anesthesia and the patients' attempts at control. *Social Behavior and Personality*, 1975, *3*, 49–51.

Rabkin, J., & Struening, E. Life events, stress, and illness. *Science*, 1976, *191*, 1013–1020.

Ramsay, R. W., & Noorbergen, R. *Living with loss: A dramatic new breakthrough in grief therapy*. New York: William Morrow, 1981.

Randolph, G. The yin and yang of clinical practice. In D. C. Sutterley & G. F. Donnelly (Eds.), *Coping with stress: A nursing perspective*. Rockville, Md.: Aspen System, 1981.

Rodin, J. Managing the stress of aging: The role of control and coping. In S. Levine & H. Ursin (Eds.), *NATA Conference on Coping and Health*. New York: Academic Press, 1980.

Roghmann, K. J., & Haggerty, R. J. Daily stress, illness and use of health care in young families. *Pediatric Research*, 1973, *7*, 520–526.

Rosa, K. R. *You and AT*. New York: E. P. Dutton, 1973.

Rosenburg, H. S. *Nutrition and stress*. New Canaan, Conn.: Keats, 1983.

Roskies, E., & Lazarus, R. S. Coping theory and teaching of coping skills. In P. Davidson & S. Davidson (Eds.), *Behavioral medicine: Changing health life styles*. New York: Brunner/Mazel, 1980.

Sadava, S. W., Thistle, R., & Forsyth, R. Stress, escapism and patterns of alcohol and drug use. *Journal of Studies on Alcohol*, 1978, *39*(5), 725–736.

Sarason, I. G., Johnson, J. H., & Siegel, J. M. Assessing the impact of life changes: Development of the life experiences survey. *Journal of Consulting and Clinical Psychology*, 1978, *48*(5), 932–946.

Sargent, J. V. *An easier way: Handbook for the elderly and handicapped*. Ames, Iowa: Iowa University Press, 1981.

Schachter, S. *The psychology of affiliation*. Stanford, Calif.: Stanford University Press, 1959.

Schachter, S., & Singer, J. E. Cognitive, social, and psychological determinants of emotional state. *Psychological Review*, 1962, *69*, 379–399.

Schmale, A. H. Giving up as a final common pathway to changes in health. *Advances in Psychosomatic Medicine*, 1972, *8*, 20–40.

Schwartz, J. *Voluntary controls*. New York: E. P. Dutton, 1978.

Scully, R. Stress in the nurse. *American Journal of Nursing*, 1980, *80*(5), 912–915.

Seligman, M. *Helplessness: On depression, development, and death*. San Francisco: W. H. Freeman, 1975.

Selye, H. The stress concept and some of its implications. In V. Hamilton & D. Warburton, (Eds.), *Human stress and cognition*. New York: John Wiley & Sons, 1979.

Selye, H. *Stress without distress*. New York: J. B. Lippincott, 1974.

Selye, H. *The stress of life*. New York: McGraw-Hill, 1956.

Shaver, K. G. Back to basics: On the role of theory in the attribution of causality. In J. H. Harvey, W. J. Ickes, & R. F. Kidd (Eds.), *New directions in attribution research* (Vol. 3). Hillsdale, N.J.: Lawrence Erlbaum Associates, 1981.

Shaw, S. E. Health education for the public: Stress and stress management. In D. C. Sutterley & G. F. Donnelly (Eds.), *Coping with stress: A nursing perspective*. Rockville, Md.: Aspen Systems, 1981.

Sheehy, G. *Passages*. New York: E. P. Dutton, 1976.

Shubin, S. Burnout: The professional hazard you face in nursing. *Nursing,* 1978, *78*(8), 22–27.

Silverman, P. R. *Helping women cope with grief*. Beverly Hills, Calif.: Sage, 1981.

Silverman, P. R. *Mutual help groups: Organization and development*. Beverly Hills, Calif.: Sage, 1980.

Sklar, L. S., & Anisman, H. Stress and cancer. *Psychological Bulletin,* 1981, *89*(3), 369–406.

Smelser, N. J. *Theory of collective behavior*. New York: The Free Press of Glencoe, 1963.

Snyder, M., & Swann, W. Behavioral confirmation in social interaction: From social perception to social psychology. *Journal of Experimental Social Psychology,* 1978, *14*, 148–162.

Sparks, L. *Self-hypnosis, a conditioned-response technique*. New York: Grune & Stratton, 1962.

Springer, T. J. Automation and office ergonomics: The promise and the problems. Proceedings of the Fourth Annual Office Automation Conference, Philadelphia, 1983, 69–77.

Staub, E., Tursky, B., & Schwartz, G. E. Self-control and predictability: Their effects on reactions to aversive stimulation. *Journal of Personality and Social Psychology,* 1971, *18*, 157–162.

Stauth, C. Nutrition for life. *New Age,* 1978, *4*(7), 46–61.

Stellman, J. M. *Women's work, women's health: Myths and realities*. New York: Pantheon, 1977.

Stewart, A. J. The course of individual adaptation of life changes. *Journal of Personality and Social Psychology,* 1982, *42*(6), 1100–1113.

Stewart, A. J., & Salt, P. Life stress, life-styles, depression, and illness in adult women. *Journal of Personality and Social Psychology,* 1981, *40*(6), 1063–1069.

Storms, M. D., & McCaul, K. D. Attribution processes and emotional exacerbation of dysfunctional behavior. In J. H. Harvey, W. J. Ickes, & R. F. Kidd (Eds.), *New directions in attribution research* (Vol. 1). Hillsdale, N.J.: Lawrence Erlbaum Associates, 1976.

Suls, J., & Mullen, B. Life events, perceived control and illness: The role of uncertainty. *Journal of Human Stress,* 1981, *7*(2), 30–34.

Sutterley, D. C. Stress and health: A survey of self-regulation modalities. In D. C. Sutterley & G. F. Donnelly (Eds.), *Coping with stress: A nursing perspective*. Rockville, Md.: Aspen Systems, 1981.

Teilhard de Chardin, P. *The phenomenon of man*. New York: Harper & Row, 1965.

Thompson, S. C. Will it hurt less if I can control it? A complex answer to a simple question. *Psychological Bulletin,* 1981, *90*, 89–101.

Veronen, L. J., & Kilpatrick, D. G. Stress management for rape victims. In D. Meichenbaum & M. E. Jaremko (Eds.), *Stress reduction and prevention*. New York: Plenum Press, 1983.

Vinokur, A., & Selzer, M. L. Desirable versus undesirable life events: Their relationship to stress and mental distress. *Journal of Personality and Social Psychology,* 1975, *32*, 329–337.

von Puttkamer, J. The future: Do we have a choice? *Educational Leadership,* 1983, *42*, 4–8.

Warren, D. I. *Helping networks: How people cope with problems in the urban community*. Notre Dame, Ind.: University of Notre Dame Press, 1981.

Weber, G. H., & Cohen, L. *Beliefs and self-help: Cross-cultural perspectives and approaches*. New York: Human Sciences Press, 1982.

Webster, S. CRTs and comfort. *Syracuse University Academic Computing Center Notes,* 1983, *96*, 14–16.

Weg, R. More than wrinkles. In N. L. Troll, J. Israel, & K. Israel (Eds.), *Looking ahead*. Englewood Cliffs, N.J.: Prentice-Hall, 1967.

Weisenberg, M. Pain and pain control. *Psychological Bulletin*, 1977, *86*, 1008–1044.

Weiss, J. M. Somatic effects of predictable and unpredictable shock. *Psychosomatic Medicine*, 1970, *32*, 397–409.

Wilder, J. F. Editorial: Recognizing burnout in health professionals. *Psychosomatics*, 1981, *22*(8), 653–656.

Williams, C. C., Williams, R. A., Grizwold, M. J., & Holmes, T. H. Pregnancy and life change. *Journal of Psychosomatic Research*, 1975, *19*(2), 123–129.

Wolff, H. G. Life situations, emotions, and bodily disease. In *Symposium on stress*. Washington: National Research Council & Walter Reed Army Medical Center, 1953.

Wolpe, J. *Psychotherapy by reciprocal inhibition*. Stanford, Calif.: Stanford University Press, 1958.

Woolfolk, R. L., & Richardson, F. C. *Stress, sanity, and survival*. New York: New American Library, 1978.

Yamamoto, K. J., & Kinney, D. K. Pregnant women's ratings of different factors influencing psychological stress during pregnancy. *Psychological Reports*, 1976, *39*, 203–214.

Zajonc, R. B. Compresence. In P. B. Paulus (Ed.), *Psychology of group influence*. Hillsdale, N.J.: Lawrence Erlbaum Associates, 1980.

Zajonc, R. B. Attitudinal effects of mere exposure. *Journal of Personality and Social Psychology Monograph Supplement*, 1968, *9*, 1–27.

Education for Contraceptive Decision Making

8

Geri LoBiondo-Wood

The use of a contraceptive method moves beyond the choice about what method to use. Choice implies one's ability to make a decision based on an independent reasoning process. The choice of a contraceptive method is not an isolated process; it reflects one's attitudes toward oneself, one's partner, pregnancy, sexuality, and intimacy. Knowledge and ability to problem solve are integral components of the decision-making process. Even though these issues may seem clear, the decision to contracept is also intertwined with social, cultural, religious, and developmental issues that exist for each individual.

Contraception has various meanings. Contraception has been defined as the prevention of conception, fertility control, birth control, and the prevention of birth by specific mechanical, chemical, or pharmaceutical means (Jaffe, 1979; Neubardt, 1967; Webster 1966). What seems to be lacking in these definitions is the role of the individual. The definition that best seems to include the individual is "the availability of an effective contraceptive, so that an individual can plan when to have or not have a child with the goal of satisfying personal desires" (Hatcher et al., 1984).

Until the early 1960s birth control was practiced by methods that carried a substantial risk of pregnancy. Many of the early methods did not require the assistance of a health care provider for procurement. With the advent of oral contraceptives, intrauterine devices, and improvements in older methods, women needed the expertise of health care providers. The need for professional assistance has added another dimension to the procurement and use of contraceptive methods. The added dimension is the knowledge, attitudes, and biases of the provider toward contraception.

Before recommending a contraceptive method, the health care professional needs to offer information about methods that are effective, safe, and economical, and ascertain which might be acceptable to both partners. The individual's life-style, family planning goals, and feelings toward sexuality also need to be considered. Contraceptive teaching should not be confined to family planning settings but should also be addressed by health care providers in primary health care settings. This chapter is designed to enhance the health care provider's knowledge about the contraceptive decision-making process and to provide guidelines for assessment and interventions that may assist individuals and their partners to make a more comfortable decision regarding contraception. Each method is reviewed and major points highlighted. Further detail on a particular method may be found in the cited references.

Before beginning the review of methods and teaching strategies, it is important to note that there are two levels of contraceptive effectiveness. These are theoretical effectiveness and use effectiveness. Theoretical effectiveness is a method's effectiveness when used without error and when used consistently. User effectiveness is the effectiveness of a method across groups of individuals, it takes into consideration inconsistency of use as well as user error. A pregnancy that results from improper method use has been termed a patient failure (Hatcher et al., 1982). No contraceptive method is 100 percent effective and without risks. Risks may be related to dangers of the method, risk of inconvenience, and risk of method failure (Hatcher et al., 1984). When suggesting a method these and other issues, which are addressed in this chapter, should be considered. (Table 8–1).

CONTRACEPTIVE METHODS

Hormonal Agents

One of the most widely used and debated groups of contraceptives are the hormonal agents. The hormonal agents include a large variety of oral and injectable agents, progestin-releasing intrauterine devices, and silastic implants. The oral contraceptive or the "Pill" is the most popular and most thoroughly tested of the hormonal agents. The other remaining hormonal agents, such as subdermal silastic capsules containing progestins and vaginal rings impregnated with progestins, are in various stages of testing and are used infrequently (Hatcher et al., 1984). The oral contraceptive contains either a synthetic progestin or a combination of progesterone and estrogen. The Pill is currently being used by 55 million women throughout the world and used by 10 million women in the United States (Ory, Forrest, & Lincoln, 1983). Only 50 to 70 percent of women who start birth control pills continue to use them after one year (Hatcher et al., 1984). The theoretical effectiveness of the Pill approaches 100 percent. The Pill affects ovulation, implantation, tubal transport, cervical mucus, and the endometrium, as well as many other body systems. There are both adverse and beneficial effects of the hormonal agents. The Pill inhibits ovulation by suppressing the effect of estrogen on the hypothalamus and pituitary. Follicle-stimulating hormone (FSH) and luteinizing hormone (LH) are consequently suppressed at midcycle. Lower estrogen dose contraceptives (50 µg or less) alone do not always suppress ovulation or progestin (Hatcher et al., 1984). Transport of the fertilized ovum is accelerated by estrogen whereas progestins seem to slow tubal transport. After ovulation, the high levels of estrogen alter the normal development of the endometrium. This results in areas of edema alternating with areas of diminished cellularity, thereby inhibiting implantation. Estrogens facilitate sperm capacitation and thereby favorably affect cervical mucus. On the other hand, progestins produce a scanty, thick, cellular mucus that hampers the transport of sperm and its ability to penetrate the cervical mucus (Hatcher et al., 1984)

Noncontraceptive benefits include protection against acne and decreased menstrual cramping and blood loss, which leads to increased iron stores (Mishell, 1982). Pill users have fewer complaints of menorrhagia and intermenstrual bleeding (Vessey et al., 1976). Various studies have demonstrated that women who have used the Pill for more than a year had approximately one-third the chance of developing acute pelvic inflammatory disease as women who used no form of contraception (Ory, 1982; Rubin, Ory, & Layde, 1981; Senanayake & Kramer, 1980). Hulka and colleagues (1982) found that women using combination product oral contraceptives had one-half the risk of endometrial cancer as

TABLE 8–1. SUMMARY OF CONTRACEPTIVE METHODS AND TEACHING CONSIDERATIONS

Contraceptive Method	Effectiveness	Advantages	Disadvantages	Other Side Effects	Teaching Considerations
Hormonal agents	100%	Decreased menstrual cramping; decreased blood loss; protection against uterine and ovarian cancer, benign breast disease, pelvic inflammatory disease (PID); no inconvenient devices; regulates menstrual cycle	Nausea; weight gain; breast tenderness; spotting between menses; requires a prescription	Increased risk of: high blood pressure, heart attack, stroke, thromboembolic phenomena	Women over 35 years have increased risk of complications: assess for history of high blood pressure, stroke, cardiovascular disease, diabetes, smoking, explain how pill works, effectiveness, advantages, disadvantages and risks
Intrauterine devices (IUDs)	97–99%	Low cost; spontaneity of intercourse; freedom from daily pill-taking and devices	Increased menstrual bleeding; anemia; spotting between menses; dysmenorrhea; IUD expulsion; lost string	Hemorrhage; uterine perforation; cervical and pelvic inflammatory diseases	Allergy to copper or other metals; advise checking for presence of string regularly, especially after each menses. Instruct patient about possible pain and bleeding upon insertion
Diaphragm	98%	Low cost; safety; no routine schedule	Increased urinary tract infections (UTI); may provide protection against STD; requires a prescription; needs available equipment, must be inserted before intercourse and remain in place for 6 hr afterward. Must be refitted after childbirth, abortion or weight gain or loss of more than 10 lb	Possible increased risk of toxic shock syndrome	Allergy to rubber or spermicides in both user and partner; advise use of a spermicide agent as well; need to teach insertion technique and care of diaphragm

226

Method	Effectiveness	Advantages	Disadvantages		
Cervical cap	Approximately 92–98%	Low cost; left in place longer than diaphragm; few side effects	Requires a prescription and examination; insertion and removal more difficult than diaphragm	Allergy to rubber or spermicide	Teaching of insertion technique can be lengthy and may be more difficult to learn
Vaginal sponge	Variable; between 73–90%	No prescription; safety; no systemic effects; protection against STD; less messy than diaphragm; can be left in longer than diaphragm; effective for 24 hr	May have some irritation or allergy to spermicide contained in sponge	Possibility of increased risk of toxic shock syndrome	Because they are purchased over the counter, women may not completely understand proper method of insertion
Condom	2 to 10 pregnancies per 100 women-years. Approaches effectiveness of pill when used with spermicide	Low cost; easily obtainable to adults as well as adolescents; protection against STD; no prescription needed	Slipping, tearing during use; complaints of decreased sensation and interruption of lovemaking	None	Allergy to rubber in both user and partner; advise use of a spermicide agent as well
Vaginal spermicidal agents	Highly variable	Increased vaginal lubrication; protection against cervical neoplasia, gonorrhea and trichomoniasis	Failure to melt in vagina	None	Allergy to spermicide in both user and partner
Coitus interruptus	Low effectivity	No cost available	Not for long-term use; male needs self-control in order to withdraw prior to ejaculation; disrupts sexual pleasure	None	Requires much self-control; watch for signs and symptoms of stress and frustration

(continued)

TABLE 8–1. (cont.)

Contraceptive Method	Effectiveness	Advantages	Disadvantages	Other Side Effects	Teaching Considerations
Sterilization	100%	Permanent	Permanent; requires surgery	Possible surgical complications	Requires a different contraceptive decision-making approach and informed consent; assess motivation, attitude and maturity of both the individual and the couple
Natural family planning (NFP)	Highly variable	Low cost; safety; acceptable to many cultural and religious groups	Requires long periods of abstinence; may decrease spontaneity in lovemaking	None	Effectiveness increased by use of multiple NFP methods; needs a motivated woman; teaches a woman a great deal about her body's changes
Others (douching; abstinence)	Low effectivity	Low cost	No systemic effects	None	Watch for signs of stress and frustration; allergic reaction to product

did nonusers. Other studies have also documented a decreased incidence of benign breast disease (Brinton et al., 1981; Paffenbarger et al., 1977) and benign ovarian cysts (Ory, 1982; Vessey et al., 1976). A decreased risk of ovarian cancer was found in women 40 through 59 years of age who had discontinued use more than 10 years previously (Cramer et al., 1982). This did not hold true for women under 40 years of age (Cramer et al., 1982).

Side effects of the Pill include minor problems as well as life-threatening complications. The minor problems are nausea, weight gain, breast tenderness, and spotting between periods. The possible life-threatening side effects include increased risk of cardiovascular complications such as stroke, myocardial infarction (MI), thromboembolic phenomena, and hypertension. Women who smoke, have diabetes, hypertension, or a history of cardiovascular disease, and those over 35 years of age have an increased risk of the cardiovascular complications. Other contraindications of the use of hormonal agents include: acute or chronic liver disease, pregnancy, malignancy of the breasts or reproductive system, and breastfeeding. Additionally, oral contraceptives can affect all other body systems including the psyche to varying degrees. These bodily responses are the same as those symptoms that occur during natural periods of hormone excess or deficiency (Fogel & Woods, 1981). Before suggesting the Pill, the health care provider should assess the woman's past and present health status, age, and habits, such as smoking. Long-term contraception intentions and the ability to follow a daily habit of pill-taking and to understand the scheduling of taking the prescribed pill also need to be considered.

Intrauterine Devices

Another popular and effective method is the intrauterine device (IUD). Approximately two million women in the United States are using an IUD (Ory, Forrest, & Lincoln, 1983). The theoretical effectivenes of the IUD is between 97 and 99 percent. The differences in effectiveness are due to variables related to the IUD such as size, shape, presence of copper or progestin, and a number of other patient variables such as age, parity, and frequency of intercourse. Use effectiveness ranges between 90 to 96 percent. Use effectiveness depends on ease of insertion, clinician experience, likelihood of expulsion by the woman, patient ability to detect expulsion, ease of reinsertion, and access to medical services (Hatcher et al., 1984). The IUD is made of inert plastic and is available in loops, seven (7), M and T shapes, and spiral coils. Some IUDs have copper or progesterone added. Each brand of IUD has its own pros and cons, as well as pregnancy and expulsion rates. The exact mode of action is unknown. It is postulated that IUDs may prevent implantation of a fertilized egg through an immune or inflammatory process or by an increased local production of prostaglandins (Hatcher et al., 1984).

Benefits of the IUD are effectiveness, cost, and freedom from daily pill-taking. The IUD does not require any equipment, and allows spontaneity of intercourse. IUDs have few noncontraceptive benefits. They are occasionally used to prevent adherence of the walls of the uterus by synechiae (Asherman's syndrome) (Hatcher et al., 1984). Side effects of the IUD include pregnancy (failed IUD), increased menstrual bleeding, spotting, hemorrhage, anemia, dysmenorrhea, IUD expulsion, lost string, uterine perforation, embedding, cervical perforation, cervical disease, pelvic inflammatory disease (PID), and ectopic pregnancy. Providers need to assess the woman's risk of PID; although there are few IUD-related deaths attributed to PID, the disease is a major cause of infertility because of scarring and blockage of the fallopian tubes. Women under 25 years of age who have more than one sex partner and wish to bear children in the future are not good candidates for an IUD because of an increased risk of PID (Ory, Forrest, &

Lincoln, 1983). On the other hand, it may be an excellent choice for older monogamous users whose risk of PID is 10 times lower than a younger woman's risk (Ory, Forrest, & Lincoln, 1983). The IUD is not recommended for women who have active or recurrent pelvic infections, ectopic pregnancy, multiple sex partners, or heavy menses and clots (Hatcher et al., 1984). The woman who has an IUD is encouraged to check for the string to make sure that the IUD is in place. Therefore, it is also not recommended for women who would find it difficult to check for the IUD string.

Mechanical Barriers

Diaphragm. The diaphragm and cervical cap are among the earliest methods of mechanical birth control. The diaphragm is a shallow, dome-shaped rubber cap made of latex rubber, with flexible edges. The diaphragm is available in a range of sizes (50–100 mm in diameter), and three rim shapes. The flex-spring rim is a delicate rim with gentle spring strength. The coil-spring rim has a sturdy rim with a firm spring strength. The third type is the arcing-spring rim, which has a sturdy rim with firm spring strength. Type used depends on parity and vaginal muscle tone (Hatcher et al., 1984). The diaphragm covers the cervix, thus preventing sperm from entering the uterus. When used correctly, an overall effectiveness rate of 98 percent has been documented for the diaphragm (Lane, Arceo, & Sobrero, 1976). For full effectiveness the use of a spermicidal agent is advised. The benefits of the diaphragm are its safety, cost, and effectivenss. The diaphragm is a favorable contraceptive option for women who cannot or do not want to use hormonal contraceptives. The diaphragm and spermicidal agent may also provide protection against sexually transmitted infections and decrease the risk of PID. The risks include an occasional allergic reaction to the rubber or the spermicide in the user or the partner, increased chance of urinary tract infection, cystitis, and the risk of pregnancy due to improper insertion. Several cases of toxic shock syndrome (TSS) have been reported associated with the use of a diaphragm (Hatcher et al., 1984). Women should be advised not to use the diaphragm during menses, to avoid prolonged placement (more than 24 hours), and to watch for the danger signs and symptoms of TSS. Women who leave their diaphragm in too long after intercourse and women who do not cleanse and dry the diaphragm properly are at higher risk for other infections as well (Hatcher et al., 1984).

The disadvantages of the diaphragm center mainly on attitude and motivation. There are psychological, social, and educational issues that may affect use. If a woman feels uncomfortable inserting the diaphragm she probably will be less motivated to use it. This method requires time, practice, and education for proper use. Some women find the method difficult and uncomfortable either psychologically or physically. This method requires a woman to have the equipment available when the possibility of intercourse exists. The carrying of equipment may not be reasonable for some women. Additionally, some women and men may find the method disruptive to spontaneous intercourse.

Cervical Cap. The cervical cap is a small thimble-shaped cup, which is widely used in Europe and its gaining in usage and acceptance in the United States. The cervical cap is made of flexible rubber or plastic. The cervical cap covers the cervix and remains in place by suction. It is usually filled with spermicide. The mechanism of action and effectiveness is similar to the diaphragm except that it can be left in place longer. The general consensus is three days but different manufacturers vary time rules for insertion and removal and their instructions should be checked (NAACOG Newsletter, 1983). The advantages of the cervical cap are: no alteration of hormonal systems, can be left in longer than a diaphragm, can be used for women with poor pelvic floor muscles, low cost, and women do not experience bladder pressure with the cap (Fogel & Woods, 1981; Hatcher et al., 1984).

The disadvantages are allergic reaction to the cap or spermicide, insertion may be more difficult to master than for the diaphragm, and the position of the cervix may make it impossible to fit a cap. The cervical cap is contraindicated for women who have cervical malformations including extremely long or short cervix, inflammation of adnexa, cervical erosion, lacerations or cervicitis, difficulty inserting or removing the cap, pelvic and vaginal infections, abnormal Pap smear, and history of toxic shock syndrome (Whartman, 1976). The cervical cap is not FDA approved and is only available through private and public health services who have FDA approved prescribing protocols. In 1981, the FDA approved monies to study efficacy rates and to fund development of the cap (NAACOG Newsletter, 1983).

Vaginal Contraceptive Sponge. The contraceptive vaginal sponge is a disposable sponge containing the spermicide nonoxynol 9 (N-9) and has been approved for use by the FDA. The sponge is smaller and thicker than a diaphragm, with an indentation on one surface (to fit over the cervix) and a woven polyester strap (to facilitate removal). It is available in one size only and without a prescription. The device acts as contraceptive in three ways: (1) it releases spermicide, (2) blocks sperm from the cervical os, and (3) absorbs seminal fluid (Hatcher et al., 1984; Medical Letter, 1983). The effectiveness has been established to be between 73 and 90 percent (Hatcher et al., 1984; Kafka & Gold, 1983; Medical Letter, 1983). Absorption of vaginal secretions and compression during intercourse causes the release of the spermicide. The advantages of the sponge over systemic contraceptive methods seem to be perceived safety and absence of health-affecting side effects (Aznar et al., 1981). It is not messy and only needs to be moistened with about two tablespoonfuls of water before use. Once inserted, it is protective immediately and for at least 24 hours. It is important to note that it should not be left in any longer than 24 hours. Like the diaphragm it should be left in place for 6 hours after intercourse, removed, and discarded (Kafka & Gold, 1983).

The negative aspects of the method include: possible allergy to polyurethane or nonoxynol 9; anatomical abnormalities, such as uterine prolapse, that may interfere with placement; the softness of the sponge may make insertion more difficult than a diaphragm; if the strap is turned the wrong way, removal may also be difficult (Aznar et al., 1981; Kafka & Gold, 1983; Medical Letter, 1983). No serious adverse effects have been reported. Some sponge users have reported allergy, vaginal dryness, difficult removal, irritation, itching and a malodor when the sponge has been left in place for long periods of time. The sponge is not recommended for use during the menstrual period (Hatcher et al., 1984; Kafka & Gold, 1983). There is currently some question as to whether use or misuse of the sponge could lead to TSS. If a woman has a history of TSS, the sponge is contraindicated (Medical Letter, 1983). The sponge is easily accessible over the counter and is likely to find acceptance as a temporary method among women changing from one contraceptive method to another.

Vaginal Spermicide Agents. Vaginal foams, creams, jellies, suppositories, and tablets are methods of contraception that should be inserted no more than 30 minutes before intercourse. These methods, if used correctly, inhibit the movement of sperm through the cervical os. Spermicidal agents consist of a chemical (usually nonoxynol 9 or octoxonol), which kills the sperm, and an inert base of foam, cream, or jelly. These preparations vary widely in their effectiveness. Failure rates of 1.55 to 29 pregnancies per woman-years of use have been reported in the past decade (Hatcher et al., 1984). When used in combination with condoms or diaphragms, these methods are highly effective. High failure rates are related to improper use. The advantages of these methods include protection against gonorrhea and trichomoniasis, increased vaginal lubrication, little physiological risk to body systems, and attainment without a prescription. Spermicides may also protect against cervical neoplasia (Hatcher et al., 1984). The most common side effect is an allergic response to the agent either in the user or partner. The major disadvantages are failure of the agent to melt in the vagina prior to intercourse, and the couple's inability to plan and incorporate the method into sexual foreplay and intercourse or to use it every time one has intercourse. Couples also complain of unpleasant taste, too much lubrication, and being messy. Even if the woman obtains a spermicidal over the counter, the health provider should explain the proper use of these methods in order to facilitate proper use.

It has been suggested that the use of spermicide at point of conception or during pregnancy only results in a higher risk of birth defects (Huggins et al., 1982; Jick et al., 1981; Rothman, 1982). The data are still inconclusive, but it is recommended that spermicide be avoided if pregnancy is suspected (Hatcher et al., 1984).

Condom. The condom, a rubber or processed collagenous tissue sheath, which fits over the penis, is probably the oldest method of birth control. The condom carries minimal risk of physiological side effects and is highly effective when used properly. When used correctly as directed the theoretical failure rate is two pregnancies per 100 women-years whereas the actual failure rate is 10 pregnancies per 100 women-years (Hatcher et al., 1984). The use effectiveness rate nears that of the Pill when the condom is used with foam.

The condom does not adversely affect or interrupt any of the body's systems. Advantages of the condom are: relatively low cost, easily accessible to adults as well as adolescents, and serves as an effective protection against sexually transmitted infections. Occasional allergic reaction to the rubber in the condom is the only known side effect. Negative aspects include: improper use, slippage or tearing during use, complaints of decreased sensation, and the interruption of lovemaking (Hatcher et al., 1984). The latter disadvantages may be prevented by the use of lubricated condoms and incorporation of putting the condom on in the couple's foreplay.

Natural Family Planning

Natural family planning or fertility awareness methods have become increasingly popular. Natural family planning methods allow freedom from adverse physical side effects, involve no equipment (except for a thermometer), are not opposed generally by religious and cultural groups, and include the partner in planning and responsibility. The natural family planning methods are rhythm or calendar method, basal body temperature method (BBT), ovulation method (mucous or Billings method), and sympto-thermal methods. The goal of these methods is to predict ovulation and fertile periods so one can avoid intercourse during these periods. The efficacy rates vary greatly in a range from 70 to 99.7 percent effectiveness. The BBT method with intercourse after ovulation is the most effective and the calender method is the least effective (Hatcher et al., 1984). All methods are based on the assumption that hormonal fluctuations in the menstrual cycle produce detectable physical signs that can be used for fertility awareness (Fogel & Woods, 1981).

The rhythm or calendar method requires a woman to calculate her fertile period by recording the length of several consecutive cycles. This method assumes that ovulation occurs on day 14 (plus or minus 2 days) before the onset of the next menses (sperms live 2 to 3 days and the ovum survives for 24 hours) (Hatcher et al., 1984). To use the calender method, a woman should record her menstrual cycle for 6 months preceding the use of this method. If a woman's cycle is irregular, cycle variability needs to be carefully accounted for and considered before implementing this method (Hatcher et al., 1984). The BBT method requires a woman to determine ovulation by recording her daily basal body temperature upon awakening and before any activity. A drop in temperature immediately precedes ovulation with a slight increase in temperature 24 to 72 hours after ovulation. The mucous or Billings method uses the changes in character and appearance of cervical secretions to assess the occurrence of ovulation. The Billings method recognizes four identifiable phases of the menstrual cycle: menstruation, early safe days, unsafe days, and late safe days. A woman is taught to recognize the changes in wetness and viscosity of the cervical secretions. A yellow, viscous mucus is normally present during the preovulatory (early safe) and postovulatory (late safe) phases of the menstrual cycle. During the ovulatory (unsafe days), the mucus becomes slippery and clear, similar to a raw egg white. This mucus can stretch without breaking into a strand that measures 6 centimeters or greater and is called good Spinnbarkeit phenomena (Billings, 1975; Britt, 1977; Hatcher et al., 1984) (Fig. 8–1). The sympto-thermal method generally involves both partners. It is based on an assessment of BBT, cervical mucous changes, and identification of secondary symptoms such as increased libido, increased fullness in the abdominal area, position of the cervix, and mittelschmerz. All of these methods require periods of abstinence from intercourse or use of another method during fertile periods. The effectiveness of these methods varies greatly and is affected by many variables. Some women use a combination of two or three natural family planning methods to increase effectiveness. Careful instructions about fertility signs and how to keep records of these changes need to be given, preferably to both the woman and her partner.

The advantages of these methods include: safety, acceptable to most religious groups, free or very inexpensive, help women learn a great deal about their reproductive system and menstrual cycle, and involve both partners. There are no physiological side effects. The disadvantages of the natural family planning methods are mainly psychological (Hatcher et al., 1984). These methods may cause frustration due to periods of abstinence, decreased spontaneity, and the necessity of keeping detailed records. Some women find it difficult to identify BBT or cervical mucous patterns or they experience irregular menses, which make natural methods a risky choice as a contraceptive method. These methods require a woman and her partner to be highly motivated and aware of physiological changes.

Coitus Interruptus

Coitus interruptus, or the withdrawal method, mandates that the man withdraw and ejaculate away from the woman's genitalia. The failure rate of this method is quite high. The theoretical failure rate is approximately 16 pregnancies per 100 women per year and 23 pregnancies per 100 women per year among actual users (Hatcher et al., 1984). The advantages of withdrawal are the lack of monetary cost and freedom from physiological side effects. On the negative side, this method requires a great deal of control, it is psychologically stressful, and couples may experience a lack of sexual satisfaction. Even if a couple uses this method correctly, ejaculatory fluid may escape before the penis is withdrawn and preejaculatory secretions may contain sperms (Hatcher et al., 1984).

234

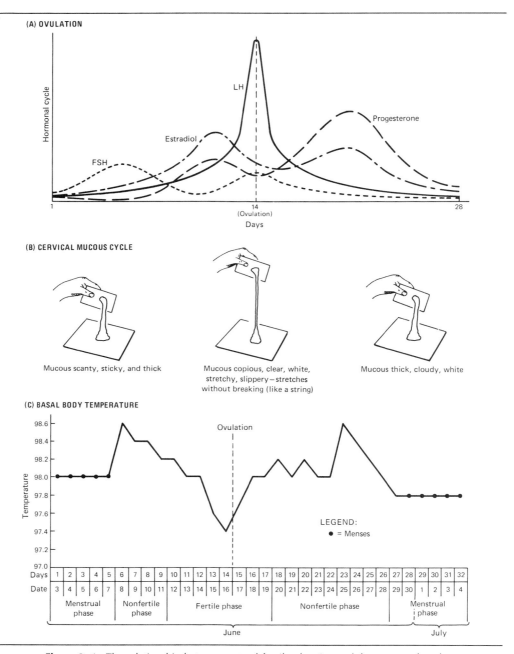

Figure 8–1. The relationship between natural family planning and the menstrual cycle.

Sterilization

For a small number of single women and an increasing number of married couples over 30 years of age, sterilization or the permanent resolution of birth control is the most commonly used method of fertility control (Hatcher et al., 1984). Approximately 11.6 million women of reproductive age have had tubal sterilization or have a male partner who has had a vasectomy (Ory, Forrest, & Lincoln, 1983). Sterilization, because of its permanence and use of a surgical procedure, requires a different contraceptive decision-making approach and informed consent. The informed written consent should include an explanation of the risks and benefits of sterilization, both physical and psychological, and possible alternative procedures. The benefits are that it is permanent, effective, and frees one of repeated decisions and costs. The risks are that surgery may lead to morbidity and mortality, expensive in the short term, not 100 percent effective (slight chance of pregnancy), and surgery to reverse the procedure is expensive and not always successful (Hatcher et al., 1984). An individual or couple who requests sterilization should be counseled on these issues and have time to ask questions and express fears about the procedure and their sexual functioning. Both partners should be included in the decision making. Whether the client is single or a couple, their motivation, attitudes, and maturity should be closely assessed. A clear explanation of the procedure and its possible side effects should be explained in detail. The woman should have written instructions, written risks, and a written signed and witnessed consent for the specific procedure to be performed (Hatcher et al., 1984). They also should be allowed several visits, if necessary, and a time should elapse between the signing of the consent and the operative procedure (usually 24 to 48 hours). This allows the client additional time for last minute mind changes.

There are many terms used to describe the various surgical techniques for female sterilization. Sterilization can be thought of as consisting of two parts—approach and method of tubal occlusion. Approaches may be done through the abdomen or the vaginal cul-de-sac. Methods of occlusion include tubal ligation, silastic ring, plastic cap, electro-coagulation, or removal of tubes, ovaries, or uterus (Porter, Waife, & Holtrop, 1983). Each procedure has its own advantages and disadvantages and should be thoroughly explored before choosing a procedure.

Ineffective Methods

Douching, abstinence, and lactation have been used as methods of birth control. Douching done after intercourse may in fact mobilize the sperm into the cervical canal. An individual using this as a method is demonstrating motivation to use birth control, but is lacking the knowledge of effectiveness. Abstinence from intercourse is effective, but may be frustrating as a long-term method. It is used by couples as part of natural planning methods. Lactation suppresses, but does not completely inhibit, ovulation after childbirth. It requires an extremely strict regimen for any level of effectiveness and is not recommended.

EFFICACY OF CONTRACEPTIVE USE

Contraceptive efficacy is defined as continuity of use, method effectiveness, user effectiveness, user comfort, knowledge, and satisfying contraceptive planning. Superficially, many methods seem effective, easy to obtain and use, yet this does not necessarily mean high efficacy.

Several million women from all age groups and backgrounds both single and married experience unplanned pregnancies every year. According to various surveys (Tietze, 1978; Zabin, Kantner, & Zelnick, 1979; Zelnick & Kantner, 1980), the number of women engaging in premarital intercourse has steadily increased. The majority of women engaging in sexual activity do not use consistent or effective means of contraception (Zabin, Kantner, & Zelnick, 1979; Zelnick & Kantner, 1979). Compared with other industrialized countries, the United States has a relatively high rate of mistimed and unwanted pregnancies; more than half of all pregnancies are reported to be unplanned (Ory, Forrest, & Lincoln, 1983). These data are troublesome for health care providers as effective methods are easily available. The selection, availability, and education in the use of a method are only part of a woman's needs when making contraceptive decisions. Reasons for continued use or nonuse are varied and complex. Before a teaching plan can be developed, a woman's motivation and needs should be closely assessed and incorporated into the planning.

CONTRACEPTIVE DECISION MAKING

How an individual makes decisions has interested many disciplines of science. Throughout one's life learning occurs by various means. As a consequence of learning an individual develops a repertoire of routine behaviors based on previous successful operations in past situations. Thereafter, when an individual encounters similar circumstances, he or she can generally apply previous behavior and feel no undue conflict. Yet as one develops and matures, new situations are encountered that require new formulations and actions. This sequence is the decision-making process (Brim et al., 1962) (Fig. 8–2). An individual's ability to make comfortable and sound personal judgments is a vital skill. Decision making can be related to one's ability to problem solve. For a discussion of factors that may affect one's ability to problem solve see Chapter 3.

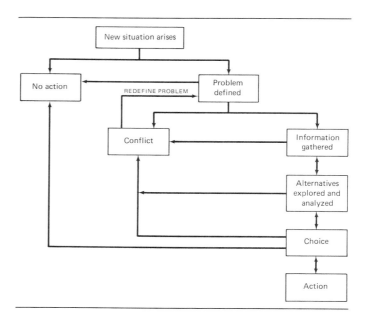

Figure 8–2. Decision-making process.

Individuals make decisions in response to a need to change either their thinking, their behavior, or both. Individual decisions occur within the context of the environment. Whether or not identified there are goals and strategies. The strategies have different weights of importance and may or may not be in line with the goals. For example, a woman may not wish to become pregnant but does not use a contraceptive method consistently. Conflict and motivation as well as personality variables brought to a situation can influence strategies depending on the importance of the goal to the individual. It seems that it is the goal itself that is central to decision processes and the value that one places on it that guides one toward a decision. Values develop over time and form a process of learning. The value attached to the goal therefore affects the strategies that one uses.

Conflict may arise depending on the complexity of a decision. It seems that if in the process of decision making one does not feel a commitment to the final decision, conflict will probably occur. The conflict, if not reduced, will draw the individual's attention away from the decision and its consequences and focus more on the conflict between the alternatives.

Contraceptive behaviors involve a complex set of variables beyond a temporal decision of which method to use or not to use. One's ability to make decisions is influenced by growth and developmental issues. Studies on adolescent sexuality highlight many points of concern; younger ages of first intercourse, low use of birth control, an increased percentage of unwanted pregnancies, and a high rate of abortions. From a developmental standpoint it is quite obvious that adolescents may have difficulty with sexual issues. Adolescence is commonly known as a time for sexual awakening, for increased curiosity, for changes in physical and cognitive processes, and a search for identity, peer approval, and a time for developing attitudes and beliefs (see Chapter 2 for a discussion on Adolescent Learning Needs). Studies on teens reveal that between 54 and 90 percent have some knowledge of contraceptive methods (Baldwin, 1977; Zelnick & Kantner, 1979). One critical factor is missing from these statements. It is not clear from these studies what the breadth, correctness, and scope of knowledge is and whether adolescents have a meaningful framework to attach to this knowledge. Younger women are also less experienced in contraception, are more fertile, and have intercourse more frequently than older women (Ory, Forrest, & Lincoln, 1983). Generally, adolescents do not easily identify with health care providers nor do they independently seek health care assistance.

With increased age comes an enlarged data base, increased experience, and time to refine beliefs, attitudes, and knowledge about one's self and the world. Fisher and colleagues (1979) and Thompson and Spanier (1978) found that contraceptive effectiveness increased among college-aged women when support from a partner was present, when relationships were more lasting, and when values and beliefs were articulated. As growth and development progress, one's knowledge and cognitive processes increase and become more specific. The knowledge one has is based on positive and negative sexual cues learned through socialization, which in turn mediate sexual behavior and attitudes. The experience of time and learning gives reference points upon which to make refined decisions. Most women tend to be more effective users as they become more experienced with a method (Ory, Forrest, & Lincoln, 1983).

Decision-making theory has been a variable used in testing how women make contraceptive decisions. Diamond and colleagues (1973) conducted a retrospective study with a group of pregnant women seeking abortions, to trace if coitus was anticipated, if pregnancy was planned, and if contraceptives were used. They found that two-thirds of the women did not use a contraceptive method even though coitus was anticipated and pregnancy unplanned. Two of the most common reasons cited for not using contraceptive measures were: "not wishing sex to seem planned" and thinking they were in a "safe period." They found that marital status, age, and religion had a significantly positive correlation to a woman's acceptance of sexuality and use of contraceptives. This study gives credence to the notion that decision making is a process whose strategies are influenced by situational factors, developmental factors, and values attached to goals.

Luker (1975) also applied decision-making theory in a retrospective study of pregnant women seeking an abortion. Her population, known as "risk takers," consisted of 50 women, 75 percent of whom had previously used contraception skillfully but who subsequently used contraceptives less effectively. She constructed a decision model of contraceptive behaviors. In Luker's model, contraceptive use is an individual process where the utilities of pregnancy and contraception are relative and not fixed. Changing life circumstances result in reevaluation of contraception and pregnancy. A once effective contraceptive user may change her view of the immediate cost and benefit of contraception versus the anticipated costs and benefits of pregnancy. Although the benefits of contraception are apparent (prevention of pregnancy), it also has costs as well. The costs include the social and cultural meanings of contraception, cost associated with maintaining contraception over time, the cost of obtaining access to contraceptives, and finally the costs associated with the physiological and medical aspects of contraception. Weighted against the costs are the utilities of being pregnant and the probabilities of becoming pregnant. A woman who takes a chance once or twice and does not become pregnant reinforces a low probability of pregnancy and encourages risk taking (Luker, 1975). In all decisions there is the option of using new information. The last step in this model is the value assigned to the likelihood of being able to reverse the situation if their appraisal of the benefits of pregnancy is in error. The reversal mechanism here was the availability of abortion. Luker saw this not as the most important part of the decision, but its availability gave contraceptive use a lower benefit and reduced long-term costs of pregnancy.

Variables Affecting Decisions

When considering human decision making, one needs to be cognizant of the fact that individuals perceive the same situations in various ways and cognitive processes are based on one's perception of the situation. Therefore, decisions are based on utility and process. It can be said that the utility and the value attached to contraceptive decision making may be related not only to knowledge of methods, but also knowledge of self. Contraceptive decisions cannot be based on a mathematical equation. This means that psychological, sociological, and situational processes warrant investigation when studying the decision-making process. Therefore, decision-making theory is valid yet limited when attempting to arrive at an understanding of contraceptive decision-making behavior. To understand the processes of contraceptive decision making psychological, sociological, and situational variables need to be considered. Research and literature exist that focus on the psychological factors of contraceptive decisions (Baldwin, 1977; Bracken & Kasl, 1975; Diamond et al., 1973; Luker, 1975). Much of the research conducted involves women who are seeking abortions. Some of this research has tended to portray women who do not use contraception as immature, impulsive, dependent women who have low self-esteem (Sandberg & Jacobs, 1971). Individual attitudes toward sexuality and one's tendency to plan and hold a future perspective have also been explored as means to predict contraceptive choices. Lack of planning behaviors can be related to risk taking or feelings of not being in control of one's life. It seems as if women, single or married, who view themselves as sexual beings tend to be effective and satisfied with their contraceptive decisions. Multiple intertwined variables operate on both the conscious and unconscious levels. These variables may add ambivalence to the decision-making process. Several of these variables can be identified.

Anxiety and Guilt. Anxiety and guilt may be related to feelings of promiscuity, fears of heightened libido, fear of method side effects, and fear of loss of future fertility. Moral and religious beliefs regarding contraception may also increase anxiety and guilt. Even though pregnancy is not desired, the use of contraceptives may be viewed as a denial of "the expected outcome" of intercourse. Finally, acceptance of self as a sexual being, whether married or single, may cause a great deal of psychological discomfort, especially when seeking contraceptive advice. Anxiety arises not only from admitting the need for a contraceptive method, but also from a lack of knowledge, and the fear of judgmental professional attitudes (Sandberg & Jacobs, 1971).

Denial. Denial influences contraceptive decision making in the following ways: (1) a belief that pregnancy will not occur, (2) a belief that contraceptives really are not effective, and (3) denial of personal responsibility for contraception, which may result in total denial between partners or a transferring of responsibility to a partner (Sandberg & Jacobs, 1971).

Lack of Knowledge. Knowledge is of critical importance in the contraceptive decision-making process. Knowledge is dynamic and changing. An individual will use and seek knowledge when it is seen as a resource. The scope of the lack of contraceptive knowledge is not well documented. Most women will admit to some knowledge of contraceptive methods, but upon careful assessment, the scope of information may be limited and questionable. The lack of knowledge includes misinterpretation, misinformation, and lack of awareness of method use, method effectiveness, and the menstrual cycle. Lack of knowledge can be found in educated as well as uneducated women.

Spontaneity. Some individuals shun the use of methods such as condoms, foams, and diaphragms because their use decreases the spontaneity of lovemaking.

Loneliness. A need for involvement and gratification despite the consequences may induce a woman to become sexually involved without considering the need for contraception. Loneliness can also be in response to a recent loss or crisis in a relationship, relative, or object.

Hostility. At times a woman may intentionally become pregnant. Hostility can be directed toward a partner or parents or self by allowing oneself to be used sexually (Sandberg & Jacobs, 1971).

Sacrifice Risk-taking. Sacrifice of self or a willingness to take risks and not use contraception may be viewed as a proof of love either by the partner or the woman herself. Risk-taking may arise when there is uncertainty in the relationship or when the possibility of the end of the relationship seems imminent.

Coital Gamesmanship. Usage of a contraceptive method may be mediated by a power struggle or need to attain control in a relationship (Sandberg & Jacobs, 1971). Either partner may resist using a more effective method if it means they will have less control of the frequency of intercourse.

Sexual Identity Conflicts. Fertility can be a symbol of womanliness, femininity, and desirability for some women. Similarly, some men see a woman as a means to demonstrate their virility through impregnation. Pregnancy then becomes a means to assert sexual ability.

Control. Control has also been linked to contraceptive decision making. Specifically, locus of control has been correlated with contraceptive behavior. Internal–external locus of control has been useful in the prediction of behavior. Internal versus external control of reinforcement refers to the extent to which one feels control over the reinforcements that occur relative to one's behavior (Rotter, 1966). Central to the locus of control theory is the perceived reinforcement value for a given behavior. Accordingly, a woman may perceive avoidance of pregnancy either as a direct result of her behavior or related to fate. MacDonald (1970) found that 62 percent of those labeled "internal" practiced some form of birth control versus 37 percent of those labeled "external." Lundy (1972) and Bracken and Kasl (1975) reported similar results.

Background and Environment. Socioeconomic variables, such as income, availability of, and accessibility to resources, affect contraceptive usage. The further constraints of culture, religious beliefs, mores, and attitudes contribute to the decision-making process. Other issues that are a part of an individual's background are educational goals, career goals, and life-style.

Individual and Partner. User comfort and acceptability of a method over time also affect decision making. A method that a couple will use accurately and continuously is more desirable than a method that one or both partners dislikes. If there is a specific partner, he should be included in the decision-making process if the woman wishes. An individual's need for an effective and acceptable contraceptive method changes over time. The implications for such flexibility necessitate both short- and long-term planning and goals. Comprehensive and systematic planning necessitates looking beyond a method to the individual who is continuously developing and interacting within the environment.

Attitude and Relationship of Care Provider to Client

Health care professionals have access to clients where contraceptive planning is routinely done or could be incorporated into a total health plan. The same contraceptive attitudes and biases that affect clients may also affect providers. For this reason those providing counseling should be cognizant of their own attitudes and values regarding contraception and sexuality. It is not always possible to know how one will react in all situations. Therefore, providers involved in contraception planning should spend time and energy assessing personal feelings, attitudes, and values toward these issues. A health counselor who experiences discomfort with these topics may easily transmit these feelings to clients. In addition to assessing one's own feelings, one should have a broad knowledge base of contraception, an ability to discuss sexual matters in an objective and supportive manner, and an accepting attitude when others' values conflict with one's own values. (See Chapter 2 for variables that may affect teaching–learning situations).

Finally, all providers cannot be equally effective with all clients. Judgment and perception are necessary to recognize when there is a conflict or an obstacle in the counselor–client relationship. If the obstacle cannot be remedied, the provider should request another member of the health team to work with the client without causing the client to feel guilty.

Impact of Improved Decisions

Viewing the use of contraception as part of the life process incorporates developmental, cultural, social, personal, psychological, and physiological variables. Process implies a systematic series of actions toward a goal. The health provider's role in issues that promote health can be significant. Positive utilization of the nursing role can assist individuals in actively planning their contraceptive future as well as building sound health habits beyond contraceptive issues.

ASSESSMENT OF LEARNING NEEDS

Before a teaching plan can be formulated, one should assess the client's learning needs and readiness to learn using the variables of decision making and efficacy. The initial information serves as the basis for planning. To assess contraceptive needs the information on Table 8–2 should be solicited.

The comprehensive information is needed to develop a sound contraceptive plan. One of the health provider's goals should be to establish a rapport with the woman over time, and to establish continuity of care. Continuity of care and an unrushed supportive approach can aid in the development of sound contraceptive practices.

Contraceptive Intentions

Generally, a woman who is seeking contraceptive advice seeks a method that is safe and effective. Safety is relative to one's contraceptive goals and past medical history. Effectiveness is also a gray area. Effectiveness is based on two issues: user effectiveness and theoretical effectiveness. Although theoretical effectiveness is generally quite high for most methods, if the user does not use the method correctly or consistently the method's effectiveness decreases considerably. No method is purely effective or without risk. Risks regarding health and inconvenience should be assessed.

A reproductive plan should be developed with an individual regardless of age or marital status. A reproductive plan is not a fixed plan but one that the woman can develop with her care provider and her partner. A reproductive plan should take into account all the variables that affect contraception. The adolescent may only wish to prevent pregnancy and may have no intentions or ideas about childbearing in the near future. A plan for an adolescent versus her older counterpart who is planning to bear children in the near future can be quite different (see Chapters 14 and 16 on Adolescents and Older Women for details). For example, a woman with a same partner relationship who plans to bear children in a few years and does not care for a hormonal preparation, may be more of a candidate for an IUD than a woman who does not have the same partner or definite plans for childbearing. Overall, a reproductive plan should take into account the woman's goals, beliefs, sexual activity, access to medical care, costs, and plans to bear children.

Inclusion of Partner

Part of continued contraceptive use is based on the cooperation of sexual partners. Certain methods such as spermicidal agents, condoms, and diaphragms, and the natural family planning methods require maturity, a stable relationship, and mutual respect.

TABLE 8–2. ASSESSMENT OF LEARNING NEEDS

Area to Assess	Information to be Gathered
1. General background	First visit or return visit When was last visit to health care provider Age Marital status Living arrangement Socioeconomic status: occupation; education; accessibility to health care Race Religion Language
2. Health history	Major illnesses, hospitalizations, surgeries especially, pelvic inflammatory disease (PID) and sexually transmitted diseases (STD) Allergies Medicatons used including contraceptives Client or family history of: diabetes, hypertension, thromboembolic problems, migraine headaches, kidney or liver problems, cardiac problems, anemia, psychiatric problems
3. Obstetrical, menstrual, and sexual history	Age of menarche Regularity and duration of menses Type and characteristics of flow Presence or absence of dysmenorrhea Number of pregnancies, abortions, and attempts to become pregnant Same partner or different partners Frequency of intercourse, pain/bleeding with intercourse
4. Physical assessment: comprehensiveness depends on specific symptoms and desire for BCP or IUD	Pelvic examination Pregnancy test Pap smear Breast examination Optional: systematic review of system Hematocrit Hemoglobin Tests for STD
5. Attitudes and beliefs	Follow through with her health care Sexuality Pregnancy planning Self-concept
6. Readiness for learning	Client expectations and perceptions Reason(s) for visit Knowledge of anatomy and physiology of reproduction and menstruation Knowledge of contraceptive methods Contraceptive preference(s) Perceived effect of contraception on her life-style Inquisitive or willing to accept any method

Methods such as the Pill and IUD do not need cooperation at the time of intercourse but do require a partner's supportive attitude. Optimally, a couple should discuss, plan, and choose a method with the assistance of a health practitioner. If the man cannot be part of the discussion at the health care setting, the woman needs to assess with the practitioner's assistance, what the partner's knowledge and attitudes are to particular methods. If the woman does not have a same partner relationship and has chosen a method that requires partner cooperation, the care provider should assess with the woman how she feels she will manage the contraceptive method with her partners.

TEACHING FORMAT

Objectives
A general framework of objectives for the contraception decision-making process is necessary. The objectives should be flexible and nonrestrictive. Objectives need alteration depending on an individual's goals. Alteration of objectives should be determined by the woman's expressed needs and feedback. Development of objectives can assist in the overall development of a reproductive plan. Examples of objectives are presented (Table 8–3).

Methods
Many methods are available that can assist the provider in developing a contraceptive decision-making plan. The specific methods chosen should reflect the individual's needs. These resources are pamphlets, booklets, films, slide-tapes, diagrams, and charts. Combining two or three methods for teaching can be effective. The overall effectiveness of any teaching plan is more but not totally dependent on its quality and structure than on its method of presentation.

Pamphlets and Booklets. Many pamphlets and booklets are available from various agencies and companies, which can be useful teaching aids. Some resources are listed in the resource list at the end of the chapter. These resources are available to both individuals and agencies. Written materials can help a woman to formulate questions and provide information. These resources cannot be depended on to answer all of an individual's questions. Some of these resources may be misleading and biased. Therefore, any infor-

---

TABLE 8–3. CONTRACEPTIVE DECISION-MAKING OBJECTIVES

Main goal:

To assist individuals in the choice of an effective and acceptable method of contraception through education, guidance, and development of a reproductive plan.

Subgoals:

1. To have the client:
    A. Identify the anatomy of the female reproductive system.
    B. Describe the physiology of the menstrual cycle, especially the hormonal changes.
    C. Identify methods of contraception: effectiveness, advantages, disadvantages, and side effects.
    D. Select a method for present use.
    E. Develop a reproductive life plan.
    F. Evaluate with the practitioner the effectiveness of the contraceptive method and reproductive plan.

---

mation given to a woman should be reviewed prior to dispensing it to clients. Additionally, not all of these resources are equally appropriate for all women. A theme-oriented catalog system should be developed that attempts to classify material according to readability, clarity, and relevance for various age groups and educational levels, for both English and non-English written material.

Diagrams and Charts. Diagrams and charts can be used to visually portray the relationship between methods and the menstrual cycle (Fig. 8–1). This method can be a useful adjunct to verbal teaching.

Films, Slides, and Physical Objects. Films, slides, models, and samples of contraceptive methods can be used in various combinations for teaching both individuals and groups. Pictorial learning is a highly effective learning method. Films and slide-tapes with contraceptives and menstrual content are available for patient teaching. Another alternative is the development of slide-tape modules. For example, a slide-tape teaching module could be developed on the various methods. Interspersed among the method slides should be slides that outline and discuss the major physical and psychological issues related to each method. The equipment needed for each method should also be available for the woman's examination.

Individual Session. Table 8–4 outlines a core teaching plan for contraceptive decision making. Each woman's goals and decision-making variables necessitate alterations of the plan. Initially, before the woman is seen by the nurse, she should be allowed a period of time to complete the self-assessment questionnaire (Table 8–5) and reproductive life plan (Table 8–6). These tools assist the nurse and the client to choose a direction for planning and teaching. The interview, assessment, and tools can aid the nurse and the woman to identify areas of concern, uncertainty, lack of knowledge, and areas that need clarification and further discussion. Once the woman chooses a method, the health care provider should use the teaching plan. The teaching session should allow time for feedback and review of the information presented.

A follow-up appointment and telephone number with the practitioner's name should be given to the woman. This confirms the need for follow-up care as well as provides the woman with an avenue for further communication. Often clients because of the stressfulness of the visit forget pieces of information gathered at the visit. For this reason, written material can reinforce what was presented during the visit. Additionally, if the woman wishes, the practitioner should arrange a telephone appointment within a week to 10 days to verify the woman's comfort with the method and to clarify any questions.

Group Method. The group approach to contraceptive decision making is a useful adjunct to individual teaching. The group approach encourages an active process of contraceptive decision making. The goal of the group approach is to emphasize the processes of contraceptive decision making rather than the details of each method. This approach is not appropriate for all women. Groups should be formed that include women with similar developmental and contraceptive needs. Groups can be designed to include adolescents, either single or with partner, adult women making a decision within a relationship, or women making a decision outside of a same partner relationship. Groups should also deal with and provide information on contraception and sexuality. A group provides a structure within which discussion can occur. Some strategies that may be used are: a review of the decision-making process; a review of values and variables that may cause conflict; and the

TABLE 8–4. TEACHING PLAN FOR CONTRACEPTIVE DECISION-MAKING

Teaching Plan	Implementation	Evaluation
A. To review anatomy of female reproductive system	1. Verbal review of structures 2. Use of diagrams, charts and models for reinforcement	1. Woman can identify the major structures
B. To review the physiology of the female menstrual cycle, especially the hormonal changes	1. Verbal review and description of menstrual cycle and hormonal changes 2. Use of diagrams, charts and pamphlets for reinforcement 3. Periodically reflect on material presented to assess if woman has questions or is unclear about information being provided	1. Woman can explain the menstrual cycle and hormonal changes
C. To review methods of contraception: a. types b. effectiveness c. advantages/benefits d. disadvantages e. side effects/risks	1. Review with woman the methods of contraception that she can choose 2. Use of films, slide-tape modules 3. Review with woman any written material she has received	1. Woman has an understanding of the various choices that are available for contraceptive use
D. To assist the woman to choose a method of contraception within the beginning framework of a reproductive life plan[a]	1. Allow woman to take self-assessment questionnaire and reproductive life plan questionnaire. Discuss these with woman (or couple) 2. Based on physical assessment, review of methods and discussion with woman (or couple), review in depth the contraceptive method chosen; administration; any common cycle variations; possible common uncomfortable reactions; any nutritional implications; possible side effects 3. Anticipatory guidance: Discuss any obstacle or problem with the method or plan the woman feels may arise 4. Follow-up appointment and telephone number 5. Follow-up telephone appointment	1. Woman aware of the implications of her answers. Provided ample time for discussion 2. Woman can describe composition and functioning of the method chosen Woman describes schedule (if one needed); possible reactions and variations in cycle that may occur related to method 3. Woman states need for vitamin and mineral supplement, if necessary 4. Woman states name of care provider, next appointment and telephone number in case questions arise

[a]Each method requires specific physical precautions and method-specific instructions.

use of hypothetical decision-making situations, both general and contraception specific that the group can use to problem solve. For example, adolescents because of their growth and developmental needs, may benefit more from a group with peers than from individual didactic sessions (Jay et al., 1984). A group whose leaders serve as role models can facilitate an adolescent's needs to make independent decisions in an area that is complicated and

TABLE 8–5. SELF-ASSESSMENT QUESTIONNAIRE

Please answer the following questions

Method of birth control I am considering.		
Have I used this method before?	Yes	No
If yes, for how long did I use this method?		
Am I afraid of using this method?	Yes	No
Will I have trouble remembering to use this method?	Yes	No
Have I ever become pregnant while using this method?	Yes	No
Have I ever become pregnant while using another method?	Yes	No
If yes, which method?		
Will I have trouble using this method?	Yes	No
I do not like a birth control method that interferes		
with spontaneity in sexual activity.	Yes	No
I still have unanswered questions about this method.	Yes	No
This method costs more than I can afford.	Yes	No
This method conflicts with my religious beliefs.	Yes	No
My partner is opposed to this method.	Yes	No
I am using this method without my partner's knowledge.	Yes	No
My partner dislikes the use of birth control.	Yes	No
Will use of this method embarrass my partner?	Yes	No
Will use of this method embarrass me?	Yes	No
I could find myself involved in an unexpected sexual situation.	Yes	No
I have a regular sexual relationship.	Yes	No
I have more than one partner.	Yes	No
Will I enjoy sexual intercourse less because of this method?	Yes	No
I do not want a birth control method with many side effects.	Yes	No
Has a nurse, doctor or friend told me not to use this method?	Yes	No
Is there anything about my personality or situation		
that would cause me not to use this method correctly?	Yes	No
Even though I don't want to get pregnant now, I		
sometimes wish to get pregnant anyway and do not use		
birth control at that time.	Yes	No
I know this method will affect my menstrual cycle.	Yes	No
There is another method I might like to use, but I		
do not have enough information about the method.	Yes	No

If yes, please check the method(s) that interested me:
_____ Pill
_____ Intrauterine device
_____ Diaphragm
_____ Cervical cap
_____ Condom
_____ Foam, creams, suppositories, jellies, tablets
_____ Natural family planning methods/fertility awareness methods

(Source: *Adapted from Hatcher, R. A., Guest, F., Stewart, G., Wright, A. H., Josephs, N., & Dale, J.* Contraceptive technology 1982–1983 *(11th ed.). New York: Irvington, 1982, by permission.)*

conflictual. The group can encourage adolescents and adult women to use the information they have and arrive at a decision appropriate for their own life-style, values, and goals. Groups can offer a secure environment in which to investigate the contraceptive decision-making process (see Chapter 3 for details regarding group process).

Inclusion of Partner. Including the partner in the decision-making process can further reinforce the decision. Some women believe contraceptive planning is their own decision. Reasons for this may be lack of a same partner relationship, or a belief that the

TABLE 8–6. REPRODUCTIVE LIFE PLAN QUESTIONNAIRE

1. Would I like to have children one day?
2. How old would I like to be when I have my first (or next) child?
3. How many children would I like to have?
4. How sad would I be if I were not able to have any (or any more) children?
5. If I were to become pregnant before I wished to be, would an abortion be a way I might approach this problem?
6. How many years of formal education would I like to complete?
7. (If not married) At what age would I like to be married if I could have this happen whenever I wanted it to happen?
8. If I do not marry, I would consider being a single parent.
9. At what point during or after this educational process would I like to become pregnant?
10. After I complete my education, I would like to establish a career before I have a child.
11. Of all the things I could do in my life, probably the most important would be to be able to accomplish this: _____
_____
12. This life goal would be affected by childbearing in the following ways: _____
_____
_____
13. How does my life plan thus far dovetail with my religious beliefs, with what I personally feel God would want me to be doing, with what I personally feel is "right" or "wrong"? _____
_____

(Source: *Adapted from Hatcher, R. A., Guest, F., Stewart, G., Wright, A. H., Josephs, N., & Dale, J.* Contraceptive technology, 1982–1983 *(11th ed.). New York: Irvington, 1982, by permission.)*

decision to avoid pregnancy is their responsibility and choice. Other women feel that the decision to contracept is the couple's choice. How a woman prefers her partner to be included should be assessed. Ideally the partner should accompany the woman to the appointment. Contraceptive planning can then be done with the dyad. It is not always possible for the partner to accompany the woman. The lack of physical presence does not discount his inclusion. Ways to include the partner are: encourage the woman to discuss the verbal and written information she has gathered with her partner; encourage them to review the reproductive life plan tool together; offer a group contraception planning session; offer the facility's telephone number so the partner can discuss any questions or concerns he may have and offer a return visit when both partners can come. Moreover, where possible, encouraging a couple's communication and joint decision making can enhance the contraceptive decision and the couple's effective and continued use of the chosen method.

Evaluation. All teaching plans require evaluation. Evaluation is an ongoing process. Evaluation of contraceptive decision making should consider the teaching plan and the process employed. The evaluation should reflect how and if goals were accomplished. An evaluation should measure by direct and indirect observation and client feedback the following points:

1. If teaching goals were met, which strategies were useful and which were problematic.
2. The woman's (or couple's) level of comfort and satisfaction with the method.
3. Knowledge of method and reproductive system.

4. The woman's (or couple's) comfort with the decision-making process and repro-ductive life plan.
5. Continued use of method.
6. If obstacles arose were they due to method side effects, dislike of method, or a need for further knowledge.
7. If problems arose, revision of the areas of concern is necessary.

SUGGESTIONS FOR RESEARCH

Health care providers are involved in teaching a wide range of health care behaviors in a variety of settings. Teaching and research are fundamental roles of the health care profes-sional. In light of the statistics related to contraceptive usage, contraceptive decision making becomes a challenge and is necessary to investigate.

Research, based on a holistic approach, needs to consider the changing needs and potentials of individuals as they progress through their reproductive lives. There is no one best method or ideal format to guide contraceptive decision making, especially in light of the ever-changing contraceptive technology. Therefore, neither research on deci-sion-making theory nor research on social and intrapersonal variables related to contra-ceptive usage can stand alone to explain or test how women decide to use contraceptive information.

Health care promoters' interests are geared toward assisting individuals to achieve a maximal level of health. Research then needs to first focus on successful users of contra-ception, to explore factors that influence not only their contraceptive beliefs and atti-tudes, but also their general health beliefs. It is important to assess how these women make contraceptive decisions before we can explore women who are uncomfortable with their decisions. A review of the literature is necessary to discover similarities between contraceptive behavior variables and those variables that are relevant to health situations requiring a commitment to a regimen. Some of the variables from other health care situations such as weight reduction programs and even programs that require one to maintain a fixed medical regimen, such as diabetics, may prove useful to contraceptive research.

The development of attitudes, values, and beliefs seems to play an important part in contraceptive resolutions. To discern new and acceptable methods of contraceptive deci-sion making, research is needed into the differences in sexual attitudes and the develop-mental of sexuality across the reproductive years. Research should not only focus on helping women avoid pregnancy, but should encourage the development of knowledge and a clear individual value system. This type of research can be generalized to other decisions that require social and interpersonal behaviors. Clinical practice and education as well as research could benefit from such exploration.

Knowledge is mentioned in many of the studies on contraception. Research has demonstrated that knowledge is available but not adequate to solve contraceptive deci-sion dilemmas. What is meant by knowledge and what level of knowledge is necessary for successful contraceptive decisions need to be established. Furthermore, an evaluation of the focus and the indices of success of past contraceptive programs is necessary. It may be that programs fail because they provide only concrete information and do not include attitudinal or developmental strategies.

In conclusion, the theories on decision making have assisted in the development of useful concepts related to contraceptive decision making. Psychological, sociological, and situational factors affect individuals differently and also mediate decision-making processes. Knowledge of self, values, and contraceptive methods also affect contraceptive behavior. An attempt has been made to extract variables from areas that contribute to contraceptive decisions. Implications for research have been drawn. Theories are used to guide and contribute to contraceptive planning. A vast majority of health care and guidance is provided by practitioners whose ideas of care need to develop into researchable questions that will foster more effective contraceptive counseling and guidance.

RESOURCES

Calderone, M. (Ed.). *Manual of family planning and contraceptive practice* (2nd ed.). Baltimore: Williams & Wilkins, 1970. *(Paperback, caringly detailed.)*

Demarest, R. J., & Sciarra, J. J. *Conception, birth and contraception: A visual presentation* (2nd ed.). New York: McGraw-Hill, 1976. *(Informative, careful book useful for clinic, school or library.)*

"The Pill" and your nutrition. Evansville, IN 47721: Mead Johnson, 1974. *(Pamphlet describes nutritional requirements needed while taking the Pill.)*

The Pill. Raritan, NJ 08869: Ortho Pharmaceutical Corp., 1978. *(Detailed description about the Pill.)*

Planned Parenthood Federation of America, Inc. *You and the Pill.* New York: Planned Parenthood Federation of America, Inc., 810 Seventh Avenue, New York, NY 10019, 1976. *(Pamphlet desribes the Pill, benefits, risks and usage of the Pill. Clinics of the agency are throughout the United States. Clinics provide contraceptive services and information.)*

Natural Family Planning Federation of America, Inc., Suite A, 1221 Massachusetts Ave., N.W., Washington, DC 20005. *(Provides information on natural family planning methods.)*

Your future family. San Juan, Puerto Rico 00936: Searle & Co., 1971. *(Careful review of contraceptive methods available, includes risk factors.)*

U.S. Department of HEW—Public Health Service, Food and Drug Administration Office of Public Affairs: HEW Publication No. (FDA) 78-3069, U.S. Department of Health and Human Services (HHS) Public Health Service, Food and Drug Administration, 5600 Fishers Lane, Rockville, MD 20857, 1978. *(Pamphlet that provides a review of contraceptive methods.)*

Many other pamphlets and resources are available from family planning organizations, pharmaceutical companies, health care agencies, Public Health Department, the Food and Drug Administration, and libraries that can be obtained from local agencies by writing or calling.

BIBLIOGRAPHY

Aznar, R., Zamora, G., Lozano, M., & Love, C. Polyurethane contraceptive vaginal sponge: Product modifications results from user experience. *Contraception*, 1981, *24*(3), 234–244.

Baldwin, W. Adolescent pregnancy and childbearing—Growing concern for Americans. *Population Bulletin*, 1977, *31*, 2–12.

Billings, J. J. *Natural family planning* (3rd ed.). Collegeville, Minn.: The Liturgical Press, 1975.

Boston Women's Health Book Collective: *Our bodies, ourselves* (2nd ed.). New York: Simon & Schuster, 1976.

Bracken, M. S., & Kasl, S. V. First and repeat abortions: A study of decision making and delay. *Journal of Biosocial Sciences*, 1975, *7*, 473–491.

Brim, O. G., Glass, D. C., Lavin, D. E., & Goodman, N. *Personality and decision processes.* Stanford, Calif.: Stanford University Press, 1962.

Brinton, L. A., Vessey, M. P., Flavele, R., & Yeates, D. Risk factors for benign breast disease. *American Journal of Epidemiology*, 1981, *113*, 203–204.

Britt, S. S. Fertility awareness: Four methods of natural family planning. *Journal Obstetrics and Gynecology Nursing*, 1977, *6*(2), 9–18.

Cramer, D. W., Hutchinson, G. B., Welch, W. R., Scully, R. E., & Knapp, R. C. Factors affecting the association of oral contraceptives and ovarian cancer. *New England Journal of Medicine*, 1982, *307*(17), 1047–1051.

Diamond, M., Steinhoff, P. G., Palmore, J. A., & Smith, R. G. Sexuality, birth control and abortion: A decision-making sequence. *Journal of Biosocial Science*, 1973, *5*, 347–361.

Fisher, W. A., Byrne, D., Edmunds, M., Miller, C. T., Kelley, K., & White, L. A. Psychological and situation-specific correlates of contraceptive behavior among university women. *Journal of Sex Research*, 1979, *15*, 38–55.

Fogel, C., & Woods, N. (Eds.). *Health care of women: A nursing perspective*. St. Louis, Mo.: C. V. Mosby, 1981.

Hatcher, R. A., Guest, F., Stewart, F., Stewart, G. K., Trussell, J., & Frank, E. *Contraceptive technology 1984–1985* (12th ed.). New York: Irvington, 1984.

Hatcher, R. A., Guest, F., Stewart, G. K., Wright, A. H., Josephs, N., & Dale, J. *Contraceptive technology 1982–1983* (11th ed.). New York: Irvington, 1982.

Huggins, G., Vessey, N., & Flazel, R. Vaginal spermicides and outcome of pregnancy: Findings in a large cohort study. *Contraception*, 1982, *25*(3), 219–230.

Hulka, B. S., Chambliss, L. E., Kaufman, D. G., Fowler, W. C., & Greenberg, B. G. Protection against endometrial carcinoma by combination-product oral contraceptives. *JAMA*, 1982, *247*(4), 475–477.

Jaffe, F. S. The need for new contraceptives. In National Academy of Sciences Symposium on Contraceptive Technology, *Contraception*. Washington, D.C.: Office of Publications, 1979.

Jay, M. S., DuRant, R. H., Shoffitt, T., Linder, C. W., & Litt, I. F. Effect of peer counselors on adolescent compliance in use of oral contraceptives. *Pediatrics*, 1984, *73*, 126–131.

Jick, H., Walker, A. M., Rothman, K. J., Hunter, J. R., Holmes, L. B., Watkins, R. N., & D'Ewart, D. C. Vaginal spermicides and congenital disorders. *JAMA*, 1981, *245*(13) 1329–1332.

Kafka, J., & Gold, B. B. Food and drug administration approves vaginal sponge. *Family Planning Perspectives*, 1983, *15*(3), 146–148.

Lane, M. E., Arceo, R., & Sobrero, A. J. Successful use of the diaphragm and jelly by a young population: Report of a clinical study. *Family Planning Perspectives*, 1976, *8*, 81–86.

LiVolsi, V. A., Stadel, B. V., Kelsy, J. L., Holford, T. R., & White, C. Fibrocystic breast diseases in oral contraceptive users. *New England Journal of Medicine*, 1978, *229*, 381–385.

Luker, K. *Taking chances*. Berkeley, Calif.: University of California Press, 1975.

Lundy, J. R. Some personality correlates of contraceptive use among unmarried female college students. *Journal of Psychology*, 1972, *80*, 9–14.

Martin, L. L. *Health care of women*. Philadelphia: Lippincott, 1978.

MacDonald, A. P. Internal–external locus of control and the practice of birth control. *Psychological Reports*, 1970, *27*, 206.

Medical Letter of Drug Therapies. *A vaginal contraceptive sponge*. 1983, (6542), 78–80.

Mishell, D. R. Noncontraceptive health benefits of oral steroid contraceptives. *American Journal Obstetrics and Gynecology Nursing*, 1982, *142*, 809.

NAACOG Newsletter. *Cervical cap use studied in U.S.* 1983, *10*(6), 1.

Neubardt, S. *A concept of contraception*. New York: Trident Press, 1967.

Ory, W. The noncontraceptive health benefits from oral contraceptive use. *Family Planning Perspectives*, 1982, *14*, 4.

Ory, H. W., Forrest, J. D., & Lincoln, R. *Making choices: Evaluating the health risks and benefits of birth control methods*. New York: Alan Guttmacher Institute, 1983.

Paffenbarger, R. S., Fasal, E., Simmons, M. E., & Kanbert, J. B. Cancer risks as related to use of oral contraceptives during fertile years. *Cancer*, 1977, *39*, 1887–1891.

Porter, C. W., Waife, R. S., & Holtrop, H. R. *Contraception: The health providers guide*, 1983. Orlando: Grune & Stratton, 1983.

Rothman, M. Spermicide use and Down's syndrome. *AJPH*, 1982, *72*(4), 329–401.

Rotter, J. B. Generalized expectancies for internal versus external locus of control of reinforcement. *Psychological Monographs*, 1966, *609*.

Rubin, G. L., Ory, H. W., & Layde, P. M. Oral contraceptives and pelvic inflammatory disease. Paper presented at the Epidemic Intelligence Service Conference, Atlanta, April 21–24, 1981.

Sandberg, E., & Jacobs, R. Psychology of the misuse and rejection of contraception. *American Journal of Obstetrics and Gynecology*, 1971, *110*, 227–242.

Senanayake, P., & Kramer, D. G. Contraception and the etiology of PID: New perspectives. *American Journal Obstetrics and Gynecology*, 1980, *138*(7, pt. 2), 852–860.

Tanis, J. L. Recognizing the reasons for contraceptive non-use and abuse. *American Journal of Maternal Child Nursing*, 1977, *2*(6), 364–369.

Taylor, D. A new way to teach teens about contraceptives. *American Journal of Maternal Child Nursing*, 1976, *5*, 378–383.

Thompson, L., & Spanier, G. Influence of parents, peers and partners on the contraceptive use of college women and men. *Journal of Marriage and Family*, 1978, *40*, 481–492.

Tietze, C. Teenage pregnancies: Looking ahead to 1984. *Family Planning Perspectives*, 1978, *10*, 205–207.

Vessey, M., Doll, R., Peto, R., Johnson, D., & Wissins, T. A long-term follow-up study of women using different methods of contraception: An interim report. *Journal of Biosocial Science*, 1976, *8*(4), 373–427.

Webster's 3rd International Dictionary. New York: Signet, 1966.

Whartman, J. The cervical cap. *Population Reports*, Series #4. Washington, D.C.: George Washington University Medical Center, 1976.

Zabin, L., Kantner, J. F., & Zelnick, M. The risk of adolescent pregnancy in the first months of intercourse. *Family Planning Perspectives*, 1979, *11*, 289–296.

Zelnick, M., & Kantner, J. Reasons for non-use of contraception by sexually active women aged 15–19. *Family Planning Perspectives*, 1979, *11*, 289–296.

Zelnick, M., & Kantner, J. Sexual activity, contraceptive use, and pregnancy among metropolitan-area teenagers: 1971–1979. *Family Planning Perspectives*, 1980, *12*, 230–239.

Health Education for the Homosexual Female

9

Geri LoBiondo-Wood

A review of the literature in the area of women's health care reveals that many of the physiological and psychological needs of women are beginning to be addressed by health care providers. There is a paucity of literature, research, and nursing care models, however, that relate to women with alternative life-styles. One such group is lesbian women. The psychological, social, and physical dimensions of the health care of those with alternative life-styles or sexual preferences need to be fully understood to deliver comprehensive health care. The majority of literature available on homosexuality deals with male homosexuality. Only recently has female homosexuality begun to be reviewed and researched. The research and literature on lesbianism has centered primarily on the etiology of the orientation and treatment. Research into sociocultural variables has largely been ignored. This omission may partially be due to a view that homosexuality is a state or condition in which all those who "suffer" from it share the same traits rather than perceiving homosexuals as a diverse group of individuals within a specific social milieu.

Recent estimates suggest that approximately 10 percent of the population is homosexual (Brossart, 1979). Estimates by the Kinsey Institute for Sex Research suggest that 4.2 percent of women have a predominately lesbian sexual and affectional orientation (Berzon & Leighton, 1979). Over and above these figures are the untold number of lesbian and bisexual women who have not "come out" to their families and friends.

Female homosexuality is still one of the most poorly understood areas in health care. Basically the health needs of lesbian women parallel those of heterosexual women. Why then a separate treatment of their health needs? Lesbians, due to biases and prejudice of others, are fearful and suspicious of traditional care settings. Some health practitioners think that the needs of lesbians are like the needs of gay men. There may be the assumption that all lesbians are promiscuous and have high rates of sexually transmitted disease. Lesbians may also stay away from traditional settings because of what is defined as heterosexism, which is the assumption that everyone is or desires to be heterosexual, and homophobia, which is defined as a rage and extreme fear reaction to homosexuals. For these reasons, some lesbians avoid health care or conceal their sexual preference to avoid prejudice, bias, inferior care, suggestions to see a psychiatrist, and negative stereotyping.

LESBIANISM

Homosexuality is a behavioral phenomenon in which one's biopsychosociological framework is such that one prefers experiencing intimacy with members of the same sex (Pettyjohn, 1979). A lesbian's gender identity is female and her sexual orientation, psychological, emotional, and intimate commitment is to another female. Lesbianism is a stigmatized life-style. Social oppression may create multiple difficulties, affect associations, and restrict basic social roles.

In the past, this stigmatized life-style resulted in beheading, castration, burning, imprisonment, and disgrace of those who admitted their preference (Hyde & Rosenberg, 1976). Homosexuals have been ostracized and avoided as social outcasts. This has resulted in the paucity of valid research and information about the homosexual life-style. Much of the early research on lesbian experiences was conducted on women who were patients in mental health facilities. Therefore, the hypothesis that lesbianism was abnormal was a logical and easily proven conclusion. Later empirical research supports the view that lesbianism is not a deviant form of behavior (Rosen, 1974). A review of the theories of lesbianism demonstrates the speculative nature of its origins.

Various theories have been developed regarding female homosexuality. One of the oldest is the biological theory. This theory postulates that homosexuality is a biological phenomenon within the individual. Research by Money (1965) and Wolff (1971) has shown that biological organic determinants of homosexuality are false. They have postulated that parental expectations and rearing with a gender role are far more important as behavioral determinants than are organic factors (Riess, 1974). The belief that homosexuality is due to a hormonal imbalance has also been the subject of research. These studies have been highly inconsistent, inconclusive, and predominately conducted on men. Meyer-Bahlburg (1977), in an extensive review of the research literature, concluded that it is premature to theorize on general mechanisms underlying endocrine disorders in adult homosexuality.

Freud was one of the first practitioners to deal with the treatment of female homosexuality. Freud developed a theory of the psychic mechanisms involved. Freud's early thinking centered around the notion that human beings were bisexual in nature, possessed of physiological and psychological components of both sexes (Hyde & Rosenberg, 1976). Over time, an increased specificity in object choice occurs during what Freud called the Oedipal stage.

> For analysis tells us that sexual wishes of the child—in so far as they deserve this designation in their nascent state—awaken at a very early age, and that the earliest affection of the girl child is lavished on the father, while the earliest infantile desires of the boy are directed upon the mother. For the boy, the father; and for the girl, the mother, becomes an obnoxious rival. (Freud, 1900/1955)

Later Freud enlarged upon his earlier theories. He postulated that lesbianism developed when a negative oedipal component was present. During the oedipal stage, the female child, realizing that there is an absence of a penis, views herself as mutilated, and though identified with the mother, blames the mother for her loss (Hyde & Rosenberg, 1976). The female child then attempts to have her father's penis, which is converted to a symbolic penis in the form of a wish to bear her father's child, thus "penis-envy." The woman's role in intercourse was seen by Freud as passive–receptive, however, and hence the development of the female is in the direction of passivity and compliance (Riess, 1974). The early, preoedipal activity components are suppressed and the passive–

compliant rewarded. The suppression of aggression results in its internalization and redirection against self, hence "female masochism" (Riess, 1974). This masochistic behavior interferes with the development of self-esteem and a secure superego. Finally, when the negative components persist, the mother and other women become the objects of love.

Both Freud (1931, 1933) and Deutsch (1932, 1947) imply that the genesis of lesbianism is the existence of and retreat from the oedipal relationship with the father. If the attachment to the father is excessive, the female later may reject men because of incestual fears that have been shunted to them, resulting in a lesbian orientation (Romm, 1965). Alternatively, Deutsch (1932) felt that lesbianism is the result of the female's failure to reject her mother as a love object and instead becomes fixated on her.

Charlotte Wolff (1971) suggests a variation of the psychoanalytical model based on her research with lesbians not involved in treatment. Wolff's theory is based on the supposition that the mother is the female child's only real love object. Throughout life the female continues to pursue the mother's love and males are loved only as a substitute. She assumes that all lesbians enter into a competitive rivalry with males and that their identification is therefore masculine. Even though research has been done that does not support that lesbians have a male identification, Wolff's research lends another view to lesbianism.

Much of the psychoanalytical work has low reliability because it is based on retrospective data. Data are based on an individual's recall of past events that are significantly influenced by their present perception of themselves. It can also be presumed to be biased because the individuals were in therapy and had been exposed to social stigmatization.

A less pathologically oriented approach to female homosexuality has been developed by behaviorists (Bermant, 1972; Ford & Beach, 1951). The behaviorist approach assumes that humans have no inborn preference for the opposite sex as a love object. Behavioral theory proposes that humans have a wide variety of sex drives that, depending on conditioning and experience, are directed into heterosexuality or homosexuality. That is, cultural and environmental experiences and pressures channel a generalized sex drive in a culturally dictated direction (Hyde & Rosenberg, 1976). This theory assumes that male and female development is basically the same. This is in keeping with the male bias within the literature. The assumption that both men and women have similar development is problematic because of the different status of men and women culturally and experientially in our society.

Another approach to lesbianism, which has gained more recognition, is existentialism. This theme is exemplified by Simone de Beauvoir (1952).

> The truth is that homosexuality (lesbianism) is no more a perversion deliberately indulged in than it is a curse of fate. It is an attitude chosen in a certain situation—that is at once motivated and freely adopted.

According to the existentialist thesis, it requires a highly integrated woman, emotionally, socially, and intellectually, to hazard the risks of social ostracism to consciously choose a homosexual relationship. Intense emotion is both risk and reward for the lesbian more than for her heterosexual counterpart (Hyde & Rosenberg, 1976). Existential thought does not consider the developmental course of a woman who chooses homosexuality; it regards lesbianism as a matter of free choice.

In 1966, publication of Masters and Johnson's research on human sexuality brought a new awareness of sexuality to the public as well as to the health care professionals. The National Institute of Mental Health (NIMH) in 1967 established a national task force to deal specifically with homosexuality. In 1972 this task force recommended provisions be made for the training and education of mental health professionals in the area of human sexuality.

Until 1974, homosexuality was listed as a mental disorder. At that time, the American Psychiatric Association removed homosexuality from its official list of disorders. "Sexual orientation disturbance" was formulated to replace homosexuality. This category excluded homosexuality itself as a disorder. Homosexuality is considered a disorder only when interests directed toward people of the same sex are disturbing, in conflict with, or include a wish to change someone's sexual orientation. This change had implications for health professionals treating women with a homosexual orientation. Many readjustments both personally and professionally had to be effected. These readjustments involved health care providers' attitudes and values clarification as well as health care education and practice.

In 1975, a report released by the World Health Organization (WHO) recognized the need for education and training in human sexuality for health professionals (WHO, 1975). This report also discussed the attitudes of health professionals and their need to understand their own sexuality as well as their awareness and acceptance of the wide range of variations in sexual behavior. The report stated:

> The need for a change in attitudes—for acceptance of sexuality as a positive component of health, for oneself, and for others—is recognized as being particularly important. Health workers at all levels share the same beliefs, myths, and superstitions that exist in the society to which they belong, and they may themselves have unresolved sexual problems. (WHO, 1975, p. 10)

This report outlines clear implications for health care professionals. To succeed in establishing health care for clients, providers need to be both affectively and theoretically educated in the sexuality of various groups.

Present research on lesbianism is beginning to fill in some of the past gaps. The available literature indicates that lesbians tend to have or seek lasting relationships more frequently than male homosexuals (Seiden, 1976). Lesbians make the same differentiation between friends and lovers as do heterosexuals. Loney (1973) compared unmarried lesbians to their heterosexual counterparts. She found that both groups had about the same percentage of transient, deepening, and co-habiting relationships that they expected to be permanent, and about the same percentage of depression and other psychiatric symptoms. Both groups, of course, were under the same familiar social pressures, e.g., to marry, to have children, and to conceal the status of their sexual relationships. These pressures may be considerably greater for lesbians and might have predicted a greater incidence of psychiatric symptoms, but this was not found (Loney, 1973). Finally, before a holistic educational health plan can be developed, some of the similarities between lesbians and their heterosexual counterparts are reviewed.

Similarities:

1. A lesbian's gender identity is female.
2. Lesbians experience similar health needs in regard to:
   a. menstruation
   b. menopause
   c. common gynecological problems (infections)
   d. breast disease and cancer
   e. cancer of the reproductive system (lesbians have a lower incidence of cervical cancer)
   f. general health problems of body systems (prevention and treatment)

3. May be victims of violence and abuse (rape).
4. Diverse in their motivation to seek health care and need for education.
5. Lesbians do become pregnant and their pregnancy needs are similar.
6. Experience similar stress and social pressure related to their gender identity.

Differences:

1. Contraceptive needs are minimal to nonexistent.
2. The way a lesbian becomes pregnant or begins a family may be different. She may elect an alternative nonmedical method of artificial insemination.
3. Parenting issues—single parenting versus couple parenting—may bring fear and anxiety that the child may be taken away or will experience negative societal attitudes. Many lesbians become aware of their orientation after marriage and birth of children. This set of circumstances also engenders fear and anxiety regarding custody and societal rejection.
4. Lesbians experience added societal pressure because of sexual orientation.

There is no known "cause" of homosexuality. It is a subject surrounded by an abundance of misconceptions. It seems, then, that women arrive at a lesbian life-style for various reasons at varying times during the life cycle. Health care practitioners should become knowledgeable about the needs of the lesbian population, learn their terminology and their resources, and become sensitized to the added stresses that the lesbian life-style can carry (Table 9–1). It is important to understand that there is a variety of life-styles that include monogamy, celibacy, multiple relationships, and open marriages. These styles, as the heterosexual styles, may vary over the life cycle.

Learning Needs

When lesbians have a health need, they require as much information and education about their bodies and their sexuality as heterosexuals. There are many resources avail-

TABLE 9–1. GLOSSARY OF HOMOSEXUAL TERMS

Butch. Connotes stereotyped masculine role.

Closet case. A person who has not accepted their homosexuality. May be sexually active or inactive.

Coming out. The process of accepting one's homosexuality.

Dyke. Female homosexual; lesbian; old term inappropriate for use.

Femme. Lesbian who plays a stereotyped female role.

Gay. Homosexual lifestyle; male or female.

Gay parent. Homosexual who has children.

Heterosexism. The assumption that everyone is or desires to be heterosexual.

Heterosexual behavior. An individual who prefers a sexual partner of the opposite sex.

Homophile. Preferred term by some to denote sexual or affectional orientation; emphasizes more than the sexual aspects of relationships.

Homophobia. An excessive fear and avoidance of homosexuals.

Homosexual behavior. Sexual relations or emotional attachments to a person of the same sex.

Homosexuality. More than a method of having sexual relationships; a way of living and loving.

Lesbian. Women whose female gender identity is female but who define themselves as having a sexual orientation for persons of the same sex.

Nongay. Heterosexual.

Straight. Heterosexual.

able through local and national homosexual associations. For selected resources see Appendix B.

The content areas for health education and prevention are:

1. Anatomy and physiology of body systems, including reproductive.
2. Knowledge of menstruation and menopause.
3. Common gynecological problems and urinary tract infections including prevention, treatment, symptoms, and transmission. The most common are vaginitis and herpes type I and type II, and the least common problems are syphilis and gonorrhea. The infections can be spread by direct vulvar contact, fingers, and vibrators. Information on how these problems affect their lovemaking should also be provided.
4. Sexuality and lovemaking. There are many diverse means of lovemaking. Health care providers are generally trained to consider only heterosexual intercourse and the related sexuality issues. Stimulation may be direct or through stimulation of breasts, vagina, anus, or other body areas such as the ears. Lovemaking includes direct clitoral stimulation by oral contact, touching, body to body rubbing, or stimulation with a vibrator. The health care provider should be familiar with these variations and be comfortable with the discussion of them.
5. Knowledge of breast self-examination—signs and symptoms of breast problems.
6. Pregnancy and parenting. Alternative methods of fertilization and physical and psychological self-care during the planning and carrying through of the process need to be addressed. Methods of artificial or alternative insemination give lesbians, who desire children yet shun a short-term sexual relationship with a man, new alternatives for bearing children. Health care providers need to be aware not only of the medical means of artificial insemination, but also alternative fertilization that some women use. The mechanics of alternative fertilization require a donor who will ejaculate into a clear small jar or condom; the woman then lying down transfers the semen to her vagina, using an eyedropper, a turkey baster, or diaphragm, or inserts the inverted condom (O'Donnell et al., 1979). These issues raise a new type of ethical, legal, and moral question for lesbians. Additionally, the added stress of single parenting, possible rejection by other lesbians, or concerns about how to parent require additional support and counseling. Further, there is some concern among lesbians that straight health care providers may not be able to render such care.
7. Alcoholism. There seems to be a higher incidence of alcoholism in the lesbian community (Fifield, 1977). Lesbians may socialize within a limited environment where they will feel accepted and among friends. The gay or lesbian bars have in the past been the main places for homosexuals to meet and socialize. Therefore alcohol and community are interrelated. Other reasons such as social isolation, stigmatized life-style, and societal pressures may also contribute to the high incidence of alcoholism. Finally, there is the unknown factor of whether the drinking developed as a response to some other unhappiness, anxiety, or a means of coping rather than as a result of a limited social environment.
8. Promotion of positive mental health strategies related to:
   a. Reduction of stress,
   b. Self-awareness and self-insight for growth towards an optimum level of development and health,
   c. Body image,
   d. Encounters with family, friends, and support systems.

A study conducted by Johnson and colleagues (1981) found that gay women experienced the gamut of both obstetrical and gynecological problems, but venereal disease and cervical dysplasia were uncommon. They noted no medical problems specific to lesbians. The prevalent concern of the lesbians was the negative attitude of their health care provider and its effect on their care.

There may be a different incidence and risk of cancer for the lesbian. Studies have demonstrated that the incidence of cervical cancer is higher in women who have had intercourse at an early age and with many different male sexual partners. Therefore, lesbians may have a lower incidence of cervical cancer. Conversely, childless lesbians may have a higher incidence of breast cancer and endometriosis that more commonly affects women who have not borne children. These are but a few possible differences that need more thorough investigation. In the past, the study of lesbian health needs was more difficult than it would currently be because of the increase in gay and feminist health care facilities.

Assessment

Deterrents. Seeking assistance for physical or psychological health concerns can be an unpleasant, frightening, and uncomfortable experience for both homosexuals and heterosexuals. Lesbians often avoid or delay seeking health care in traditional settings due to anxiety and fear. This avoidance may also be due to the potential need to disclose sexual orientation. Therefore, the health care provider who is working with any woman should not assume a heterosexual or a homosexual orientation. This may ease a woman's initial fears. Establishment of a trusting and comfortable provider–client relationship is essential for optimal care. Establishment of confidentiality is also essential to the provider–client relationship. Confidentiality may be especially important when dealing with a woman who has not yet chosen to disclose her orientation.

Comfort and Attitudes. A lesbian's acknowledgment of her sexual orientation may occur at any point in the woman's life cycle. An individual's comfort and attitude toward her acknowledgment or "coming out" is a complex issue. There are three intertwined stages in the coming out process that she may or may not complete:

1. Coming out to oneself—starting to see oneself as homosexual;
2. Coming out in the gay world—starting to meet other gay people;
3. Coming out in the straight world—starting to be open to non-gays about one's gayness. (Hart & Richardson, 1981)

Knowing where an individual is in this process can help in the assessment of the woman's level of comfort with her self. A woman can be at any age when she first sees herself as gay. The age when she first saw herself as homosexual, her coping mechanisms, situational supports, and past successful life experiences may affect the woman's comfort level with her sexual orientation and consequent openness to health care.

Knowledge and Motivation. Knowledge and motivation to enhance one's own knowledge base can affect behavior. To reinforce the concepts of learning, as outlined in Chapters 2 and 3, before a specific health education plan can effectively be taught, the practitioner should assess:

1. The client's ability and desire to learn.
2. The client's level of knowledge of the specific area and any past experiences related to it.

3. Any factors that may alter learning. These factors include age, education, readiness or interest in topic, motivation, past experience with the health care system, and physical and psychological state.

Methodologies

Interview and Sexual History. An important aspect of the interview is to determine a woman's sexual orientation. This is necessary for the practitioner to provide holistic and comprehensive care. This is especially true in the area of obstetrics and gynecology with its psychosocial implications. It is in the area of contraception where the lesbian's needs differ most from those of the heterosexual woman. Incorrect identification of sexuality can lead to misunderstanding and blockage of further care. A sexual history is an integral part of the general health history. It should be taken to gain information about sexual and psychosocial growth of the woman and developmental issues as they relate to the woman's overall health status. Sexual issues affect an individual's self-concept in both physical and psychological illness. The depth of the interview should be modified depending on the type and nature of the problem presented. To accomplish this the health care provider needs to have gained some mastery of interviewing skills in sexual matters.

A question such as "Do you have intercourse?" requires a yes or no response, and may preclude further communication. Using an open-ended question such as "Tell me about your sexual activity" at an appropriate time during the interview may help to elicit more information (Good, 1976). Interviewers should be cognizant of their own feelings and reactions. Questions about sexuality should be expressed with as much concern and comfort as questions related to less stressful topics. It is generally useful to begin in an area that is less stressful such as menstruation and progress to areas that may produce more anxiety.

Educational information should be incorporated into the interview. An example of this is menstruation. The interviewer can educate and decrease apprehension by suggesting that "We have all heard many stories and myths about menstruation which can be confusing. Can you think of any such stories that have affected you?" Similar questions on other topics such as masturbation or sexuality can open up areas for discussion. Furthermore they may help to identify leaning needs, problem areas, or areas that the client would like to discuss with the health care provider. Before the practitioner opens up an area, it is important that she be aware of not only her comfort level but also her knowledge base. It is possible that the practitioner may not have all the necessary information required for an extended discussion, but she should be able to provide appropriate referrals. Finally, do not dismiss unanticipated responses. If a woman says she does not use or need contraceptives, she may be telling the truth (Brossart, 1979). Answers such as these need further investigation. It would be important to assess if she is celibate or has sexual relations with men and wishes to become pregnant or if she is infertile or sterilized. If the answer to these questions is "no," then the practitioner should ask if she has sexual relations with women. Sexual preferences should be established prior to development of a health education plan so that the woman's individual needs may be met.

Care Settings: Inpatient and Outpatient

When seeking outpatient services, lesbians can choose between traditional care settings or gay health clinics. But for inpatient care, the only choice is the traditional hospital setting. Physical care of the lesbian in the hospital does not differ from that of the heterosexual client. Psychologically, the experience may be overwhelming and can overshadow any teaching. Legally, the lesbian is denied her strongest support system. Hospital guidelines and health insurance plans do not recognize a lesbian lover as a family member. Displays of affection so often seen in hospitals between heterosexual couples are frowned upon, or draw curious and unaccepting attention, when displayed by homosexual couples. Staff may avoid or covertly ridicule such couples. Because of these responses, increased psychological pain may be imposed upon clients. During hospitalization the health care provider is in an important position to be the client's advocate. Accordingly, during hospitalization and when doing discharge planning, the loved one should be included in the plans and informed of the client's progress and needs.

Many large cities have outpatient clinics for homosexuals. These clinics are especially geared to the physical and psychological needs of their clients. Gay clinics grew out of negative experiences with traditional settings. This may be a better alternative for some women, but not all lesbians have access to such a setting or will go to a gay clinic for fear of being discovered. Traditional settings need to address the issue of providing comprehensive physical and psychological services for homosexuals.

Objectives. The major objective is to deliver flexible and nonrestrictive comprehensive care for each woman's expressed needs and goals. The objective of education should meet the woman's physical and psychological needs as a whole. Generally the teaching objectives for the lesbian and the nonlesbian are the same.

1. Comprehensive health care: Maintenance of both physical and psychosocial well-being.
2. Knowledge and information on health issues that affect them as women, such as menstruation, pregnancy, childbirth, parenting, breast care, menopause, and demystification of routine gynecological care.
3. Inclusion in the decision-making process regarding health care.
4. Inclusion of partner in health care planning.

When approaching these objectives one must be cognizant of the following facts. Lesbians do not wish to be urged toward heterosexuality when seeking health care, and they do not wish their health care problems or needs to be "blamed" on their lesbianism. Lesbians, like all women, deserve respect for their life-style. Other areas in which care planning may differ are listed in Table 9–2.

TABLE 9–2. EDUCATIONAL OBJECTIVES FOR THE POSSIBLE SPECIAL NEEDS OF THE LESBIAN CLIENT

The woman will:

1. Be able to describe the symptoms of urinary tract and vaginal infections, how to procure and use treatment.
    Rationale: Lesbian women have an extremely low rate of venereal disease and cervical dysplasia, but do experience other common urinary and gynecological infections.

2. List the options that exist for alternative fertilization, and understand the means of alternative fertilization if she wishes to bear children.
    Rationale: Choosing a lesbian sexual orientation does not preclude bearing children. A woman's wishes in this area should be assessed and supported.

3. State the incidence, prevalence, and symptoms of alcoholism.
    Rationale: The high incidence of alcoholism in the gay community requires special education. Traditionally the lesbian bar has been the setting for social activities, and the social isolation of a gay life-style due to discrimination may be a factor in the high rate of alcoholism. Education should focus not just on alcoholism, but on the positive aspects of building support systems within the community.

The Coming Out Process. Strategies for assisting the lesbian in the coming out process may be accomplished in traditional health settings, alternative health settings, and community settings such as churches and schools. These strategies can be for individuals, groups, the lesbian's biological family, or the lesbian couple. The health care provider' may not see a lesbian in the early stages of "coming out" or at a time when assistance is not necessary in this area. This section is included to help raise the health provider's consciousness to this period and to provide information if the woman is in this process.

Before any teaching strategy is used, assessment of the woman's goals and needs is important. Coming out is the process of accepting one's lesbian orientation just as other women accept their heterosexuality. For some this can be a lifelong process. Coming out may be a critical point of reference for some women. The process can be positive or negative, but is always highly stressful. Each person's experience is unique and highly dependent on the situation and one's support systems. Coming out usually begins when one feels that she has erotic feelings toward other women. After one admits these feelings to oneself, then comes the decision to tell someone, to act upon the feelings, or to deny them. In the process of coming out one decides how, when, and to whom she will reveal her preference.

The decision to come out requires action. This action can create mild to severe anxiety, a reconsideration of self, and a search for what it means to be gay. Coming out does not occur in a predictable pattern. That is, once a woman admits her preference to herself, she may choose to tell her closest friends, but not her family or employer.

At any time during this process a woman may present for assistance whether for concerns directly related to sexual orientation or indirectly through other health concerns. Commonly, problems are related to finding acceptable outlets for socialization and accepting support networks. Several factors should be assessed and explored with the woman before any intervention is begun. According to Woodman and Lenna (1980), these are:

1. Greater sexual arousal by women than men, including masturbation fantasies.
2. Preference for initiating and enjoying same-sex experiences.
3. More or only sexual experiences with women. During the coming out process the woman may be having heterosexual and homosexual experiences but prefers homosexual experiences.
4. Consistency in number, duration, and intensity of relationships with women. This includes a pattern of same-sex relationships.
5. Expectations and fantasies of the future revolve around partners of the same sex.
6. Preference for same-sex social interaction.
7. Describing self with terms indicating a homosexual identity.
8. Level of tolerance for heterosexist situations and pressures. For example, jokes about gays or pressure from others to give up their "crazy ideas."

A woman may display varying degrees of comfort with these areas but still requires some assistance. The health care practitioner should be equipped to intervene on any of these points. These issues can be addressed by short-term and crisis intervention techniques (Table 9–3). Another method is to develop an alliance with a gay health care facility. The provider, therefore, needs to be aware of the community's organizations for homosexuals and be able to function as the woman's advocate and facilitator. In many instances, a woman may feel that the coming out process is best facilitated by a gay health care provider who can be a model.

Whether or not the woman attends a gay health care facility, the health care pro-

TABLE 9–3. EXAMPLES OF CRISIS TECHNIQUES

Assessment	Intervention
Assessment of immediate problem	Process precipitating event
1. Allow client to identify problem	Identify with client ideas and feelings about the problem and its consequences
2. Allow client to define the event that lead to the seeking of assistance	Promote self-image
3. What does the event or problem mean to the woman	Promote strengths
4. How does she feel it will affect her or her support systems	Provide education on relationship between the crisis and event
5. Assess any recent changes in work, living situation, or losses or fears	Provide education on alternatives, explore possible variations of life-style
	Encourage woman to participate in activities that may assist to build her self-esteem
	Develop a trusting relationship with client
Availability of support systems	Evaluate how one views self in relationship to family, friends, and community
	Evaluate who the woman feels that she can depend on, and are they readily available
	Problem solve with client around her ability to use support systems or to develop new ones
	Assess her interest in joining a self-help group or organizations that are appropriate to her needs
	Problem solve with client to examine alternatives
Growth and developmental stage	Evaluate where client is in growth and developmental stages: does she give evidence of work record or educational pursuits, or social outlets
	Have her summarize where she feels she is in relationship to current situation
	Assist her to ventilate concerns
Coping mechanisms	Problem solve with client to identify "problem" areas
	Evaluate with client which coping mechanism she uses either successfully or poorly, and has she used them in this situation
	Problem solve with the woman to explore alternative coping strategies to deal with concerns
	Reinforce any positive coping mechanisms and strengths
Evaluation	Evaluate all interventions; are outcomes useful to client and meeting her needs

vider should complete the contract with the woman to help her gain an understanding and exploration of feelings regarding her experiences, fears, relationships, and concerns. The woman should also be helped to understand that a personal sexual choice is a right and not an illness, by pointing out the client's strengths and abilities. Religious guilt may also be experienced. Referrals to pastoral counselors known to be sensitive to the needs of homosexuals may also be beneficial.

Group therapy or discussion groups during the coming out process can also be a means of both short- or long-term therapy. The milieu is extremely important. An atmosphere of openness, compassion, honesty, and acceptance is important. This can lead to universality, catharsis, and sharing of hopefulness. The group leader should be equipped and prepared to deal with the usual spectrum of emotional concerns as seen with most groups. These, of course, will differ in degree. Depression, guilt, anger, anxiety, denial, doubting, indecision, and listlessness are common causes of complaint (Gershman, 1975). After the atmosphere has been established the group leader should encourage group interaction. Groups for lesbians can help to resolve interpersonal relationship concerns and provide a format for sharing experiences common to most in the lesbian community.

Family interventions can also be an effective therapeutic method. This may not include the family in the traditional sense. This may include the immediate group of people that the woman is living with or her biological family. The health care provider who renders this type of care should be trained in family therapy. The provider may help the client and her loved ones to clarify concerns and offer support, guidance, and education. If the client is experiencing interpersonal relationship difficulties with those she lives with, the therapist can intervene to clarify the issues that are causing distress in the family and offer support and guidance in their resolution. In summary, the coming out process can be a time in which the health practitioner can help the lesbian develop her potential and foster a sense of self-esteem as a person with individual preferences rather than exclusively as a homosexual.

Many large communities have gay support groups within gay clinics or other community settings. Health providers should be aware of the scope of these services. Generally these alternative clinics have the benefit of health professionals within their organizations who are trained in counseling. Other clinics and lesbian groups that do not have this benefit do have interested members who are willing to receive training so they may help others. An exchange of professionals or a series of gay community workshops could be a valuable way to educate, guide, and exchange information between straight health care workers and the gay community. Also a liaison service for the homosexual paraprofessional with a heterosexual care provider could be an alternative to aid in health problem solving.

Health Care Provider. Quality health care requires a holistic view of clients. The role of the health care provider is consistent with providing health education for the lesbian. For an in-depth review of learning strategies and health provider role in education see Chapter 3. Following the same general recommendations, the provider may assume a number of roles when teaching health care for lesbians:

1. Provider of anticipatory guidance
2. Educator (including physical and psychosocial dimensions of health)
3. Role model and consultant to other health care providers
4. Counselor and client advocate
5. Validator of normalcy (Woods, 1979)

Many clients have either personally experienced or heard about negative experiences at traditional health care facilities. This fact calls for more knowledge and education of health professionals on homosexual life-style, feelings, concerns, and community support systems.

To carry out these roles the provider requires a broad knowledge base, including information on various sexual behaviors and life-styles of lesbians. One should also have an awareness of the correlation between age-related needs, life events, and sexuality. A priority equal to knowledge base is awareness of one's attitudes and value system. One's attitudes and value system reflect beliefs and biases toward sexuality. For these reasons providers must first understand their feelings, values, and attitudes toward their own sexuality. It may be helpful for health care providers to answer the following questions: (1) What does sexuality and its various forms mean to me? (2) How do I feel about sexual behavior that differs from mine? (3) What do I think is normal? After one begins to understand one's own sexuality then one can begin to explore her acceptance level and attitudes toward alternate life-styles.

Part of the provider's responsibility is to respect and relate honestly with clients. Development of communication skills and awareness of social and health issues that may affect health care, goal setting, and problem solving are important assets. It is important to note that not all health care providers are heterosexual either in traditional or gay health care settings. Additionally, a lesbian may not be comfortable with a straight health care provider. When a woman's life-style preference is known to be lesbian it is important to determine with her who the best provider would be dependent on her needs.

Health Education. A review of the literature related to lesbian health teaching reveals that few curricula include information specific to lesbians. There are courses related to human sexuality that contain general information on homosexuality. Studies done by Mims and Swenson (1978) and Turner (1977) suggest that there is a lack of information or, in some cases, misinformation regarding human sexuality especially in nursing curricula. As nurses expand their role in counseling individuals and families, so must their preparation be enhanced to meet clients' needs. Both undergraduate and graduate curricula need to provide a knowledge base of sexuality with its attendant physical, psychosocial, and sexual implications. Education on communication skills and interviewing techniques involving human sexuality is a vital part of health education. Human sexuality education focusing on specific life-style patterns should be integrated in all areas of health care reflecting the needs of a lesbian woman throughout her life cycle.

Continuing Education. In-service education in outpatient facilities, general hospitals, and psychiatric settings needs periodic update and review of the needs of all types of patients, including lesbians. This can be accomplished by offering seminars with both didactic information and discussion time. In addition, the inclusion of members of the homosexual community is an important resource of information and education.

This exchange of education can extend into the homosexual community. Practitioners should go to gay community meetings and teach aspects of preventive physical and mental health care in areas such as breast self-examination, nutrition, alcoholism, as well as other care related to maintaining a positive health status.

Health care provision strives toward equal, accountable, and quality client care for all groups. Lesbians are no exception. In the past, ignoring the lesbians' needs as individuals and as a group has not been in line with stated health care goals. To assure quality holistic care, upper division health care programs and continuing education programs should include a greater depth of sexuality education. Providers need to rethink their biases regarding lesbianism. Additionally, research on the health education and health care needs of the lesbian must be undertaken.

Health practitioners need to act as role models to the community in gaining education, acceptance, and respect for the lesbian's life-style and relationships as healthy alternatives to heterosexuality. In response to community needs the practitioner needs to maintain a current knowledge of services available and an openness to an exchange of information and services.

There are an estimated 20 million homosexuals in the United States, including many health professionals, as well as clients. To meet the challenge of serving their needs with dignity, health care providers should be aware of the needs of homosexuals and clarify their own values so that they may care for lesbian clients or refer them to gay health facilities and gay providers.

RESOURCES FOR CLIENTS

Abbott, S., & Love, B. *Sappho was a right-on woman: A liberated view of lesbianism*. New York: Stein & Day, 1972. Cloth and paper editions.

Clark, D. *Loving someone gay: A gay therapist's guidance for gays and people who care about them*. Celestial Arts, 1977.

Johnston, J. *Gullibles travels*. New York: Links Books, 1974.

Johnston, J. *Lesbian nation: The feminist solution*. New York: Simon & Schuster (Touchstone), 1973.

Katz, J. *Coming out: A documentary play about gay life and liberation in the USA*. New York: Arno Press Series on Homosexuality, 1975.

Katz, J. *Gay American history*. Crowell, 1976.

Klaich, D. *Woman + woman: Attitudes toward lesbianism*. Morrow, 1974.

Journal of Homosexuality. 130 W. 72nd St., New York, NY 10023. Quarterly/year. Scholarly and psychological research in mental health field.

Martin, D., & Lyon, P. *Lesbian women*. New York: Bantam Books, 1972.

O'Donnell, M., Pollock, K., Loeffler, V., & Saunders, Z. *Lesbian health matters!* Santa Cruz, Calif.: Santa Cruz Women's Health Collective Publication, 1979.

Sex Information and Education Council of the United States. *Homosexuality*. SIECUS Study Guide No. 2. (rev. ed.) Behavioral Publications, 72 Fifth Ave, New York, NY 10011. $1.00 prepaid.

The lesbian feminist. Lesbian Feminist Liberation, 243 W. 20th St., New York, NY 10011.

Vida, G. (Ed.). *Our right to love: A lesbian resource book*. Englewood Cliffs, N.J.: Prentice-Hall, 1978. Covers many topics and has an extensive resource list.

Weinberg, G. *Society and the healthy homosexual*. New York: Doubleday/Anchor, 1972.

RESOURCES FOR HEALTH CARE PROVIDERS

American Association of Sex Educators, Counselors & Therapists. Gay, Lesbian and Bisexual Caucus, P.O. Box 834, Linden Hill, NY 11354.

American Psychological Association, Task Force on the Status of Lesbian and Gay Psychologists. Committee on Gay Concerns, c/o APA Office of Social and Ethical Responsibilities, 1700 17th St. N.W., Washington, DC 20036.

Bibliography of lesbian related materials. 1974. Lesbian Resource Center, 2104 Stevens Ave. South, Minneapolis, MN 53404. Free.

Dignity. A Catholic bibliography on homosexuality. 1975. Dignity-National, 775 Boylston, Rm. 514, Boston, MA 02116. Free.

Dykes & Tykes, Assistance for Gay Parents. New York Chapter, Box 621, Old Chelsea Station, New York, NY 10011.

Fairchild, B. *Parents of gays*. Revised 1975. Lambda Rising, 1724 20th St., N.W., Washington, DC 20009. $1.00 plus 35¢ for postage.

Grammick, J., et al. Catholic homosexuals: A primer for discussion. Dignity, 1975. Dignity National, 775 Boylston, Boston, MA 02116. $1.50 prepaid.

Gay and lesbian-feminist organizations list. Complete United States, updated monthly. National Gay Task Force, 80 Fifth Ave., New York, NY 10011.

Gay Nurses' Alliance, c/o St. Mark's Clinic, 44 St. Mark's Place, New York, NY 10003; or P.O. Box 673, Randolph, MA 02368; or Box 1015, Brownsville, TX 78520.

Gay parent support packet. National Gay Task Force, 80 Fifth Ave., New York, NY 10011. $1 prepaid. Statements on gay parents' custody and visitation rights.

National Association of Gay Alcoholism Professionals. P.O. Box 376, Oakland, NJ 07436.

National gay health directory. National Lesbian and Gay Health Conference, P.O. Box 6189, San Francisco, CA 94101. Gay resources listed for all United States and Canada.

National Gay Task Force, 80 Fifth Avenue, New York, NY 10011.

BIBLIOGRAPHY

Beauvoir, Simone de. *The second sex*. New York: Knopf, 1952.

Bermant, G. Behavioral therapy approaches to modification of sexual preferences: Biological perspective and critique. In J. Bardwick (Ed.), *Readings on the psychology of women*. New York: Harper & Row, 1972.

Berzon, B., & Leighton, R. (Eds.). *Positively gay*. California: Celestial Arts, 1979.

Brossart, J. The gay patient—What you should be doing. *RN*, 1979, *4*, 50–52.

Deutsch, H. On female homosexuality. *Psychoanalytic Quarterly*, 1932, *1*, 484–510.

Deutsch, H. *Psychology of women* (Vol. 1). London: Research Book, 1947.

Fifield, L. *Alcoholism in the gay community: The price of alienation, isolation and oppression*. Los Angeles, Calif.: Gay Community Services Center, 1977.

Ford, C. S., & Beach, F. A. *Patterns of sexual behavior*. New York: Harper & Row, 1951.

Freud, S. *The interpretation of dreams* (J. Strachey, Ed. and trans.). New York: Basic Books, 1955. (Originally published, 1900)

Freud, S. *Psychology of women: New introductory lectures on psychoanalysis*. London: Hogarth Press, 1933.

Freud, S. *Female sexuality. The complete psychological works of Sigmund Freud* (Standard edition, Vol. 21). London: Hogarth Press, 1931.

Gershman, H. The effect of group therapy on compulsive homosexuality in men and women. *American Journal of Psychoanalysis*, 1975, 35, 303–312.

Good, R. S. The gynecologist and the lesbian. *Clinical Obstetrics and Gynecology*, 1976, *19*(2), 473–482.

Hart, J., & Richardson, P. *The theory and practice of homosexuality*. London: Routledge & Kegan Paul, 1981.

Hedblom, J. Dimensions of lesbian sexual experience. *Archives of Sexual Behavior*, 1973, *4*, 329–341.

Hyde, J., & Rosenberg, R. G. *Half the human experience*. New York: D.C. Heath, 1976.

Johnson, S. R., Guenther, S. M., Laube, D. W., & Keettel, W. C. Factors influencing lesbian gynecologic care: A preliminary study. *American Journal of Obstetrics and Gynecology*, 1981, *140*(1), 20–28.

Loney, J. Family dynamics in homosexual women. *Archives of Sexual Behavior*, 1973, *2*(4), 313–350.

Meyer-Bahlburg, H. F. L. Sex hormones and male homosexuality in comparative perspective. *Archives of Sexual Behavior*, 1977, *6*(4), 297–325.

Mims, F., & Swenson, M. A model to promote sexual health care. *Nursing Outlook*, 1978, *26*, 121–125.

Money, J. Sex hormones and other variables in human eroticism. In W. C. Young (Ed.), *Sex and internal secretions* (Vol. 11). Baltimore: Williams & Wilkins, 1965.

O'Donnell, M., Pollock, K., Loeffler, V., & Sanders, Z. *Lesbian health matters*. Santa Cruz, Calif.: Santa Cruz Women's Health Collective Publication, 1979.

Pettyjohn, R. D. Health care of the gay individual. *Nursing Forum*, 1979, *18*(4), 366–393.

Riess, B. New viewpoints on the female homosexual. In V. Franks & V. Burtle (Eds.), *Women in therapy*. New York: Brunner/Mazel, 1974.

Romm, M. E. Sexuality and homosexuality in women. In J. Marmor (Ed.), *Sexual inversion: The multiple roots of homosexuality*. New York: Basic Books, 1965.

Rosen, D. H. *Lesbianism: The study of women's homosexuality*. Springfield, Ill.: Charles C. Thomas, 1974.

Seiden, A. Research on the psychology of woman: Women in families, work and psychotherapy. *American Journal of Psychiatry*, 1976, *133*(10), 1111–1123.

Turner, M. *Attitudes of nursing students toward homosexuality*. Unpublished thesis, University of Rochester, 1977.

Wolff, C. *Love between women*. New York: Harper & Row, 1971.

Woodman, N. J., & Lenna, H. R. *Counseling with gay men and women*. San Francisco: Jossey-Bass, 1980.

Woods, N. F. *Human sexuality in health and illness* (2nd ed.). St. Louis, Mo.: C. V. Mosby, 1979.

World Health Organization. *Education and treatment in human sexuality: The training of health professionals*. Report of a World Health Meeting (Teaching Report Series No. 572), 1975, 5–33.

Education for Disabled Women

10

Mary Sprik

As the health and wellness movement gains impetus, society is increasing its emphasis on health teaching and learning. More and more individuals are learning how to promote mental and physical well-being via the media, the classroom, self-help groups, community health services and agencies, and even their health providers. In addition the women's movement has brought together groups of women to promote their mutual mental as well as physical health. Core groups forming the movement have been consciousness raising, assertiveness training, and gynecological self-help. Furthermore, as women gained independence and self-confidence, other groups arose to assist women with specific problems, such as divorce, single parenthood, menopause, and alcoholism. Women are also participating with men to gain skills in maintaining wellness through the health related topics of nutrition, meditation, exercise, and relaxation. The option to experience the women's and the wellness movement through health educational experiences needs to be available also to disabled women.

Architectural designs, transportation difficulties, lack of money, and stereotypical attitudes may all act as barriers to full participation of the disabled woman in the health education experience. The purpose of this chapter is to identify the special needs and circumstances of disabled women that will impact any plan for health education. Special emphasis is placed on interventions to enhance accessibility of disabled women to community groups. A framework is presented for the adaptation of the teaching–learning process to include the unique needs of women who have a disability. Modeling of the framework is achieved by specific teaching–learning interventions for women with hearing impairments. Lastly, a guide of related bibliographies, audiovisual aids, and other resources to teach women with mobility, sensory, and mental impairment is presented.

Promoting Accessibility

Methods used successfully by others to promote accessibility of disabled individuals to their services are reviewed here. This portion relies heavily on the germinal work in this area, *Who Cares?*, a product of the Sex and Disability Project (Cornelius et al., 1982). The book was written by project members specifically to promote community sex education and counseling services to meet the needs of disabled persons. With adaptations, suggestions are just as relevant for women's health education.

Barriers for disabled women participating in health education services can be categorized as environmental, financial, and attitudinal. Barriers are outlined below along with specific intervention strategies for their dissolution.

Attitudinal Barriers. The attitude of the teacher–health educator is crucial in facilitating the process of health education. Rodgers (1969) emphasizes prizing, acceptance, and trust as critical components of the teacher in the teaching–learning process. Rodgers further clarifies that the teacher needs to accept the learner's imperfections as well as abilities. For the health educator, working with a disabled person may be especially difficult if they have had no prior experience with disablement or they subscribe to prevalent myths about disability. Therefore, at the outset it seems prudent to explore some of the common myths about disability as they relate to this group of women.

Disabled Persons Are Dependent or Ill. People who have disabilities are often regarded as childlike. This concept may be fostered by significant others and health providers, as well as the disabled themselves. Our society accepts dependent roles for children and women but has little tolerance for this trait in men. The tendency of some parents of children with disabilities is to overprotect, thus inhibiting the child's ability to master the developmental task of independence. Women with disabilities, because they are chastized less for dependency behavior, are at greater risk of never achieving independence. Because independence contributes to self-esteem and the ability to reach one's highest potential, fostering dependency violates women's basic human right of self-actualization (Dowling, 1981). People with disabilities are a heterogenous group. Various disabilities will handicap the individual totally, not at all, or only in certain function(s). The goal is to provide maximum independence as defined by the individual's limitations. Women's groups favor andragogical learning approaches and are more concerned with the growth of the learner than the content presented. Therefore, participation in women's groups offers an advantage to the disabled woman who has experienced little independence.

The "spread" theory accounts for the perception of disablement as illness. The theory states that if one part of the body or body function is impaired, then other parts or functions are also affected (Wright, 1960). Thus a woman with impaired mobility due to a spinal cord injury may be perceived also to have impaired sexual functioning. The danger of accepting the spread theory is that women with a spinal cord injury may not receive appropriate health services such as birth control counseling, or testing for venereal disease or pregnancy. Some evidence exists that shows that disabled women do in fact receive less routine health screening than their nondisabled counterparts (Hale-Harbaugh et al., 1978; Natale & Sprik, 1980). Further, the belief that the disabled are sick often precludes their involvement in health-oriented activities, such as health education.

Disabled people raised to think of themselves as ill adopt a sick role. The advantages of assuming a sick role include limiting the expectations of others, excusing failures, and offering legitimate barriers to success.

> Vicki, a 24-year-old woman with cerebral palsy, attended the University for a Special Education Degree. Prior to course exams she routinely appeared at the University's Health Services with vague symptoms. If her exams went well, she wasn't heard from until the next examination session. If exams went poorly, she presented with more vague symptoms resulting in a note to her instructor that she was having health problems. By playing the sick role, Vicki could excuse her failures.

Women with Disabilities Are Asexual. The statement that because a person has a disability she is not a sexual being sounds ludicrous. However, countless blatant as well as subtle actions attest to the perception that when one part of the body does not work, all parts malfunction.

- The first words spoken to a young woman with cerebral palsy who was obtaining a routine Pap smear were ". . . did she want her tubes tied?"
- A body brace that didn't change to allow breast development as a girl went from childhood to womanhood . . .

Another facet of this myth is our society's emphasis on the "perfect body." The implication is that the more perfect a woman's body, the more desirable she is as an intimate partner. This line of reasoning results in other destructive myths.

- Disabled women are only desirable to disabled men.
- If a nondisabled man is dating a disabled woman it's because he can't get anyone else or he feels sorry for her.

Women in our culture experience more dissatisfaction with their bodies than do men (Johnson, 1956; Jourard & Secord, 1955; Plutchnik, Weiner, & Conte, 1971; Secord & Jourard, 1953). The cover girl standards of our society have caused women to have needless anxiety and insecurities, and even needless surgery. In studies designed to test body image, children with disabilities demonstrated more alteration in their body images than did children without disabilities (Weininger, Rotenberg, & Henry, 1972). Studies are needed that explore and contrast body image variables of men and women who have disabilities with men and women who are not disabled.

Much of our sexuality is defined by society's roles for us. Until recently, women were expected to be wives and mothers. Consider the hopelessness a disabled woman might experience if she perceives herself as unable to achieve the independence afforded by a job or a career while also believing she cannot be "rescued" by Prince Charming because she is not a desirable partner. The feminist movement created a climate in which women could approach society, their perceptions of themselves, their bodies, and their roles more realistically. This redefinition, while benefiting many women, may be particularly critical for disabled women who have not reached these levels of growth.

Covert attitudinal barriers are more difficult to identify than structural and financial impediments. Stensrud and Stensrud (1981) organized a useful framework for exploring attitudes by looking at negative and positive prejudices. Prejudice is defined as a favorable or unfavorable feeling toward a person with a disability prior to or not based on actual experiences (Stensrud & Stensrud, 1981, p. 43). For the disabled woman negative prejudices may cause inappropriate limitation of a whole range of normal activities and roles, such as physical exercise, sexual expression, marriage, and parenthood. Positive prejudice is demonstrated in behavior that is overly solicitous or apathetic. Over-solicitousness causes the disabled woman social embarrassment, awkwardness, and dependent behavior. Apathy or ignoring a woman's disability is a two-edged sword. It can be positive if it gives a pregnant woman who is also blind acceptance in a mother role. It can also be disastrous if this woman's handicap is ignored and her unique needs are not managed.

Attitudinal Accessibility. Attitudinal barriers are difficult to eradicate. The subtleness and variability of negative as well as positive prejudices preclude easy recognition.

- While assuming a woman with mental impairment is not sexually active . . . a health professional does not perform a cervical gonorrheal culture.
- A childbirth educator perceives a blind woman to be disinterested in course content . . . because of her lack of facial expression.

Consciousness-raising and experience with disablement are keys to dispelling social stereotypes. E.A.S.E. is an acronym developed by the author to outline four steps designed to "ease" the health educator into a comfortable attitude toward disablement: Education–Awareness–Sensitization–Experience.

Education. This step seeks to increase the base of knowledge regarding disability. It may be useful to invite experts on disability to come and speak to your group or attend a continuing educational offering that deals with some aspect of disablement. It may also be useful to read appropriate material from the bibliography at the end of this chapter. Stensrud and Stensrud (1981) remind us, however, that educational efforts by themselves have had little success in altering stereotypes.

Awareness. The value of this step is recognized by many groups that have conducted a Mobility Awareness Day. Heightened awareness of mobility and communication difficulties encountered with some disabilities is accentuated when the able-bodied assume the role of the disabled individual. Participants are assigned to complete daily routine activities using a wheelchair, crutches, blindfolds, or sound mufflers. Further insights and empathy result when disabled and able-bodied discuss the experience. You may want to participate in Mobility Awareness Experiences Days that are conducted on many college campuses or you may want to develop your own.

In one setting participating clinic staff were assigned to role play a mobility impairment for a day. Staff carried out their usual functions, making adaptations where necessary. From this experience, staff rearranged several clinic procedures to more easily accommodate individuals with mobility impairment (Natale & Sprik, 1980).

Sensitization. Individuals are often unaware of their personal attitudes, beliefs, and values toward issues in disablement. Sensitizing techniques have been used to assist individuals in clarifying their value system. These exercises are particularly suited to facilitate the individual in confronting myths and prejudices held about women with disabilities.

One effective sensitizing exercise employs films that depict how social stereotypes impact on everyday activities of disabled women. A study by Abroms and Kodera (1979) employed a similar technique for sensitization. College students were asked to rank the personal acceptability of various disabling conditions. Nonvisible organic impairments amenable to medical intervention (e.g., asthma or diabetes) were ranked as most acceptable whereas sensorimotor impairments were moderately acceptable. Mental and physical impairments not responsive to medical intervention were least acceptable for these students.

Sensitizing occurs when values clarification exercises and films allow the individual an opportunity to recognize what values are prized. When sensitizing occurs in a group, prizing values of others is considered in relationship to self and confirmation or change of value stance may occur.

Experience. Fears, anxieties, and misconceptions about disability held by able-bodied persons fade quickly as the two groups interact. Meaningful exchange illuminates the fact that disabled people are individuals and therefore are subject to the same variety of characteristics and emotions as the general population. Furthermore, professionals who have little expertise with disablement frequently experience performance anxiety and conclude that they are not qualified to service people with disabilities even when their services are unrelated to the person's disability. Experience is our best teacher. Participation of both disabled and nondisabled women in women-focused groups has the potential to dispel myths, clarify values, identify common problems, and promote mutual problem solving.

Environmental Barriers—Accessibility. National legislation in 1977 (Rehabilitation Acts 503 and 504) was intended to provide access to services used by the general community. The outcome of this legislation was to create equality and normalization for individuals with disabilities. This normative approach, called "mainstreaming," allows the disabled person to establish or maintain personal behaviors, appearances, and characteristics that are culturally normal and valued, hence promoting social integration and acceptance (Flynn & Sha'ked, 1978).

The removal of access barriers to the community has begun but is by no means complete. Although new buildings are accessible, older buildings often are not. Beyond parking and curb access, internal environments are all too often prohibitive. Environmental barriers include thick carpets, cluttered hallways, high elevator controls, lack of braille signs for the blind, absence of alternative communication systems for the hearing-impaired, and no planning for alternative fire escape routes. Table 10–1 gives the general assessment and suggested management of environmental barriers. Additional suggestions are:

TABLE 10–1. ASSESSMENT AND MANAGEMENT OF ENVIRONMENTAL BARRIERS FOR HEALTH EDUCATION FACILITIES

Assessment	Management
No accessible mass transportation to your facility	Consider offering service in a convenient setting, i.e., independent living center, rehabilitation facility, etc. Contact and lobby community service groups to provide alternatives or provide bus lines with lifts.
Prohibitive building entrance access	Review governmental regulations.
Consider:	
parking	Provide adequate parking spaces designated for use by disabled persons.
walkway	Clear obstacles, keep surface level and in good repair.
doorway	Widen to 32 inches, lower door handles so that they are within reach of wheelchair users. Provide pull ropes on door handles. Eliminate or modify curbs, build ramps.
Internal building obstacles	Include disabled consumers in evaluation and planning of your facility.
Consider:	
stairs	Modify steps to no more than 7 inches high, build handrails, provide alternatives (e.g., elevator or ramps).
elevators	Provide control buttons in braille, place control panel at no more than 4 feet from the floor or provide a hanging stick from a chain that can be used to press the buttons.
floors	Make sure surface is nonskid; if there is carpeting avoid thick shag or scatter rugs.
phone, restrooms and fountains	Modify for wheelchair user.
emergencies	Install both sound and visual (e.g., flashing light) alarms, provide alternative emergency exits.

(Source: Chipouras, S., Cornelius, D., Daniels, S., & Makas, E. Who cares? A handbook on sex education and counseling services for disabled people. Washington, D. C.: George Washington University, 1978, by permission.)

- Obtain local government regulations regarding your facility.
- Review regulations and items above to evaluate accessibility.
- Organize and meet with a panel of disabled women to get suggestions on how to make your facility more accessible.
- Include disabled women in all aspects of service planning.
- The Task Force on Concerns of Physically Disabled Women also has a very helpful handbook *Within Reach*, on architectural and environmental accessibility, which includes illustrations, dimensions, and specific information on making services barrier-free. (Hale-Harbaugh et al., 1978)

Financial Barriers—Accessibility. Financial barriers represent another major dynamic force limiting access of the disabled to the community. According to the national census, people with disabilities have less income, less employment, and subsequently more poverty than the nondisabled (Hale-Harbaugh et al., 1978). Furthermore, in this country where women make 59¢ to every dollar a man earns, what must a disabled woman earn?

Lack of money, for both service provider and recipient, is a pervasive problem in human services. Books, films, and other resources are often costly. Consultants, staff pay, overhead, and rent seem to prohibit ideal provision of services. The reaction of many service providers, coordinators, and policy makers to these high expenses is to raise the price of the service, to discontinue the service, or to offer the services primarily to professionals who are sponsored by their employers.

But what about disabled women? How do they obtain the necessary resources to attend available programs? Should the availability of appropriate services depend upon the potential recipient's financial status? Cornelius and colleagues (1982) suggest several ways to enable less affluent people to use services without reducing the quantity or quality of the services.

- Consider a sliding scale based on an individual's income.
- If your services are sometimes offered to people who are sponsored by agencies (e.g., in-service training participants), charge them more for the service than non-sponsored people (e.g., sponsored medical and rehabilitation professionals $60; nonsponsored professionals $35; students $20).
- Take a good hard look at your services to see if excess money is being spent and trim your budget where appropriate.
- Assess your budget and cut unnecessary expenditures.
- Research outside funding assistance. Start by checking with the Division of Vocational Rehabilitation, the Office of Rehabilitation Services Administration, social and civic organizations (e.g., United Way, Kiwanis Club), the National Institute of Mental Health, the Bureau of Education for the Handicapped, and community health centers.

Once major barriers have been managed, women who have a disability will need to know about your efforts. Take a look at your public relations network and expand it to reach the disabled community. Consider the following tactics used by others:

- Make a statement in your program announcement about your accommodations for handicapped women, i.e., barrier-free access and sign interpretation.
- Consider advertising your program through multiple media. Television *and* radio media provide information to visually- and hearing-impaired.

- Send program announcements to rehabilitation staff, physical therapists, and other appropriate professionals.
- Send program announcements to pertinent social and civic organizations, i.e., Cerebral Palsy Foundation, Kiwanis.
- Post program announcements in independent living centers, residential facilities, and disabled organization centers.
- If you normally advertise your program in professional journals, consider disability-related journals listed in the resource section.
- Make contact with local experts in the field of disability and ask for their program awareness suggestions. (Adapted from Cornelius et al., 1982)

Once you have invited disabled women to participate in your group, you need to consider each woman's individual needs. As in all teaching, the learner's unique needs must be considered. Disabled women, like able-bodied women, are a heterogenous group and need individual attention. For disabled women, however, the woman's disability must be considered for its effect on the learning process and course content. Aspects of the woman's disability that inhibit cognitive, communicative, and social function need to be evaluated and managed.

Adaptation of the Teaching–Learning Process

Cognitive inhibitors are aspects of the disability that limit usual modes of processing information and learning. For a woman with a visual impairment it will mean substitution of visual instructional materials with those that are auditory or tactile. A group of mentally retarded women will need concepts presented simply, clearly, and slowly. *Communication inhibitors* are those that block the usual means the woman has of giving and receiving information. Communication inhibitors exist for women with sensory impairments, because so much of our language is visual and auditory. Those women whose speech is difficult to perceive will also experience communication difficulties. Consideration of possible *social inhibitors* is also important for successful group interaction. High rates of parental overprotectiveness, institutional living arrangements, and self- or environmentally-imposed isolation may contribute to the disabled woman's lack of group socialization. Identification and creative problem solving of these inhibitors will eliminate barriers to the woman's full participation in your group. For illustration, an example of this process carried out for hearing-impaired women follows.

Teaching Strategies for Hearing-impaired Women. Hearing-impaired women have in common both the alteration in hearing and in understanding the spoken word. In other ways they are very individual. The woman's hearing loss may have occurred before or after language skills were acquired, the loss itself may vary from hard of hearing to complete deafness, and women will differ on how they choose to communicate. Successful accommodation of the hearing-impaired woman into the group is dependent upon the health care professional's attention to individuality when using the teaching strategies presented here.

Cognitive Inhibitors. It is a common misconception that deaf individuals are intellectually inferior to the hearing population. When the intelligence of deaf individuals has been tested, the findings have been mixed and nondefinitive. What needs to be considered is that loss of hearing affects cognitive functions that require hearing for reception and processing but does not affect functions that depend on other senses (Boyd & Young, 1981). For example, a woman with a hearing impairment may not be knowledgeable about her body if in her environment information about her body is transmitted primarily by media and word of mouth. Her lack of knowledge does not mean she cannot learn this information if it is properly presented. Table 10–2 is presented to assist in identification and management of possible cognitive inhibitors to hearing-impaired group participants and learners.

Communication Inhibitors. Communication barriers presented by deafness are the most critical factor affecting the deaf woman's group participation. Women with hearing impairment use a wide range of communication modalities. Table 10–3 familiarizes the health educator to the basic concepts needed to effectively communicate when sign language, lip reading, oral skills, or hearing aids are used.

Social Inhibitors. As deaf individuals are mainstreamed and the deaf culture strengthens, it will be interesting to see if previous deviations from the social norm will continue. Currently as a result of language deprivation and isolation from the mainstream culture, deaf individuals may fall below the socialization norms found in the general population.

Deaf adolescent women's traditional attitudes toward their sex role resulted in their

TABLE 10–2. ASSESSMENT AND MANAGEMENT OF COGNITIVE INHIBITORS IN HEARING-IMPAIRED WOMEN

Assessment	Management
Terms and concepts related to body, health, and sex are lacking or vary from the group norm	Clarify key words and concepts prior to their introduction.
	Group members can contribute their knowledge of naming body parts and functions. This exercise is useful to arrive at a group consensus of terminology to be used and the meaning the term will convey.
	Supplemental (tutorial) educational opportunities. Consider if nonmainstreamed groups are appropriate.
Low English proficiency	Provide outlines and new terminology list prior to the group meeting where they will be used.
	Provide simply written handouts showing key concepts.
	Use materials that are highly visual with little or no narration.
	Increase use of body language, facial expression and pantomine.[a]
	Slow down pace and allow extra time for the woman to assimilate information and respond. Remember while the woman is writing she will not be "hearing."[a]
	Write out any changes in meeting time or place.[a]
	Allow time for questions, use frequent repetition of basic important concepts.[a]
	If you are having difficulty sending or perceiving an idea, rephrase a thought or restate a sentence.[a]

Note: Non-footnoted managements are the author's.
[a]Excerpted from National Technological Institute for the Deaf (NTID). Undated printouts.

TABLE 10–3. ASSESSMENT AND MANAGEMENT OF COMMUNICATION IN HEARING-IMPAIRED WOMEN

Assessment	Management
You are unsure of what communication mode the hearing-impaired woman uses.	Consult the woman who has the hearing impairment as she is the best judge of what adaptations she will require.
The primary communication mode is *Sign Language*	Make arrangements for a sign language interpreter (SLI). If your group does not have access or funds for an interpreter, discuss options with the woman. Women who sign frequently have access to interpreters but less often have funds to pay an interpreter.
	Arrange to talk with the interpreter prior to the group meeting to ascertain any difficulty the interpreter may have with vocabulary or process.
	Stand next to the interpreter and talk directly to the hearing-impaired woman. Do not speak to the interpreter.
The primary communication mode is *Lip Reading* Works best in small groups or one-to-one	Speak normally; do not slow down or exaggerate mouth movements.
	Make your face visible: light sources behind you and hair in your face will decrease visibility.
Do not assume all deaf women have this skill. It is very difficult, as only 26 percent of speech is visible on the lips (NTID, undated)	Minimize distracting habits like smoking, gum chewing, and putting your hands in front of your face (NTID, undated).
	Do not speak while your head is turned, e.g., talking and writing on the board simultaneously.
	Write out unfamiliar terms.
The primary communication mode is *Oral* Deaf women have normal voices; some choose not to use them if they think their speech is difficult to understand.	Listen for a while to become attuned to the woman's voice; usually her speech will become clearer, as one becomes accustomed to a foreign accent.
	If you do not understand, do not pretend understanding; ask for clarification, suggest she rephrase or write. Let her know you want to understand her fully and you will keep trying as long as she is willing.
	Remember there is no correlation between a deaf woman's speech abilities and her intelligence.
The primary communication mode is *Hearing Amplification*	Hearing aids do not restore normal hearing. They only amplify sound. Background noise is amplified as is speech. This may produce problems in a crowded room (Holder, 1982).
	Speak slowly and clearly. If the woman does not understand, rephrase the statement. To verify her understanding, ask her to repeat what you have said or ask her a relevant question.

choosing traditional courses geared toward "homemaker" roles (Cook & Rossett, 1975). In addition, Grossman (1972) found deaf college students, although they were more sexually active, had less sexual knowledge and were more accepting of sexual myths. Past studies have found that deaf men and women marry less, have more paranoia, dependency behavior, lower self-esteem, and impulsive behavior. It is now suggested that the negative results of these studies are not a result of the intrinsic deafness, but rather a result of extrinsic social environmental factors (Table 10–4) (Emerton, Hurwitz, & Bishop, 1979).

Resource Guide. The resources in this guide are intended to facilitate inclusion of disabled women into existing women's groups, as well as ease the formation of groups exclusively for disabled women. It is assumed that the content and the objectives for the group are already developed, therefore resources for curriculum development of various women's groups are not included. An attempt has been made to list resources of particular importance to disabled women, but the state of the art puts heavy emphasis on sex education and on male disability. These resources were included when the materials' adaptation to women in groups appeared feasible.

TABLE 10–4. ASSESSMENT AND MANAGEMENT OF SOCIAL INHIBITORS IN HEARING-IMPAIRED WOMEN

Assessment	Management
Unfamiliarity with group process	Assist the woman's integration into the group. Use introductory games and exercises that facilitate cohesiveness.
	Clarify group goals and objectives.
	Reassess the woman's comfort level frequently.
Discomfort with andragogical learning	Clarify approach at the onset. Discuss the advantages and disadvantages of approach used.
	Give anticipatory guidance for possible feelings, e.g., anxiety from uncertainty, fear of self disclosure, etc.
	Recognize and support all efforts. Acknowledge the woman's feelings and discomfort.
Difficulty in expressing feelings	Have the group develop a list of words that expresses different emotions, i.e., happiness and unhappiness, anger, fear, anxiety. Explore emotional situations and expressions in which different feelings were experienced (Blum & Blum, 1977).
	Be a role model by expressing and sharing in the group personal feelings and responses.
Passive group behavior	Teach assertiveness skills.
	Role model assertiveness skills.
	Recommend assertiveness training books or groups.
Values in high variance with the majority of group participants or to the course content	Respect individual values. Do not assume to know the woman's value structure; find out.
	Use value clarification techniques.
	Remember that there is no right or wrong value.
	Use the principles of consciousness raising.

RESOURCES

General Disability

Resources

Dahl, P. R., Appleby, J. A., & Lipe, D. *Mainstreaming guidebook for vocational educators: Teaching the handicapped*. Utah: Olympus Publishing, 1978. *(Extremely useful text. Discusses the concept of mainstreaming as well as strategies to overcome attitudinal and environmental barriers. Provides a useful framework for modification of curriculum dependent on the individual disability. Geared for vocational educators.)*

Gay Care, 84 Burton Road, London SW9 6TQ offers supportive counseling and helps disabled homosexuals, of both sexes and all ages, to establish social contacts.

Gemma, BM Box 5700, London WC1 V6XX, a group for disabled lesbians.

Sex Information and Educational Council of the United States (SIECUS), 1855 Broadway, New York NY 10023. Write to Human Science Press, 72 Fifth Avenue, New York, NY 10011 for publications catalog that includes books of particular interest to people with disabilities.

Task Force on Concerns for Physically Disabled Women. Female sexuality and physical disability. Bibliography available from Planned Parenthood of Snohomish County, 2370 Hoyt, Everett, WA 98201.

Sister Kenny Institute. Chicago Avenue, 27th Street, Minneapolis, MN 55407. *(Publications pertaining to education of individuals with disabilities. Publication list of literature and audiovisual materials.)*

Readings

Adams, V. R., & Stevens, B. M. Baby management for a disabled mother. *Occupational Therapy*, 1973, *10*, 510–511.

Bigge, J. L. (Ed.). *Teaching individuals with physical and multiple disabilities*. Columbus, Ohio: Charles E. Merrill, 1976. *(Practical guide for professionals who want to teach children and young adults skills and adaptive behaviors needed for self sufficiency. Good bib and resource section.)*

Blum, G., & Blum, B. *Feeling good about yourself*. San Rafael, Calif.: Academic Therapy Publications, 1977.

Bullard, D. O., & Wallace, P. H. Peer educator–counselors in sexuality for the disabled. *Sexuality and Disability*, 1978, *1*, 147–152.

Canter, R. C. *Toward fitness: Guided exercise for those with health problems*. New York: Human Science Press, 1980. *(Educational and rehabilitation techniques.)*

Comfort, A. *Sexual consequences of disability*. Philadelphia: George F. Stickley, 1978.

Edmonson, B. Sociosexual education for the handicapped. *Exceptional Education Quarterly: Special Issue on Special Education for Adolescents and Young Adults*, 1980, *1*(2), 67–76.

Griffith, E., Trieschmann, R. B., Hohmann, G. W., Cole, T. M., Tobis, J. S., & Cummings, V. Sexual dysfunctions associated with physical disabilities. *Archives of Physical Medicine and Rehabilitation*, 1975, *56*, 8–13.

Grosse, S. Organizing and implementing sex education programs for students with handicapping conditions. *Practical Pointers*, 1980, *4*(4).

Hale-Harbaugh, J., Norman, A., Bogle, J., & Shaul, S. *With-in reach: Providing family planning services to physically disabled women*. New York: Human Science Press, 1978.

Hale-Harbaugh, J., Norman, A., Bogle, J., & Shaul, S. *Toward intimacy: Family planning and sexuality concerns of physically disabled women*. New York: Human Science Press, 1978.

Hamilton, E. A. The problem of period control in disabled women. *Annals of Physical Medicine*, 1968, *9*, 288–294.

Helleman, R. A. *Library services for the handicapped: A course outline and bibliography*. New York: Long Island University Palmer Graduate Library School, 1980.

Hopper, C. E. *Sex education for physically handicapped youth*. Springfield, Ill.: Charles C. Thomas, 1980.

Latlin, D. President's committee on employment of the handicapped: Images of ourselves, women with disabilities talking. *Disabled USA*, 1981, *4*(7), 22.

Johnson, W., & Kempton, W. *Sex counseling of special groups: The mentally and physically handicapped, ill and elderly*. Springfield, Ill.: Charles Thomas, 1981.

Lindemann, J. E. *Psychological and behavioral aspects of physical disability*. New York: Plenum Press, 1981.

MacGugan, K. *Ki-Ackido for handicapped students at Leeward Community College: Theory and practice*. January 1979, Ed.D. Practicum, Nova University, Hawaii. *(Education document (ERIC). Good example of the positive effects of including women who are disabled in able body activities.)*

Mayers, K. S. Sexual and social concerns of the disabled: A group counseling approach. *Sexuality and Disability*, 1978, *1*, 100–111.

Metcalf, W. Social problems of disabled women. In E. Chigier (Ed.), *Annals of Israel National Society of Rehabilitation of the Disabled*. Tel-Aviv, Israel: Meretz, 1977.

Ryerson, E., & Sundem, J. M. Development of a curriculum on sexual exploitation and self-protection for handicapped students. *Education Unlimited*, 1981, *3*(4), 26–31.

Sapienza, B., & Thornton, C. Curriculum for advanced family life for the physically disabled. *(Available at McAtker High School, San Francisco United School District, San Francisco, CA)*

Sha'ked, A. *Human sexuality in physical and mental illness and disabilities: An annotated bibliography*. Bloomington, Ind.: University Press, 1978.

Skipper, J., Fink, S., & Hollenbeck, P. Physical disability among married women: Problems in the husband–wife relationships. *Journal of Rehabilitation*, 1968, *34*, 16–19.

Smigielski, P. A., & Steinmann, M. J. Teaching sex education to multiple handicapped adolescents. *Journal of School Health*, 1981, *51*(4), 238–241.

Stensrud, C. Recreations, role in meeting, the sociosexual needs of special populations. *Therapeutic Recreation Journal*, 1976, *10*(3), 94–98.

Szasz, G., Miller, S., & Anderson, L. Guidelines to birth control counseling of the physically handicapped. *Canadian Medical Association Journal*, 1979, *120*(11), 1353–1368.

Tabeek, E., & Conroy, M. Teaching sexual awareness to the significantly disabled school-age child. *Pediatric Nursing*, 1981, *7*(5), 21–25.

Vash, C. L. *The psychology of disability*. New York: Springer, 1981.

Wehman, P. *Curriculum design for the severely and profoundly handicapped*. New York: The Human Science Press, 1979. *(Contains extensive selection of sample programs and instructional guidelines for implementing training programs in self-help, motor, language, vocation and functional academics.)*

Hearing Impairment

Resources

Captioned Films and Telecommunications Branch, Bureau of Education for the Handicapped, U.S. Office of Education, DHEW, 400 South 6th St. S.E., Donahue Bld., Washington, DC 20202.

Council of Organizations Serving the Deaf. P.O. Box 894, Columbia, MD 21044. *Publication list available.*

Gallaudet College, Washington, DC 20002. *(Bookstore with audiotapes, a national registry of sign language instruction and interpreters.)*

Into Womanhood. Captioned filmstrip. Stanfield House, 12381 Wilshire Blvd., Suite 203, Los Angeles, CA 90025.

Perennial Education Series. 477 Roger Williams, P.O. Box 855 Ravinia, Highland Park, IL 60035. *Three films/16-mm/color/no sound: About conception and contraception; About puberty and reproduction; About venereal disease.)*

National Association of the Deaf, 814 Thayer Avenue, Silver Spring MD 20910. *(The main organization of deaf Americans.)*

National Technical Institute for the Deaf at Rochester (NY) Institute of Technology. *(Public information office and a national registry of interpreters.)*

Sex Education for Persons with Communication Impairments. Workshop to provide training in sex education to professionals who work with hearing-impaired or mentally disabled individuals. Sponsored by the Institute for Family Planning, Planned Parenthood of Southeastern Pennsylvania, 1220 Sansom Street, Philadelphia, PA 19107.

Readings

Bond, D. E. Aspects of behavior and management of adolescents who are hearing-impaired. *Teacher of the Deaf*, 1981, 5(2), 41–48.

Culhane, B., & Williams, C. (Eds.). Social aspects of educating deaf persons. Unpublished manuscript, Gallaudet College, 1982.

Gerber, B. M. Interpreter effects with deaf patients (letter). *American Journal of Psychiatry*, 1979, 7, 990.

Kyle, J. G., & Allsop, L. Communicating with young deaf people—some issues. *Teacher of the Deaf*, 1982, 6(3), 71–79.

Laitmon, E. Group counseling: Sexuality and the hearing-impaired adolescent. *Sexuality and Disability*, 1979, 2(3), 169.

Lewis, K. J. Health education in schools and units for the deaf. *Teacher of the Deaf*, 1981, 5(2), 34–40.

Moores, D. *Educating the deaf: Psychological principles and practices.* Boston: Houghton Mifflin, 1978. *(Basic resource text that covers educational techniques as well as social and psychological characteristics of the deaf and their families.)*

Neyhus, A. I. Deafness and adolescence. *Volta Review*, 1978, 80(5). *(Collection of original papers focuses on understanding and managing the impact of real life issues on the adolescent with hearing impairment.)*

Schein, J., et al. *Continuing education of deaf adults.* New York: New York University, 1976. *(A report of a government-sponsored survey conducted to delineate barriers and facilitators to participation of the deaf adult in adult learning.)*

Sussman, A. E., & Stewart, L. G. *Counseling with deaf people.* New York: New York University School of Education, 1971. *(A still relevant text that delineates problems and provides solutions to the barriers of providing counseling services to individuals who are deaf.)*

Withrow, F. B. Learning technology and the hearing-impaired. *Volta Review*, 1981, 83(5). *(A whole issue devoted to the application of telecommunications technology, e.g., computers, educational media and video disc teaching strategies.)*

Woodward, J. *Signs of sexual behavior: An introduction to some sex-related vocabulary in American Sign Language.* Silver Spring, Md.: T. J. Publishers, 1979.

Mental Impairment

Resources

Birth control methods: A simplified presentation. Perennial Education, Inc., 477 Roger Williams, P.O. Box 855, Ravinia, Highland Park, IL 60035. *(A kit that may be used in presenting information on birth control methods and sexual responsibility to mentally retarded individuals.)*

Ease (Essential Adult Sex Education) Curriculum. Madison Opportunity Center, 601 E. Main Street, Madison, WI 53703. *(Instructional aids specifically designed to be used in presenting information to mentally retarded adults on physiology, sexual behavior, health, and interpersonal relationships; includes menstrual and birth control materials.)*

Feeling good about yourself. Perennial Education, Inc., 477 Roger Williams, P.O. Box 855, Ravinia, Highland Park, IL 60035. *(A teacher training film that demonstrates a dynamic method of assertiveness training, covers issues of victimization, making yourself understood, self-esteem and sexuality.)*

Girl to woman. Churhill Films, 622 North Robertson Blvd., Los Angeles, CA 90069. *(A film designed to teach mentally retarded individuals about changes that occur in the female body at puberty.)*

Gloria J. Blum, M. A. Educational Consultant for the Development of Disabled/Nondisabled People, 507 Pama Way, Mill Valley, CA 94941.

Planned Parenthood of Southeastern Pennsylvania, 1220 Sansom Street, Philadelphia, PA 19107. *(Sex education resources for the mentally handicapped. Parent and teacher guides, filmstrips and slides in English and Spanish.)*

Sex education for the mentally handicapped. Education Division: Hallmark Films and Recordings, 51–53 New Plant Court, Owings Mill, MD 21117. *(Set of three 16-mm films/18–20 mins: The ABC of sex education for trainable persons; The how and what of sex education for educable persons; Fertility regulation for persons with learning disabilities.)*

Sexuality and the mentally handicapped. Stanfield House, 12381 Wilshire Blvd, Suite 203, Los Angeles, CA 90025. *(Slides for the teaching mentally handicapped by Winifred Kempton.)*

Sex education for persons with communication impairments. Workshop to provide training in sex education to professionals who work with hearing impaired or mentally disabled individuals. Sponsored by the Institute for Family Planning, Planned Parenthood of Southeastern Pennsylvania, 1220 Sansom Street, Philadelphia, PA 19107.

Readings

Amary, I. *Social awareness, hygiene, and sex education for the mentally retarded—developmentally disabled.* Springfield, Ill.: Charles C. Thomas, 1980.

Bender, M., & Valletutti, P. J. *Teaching the moderately and severely handicapped: Curriculum objectives, strategies and activities* (3 vols). Baltimore: University Park Press, 1976.

Caparulo, F., & Kempton, W. Sexual health needs of the mentally retarded adolescent female. *Issues in Health Care of Women*, 1981, *3*(1), 35–46.

Craft, A., & Craft, M. *Sex education and counseling for mentally handicapped people.* Baltimore: University Park Press, 1983.

David, H. P., Smith, J. D., & Freeman, E. Family planning services for persons handicapped by mental retardation. *American Journal of Public Health*, 1976, *66*, 1053–1057.

Davis, V. S., & Davis, W. Q. (Eds.). *Sexuality and the mentally retarded.* New York: Planned Parenthood of Northern New York, 1975.

Edmonson, B., McCombs, K., & Wish, J. What retarded adults believe about sex. *American Journal Mental Deficiency*, 1979, *84*(1), 11–18.

Hartman, S. S., & Hynes, J. Marriage education for mentally retarded adults. *Social Casework*, 1975, *56*(5), 280–284.

Hyatt, R., & Rolnick, N. (Eds.). *Teaching the mentally handicapped child.* New York: Human Science Press, 1974.

Hunt, A. A nurse's in-depth look at needs of disabled: Sex and the developmentally disabled. *California Nurse*, 1981, *77*(1), 6–7.

Kempton, W., Bass, M. S., & Gordon, S. *Love, sex and birth control for the mentally retarded: A guide for parents.* Philadelphia: Planned Parenthood and Syracuse: Institute for Family Research and Education, 1978.

May, D. Survey of sex education course work in special education programs. *Journal of Special Education*, 1980, *14*(1), 107–112.

Moon, M., & Renzaglia, A. Physical fitness and the mentally retarded: A critical review of the literature. *The Journal of Special Education*, 1982, *16*(3), 269–287.

Rinckey, D. J. *A curriculum for teaching human sexuality for mentally impaired adolescents.* Master's Thesis, Central Michigan University, 1975.

Ryerson, E., & Sundem, J. Development of a curriculum on sexual exploitation and self-protection for handicapped students. *Education Unlimited*, 1981, *3*(4), 26–31.

Smigielski, P. A., & Steinmann, M. J. Teaching sex education to multiple handicapped adolescents. *The Journal of School Health*, 1981, *51*(4), 238–241.

St. Clair County (MI) Intermediate School District, Syllabus: Human Sexuality and the Retarded: A training course based on sessions developed by Winifred Kempton, 1977.

Watson, G. Sex education surveyed. *Special Education: Forward Trends*, 1980, *7*(3), 11–14.

Mobility Impairment

Readings

Abrams, K. The impact on marriages of adult-onset paraplegia. *Paraplegia (Review)*, 1981, *19*(4), 253–259.

Becker, E. *Female sexuality following spinal cord injury*. Bloomington, Ill.: Cheever Publishing, 1978.

Blanchard, M. G. Sex education for spinal cord injury patients and their nurses. *Supervisory Nurse*, 1976, *7*(2), 20–22, 24–26, 28.

Bregman, S. *Sexuality and the spinal cord injured women: Guidelines concerning femininity, social, and sexual adjustment*. Minneapolis: Sister Kenny Institute, 1975.

Cole, T. M. Sexual counseling of the physically disabled. *Postgraduate Medicine*, 1975, *58*, 117–126.

Comarr, A., & Visue, M. Sexual counseling among male and female patients with spinal cord and/or cauda equina injury. Part II. Results of interview and neurological examinations of females. *American Journal of Physical Medicine*, 1978, *57*(5), 215–227.

Eisenberg, M. G., & Rustad, L. C. Development of a sex counseling education program on spinal cord injury service. *Archives of Physical Medicine and Rehabilitation*, 1976, *57*, 135–140.

Fitting, M., Salisbury, S., Davies, N. H., & Mayclen, D. K. Self-concept and sexuality of spinal cord injured women. *Archives of Sex Behaviors*, 1978, *7*, 143–156.

Goller, H. Our experiences about pregnancy and delivery of the paraplegic woman. *Paraplegia*, 1970, *8*, 161–166.

Gordon, S., & Snyder, C. Family life education for the handicapped. *Journal of School Health*, 1980, *50*(5), 272–274.

Laboy, P. Pregnancy in the spinal cord patient. *Paraplegia Life*, 1976, *6*(1), 17–24.

McCarthy, B. Menstruation: The management of menstrual flow in disabled women. *Nursing Times*, 1980, *76*(10), 409–411.

Melnyk, R., Montgomery, R., & Over, R. Attitude changes following a sexual counseling program for spinal cord injured persons. *Archives Physical Medicine Rehabilitation*, 1979, *60*(12), 601–605.

Ohry, A., Peles, D., Goldman, J., David, A., & Rozin, R. Sexual functions, pregnancy and delivery in spinal cord injured women. *Gynecol-Obstet-Invest*, 1978, *9*(6), 281–291.

Peters, L. Women's health care: Approaches in delivery to physically disabled women. *Nurse Practitioner*, 1982, *7*(1), 34–37.

Romano, M. O. Sexuality and the disabled female. *Sexuality and Disability*, Spring 1978, 27.

Rohme, M. W. The public health nurse as sexual counselor for spinal cord injured men. *Sexuality and Disability*, 1979, *2*(1), 8–15.

Sargent, S. Growing up with a physical handicap. In C. B. Knapp (Ed.), *Becoming female: Perspectives on development*. New York: Plenum Press, 1979, 67–88.

Ziff, S. The sexual concerns of the adolescent woman with cerebral palsy. *Issues in Health Care of Women*, 1981, *3*(1), 55–63.

Visual Impairment

Resources

AASECT TAPES. American Association of Sex Educators, Counselors and Therapists. Suite 304, 5010 Wisconsin Ave., N.W., Washington, DC 20016. *(A series of tapes giving advanced sexuality and related information (e.g., homosexuality and sex roles).*

American Foundation for the Blind, 15 West 16th Street, New York, NY 10011.

American Printing House for the Blind, 1839 Frankfort Avenue, Louisville, KY 40206.

American Telephone and Telegraph Company, Services for the Blind, 295 North Maple Avenue, Basking Ridge, NJ 07920.

Braille Book Review, Division for the Blind and Physically Handicapped, Library of Congress, Washington, DC 20542.

Strictly Feminine. Booklet available in Braille or large print. Personal Products, P.O. Box 117, Ridgefield, NJ 07657. *(A pamphlet designed for visually-impaired adolescents that discusses menstruation, puberty and feminine hygiene.)*

Talking Book Topics, Division for the Blind and Physically Handicapped, Library of Congress, Washington, DC 20542.

Your Changing Body. Audiocassettes. Perennial Education, 477 Roger Williams, P.O. Box 855, Ravinia, Highland Park, IL 60035. *(A guided program of body self-exploration designed for visually-impaired children and adolescents.)*

Readings

Allen, P., & Lipke, L. A. *Your changing body: A guided self-exploration*. Grand Rapids, Mich.: Institute for the Development of Creative Child Care, 1974.

American Foundation for the Blind. *Sex education and family life for visually behavioral handicapped youth: A resource guide*. New York, 1975.

Dalton, K. Sexual and menstrual problems in the blind. In E. Chigier (Ed.), *Annual of Israel National Society for Rehabilitation of the Disabled*. Tel-Aviv: Meretz, 1977.

Elliot, B. Look but don't touch: The problems blind children have learning about sexuality. *Disabled USA*, 1979, *3*, 15–17.

Foulke, E., & Uhde, T. Sex education and counseling for the blind. *Medical Aspects of Human Sexuality*, 1976, *10*(4), 399–403.

Inana, M. You and your body: A self-help health class for blind women. *Visual Impairment and Blindness*, 1978, 402–403.

Neff, J. *Behavioral objectives and learning activities in human sexuality for the visually handicapped*. New York: American Foundation for the Blind, 1976.

Smigielski, P. A., & Steinmann, M. J. Teaching sex education to multiple handicapped adolescents. *Journal of School Health*, 1981, *51*(4), 238–241.

Selvin, H. C. Sexuality among the visually handicapped: A beginning. *Sexuality and Disability*, 1979, *2*(3), 192–199.

Torbett, D. A humanistic and futuristic approach to sex education for blind children. *The New Outlook for the Blind*, 1974, *69*, 210–215.

Toit, P., & Kessler, C. The way we get babies: A tactual sex education program. *The New Outlook for the Blind*, 1976, *70*, 116–120.

Van T. Hooft, F., & Heslinga, K. Sex education of blind-born children. *Sex education for the visually handicapped in schools and agencies*. Selected papers. New York: American Foundation for the Blind, Inc., 1975.

Wore, M. A., & Schwab, L. O. The blind mother providing care for an infant. *The New Outlook for the Blind*, 1971, *65*, 169–174.

BIBLIOGRAPHY

Abroms, K., & Kodera, J. Acceptance hierarchy of handicaps. *Journal of Learning Disabilities*, 1979, *12*(1), 15–20.

Blum, G., & Blum, B. *Feeling good about yourself*. San Rafael, Calif.: Academic Therapy Publications, 1977.

Boyd, R., & Young, N. Hearing disorders. In J. Lindemann (Ed.), *Psychological and behavioral aspects of physical disability*. New York: Plenum Press, 1981, 389–390.

Cook, L., & Rossett, A. The sex role attitudes of deaf adolescent women and their implications for vocational choice. *American Annals of the Deaf,* June 1975, 341–345.

Chipouras, S. Cornelius, D., Daniels, S., & Makas, E. *Who cares? A handbook on sex education and counseling services for disabled people.* Washington, D.C.: George Washington University, 1978.

Cornelius, D., Chipouras, S., Makas, E., & Daniels, S. *Who cares? A handbook on sex education and counseling services for disabled people* (2nd ed.). Baltimore: University Park Press, 1982.

Dowling, C. *The Cinderella complex: Women's hidden fear of independence.* New York: Pocket Books, 1981.

Emerton, G., Hurwitz, A., & Bishop, M. Development of social maturity in deaf adolescents and adults. In L. Bradford and W. Hardy (Eds.), *Hearing and hearing impairment.* New York: Grune & Stratton, 1979, 451–460.

Flynn, R., & Sha'ked, A. Normative sex behavior and the person with a disability: Assessing the effectiveness of the rehabilitation agencies. *Journal of Rehabilitation,* 1977, *43*(5), 34–36.

Grossman, S. *Sexual knowledge, attitudes and experiences of deaf college students.* Unpublished Master's thesis. Washington, D.C.: George Washington University, 1972.

Hale-Harbaugh, J., Norman, A., Bogle, J., & Shoul, S. *Within reach: Providing family planning services to physically disabled women.* New York: Human Science Press, 1978.

Holder, L. Hearing aids: Handle with care. *Nursing '82,* April, 1982, 64.

Johnson, L. Body cathexis as a factor in somatic complaints. *Journal of Consulting Psychology,* 1956, *20,* 145–149.

Jourard, S., & Secord, P. Body-cathexis and the ideal female figure. *Journal of Abnormal and Social Psychology,* 1955, *50,* 243–246.

Natale, P., & Sprik, M. Adaptation of a primary care nursing service to provide health care for women with disabilities. *New Directions for Nursing in the '80's.* Kansas City: American Nurses' Association, 1980, 29–35.

National Technological Institute for the Deaf (NTID). Misconceptions about deaf people; The meaning of deafness; Communication: What's it all about? Undated printouts.

Plutchnik, R., Weiner, B., & Conte, H. Studies of body image. 1. Body worries and body discomforts. *Journal of Gerontology,* 1971, *26*(3), 344–350.

Rodgers, C. *Freedom to learn.* Ohio: Charles E. Merrill, 1969.

Secord, P., & Jourard, S. The appraisal of body-cathexis; body cathexis and the self. *Journal of Consulting Psychology,* 1953, *17,* 343–347.

Stensrud, R., & Stensrud, K. Interpersonal stress as a consequence of being disabled. *Journal of Rehabilitation,* 1981, *47*(2), 43–46.

Weininger, O., Rothenberg, G., & Henry, A. Body image of handicapped children. *Journal of Personality Assessment,* 1972, *36,* 248–253.

Wright, B. *Physical disability—A psychological approach.* New York: Harper & Row, 1960.

Alternatives for Birthing

11

Dona J. Lethbridge

Childbirthing can be a rich and positive experience or it can be negative and upsetting depending on how well pregnancy, labor, and delivery health care meets the needs of the client's situation. There is now more than one mode of health care available for childbirthing. Although the majority of women and their partners/husbands choose the traditional hospital system, some families are now seeking alternative, less traditional modes of care. More conventional methods of childbirthing may interfere with preferences, needs, and goals of women who want to be in control, participate in decisions regarding their care, and have maximum involvement of their families in the birth of their babies.

This chapter describes the childbirthing matrix, which is made up of four quadrants, each representing one style for the birthing experience. Health care practitioners are often in the position of helping a client to select a birthing option. Although each health care provider holds values and beliefs about various birthing options, the premise in this chapter is that the client should be aided in choosing the method that best fulfills her own criteria for a birthing experience. The childbirthing matrix can be used to help clients and providers make an informed decision.

The Childbirthing Matrix
There are two major parameters that influence decision making as to type of childbirthing experience preferred. One parameter determines the degree of authority of the client versus that of the health care practitioner. The other parameter is the philosophy about the nature of childbirth, whether childbirth is a normal or pathological process. Although there may be a relationship between these parameters, or some areas of commonality, there are also differences that provide the basis for rather different perspectives on childbirthing. The two parameters may be viewed as continua and connected to form a matrix that is useful in outlining the various alternatives in childbirthing (Fig. 11–1). The quadrants of the matrix can then be used to describe the norms pertaining to health care for pregnancy and delivery, and the nature of the relationship between the health care practitioner and the client.

The first continuum, pertaining to the nature of the practitioner–client relationship, is termed professional-orientation—community-orientation continuum. At one end of the continuum the practitioner is in authority over the client and childbirthing events. This

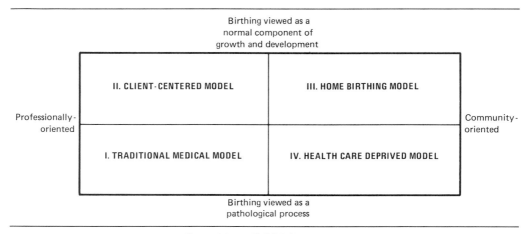

Figure 11–1. Childbirthing matrix.

view holds that the practitioner has the knowledge and the skills that the client needs to cope with the experience. The client therefore comes to the practitioner for "help." The practitioner is also considered able to control events so that untoward outcomes of the process can be prevented or thwarted.

The other end of the continuum promotes a relationship of equality between the practitioner and the client. The practitioner is considered to have knowledge and skills that are to be shared with or given to the client. The client is helped to move through the childbirthing experience, but the client has authority over the conditions of the event. There is little emphasis on risk factors at the extreme end of this continuum. Outcomes, whether positive or negative, may be given over to the authority of a supreme being, chance, nature, or may be dealt with through a philosophy of acceptance.

The second continuum describes the philosophical view of the childbearing experience and is termed pathology–growth and development. Throughout history, childbirthing has been viewed from both perspectives. Although childbirth was considered a natural event in some cultures, allowing women to deliver unattended during the course of their workday, there has also been an aura of pathology around childbirth that led to taboos and sequestration. For example, there were beliefs that "others" had to be protected against pathology arising from contact with the childbearing woman. Childbearing was also seen as punishment for women.

On the pathology end of this continuum childbirthing is looked on in terms of pathology; the client is unwell or in crisis and must be treated so that she may be returned to health or her normal state. The focus of health care is treatment, with emphasis placed on the potential development of problems.

The other end of this continuum describes childbirthing as a normal stage in growth and development. Women have always become pregnant and borne children and in fact their body is designed for doing just that. Therefore, health care, if considered relevant at all, is geared to health teaching and assisting the client to cope with this particular change in life.

The four quadrants emerging from the intersection of these two continua are: (1) traditional–medical perspective, (2) client-centered perspective, (3) home birthing, and

(4) health care deprived (see Table 11–1). Each of these quadrants may also be described in terms of the implications for childbirthing health care and the nature of the relationship between client and practitioner. Table 11–1 summarizes these differences.

Traditional–Medical Perspective. It is perhaps appropriate to discuss the traditional–medical perspective first because it is still the dominant perspective of health care in North American society. It can be misleading to use the term traditional to discuss this form of health care because it has chiefly gained acceptance during the twentieth century.

The current "medical" model, although having roots in early Greek society under the leadership of Hippocrates, developed its predominant theme during the seventeenth

TABLE 11–1. CHILD-BIRTHING QUADRANTS: HEALTH CARE

	Prenatal	Labor	Delivery	Post-partal
Traditional–medical model	Periodic monitoring by physician; focus of care is identification of risk factors	Perineal shave; enema; attended by hospital labor room nurse(s); use of analgesia; bed-centered care; I.V.; fetal monitor	Attended by own physician; delivery room; delivery table; lithotomy position; Use of anesthesia; episiotomy; emergency equipment present	Infant in nursery; infant schedule fed
Client-centered model	Care by physician or nurse midwife; risk factors identified; focus of care is teaching and planning for delivery and childcare	In a hospital or birthing center; may be no shave and/or no enema; attended by labor room nurse or midwife; care oriented to laboring; woman and mate use of relaxation and breathing techniques for control of discomfort	Labor room or birthing room; various positions for 2nd stage; mate present at delivery; delivery by physician or nurse midwife; emergency equipment present	Infant rooming in; infant demand fed; flexible visiting times for mate
Home birthing model	Care by nurse midwife or lay midwife; focus of care is support, teaching, planning for delivery	No attendant (client attended) or midwife at home; mate, family, and/or friends may be present; client ambulatory; relaxation and breathing techniques used for discomfort	Delivery in bed; various positions in second stage	Mother, infant and family in own home; may be periodic monitoring by midwife
Health care deprived model	Sporadic or no prenatal care	Attended by emergency room staff; same as traditional–medical model	Attended by hospital staff physician; same as traditional–medical model	Same as traditional–medical model

century with the influence of Descartes. Human beings, during the time and henceforth to the current day, were seen as machines, comprised of many parts, and with the mind and body being considered separate. Ill health or pathology was interpreted as the dysfunctioning of one part of the machine. It was the task of medicine to repair diseased parts.

With this view of human beings, medicine, in the nineteenth century, gained predominance in childbearing. The practice of obstetrics was established. Earlier, trained midwives or lay people had assisted with birthing. The norm in the nineteenth century and today is to be attended at birth by a physician, with conformity to the values and beliefs that the medical profession holds. Midwifery lost ground in attending births because the practice of midwifery was unregulated and had few programs of formal education (Hiestad, 1978). In addition women midwives were reluctant to seek training in forceps delivery due to modesty (Chaney, 1980). In 1898, the medical profession advocated abolition of midwifery, as well as the provision of a single standard of care, which was that all deliveries would be by obstetricians (Perry, 1980). Although medicine was still largely ineffective in healing disease, the twentieth century brought major technological advances. Medicine's new success as well as the social appreciation of the new technological culture changed perceptions and expectations of health care. This view extended to perceptions of the childbirthing experience. Physicians became the dominant practitioners, and therefore their view of the client and the purpose of health care dominated the health care system.

Until the twentieth century, childbearing was indeed frought with danger for both mother and child. For example, in 1915, the maternal mortality rate was 727.9 per 100,000. In 1978, the maternal deaths were 9.9 per 100,000 (National Center for Health Statistics, 1979). The infant mortality rate in 1900 was 200 per 1000 births in those states reporting statistics. In 1978, infant mortality was 13.6 per 1000 (Clark & Alfonso, 1979; National Center for Health Statistics, 1973). Therefore, it can be seen that there is a basis for the pathological viewpoint. Until the advent of sterile technique and the use of antibiotics, many women, for instance, succumbed to puerpural sepsis (postpartum septicemia). With surgical accessibility and sophisticated fetal monitoring many infants have been saved from intrauterine death or birthing injury.

Many of the procedures and policies of the past have been continued into today's traditional care for childbirth. Moreover, for many women and their families, this is the expectation they have for their own personal experience. Childbirthing lore is passed down from mother to daughter. Birthing may be viewed as a negative, painful process, and an experience to be survived. Women with this expectation may say things such as "I just want to be put to sleep until it is all over," or "I don't want to feel anything." Expectations may be such that the father of the child has no intention of seeing the birth, and the laboring mother will agree that she does not want him "to see her like that."

Additionally, some women want to be able to have complete confidence and faith in their physician. They feel safe it they know he or she has authority over them, over other health care personnel, and certainly over the outcome of events. For some women concerned over the possible negative outcomes of their pregnancy and delivery, use of medical technology is reassuring. In a research study investigating reactions to electronic fetal monitoring, for instance, some women had totally positive responses to the monitoring process, claiming that they saw it as a source of comfort and protection, an extension of the physician's "protective power." This response was especially present in women who had suffered previous fetal losses (Starkman & Youngs, 1980).

Childbirthing norms are changing. Many health care providers, especially nurses, and many physicians, no longer subscribe to a strict traditional–medical perspective. These providers are joined by many women, families, and lay groups. There is a push to establish family-centered, client participatory care in traditional settings. It must be remembered, however, that the traditional–medical mode of birthing may still be most consistent with some client's beliefs and needs.

Client-centered Perspective. The client-centered perspective is gaining strength in the health care system today. Many hospitals are using a more "family-oriented" approach. This approach assumes the childbirthing process is a normal part of the life process and more aligned to health.

In the client-centered mode of care the role of the health care provider could be likened to that of a consultant. The physician or perhaps the nurse midwife is considered to be an expert contracted by the family to provide the means by which the childbearing process will proceed. Childbirthing itself may be considered either a natural, although complex, event, or a developmental crisis, one of a number of crucial turning points in the life process. Emphasis in this orientation is on teaching and planning for labor and delivery and for childbearing. Family changes will be dealt with as well.

Although possible complications are not focused on, the health care provider is considered to have the knowledge to monitor or predict the onset of possible risk factors. If an "out of the ordinary course of events" occurs referral will be made to the obstetrician, and the childbearing process will be considered more in pathological terms. Care is more likely given by either the physician (often the family practitioner) or a nurse midwife.

Client-centered care may occur in a hospital or a birthing center. Birthing centers are generally staffed by nurse midwives and offer prenatal and birthing care in a facility geographically separate from a hospital. They provide a homelike setting so that birthing may take place in a comfortable, informal atmosphere, but have emergency equipment unobtrusively available.

A number of studies have been performed comparing the outcomes of deliveries by midwives to those by physicians. Two studies (Dillon, 1978; Slome, 1976) found either that there were no differences in the outcome of deliveries by midwives and by obstetricians, or that instrumental deliveries were more common in the physician group. Haire (1981) reported that in a hospital in a socially depressed section of a large metropolitan area, midwives cared for 2608 high- and low-risk mothers, with 88 percent of their deliveries normal, spontaneous, and vaginal. Another study (Mehl et al., 1980) obtained comparable results. These research studies have shown that the absence of a physician in the birthing process is not necessarily a problem and may lead to very positive outcomes.

In the client-centered approach the perineal shave and the enema may be omitted; the laboring woman will be encouraged to walk during labor and she may select the diet she prefers. The woman's partner is encouraged to be present, and a form of psychoprophylaxis such as the Lamaze method is taught. The use of analgesia for labor is discouraged by the attendant; emphasis is placed on breathing and relaxation techniques for the alleviation of discomfort. In the hospital, the delivery may be in the labor room or in a birthing suite, a pleasantly decorated room with a bed rather than a delivery table. Delivery position may be merely supine position with knees flexed, or sidelying. Some facilities offer birthing chairs or beds that may become birthing chairs. These capitalize on gravitational force to facilitate delivery. The episiotomy may be used, but may be eschewed if the delivery attendant believes a normal delivery will be possible without one.

During the postpartal period in client-centered care, the relationship between the mother and the infant is central. The mother and father will be able to spend time with the infant shortly after delivery to promote bonding. Rather than staying in the newborn nursery, the infant will room with the mother, at least in the daytime. Breast feeding will be encouraged, on an infant-determined or on-demand rather than a scheduled basis. The father may be allowed round the clock visiting hours. Siblings of the new infant are also allowed to visit. Health care is aimed at teaching and counseling as the new member is integrated into the family. To test the safety of sibling visitation, Umphenour (1980) studied the incidence of bacterial colonization in neonates after their siblings visited and found no differences from those having no young visitors.

Home Birthing Model. In the home birthing perspective, childbearing is viewed solely in the sense of normality and development. A pathological perspective is eschewed and may be considered harmful to the pregnancy and the birthing process. The centering of childbearing within a perspective of pathology is seen as a result of the current medical domination of health care. Physicians who participate in home birthings are those who are willing to practice outside the hospital setting. Much more frequent are deliveries by midwives or the family.

In the home birthing model, the health care attendant may be a physician, a nurse midwife, a lay midwife, or the woman and her partner themselves. The health care attendant acts as a facilitator where control of the relationship rests with the client. The practitioner may have expertise but the purpose of the relationship is to effect the sharing of knowledge and skill. Practitioners may be prepared to act immediately if an emergency situation should occur, or may hold to a philosophy of nonintervention (as, for example, in the case of childbearing within a Christian Science philosophy).

Prenatal care emphasizes teaching and preparation for birthing. Meetings may take place within the home. The family may need help in preparing their home and gathering equipment as well as learning techniques for the labor and delivery.

During labor, the attendant's care will focus on support measures. It may be a very private event with the mate, other children, and perhaps friends providing support through labor, and help at the time of the birth. The laboring woman will be encouraged to behave in ways that are comfortable to her, whether walking indoors or out, reclining in a warm water bath, or taking to her bed. There is much less emphasis on formal procedures such as sterile technique. An atmosphere of cleanliness is much more common.

In the event of complications, an emergency vehicle may be summoned to provide care and transport to an acute care facility. If only family and friends are present and a complication occurs, emergency treatment may be impossible. Therefore, with home deliveries, a philosophy of acceptance and accedance to any outcome may be a component of this mode of birthing.

Health Care Deprived. This quadrant of childbearing describes those who do not easily fit into the traditional health care system but whose norms and beliefs are similar to it. Families who are health care deprived are not able to obtain adequate health care either because it is not accessible or because their own style and mode of living make them uncomfortable with health care providers.

During pregnancy, individuals of the health care deprived group often do not have any or minimal formal prenatal care. Such care and help as they receive come from family or community members. As long as striking complications do not occur, pregnant women may not seek formal treatment until late pregnancy or the onset of labor.

Labor and delivery will take place in a fashion similar to the traditional medical model except that no previous relationship will exist between the various health care providers and the client. Because these women are often alone, fearful, and unknowledgeable about the birthing process, the lack of an established relationship with a caregiver is especially unfortunate.

Labor and delivery without analgesia and anesthesia is often not possible because of the lack of preparation for birthing. Lack of knowledge and fear may make an unassisted delivery in a birthing bed impossible as well. If the pregnancy was not completely welcomed or social and family constraints are present, bonding may be minimal.

In short, there are few benefits to being in the health care deprived group. These individuals have difficulty taking advantage of traditional, client-centered, or home birthing modes of health care. If they are fortunate, they emerge from the childbirthing experience physically unscathed.

Childbirthing Decision Making

To assist the client in deciding on a birthing option a questionnaire was developed for use by the health care provider. This questionnaire (Table 11–2) asks critical questions and allows the health care provider to class each client as to the traditional–medical, client-centered, or home birthing model. An assessment as to the availability of various options in a community can also be evaluated, allowing the preferences of an individual client to be determined.

This questionnaire could be used as a self-scored assessment tool by many clients. Then the actual options available could be described and/or visited. Table 11–1 could be used as a handout so the client may recognize the different options. The client then could see how her preferences could be met and how she has come to her decision concerning her birthing experience.

Many health care providers would guide the individual toward client-centered care. It can be considered an evolution from the traditional–medical model, reflecting changing social mores about the role of professionals and the need for informed consent. Nevertheless, the health care provider who subscribes to the client-centered approach must remember that the practitioner's own value judgment is operative in this preference. Client-centered care can be described as an American middle-class custom, used by those clients who are educated and perceived by themselves as being able to control events in their lives. Clients of other cultures, for instance, may not have this orientation (see Chapter 2, Culture/Value section). Some clients may not be motivated to learn about the birthing process, and the traditional hospital delivery methods may be more suitable for them.

Differing values and beliefs about childbirthing will cause the practitioner to view health care practices as positive or negative. If the provider prefers birthing in the traditional–medical model then birthing care that is aggressive or invasive (such as the use of intravenous and fetal monitoring) will be provided. Interventions are thus justified. An advocate of another perspective, however, could argue that these interventions are unnecessarily uncomfortable for the client. This, then, results in two orthogonal positions—the importance of comfort versus problem prevention. As health care practices become more grounded in research, the beliefs within each model will be either validated or relegated to the place of myth or dogma. In the traditional–medical model, some research questions that must be asked are: Does an enema during labor facilitate the effectiveness of contractions? Does the perineal shave lessen the incidence of postpartal infection? Does the use of an episiotomy reduce the chance of occurrence of

TABLE 11–2. BIRTHING DECISION AID

	Traditional–Medical	Client-centered	Home Birthing
1. Is the client knowledgeable or open to learning about pregnancy and birthing?	no[a]	yes	yes
2. Does the client have an established and comfortable relationship with a traditional physician?	yes[a]	no	no
3. If birthing facilities are limited to traditional–medical care, is the client comfortable with challenging the traditional health care system?	no[a]	yes	yes
4. Does the client have a client-centered practitioner or is she open to establishing a new relationship with one?	no	yes[a]	yes
5. Are client-centered care facilities available?	no	yes	—
6. Does the client hold the attitude that pregnancy and birthing are a normal stage of life?	no	yes	yes
7. Is the client aware and fearful of complications of birthing?	yes[a]	yes[a]	no
8. Regarding control over decision making:			
a. Does the client have the need to give responsibility to a knowledgeable expert?	yes[a]	no	no
b. Does the client have the desire to participate in decision making?	no	yes[a]	yes
c. Does the client wish to have complete control over all decision making?	no	no	yes[a]
9. Does the client have specific desires regarding:			
a. Labor routines?	no	yes	yes
b. Birthing routines?	no	yes	yes
c. Family and friends' attendance at the delivery of the infant by the mate	no	no	yes[a]
d. Postpartal infant care	no	yes	yes
e. Delivery in the home	no	no	yes[a]
10. Is the client willing to accept with equanimity any outcome, positive or negative, of the birthting experience?	no	no	yes[a]

[a]Indicates a critical determinant in the birthing decision.

vaginal cystocele or rectocele? There are initial research findings regarding these questions (Brendsel, Peterson, & Mehl, 1980; Rommey & Gordon, 1981), but no finding from studies sufficiently controlled to encourage all providers to abandon a belief in the effectiveness of various interventions they value.

For example, emphasis on the importance of the bonding process between parents and infant comes from a body of research performed on animals (see, for instance, Rheinfolds, 1963). Extrapolations have been made to the presence of bonding in human beings, with support from studies investigating the effects of mother–infant separation

(Klaus & Kennell, 1976). Conclusive research findings are still needed on this topic. The debate about liberal contact between newborn, mother, and family continues.

As health care evolves, those practices that may not be validated by research may be found questionable or false. Beliefs that are truly values, however, can never be tested and can only be accepted as being held by a client and/or a practitioner. Some factors for birthing decision making may change or may be argued in the future, but those factors that are values will change as social norms and practices evolve. The health care provider is really only justified in questioning a client's informed decision if it rests on a belief about practice that has been found to be false or harmful. However, these and other beliefs and wishes of the client should be respected. A number of factors that should be considered for assisting clients in choosing an appropriate childbirthing option will be explained.

Deciding for the Traditional–Medical Model. First and foremost, an assessment should be made as to whether a normal spontaneous delivery is likely. Are there risk factors already apparent such as preexisting health problems? Such conditions as cardiovascular or renal disease, diabetes mellitus, or malignancy would warrant close medical attention throughout pregnancy, labor and delivery, and the postpartal period. If a woman has had a previous cesarian section and desires a vaginal birth, she should of course be under the care of an obstetrician because uterine rupture is a possibility during labor.

A second focus of the assessment is whether the client is concerned with the possibility of complications and prefers that every measure be taken to avoid these complications. Would the client feel more assured with the perineal shave and the enema to ward off infection, intravenous fluids to alleviate dehydration, the fetal monitor to assess fetal condition, and the availability of analgesia for pain? Certain clients may feel comforted by giving control and the decision-making power to an expert. This client may not feel panicked at loss of control so much as grateful that someone else, an expert with whom she is familiar, appears to be in control.

An additional factor in selecting this perspective of care is the nature of the relationship with the practitioner. Does an established relationship already exist, and if so, what is the perspective of that practitioner? If it is a physician who is traditional and medical in approach, then the client will perhaps feel more comfortable adhering to the wishes of this known provider. It may be more upsetting to change providers than to seek a different mode of care.

In one study that investigated women's interests in alternative maternity facilities, of those women who had previous birth experiences, 68 percent stated they would use the same physician and 70 percent the same facility (Mather, 1980). Eighty-six percent of the women in this study chose the physician first and went to the facility she or he preferred. "It was also found that whether or not a woman has had a negative or neutral birth experience does not increase the likelihood of her seeking an alternative health care provider or facility" (Mather, 1980, p. 6).

Finally, if health care services are limited as in a rural area or where hospitals are smaller, the client may have little choice as to the mode of care rendered. It was found in a study of New York City hospitals, for instance, that those hospitals with fewer than 2000 beds are less likely to provide client-centered birthing experiences (Turnock & Pakter, 1979).

If it seems that the client may be more suited to a client-centered approach and only the traditional–medical approach is available, the client may need an advocate. This would be someone to represent her and her family to the health care system, and who is knowledgeable and able to aid the client in obtaining concessions in routine care. Should the client, however, not wish to challenge the health care system through fear of disapproval or repercussions, this also must be respected. This client, even though privately desirous of a client-centered approach, will accede to traditional–medical care rather than making problems or creating conflict with health care providers.

In a study of randomly selected women who intended to become pregnant within the next 10 years, it was found that many lacked awareness of hospital birthing suites or birthing centers. Before reading descriptions of these centers, 62 percent of the women studied ranked the traditional method as their most preferred choice. After reading about the alternatives, 62 percent ranked nontraditional methods as their first choice (Mather, 1980).

Because this study seems to indicate that clients choose what they are familiar with, clients should be given full knowledge concerning all options available. The woman should also know that she can refuse to have a perineal shave, or that fetal monitoring need only be used it there is a suspected problem with the fetal condition.

Recognizing the various health care providers that provide a different type of care can also help the client select a provider that supports the philosophy of care nearest her own and her partner/husband's philosophy. Interviewing potential providers may be helpful.

Deciding for Alternative Birthing. Some clients actively wish to avoid any acute care facility, or truly want to have their baby in their home. This may pose problems for the provider because physicians and nurse midwives who attend home births may be in jeopardy. In some states, home deliveries are unlawful; physicians may risk losing their license through "negligence." Nurse midwives may be taking risks with their license to practice midwifery. Lay midwives may be charged with practicing medicine without a license, or if a complication occurs, more serious offenses.

The practitioner who is an advocate for the client using an alternative outside of a health care facility may also be in a difficult position. One physician, chairman of the obstetrics department of a large city hospital, was quoted as describing home birth as "the earliest form of child abuse" (United Press, 1981). Therefore, the provider defending the client's rights to this choice may receive a share of condemnation. As discussed by Kohnke (1982), the client advocate must ensure his or her own legal ground and must be prepared to risk disapproval when taking an unpopular stand.

The client desiring an alternative may feel uncomfortable in a client-centered facility if her criteria cannot be met anywhere but in the home. Some religious persuasions are more consistent with home births. Those practicing Christian Science, some forms of Buddhism, and Jehovah's Witnesses may have beliefs about nonintervention that are more easily followed outside of a care facility. Such religions offer the faith and support that allow parents to accept a negative outcome if it should occur.

The Situation of the Health Care Deprived

Some providers work with those clients considered to be health care deprived. Often they do not enter the health care system until delivery is imminent. However, if they come to the attention of a health care provider, either through community care or inadvertently through a need for acute care, they can be helped to obtain birthing care that is consistent with their beliefs and life-style.

Some clients are uncomfortable in the presence of a traditionally-oriented physician, with the concomitant clash in social status, values, and culture. Such a client may be more amenable to seeing a nurse midwife who has the knowledge base to teach and support clients of different life-styles, and the time to develop an interpersonal relationship. A nurse midwife in conjunction with a community health nurse may help this client to obtain appropriate prenatal care.

Health care deprived clients, though, may have difficulty in meeting the demands of a client-centered labor and delivery approach. Those holding cultural values other than middle class values may perceive labor and delivery as painful, and may desire analgesia and anesthesia throughout. Such clients may also not wish to participate in decision making throughout the birthing process. These clients would rather be helped through it.

In the study of 2608 women delivering in a socially depressed city hospital, however, nurse midwives used analgesia and anesthesia in less than 30 percent of all labors, no shave preps or enemas were used, and 45 percent of the deliveries were with an intact perineum (Haire, 1981). This study suggests that if the proper orientation and approach is available to the health care deprived woman, client-centered care can be provided. Unfortunately, in many areas the health care deprived woman has only the option of the traditional–medical model of birthing.

Educational Orientation

The reader will recognize a similarity between andragogical (adult) educational approaches and client-centered approaches to the birthing experience. In both, it is the client–learner who is in control, who decides what is needed and when goals have been met. The health care provider–teacher facilitates versus controls and directs the experience. It seems logical that those individuals who prefer client-centered care may prefer andragogical approaches to learning. Thus andragogical approaches are appropriate for teaching about all aspects of pregnancy and delivery and to use with those clients who want to make decisions about birthing options. A more direct educational orientation seems appropriate for clients who prefer others to decide, be expert, and know what is best. The learning style of the client may thus determine how the options are presented and how direct the care provider is in assisting the client to make decisions regarding how she delivers her baby.

Offering information concerning the alternatives is critical. Adult learners have demonstrated that they will choose options with which they are familiar (Cross, 1978). If the available options are not shared with childbearing women and their families, many will miss more satisfying alternatives. Sharing the concept that there *is* a decision to make in childbirth classes is helpful in matching the client to the most appropriate mode of care.

Certainly, perpetuating the health care deprived model is not desirable. Perhaps the problem here is that health care providers do not know what this group of women want. Using andragogical approaches to teaching–learning with this group of women may allow health care providers to learn from clients. How can their preferences and needs be met? How can other alternatives be created? How can some of our current alternatives be *altered* to fit these clients? These questions may only be answered when the teacher–provider considers clients expert and knowledgeable.

The decision-making process described in Chapter 3 is useful for clients who want to decide on various childbirthing options. Weighing costs and benefits of available options when the client's preferred choice is unavailable may facilitate the client feeling she has some degree of control when she wants more control than is available (see Chapter 3 for more detail). Three case studies are presented to highlight various client preferences and how these clients made decisions regarding childbirthing.

Case Studies

Linda and Bill are a professional couple, Linda being a nurse and Bill a computer specialist. This couple is knowledgeable about pregnancy and birthing and live in a city where both traditional and alternative modes of care are available. They chose, however, to deliver their first child in the hospital with the help of their traditionally-oriented physician. Linda explained that she feels very comfortable in a hospital because she works in one and understands the intricacies of the system. She and Bill had an established relationship with their physician and shared his views on the merits of a problem prevention approach to delivery. Linda had a pudental block to provide anesthesia during labor and pronounced it an excellent method for controlling pain. They felt satisfied with their birth experience.

Two critical factors were operative in this couple's decision making. They had an established relationship with their practitioner that they wanted to preserve, and they were aware of and concerned over possible complications of childbirthing. Because they had no aversion to the hospital environment, the traditional–medical model of birthing was their choice. This mode met their needs.

Sandra and Winston were another couple planning for the birth of their second child. They too were knowledgeable about birthing options and visited a birthing center to see whether it would be an appropriate environment for their delivery. They interviewed the nurse midwife, and after a tour, decided to use a more traditional hospital setting. They reported that the birthing center attendant had stressed the homelike atmosphere and had deemphasized the presence of emergency equipment. Sandra and Winston explained later that their first child needed resuscitative measures after delivery and that they therefore received more reassurance from the presence of emergency equipment than the factors relating to a "homelike" atmosphere.

This couple also was guided by the critical factor of their fear of birth complications. Other factors had less significance when examined in the light of their first birthing experience and expectations of the second one.

Jennifer and Sol had had two children and were expecting their third. Jennifer stated vociferously that she hated hospitals and had had unpleasant experiences in her previous deliveries, especially in interacting with hospital physicians and staff. The first two deliveries had been relatively free of complications and this couple planned to deliver their third baby at home by themselves with the help of friends. The community health nurse in contact with them ascertained their intent and provided teaching regarding labor and delivery and information about available emergency facilities.

Because Jennifer and Sol had had unpleasant experiences with health care professionals during their previous deliveries and decided that the third time they would maintain complete and sole control over events, the nurse respected their decision and provided as much assistance as their situation allowed.

Summary

Allowing women and their partners to make a decision as to how they deliver their baby has been viewed as a right and responsibility. This chapter has provided information and instruments to assist health care providers to facilitate such decision making. Presenting options to childbearing women is considered a responsibility of today's health care providers. Denying options should *only* be done when such options place the client at great risk or when the client requests the health care provider to make decisions for her.

BIBLIOGRAPHY

Brendsel, C., Peterson, G., & Mehl, L. E. Routine episiotomy and pelvic symptomatology. *Women and Health*, 1980, *5*(4), 49–60.

Chaney, J. A. Birthing in early America. *Journal of Nurse Midwifery*, 1980, *25*(2), 5–13.

Clark, A. L., & Alfonso, D. D. *Childbearing: A nursing perspective* (2nd ed.). Philadelphia: F.A. Davis, 1979.

Cross, K. P. The adult learner. Address presented at the 1978 National Conference on Higher Education, American Association for Higher Education, Chicago, March 20, 1978.

Dillon, T. Midwifery, 1977. *American Journal of Obstetrics and Gynecology*, 1978, *130*, 917–922.

Haire, D. Improving the outcome of pregnancy through increased utilization of midwives. *Journal of Nurse Midwifery*, 1981, *26*(1), 5–8.

Hiestad, W. C. The development of nurse-midwifery education in the United States. In M. L. Fitzpatrick (Ed.), *Historical studies in nursing*. New York: Teachers College Press, 1978.

Klaus, M. H., & Kennell, J. H. *Maternal–infant bonding: The impact of early separation or loss in family development*. St. Louis, Mo.: C. V. Mosby, 1976.

Kohnke, M. F. *Advocacy: Risk and reality*. St. Louis, Mo.: C. V. Mosby, 1982.

Mather, S. Women's interest in alternative maternity facilities. *Journal of Nurse Midwifery*, 1980, *25*(3), 3–10.

Mehl, L. E., Remiel, J. R., Leininger, B., Heff, B., Kronenthal, K., & Peterson, G. H. Evaluation of outcomes of non-nurse midwives: Matched comparisons with physicians. *Women and Health*, 1980, *5*(2), 17–29.

National Center for Health Statistics. Annual Summary for the United States, 1978. Monthly Vital Statistics Report, August 13, 1979, *27*(13), DHEW Pub No. (PHS) 79-1120.

National Center for Health Statistics. Vital Statistics of the United States, 1973. Hyattsville, Md.: National Center for Health Statistics.

Perry, H. B. Role of the nurse-midwife in contemporary maternity care. In D. D. Youngs & A. A. Ehrhardt (Eds.), *Psychosometric obstetrics and gynecology*. New York: Appleton-Century-Crofts, 1980.

Rheinfolds, H. L. (Ed.) *Maternal behavior in mammals*. New York: John C. Wiley, 1963.

Rommey, M., & Gordon, H. Is your enema really necessary? *British Medical Journal*, 1981, *282*, 1269–1270.

Seashore, M. J., Leifer, A. D., Barnett, C. R., & Leiderman, P. H. The effects of denial of early mother–infant interactions on maternal self-confidence. *Journal of Personality and Social Psychology*, 1973, *26*, 369–378.

Slome, C. Effectiveness of certified nurse midwives: A prospective evaluation study. *American Journal of Obstetrics and Gynecology*, 1976, *124*, 177–182.

Starkman, M. N., & Youngs, D. D. Reactions to electronic fetal monitoring. In D. D. Youngs & A. A. Ehrhardt (Eds.), *Psychosometric obstetrics and gynecology*. New York: Appleton-Century-Crofts, 1980.

Turnock, B., & Pakter, J. Family centered care activities by size of maternity service. *Women and Health*, 1979, *4*(4), 373–384.

Umphenour, J. H. Bacterial: Colonization in neonates with sibling visitation. *Journal of Gynecological Nursing*, 1980, *9*(2), 73–75.

United Press International. Home birth: Still controversial. *New Hampshire Sunday News*, Manchester, N.H., September 13, 1981.

Health Education for the Childbearing Experience: A Guide for Continuity

12

Vivian M. Littlefield

Continuity and consistency in education for the childbearing woman and her family is a major problem. The shortened hospital stay, the numerous staff from several units (labor and delivery, postpartum, and nursery), and the multiple professionals giving information, handing out literature, and evaluating what is learned makes consistency seem next to impossible. Also, varying opinions as to specific instructions for perinatal care exist between and among professionals.

The patients' readiness to learn, the staff's commitment to teaching, and the multiple patients taught makes comprehensive perinatal education seem like an unachievable goal. The increasing requirements for complete documentation coupled with shorter hospital stays also pose special problems for the obstetrical care provider. Some method is needed that provides standardization of what content is to be taught, allows one care provider to know what the other taught, and promotes easy, efficient documentation.

Nurses working in a large perinatal service were frustrated with these complexities and decided to propose a "tool" that would help improve the quality of education and make the teaching process easier.

When data were collected in this center, concerns about the content, completeness, and continuity of the teaching arose. There was also a significant amount of repetition of material being taught, often resulting in the exclusion of other valuable material. Clearly, there was a need to identify what material should be taught antepartum versus postpartum and to communicate what each professional had taught.

It was suggested that the best way to ensure continuity of teaching and decrease the amount of repetition was to have one form on which all perinatal teaching would be documented. This form would "follow" the woman throughout her pregnancy and postpartum. This form was called the teaching tool (see Appendix A). Previous knowledge and repetition of material would thus be less likely and continuity of teaching between the in- and outpatient areas, hopefully, would be ensured.

The need for uniformity in teaching was met by identifying the topics that would be taught antepartum versus postpartum, and writing guidelines and behavioral objectives for the information to be taught for each topic. Guidelines were compiled and made available to various staff and professionals in a reference folder. To meet JCAH (Joint Commission on the Accreditation of Hospitals) standards for documentation, the teaching tool was made a permanent part of the client's hospital record. The guidelines were placed on file in medical records. The tool was thus brief and saved time in repeated documentation.

DESCRIPTION OF THE TEACHING TOOL

The Obstetric and Perinatal Teaching Needs form (teaching tool) is a written record of patient teaching done. The form consists of two major sections: antepartum and perinatal. The antepartum section, which is completed during the prenatal period, is subdivided into selected common teaching needs. These are physical and emotional changes; fetal growth and development; sexuality; nutrition and weight gain; activity; potential impact of substance use; and danger signs (Fig. 12–1). Generally, the ambulatory nurse has

SMH **477**

OBSTETRIC AND PERINATAL
TEACHING NEEDS

Patient Name _____

Unit Number _____

	Date	Signature	Written Mat'l Given	Assessment	Plan
ANTEPARTUM					
Physical/ Emotional Changes					
Fetal Growth/ Development					
Sexuality					
Nutrition/ Weight Gain					
Activity					
Potential Impact: Substance Use					
Danger Signs					

Figure 12–1. Obstetric and perinatal teaching needs form. *(Source: University of Rochester, Strong Memorial Hospital, Rochester, N.Y., by permission.)*

primary responsibility for antepartum and initial assessment of perinatal teaching needs. The nutritionist, social worker, physical therapist, and physician, however, can document their teaching on the form also. The inpatient nurse may also document on the antepartal section when an obstetrical patient is admitted to the hospital antepartally.

The perinatal section is subdivided into other areas such as physical and emotional changes; nutrition and exercise; sexuality and contraception; infant care at home; infant development and sibling preparation; bath demonstration; infant feeding; temperature taking; circumcision care; pre- and postoperative teaching; jaundice; and danger signs.

After the client is taught and evaluated for learning, the health care provider writes an assessment of the client's understanding of the teaching done as well as a plan for follow-up, if indicated. Each entry on the form is dated, initialed, and any written material given is recorded (Fig. 12–2). If a particular subject is problematic and requires extra documentation, a progress note is written in the chart.

Upon delivery, the teaching tool, which was begun in the antepartal period, is pulled from the prenatal record and the perinatal section is completed by the inpatient nurse during the postpartum period. Using one form throughout the pregnancy and postpartum period enhances continuity of client teaching and necessary follow-up. Also, a discussion of some perinatal subjects, i.e., birth control, circumcision, and infant feeding, is begun prenatally.

The guidelines identify critical content to be taught around each subject on the teaching tool. Behavioral objectives were developed to clarify as specifically as possible what the patient needs to know. In addition, the guidelines provided information needed by the teacher to assist the client's learning, references for the content area, and a listing of pamphlets to assist clients' learning the specific topic. Table 12–1 is a selected sample

---

SMH 477

OBSTETRIC AND PERINATAL TEACHING NEEDS

Patient Name: Mary Jones

Unit Number: 18-20-190

	Date	Signature	Written Mat'l Given	Assessment	Plan
ANTEPARTUM Physical/ Emotional Changes	8/24/83	Mrs. Dale, R.n.	Sm H Common Discomfort of Preg.	Taught as per guidelines N & V c̄ day – Reviewed ways to ↓ N & V.	1. ✓ if N & V decreased 2. See note 1/19/84
	1/19/84	Mrs. Dale, R.n.			N & V resolved
Fetal Growth/ Development	8/24/83	Mrs. Dale, R.n.		Saw film A&P of preg – Taught as per guidelines limited – very limited knowledge	1. Review next week 2. See note 1/19/84
	1/19/84	Mrs. Dale, R.n.			
Sexuality	8/24/83	Mrs. Dale, R.n.		Taught as per guidelines bleeding p̄ intercourse – Instructed to call if continues	1. Review & ✓ re: bleeding 2. No further Ed needed
	1/19/84	Mrs. Dale, R.n.		Bleeding has stopped	
Nutrition/ Weight Gain	8/24/83	Mrs. Dale, R.n.	Basic 4 Food Groups	Very limited appetite – much asepsis, diarrhea, & nausea. Discussed other forms of Calcium – advised to keep diet record – Interested in WIC	1. Review next visit 2. Furnish WIC form see note 1/19/84 3. Is on WIC
	1/19/84	Mrs. Dale, R.n.			

Figure 12–2. Sample of completed obstetric and perinatal teaching needs form. (*Source: University of Rochester, Strong Memorial Hospital, Rochester, N.Y., by permission.*)

TABLE 12–1. NUTRITION AND WEIGHT GAIN

Behavioral Objectives

The patient will:

1. Relate that her prenatal nutritional status affects both the way she feels during pregnancy and the outcome of her pregnancy.
2. Name the four basic food groups and the amount of each that are required during pregnancy.
3. Relate the appropriate rate or amount of weight gain needed during pregnancy and the rationale for gaining weight consistently.

of the guidelines for one topic area. Appendix A contains the entire set of guidelines and a detailed description of how to record teaching done and client learning. Obviously, if patients know the content, no teaching in that area needs to be done. If the client fails to learn, repeated teaching sessions will be held prior to documenting learning.

In-service Training for Using the Teaching Tool

The teaching tool and the teaching guidelines were introduced to the professional staff in a formal in-service program. Teaching–learning theory (as per Chapter 2 and 3) was presented in an organized and scheduled time frame so that the staff on all shifts could attend. Lectures and a variety of visual aids were used to present the information. At the end of each in-service class a question and answer session was offered. Afterward, the teaching tool and guideline booklets were distributed to each patient care unit. Staff were asked to use them for 3 months and to get a feel for the usage of the tool in their daily ongoing teaching plans. At the end of the trial period both informal communication and written feedback concerning the effectiveness of the tool were sought from staff members.

Evaluation

The majority of the responses by the staff were quite positive. In fact, there were only three major concerns and they were easily rectified. One concern was where to place the teaching tool. First, it was agreed to keep this tool at the patient's bedside so that the patient could be involved in her teaching assessment and education. Unfortunately, when the tool was kept at the bedside, visitors or family members would also review the teaching tool that contained some private information (i.e., sexuality and contraceptive use). Therefore, the teaching tool was kept in a folder with the patient's Kardex. Then, when care providers planned to do some teaching, they could pull the tool from the Kardex folder, take it to the bedside, involve the patient in assessing teaching needs, document all teaching done, and return it to the Kardex folder. This way the patient's privacy was maintained but involvement in identifying learning needs and progress toward meeting these needs was maintained.

A second problem was some confusion as to what to put under each heading such as assessment, plan, and evaluation. Further in-service programs were provided to clarify what documentation was necessary to record under what heading. This decreased confusion and increased consistency in recording. Clearer directions were developed and distributed to staff using the tool.

The third concern was that at times the tool would get misplaced or lost due to several hospitalizations resulting in the removal of the tool from the old chart or previous record. Consequently, new tools would be started and a record of what was taught would have to be reviewed with the patient whenever the health care provider tried to get a baseline of knowledge. An effort was made to reinforce the need to pull out the teaching tool from the old records and return it to the chart after discharge.

SUMMARY

In conclusion, the teaching tool and guideline booklets were found to be of great benefit. New nurses less familiar with obstetrics were able to contribute to the teaching efforts for each patient by glancing over the booklet of guidelines. Other health team members could identify what was taught and have an idea of the clients' baseline knowledge. Physicians found the tool helpful also and relied on nursing to do the teaching indicated. Clients, as a result of more complete and consistent teaching, felt more confident and secure in their ability to care for themselves and the baby upon discharge. Consistency from care provider to care provider increased patients' confidence in their care. The professional staff recognized the minimal amount of actual charting required in this methodology.

The unique contributions made by the teaching tool were threefold. First, it improved continuity, consistency, and quality of patient education. Second, it made the professional staff accountable for client teaching by more clearly defining areas of responsibility. And third, it efficiently documented patient teaching done. The tool allowed the interdisciplinary staff to achieve a goal of insuring the right of the patients to be informed.

Education for the New Mother and Her Family

13

Margret Banton and Barbara Lum

The transition to the parent role is identified by many authors as a crisis (Donaldson, 1981; LeMasters, 1965). When health professionals are aware of the elements of crisis with which a maternity client must deal they are in a position to effectively support a new mother and assess her readiness for learning. What are some of the crisis issues present in the postpartum period? Role conflict, lack of societal support, body image, and self image are the broad categories that emerge in the literature.

Role conflict can be a basis for crisis in the postpartum family. New parents may not initiate a telephone call for help and support because of a sense that society might disapprove of parents who admit feelings of stress or unhappiness (Cooksey & Goetting, 1982). Rossi (1980) discussed the historical cultural pressure to assume the parental role, and noted that the greater the cultural pressure to assume a given role, the greater the tendency toward covert rather than open expression of negative feelings about the role. Thirty-eight out of 46 first-time parent couples studied by LeMasters (1965) characterized themselves as in "severe or extensive crisis." They felt unprepared for the role of parent. Loss of sleep, confinement to home, additional housework, guilt about falling short of their idealized parent role, and distress over postpartal appearance all were reported by the mothers. Fathers' adjustments were similar. Additionally, fathers were concerned over their wives' decline in sexual response, reduction to a single income at the time another individual was added to the family, possibility of an imminent repeat pregnancy, and disillusionment with the role of parent. New parents reporting crisis in LeMasters' study had "almost completely romanticized parenthood" (LeMasters, 1965, p. 114). They felt they had little or no preparation for parenthood. Based on crisis theory and the stresses common to fourth trimester mothers, Donaldson (1981) developed a role for a postpartum follow-up nurse clinician. LeMasters and Donaldson both concluded that preparation and anticipation for what to expect could lessen the intensity of the parental role crisis.

Meeting the educational needs of the postpartum family is a complex task. The increasing national mobility has placed more and more families in communities without the traditional support of relatives. This, in turn, increases the need for community-based support services. Additionally, the fragmentation of medical services, particularly for the childbearing family, hampers patient teaching programs. The trend toward early hospital discharge further shortens the time for the in-hospital nurse to offer information and guidance. All of these factors place an increased burden on extra-hospital sources to meet the educational needs of the postpartum family. The purpose of this chapter is to look at postpartum parents as learners and discuss some ways to address their learning needs.

ORGANIZING A COMPREHENSIVE PROGRAM

Childbirth is not only an important time for health care education but also an opportune one, for it is a period when families actively seek information and support. A comprehensive educational offering during pregnancy and the early postpartum period can often provide new families with a firm foundation to begin the challenge of parenthood. Yet, current health care practices frequently fragment the services provided to these families who may see obstetricians, pediatricians, and nurse practitioners, along with interns, residents, labor and delivery nurses, postpartum nurses, and public health nurses. They see still another set of nurses or lay people during childbirth education classes. Maternal–child nurse practitioners, as described by Brown, O'Meara, and Krowley (1975), offer families a more comprehensive program of both education and support throughout the childbearing period. Midwives and obstetrical nurse practitioners may also fill this role. However, many families do not receive these latter services and the coordination of their care tends to vary a great deal.

There is a great deal of information that can support a new family, but it cannot be presented appropriately in a few days in the hospital. It must be provided in a comprehensive long-range program to be most helpful to families. This means that nurses in all areas of perinatal care must work together to organize such programs. Dickson (1982) has reported a program that utilizes a primary nurse who visits the prenatal family, devises a plan of care, and assists the family through pregnancy, the in-hospital stay, and the initial home period. Similarly, other groups have established programs where in-hospital nurses provide childbirth education, offering continuity to the educational program. It may be necessary to establish a coordinated network in the community designed to best serve the needs of clients and utilize available resources. Other approaches may utilize lay mothers, sponsor a newsletter, or reorganize postpartum care to provide time for telephone calls and office visits.

A creative solution to coordinating communication about patient education is the comprehensive teaching tool described in Chapter 12. Using the teaching tool, nurses who see patients only prenatally receive feedback from those who see patients postpartally to discover how effective was their teaching program and what alternative methods they might use. Equally, nurses seeing clients in-hospital or at home can use the tool to determine what information patients have been receiving prenatally so that they do not duplicate or confuse information previously given.

With the advent of early discharge, programs have been developed to provide additional means of support and education, such as homemakers and visits from public health nurses. Examples of such programs are described by Avery and colleagues (1982) and, in the authors' community, the Home Care Association (1981). Clients electing early discharge (8 to 24 hours postpartum) need to be carefully monitored both prenatally and in-hospital to establish that they are going to benefit from the program. Because early discharge limits the new family's time in the hospital, the program must include a way of providing the necessary teaching (Carr & Walton, 1982; Scupholme, 1981). This may be accomplished by using the mother's social support system and written instructions, as well as postpartum programs that provide postpartum teaching and support such as community health nurse visits, daily telephone calls, or an organized lay support group in the neighborhood.

Prenatal Planning

Preparation should be made, not only for the birth experience, but also for the postpartum period. Prenatal education programs should include dietary counseling, birth control information, newborn behavior and appearance, and a discussion of sexual needs during and after pregnancy. The postpartum period may then be better utilized for review and discussion as needed. Complex decision making requires that the patient have stress-free time to consider alternatives. The family requires information about the mother's need for rest and the family's need for time to become acquainted with their new member. In addition, a plan of exercise provided prenatally will allow, for example, Kegel exercises to be started immediately. Knowledge of options such as early discharge and community health nurse visits is helpful. Information about community resources and support groups should be provided both verbally and in writing. For mothers with little substantive experience with children, this may be an appropriate time for pairing new mothers with experienced lay mothers.

Breast-feeding

Mothers who have elected to breast-feed their infants need to receive information on breast-feeding, including a choice of several reference books on the subject. Office loan copies may be helpful for indigent mothers. Health care professionals might also provide some information about La Leche League or other breast-feeding support groups in their area. The name of a contact person, for instance an experienced breast-feeding mother known to the nurse and convenient to the mother, may also be helpful.

THE EARLY POSTPARTUM PERIOD

The New Mother

There is a great deal of information to be offered postpartally (Jennings & Edmundson, 1980), yet your time is limited and the mother's need for rest and acquaintance with her infant must be considered. A bombardment of teaching materials may overwhelm some families. Great care must be taken, therefore, to optimize learning without diminishing the family confidence. As much information as possible should be provided to the maximum number of family members. The adult learning principles developed in Chapter 3 apply to the family. The concept of correct "dosage" is especially important as the new mother moves through the psychological changes of the first few postpartum days.

Psychological Set of the Mother. The mother is particularly receptive to information about her changing self and her newborn in the immediate postpartum period. Your role is to provide an environment and a climate in which the mother can begin taking on her new role as well as regenerating physically and psychologically. The professional's interaction with the mother's support person influences her ability to work on maternal role attainment (Dunn & White, 1981).

Taking-in. The length of time since birth as well as the assessment of maternal behavior can be used to evaluate the mother's progress through Rubin's (1961b, 1984) three phases of postpartum emotional development and tailor teaching to her immediate needs. In the "taking-in" phase, the mother will act in a passive, receptive, oral mode. Sleep and food are paramount. Lack of sleep will delay her progression to the next phase, as well as inhibit her ability to learn. She is verbal and talks continuously to nurses or visitors about her experience. Otherwise she is engaged in constant telephone conversation. Relieved and reassured that she has indeed had safe passage for herself and her infant through labor and delivery, she spends the first 24 to 48 hours taking-in. Her sphere of interest is narrow, encompassing herself and the baby. She identifies the baby in terms of gender, weight, and length. She spends time claiming the infant, bringing the baby into her social fabric as being "like" the father or other relatives. It is well to discuss the development over time of maternal feelings to insure that mothers are aware that not everyone experiences a total release of maternal emotion at the first contact with her infant.

Cognitively, the new mother is very active, even during the first, "taking-in" days. An adult learning approach can support her previous knowledge and focus on her here-and-now state. The most effective teacher at this time identifies her learning need for help to "see" her infant in greater detail and to learn her baby's capabilities for interaction. Mother–infant interaction is frequently initiated by the infant and commented upon and elaborated by the mother. Her receptive state is again noticeable as she holds herself ready for the infant's activity and makes possible a dialogue between them (Shaffer, 1977). The infant's individuality and unfolding interactions are perhaps supported by the passive–receptive state of the new mother in the first postnatal days. A cycle is begun in which the mother's passivity and receptivity to infant-initiated behavior facilitates the infant's contribution to the relationship, which in turn stimulates response from the mother (Dunn & White, 1981).

An adolescent mother typified this passive–receptive state as she searched her infant's face for a response as he lay under a warming light in the nursery. The pediatric resident who explained the reason for the baby's low temperature was frustrated as his explanation seemed to fall on deaf ears. The young mother appeared at the moment only able to "take-in" the existence of the baby and his ability to return her gaze.

Taking-hold. The "taking-hold" phase of postpartum emotional development is usually under way by the third postpartum day. Autonomy, independence, and a focus on accomplishing what must be done are characteristic for approximately the next 2 weeks. Rubin identified the taking-hold phase as "a stage of maximal readiness for new learning" (1961b, p. 755). Hall (1980) reported a positive influence on mothers' perceptions of their infants when information about normal newborn behavior was presented during the taking-hold phase of the puerperium. Additional impetus to her desire to learn comes as she again masters her own body's functioning and feels able to "take hold" of some of the tasks of mothering (Martell & Mitchell, 1984; Rubin, 1961b). This optimal time for learning usually coincides with the mother's discharge from the hospital, thus putting greater pressure on extra-hospital sources for postpartum education.

Letting-go. The final phase of maternal role attainment begins about 2 weeks into the postpartum period. The mother begins letting-go or separating herself from the symbiotic relationship she and her infant have enjoyed during the earlier postpartum period (Rubin, 1977). That the mother, during the overall 6 weeks postpartum, is still receptive to learning opportunities is evident in several studies. Sumner and Fritsch (1977) report maternal telephone inquiries about their own recovery and problems with their newborn. Of 2081 telephone calls to a medical center ambulatory pediatric unit, 153 were for infants 1 month or younger. Among the most frequent calls from parents of newborns were those about formula, gastrointestinal problems, and breast-feeding (Overton, 1981).

Body Image. Body image, symbolized by the woman's concern for return of her figure to normal, is a major concern (Gruis, 1977; LeMasters, 1965). This concern over their own bodies was intense and caused women in Grubb's (1980) study to feel they were somewhere between pregnant and not pregnant. Review of the labor experience helps her comprehend what happened and enables her to move on to her present role and its requirements. Affonso (1977) substantiates the importance of this review. Her self-image requires that she integrate the experience of her labor and delivery to make it a cognitive whole in order to "own it" (Mercer, 1981; Rubin, 1961a). Croog and Zigrossi (1983) found a format that permitted small groups of mothers to share their review with a nurse discussion leader on hand to clarify as needed. They assembled mothers on the postpartum unit for parenting luncheons. They found mothers consistently needed to review their labor before moving on to sharing concerns and problems and anticipating the early weeks of parenthood.

Self-image. A blow to the new mother's self-image may come as she perceives the shift of attention of well-wishers. During pregnancy, the focus was on her. In the postpartum period the focus shifts to the baby. At a time when demands on her are increased and her supply of energy and well-being is depleted, she often feels ignored. The new mother often finds it difficult, too, to achieve a stable concept of her rapidly growing, changing infant. This makes it all the more difficult for her to achieve a stable self-image as mother (Grubb, 1980). Chao (1979) studied mothers' cognitive activities during three consecutive days following delivery. She noted that one-third of their activity was devoted to their self-concept related to care-giving activities and incorporating the new baby into the family constellation.

The emotional ups and downs of the newly delivered mother reflect the sudden physiological and psychological changes she has undergone (Rubin, 1961b). The maternal–infant nurse requires a broad knowledge base of the physiological and psychosocial aspects of both the postpartum and the newborn periods. The unique psychoemotional set of the postpartum mother will direct your postpartum educational program.

Physical Care. Studies (Bull, 1981; Sumner & Fritsch, 1977) demonstrate that a major concern of many women in the first week postpartum is their physical self; therefore, it is important to offer her sufficient support and information about her own bodily changes. Much of the information about the mother's physical care can be provided incidentally during routine postpartum checks. Nurses can influence the new mother's body image and self-image as they perform the postpartum assessment. The eight-point postpartum assessment described by Kilker and Wilkerson (1973) has proved useful. Positive statements during the assessment about the status of the mother's breasts, fundus, or lochia, and information about what to anticipate relieve her anxiety about her intactness and enhance her body image. Use of a mirror for mothers who want to see what their episiotomy really looks like may also be welcomed.

Transition. "Mothering the mother" is an important step in helping her prepare to learn about and nurture her infant. Helping her proceed at her own pace can often be of the most benefit. A mother's entire attention was absorbed in the discomfort of her episiotomy, a hemorrhoid, and inability to have a bowel movement. Her behavior was very passive and she requested that her baby be fed in the nursery. After a Sitz bath and perineal spray she relaxed enough to have a bowel movement with the help of a suppository. The mother then asked for the baby. When she arrived the mother commented, "She probably has a full diaper. I'll change her." At the return of some feeling of comfort and control over her body, she moved in a few minutes from the taking-in phase to the talking-hold phase. The nurse's directive, care-giving intervention then changed to a more collaborative, adult-oriented teaching role. The mother then comfortably participated in her infant's care, ready to begin looking at her baby's behavior and needs because her own physical needs were met.

Breast-feeding. The decision to breast-feed may arise from discussion with peers, family, health care professionals, or information gleaned from the media. Mothers who are breast-feeding require factual information about breast care in addition to suggestions for positioning and assistance with beginning nursing. Information on breast-feeding can be found in a large number of sources (see Supplemental Bibliography). The eagerness with which breast-feeding mothers seek and implement suggestions such as avoiding soap on their nipples, exposing their nipples to air, increasing fluids, and obtaining adequate rest to promote lactation makes this a rewarding area of teaching. A mother who came home from the hospital breast-feeding without these instructions experienced problems with sore nipples. At the advice of one of the authors she stopped using alcohol to clean her nipples and began exposing them to air. Her difficulties disappeared and she felt very successful breast-feeding.

Some mothers may find a discussion group of breast-feeding mothers on the unit helpful, particularly if this is attended by some experienced mothers. If a group is not possible, then a breast-feeding consultant, an experienced breast-feeding nurse or mother on the unit, may be helpful to the mother. Such support needs to be continued throughout the early postpartum period. This seems to be the critical period for breast-feeding success. Postpartum telephone calls and/or home visits are very useful in this regard.

Despite many helpful books and articles, comprehensive support for breast-feeding mothers is often sporadic. Familiarity with the available information and community resources which support breast-feeding is invaluable in guiding new mothers. A hospital or childbirth education-based telephone consultation service for breast-feeding mothers can be developed if one is not already available in the area. A list of other breast-feeding mothers willing to communicate could be helpful and supportive to new mothers. Such neighborhood support is often most effective. Women who had wished to breast-feed and who are unable to or unable to continue to nurse their infant may need support to deal with feelings of guilt.

Bottle-feeding. A woman may choose to bottle-feed her infant for a variety of reasons. These include her level of comfort with her body, social reasons such as her husband's feelings, life-style, need to return to work, physical problems such as inverted nipples, medication, and a previous unsuccessful breast-feeding experience. She may need help to deal with proponents of breast-feeding, from well-meaning neighbors to talk show guests. Mothers who are bottle-feeding need to know how to prevent overfeeding by recognizing infant cues of hunger and satiety, as well as needing information about burping, positioning, and variations in eating patterns. Breast-feeding as well as bottle-feeding mothers need to learn about formula preparation and use. Families should be reminded not to begin using whole milk with their infant prior to 6 to 12 months to prevent enteric blood loss. They should be discouraged from beginning solids prior to 4 months of age as this appears to affect eating habits and encourage the development of allergies (Fomon, 1979).

Birth Control. After making an assessment of a woman's contraceptive status, the nurse can present information that corresponds to her need. She may need to choose a method, increase her knowledge of the method she has used, or simply review the method she is satisfied using. Written information is helpful. For beginners, the opportunity to see and handle materials is useful. Natural family planning groups in many cities offer information and classes. Many women's health care texts describe instruction about each method's effectiveness, safety, and special instructions for the user.

The teaching tool initiated antepartally can provide helpful information about the postpartum mother's need for birth control information. Often it is sufficient to confirm with the mother her plans and review her knowledge of the method she has chosen. A nurse faculty member who as a postpartum mother was asked by her nurse what method of birth control she planned to use felt her obstetrical background and knowledge were disregarded. An adult-oriented learning approach that acknowledged her competence and offered her support might have resulted in identification of areas of concern regarding her new role and the life changes she could anticipate.

Rest and Blues. Postpartum mothers name fatigue as a major experience (Mercer, 1981). Most postpartum mothers need encouragement to get adequate rest both in and out of hospital. The family should be helped to understand the mother's need for rest and the potential for postpartum depression. It may not alter her fatigue or her depression but it will help her and her family to accept it, identify it, and deal with it. Often knowing that it is common and time-limited makes it a bit easier to handle. The prenatal checklist devised by Petrick (1984) to help identify mothers at high risk for postpartum depression may be useful in assessing emotional state postpartum. The topic of emotional changes postpartum is included in the teaching tool to prepare new mothers and their families in the event that the "blues" occur.

THE INFANT

Interaction with the Family

The most important aspect of the in-hospital stay is the opportunity for all of the family members to get acquainted with the infant. Encouraging rooming-in or modified rooming-in and promoting the philosophy of family-centered maternity care have proved very helpful in fostering a positive child–parent relationship. This is particularly true when it is individually tailored to meet the needs and desires of each family. Studies by a number of investigators suggest that increased postpartum contact between mother and child has a positive influence on that relationship (deChateau & Wiberg, 1977; Klaus & Kennell, 1976). Parents need an awareness of the unique capacity of their infant to relate to them (Affonso, 1976).

The newborn is capable of social interaction from the moment of birth. His or her ability to interact with the environment needs only to be activated by stimulation from that environment. There are a number of elements that influence an infant's behavior. The infant's state will largely determine his or her responses with the quiet–alert state being the most appropriate for optimal interaction. The characteristics of the stimuli also play an important part. A favorable combination of frequency and variety of stimuli can arouse an infant and cause him or her to interact with this environment whereas an unfavorable combination can cause a withdrawal. Infants provide a feedback mechanism to the stimuli to indicate a desire for more stimuli and withdraw when overstimulated. The child also learns how the environment responds to him or her—how soon a cry is responded to, how he or she is spoken with, fed, and touched.

These behaviors are extremely important for they create environmental interactions that help the newborn to define him or herself and the world. Infant development can be facilitated by helping parents to become aware of their newborn's potential for interactions, recognize when their infant is best able to receive stimuli, appreciate the interactive behaviors of the newborn, coordinate their responses with the infant's cycle and state needs, and provide appropriate kinds of feedback to the infant (Affonso, 1976).

Infants' interactions are comprised of three parts: (1) receiving stimuli (sights, sounds, odors, tastes, textures), (2) maintaining stimulation (rooting reflex, grasp reflex, suck reflex), and (3) initiating (gestures, vocalization) stimulation. Some of this information can be offered to the family unobtrusively as part of the daily interaction with them. In the room with the family and the infant, health professionals can speak to the infant, demonstrating both the manner and the appropriateness of doing this. For example, the family can gather information about the seeing and hearing preferences of the infant by observing professionals speaking to the infant about the things he or she is seeing or hearing, or seeing them demonstrate his or her visual following of an object. Helping parents to respond to their infant's cues gives them a greater sense of confidence with the new child and eases their concerns about the many things they have to learn in order to raise this child.

Positive interactions require a recognition by both parties of the reciprocal nature of behaviors. Each member affects the other. Osofsky (1976) looked at the relationship between infant temperament and mother–infant interaction. Although he found that the more alert babies had very responsive mothers, it is not clear whether the mothers' offering of more stimuli created the alert behavior or the alert behavior created the offering of more stimuli. This reciprocity is extremely important. Shea, Klatskin, and Jackson (1952) found that maternal tensions created fussy babies, which increased maternal tensions which, when allowed to persist, often created behavior disorders and maternal deprivation syndromes. Prechtl (1958) suggests that mothers' abilities to anticipate and react to their child's responses can be facilitated by an increase in early contact and care giving.

Gottlieb (1978) has suggested a number of ways to facilitate the discovery and attachment process: First, the provision of information about the interactive capabilities of infants; second, the provision of praise to increase maternal confidence, including the allaying of fears about mothering capabilities and the normalcy of the child; third, personalized mother–infant contact so that the individual needs of the pair can be met and the quality of the time can be maximized; and fourth, as far as possible, provision for the physical well-being of the pair so that pain or discomfort are not distorting the relationship.

Four studies verify the importance of the suggestions of Gottlieb (1978). Reisch (1979), by assessing 30 infants' interactive capacities using the Brazelton assessment scale and interviewing their mothers, determined the maternal perception of her infant's interactive potential. She found that although mothers expected and observed these behaviors they were unaware of the purposeful nature of these behaviors.

Snyder, Eyres, and Barnard (1979), by evaluating 193 mother–child pairs prenatally, early postpartum, and at 1, 4, 8, and 12 months of age (infant), were able to evaluate the relationship between maternal expectations and infant behaviors. They found that many mothers had little prenatal knowledge of their infants' interactive abilities. In addition, they found that those mothers with high prenatal knowledge correlated with the more interactive infants, a correlation that continued in the 4-, 8-, and 12-month evaluations.

Banton (1980) studied the efficacy of providing some information about the interactional capabilities of newborns on early postpartum maternal–infant attachment. The film *The Amazing Newborn* (Health Sciences Communication Center, 1976) was shown to subject mothers, half of whom also participated with the researcher in an individual discussion of newborn capabilities. Observations of mother and infant a day or two later were used to measure interaction. The author found the nursing intervention increased maternal and infant interactive behaviors in a positive fashion. Furthermore, the addition of discussion that served to personalize and provide understanding of the knowledge presented in the film increased the interactive behaviors more than showing the film alone. Although the author does not recommend the general use of this particular film (because of its somewhat technical nature), similar films or group presentations would surely be equally or more effective.

Dean, Morgan, and Towle (1982) designed a program wherein the nurse provided a one-on-one teaching session with parents and their newborn directed solely to an examination of their infant and a discussion of his or her characteristics, including any common variations. The infant's unique ability to interact was also demonstrated as were relevant reflexes. An information sheet geared to their infant was given to the parents at the conclusion of the session. Perhaps the most significant finding was the dramatic reaction of the parents to the session. They responded with a great deal of enthusiasm and did not wish to conclude the session—continuing to explore and talk with their infant.

In addition to providing information about behavioral characteristics to the parents, assessment of the newborn (perhaps using the Brazelton assessment scale, 1973) can provide a guide for planning parent–infant care. Buckner (1983) has clustered infant behavior for evaluation and described nursing interventions appropriate for low-risk and high-risk parent–infant pairs. Helping parents with a "difficult" or hard to care for infant adjust their behaviors and more appropriately plan for the infant's care can make the family adjustment smoother. For example, small for gestational age infants are often characterized by their parents as difficult to live with, unpredictable, and very active (Als et al., 1976). Providing anticipatory guidance, such as suggestions to limit extraneous stimulation during feedings, and ongoing support, can truly help these parents cope in a positive, loving way with this child.

Physical Care of the Infant. Rooming-in or extended visiting of the infant when appropriate for and desired by the family can be helpful to new parents in gaining confidence in their abilities to perform routine care. It also provides them with the opportunity to begin to make decisions about their newborn such as when to feed, how to dress, and how to soothe, while receiving reinforcement of their choices from professionals. This fosters confidence and encourages further role-taking by parents. However, parents should not be made to feel obligated to keep the infant in the room at all times.

Information about the physical care of the infant can be offered both formally and informally. A baby bath demonstration is frequently used on postpartum floors during which many of the physical aspects of the newborn are discussed. It is helpful to explain that touch and interaction with the infant are essential to the infant's organization of learning behaviors and development of trust. If done in a group, the demonstration and comments may stimulate questions and discussion useful to all the mothers present.

Participation by an experienced mother can enhance the group discussion. It is important to emphasize that except for a few things, such as not leaving the baby unattended and not soaking the cord prior to its healing, there is no right or wrong way to bathe a baby and there is a great deal of room for variation in the procedure. Eye contact, smiling, and talking to the baby during the bath can model parenting behaviors as well as elicit attending responses from the infant. The nurse can demonstrate that this is a time to enjoy your baby—it is not an unpleasant chore.

Fathers. There has been an increasing involvement of fathers in child rearing. They have been taking a more active role in the prenatal and birthing process. Most hospitals offer open visiting for fathers but frequently they are not included in the teaching program. Their need for information about their infant and assistance with child care practices is at least as great as the mother's—possibly greater. Many fathers have not had previous experiences with children, nor have they had a role model for this type of fathering. Every effort should be made to facilitate his acquaintance process and prepare him for the role he has chosen. Community groups (such as YMCA or JCC) are beginning to offer father and child "play programs" to provide a support for the importance of the father in parenting. They also offer couple support groups for new parents and for parents with new siblings that help with the adjustment process. Prenatal classes can include special sessions for fathers to discuss their feeling about fatherhood and to learn some fathering skills.

Fathers' involvement in the care of their infants will facilitate bonding (Bills, 1980; Taubenheim, 1981). Including the father in discussions with the mother and scheduling teaching video tapes for his visits will assist him in feeling an equal partner in parenting. Giefer and Nelson (1981) devised a formal program of fathering classes. They used group discussions, lectures, demonstrations, and audiovisual materials to conduct the classes. Fathers brought their child to a common room for the presentations. The program included physical, psychological, and intellectual development and needs of infants with discussions about ways of meeting these needs. An emphasis was placed on the behavioral aspects of the newborn and information on ways to stimulate newborns through play. They also included discussions of fathering. Fathers might also benefit from post-hospital follow-up by telephone or community groups.

Siblings. A sibling's reaction to the new member has direct influences on the infant and indirect influences on the parents (Vestal, 1979). If a sibling has a lot of difficulty adjusting to a new member, the parents will be expending a great deal of time and effort dealing with these problems. Each sibling will bring a unique set of variables to the adjustment of a new addition, such as age, parent's attitudes, family size, personality, and preparation for the change.

Preparing the child for the new member is designed to mitigate the impact of this experience. Prenatal preparation may include involving the child in the planning for the new child, reading topical books, touring the hospital facilities, and group demonstrations (Sweet, 1979) or films about newborns. Some parents include the sibling in the birth process.

Sibling visitation on the postpartum floor is designed to further assist the acquaintance process. Studies by Jordan (1973) and Trause (1978) report that limited sibling visitation (1 or 2 brief visits) had little effect on sibling rivalry behaviors such as sleep disturbances and clinging. Thus, liberal visitation times and facilities for visits can be helpful. The optimal time for each visit can range from 15 minutes to 3 hours, depending on the family and the child. In addition, facilitating visits may prove helpful. Video tapes on infant behavior can be shown. Children, if old enough, may help with diapering and feeding. Most children can be helped to hold a new baby. Puppets or dolls can be used to help children verbalize their reactions to the new baby and possibly dispel misunderstandings. Books designed for children can be very helpful. Gates (1980) has described this use and has included an annotated list of selected readings. These programs can be continued in the community post-discharge.

Special Considerations

Multiparas. Multiparas should not be overlooked in your teaching program. Not only will they provide insights and practical tips for new mothers, but they, too, may have many concerns and questions (Mercer, 1979). Although few of their questions are about infant's physical care, multiparas are interested in infant growth, development, and behavior. Moss (1981) and Grubb (1980) have reported that their major concerns center around family adjustment and sibling response, as well as interest in personal changes and meeting the increasing demands placed on their time by the new member. Groups for multiparas on the postpartum unit can prove very helpful.

Educational Level. Mothers with master's and doctoral degrees have nearly as many concerns as those not completing high school. Moss (1981) points out that nurses sometimes feel intimidated relating to mothers who have more education than they. Self-awareness and problem solving with other nurses, as well as further education, can assist in approaching these mothers with confidence to offer supportive care. A professional woman who has read a great deal may only need more practical information. If she has no familiarity with childbearing and infants, however, a physician, a lawyer, or any professional may need factual as well as practical information. A well-informed mother may only need support. A nurse midwife felt postpartum staff avoided her after the birth of her first child. Her progression into the new parent role was only partially familiar, because previously her knowledge was theoretical. She would have benefited from the opportunity to review her labor and feel support and appreciation for herself and her new infant.

A new mother who is a ninth grade dropout may have much practical experience caring for siblings. Her learning needs are perhaps for some more factual information, as well as for support of her experience.

Older Primipara. The older primipara is often a professional or semi-professional woman who has read widely about her pregnancy and her body. She needs your emotional support and assistance in recognizing her needs as a new mother. Articles such as those of Howley (1981) may prove helpful to the professional in aiding both parents in understanding their situation. They usually have the resources to deal with problems once these are sorted out and identified.

High-risk Families. Parents whose status is high risk, whether related to medical or obstetrical complications, an ill neonate, psychosocial problems such as unstable family/social situations, or lack of finances, require greater tact and skill from you. Dealing with the issues presented and awaiting more auspicious moments to present formal teaching will be helpful. These parents need support and guidance on a continuing basis during the childbearing period. The wide variety of high-risk problems are beyond the scope of this chapter. Some articles specific to high-risk families are included in the supplemental bibliography.

Culture. One needs to be aware of the variations in culture regarding a number of infant care issues. Such practices are too numerous to include in detail here, but those practices common to your area can be considered so that the health of the infant is maintained. This may require considerable discussion with experienced lay people and health care providers in any given locale. See Chapter 2 for further discussion about including an individual's value and cultural orientation in the learning assessment. The supplemental bibliography includes a number of articles related to culture and childbearing.

PREPARING FOR DISCHARGE

Mothers and their families need information about the first few weeks at home. Films such as *Are You Ready for the Postpartum Experience?* (Parenting Pictures, 1975) may be used. It is important to carefully assess the mother's support systems to assure that the family has adequately planned for the needs of all concerned during the first few weeks at home. Arising nightly to feed an infant may deplete a mother more than she expects. Help at home should offer her an opportunity for rest, particularly if there are other small children at home. Are there family, neighbors, or friends who can be called upon to anticipate a mother's need for a nap or a planned meal? If the family is without resources, can some be established? Each mother needs to feel she knows someone to call for help during the first few weeks postpartum. A postpartum telephone call system, either through the in-hospital nurse, nurse practitioner, or some other coordinating system, can be most helpful. An experienced lay mother may be the ideal bridge for the new family. Brown (1982) has described a program of patient teaching and discharge planning used at Mount Carmel Medical Center that used a full-time planning coordinator. They developed a method of providing patient education as a part of the postpartum care plan. It included individualized instruction, group demonstration, and audiovisual presentations. Pre-hospital preparation included the distribution of an orientation manual and in-hospital tours. The use of post-discharge telephone calls by nurses to mothers not only assisted the new family but helped the staff evaluate their program.

Because many parents are distracted and so much material is presented, written materials in the language and reading level of the mother can be helpful. These handouts might include a range of expectations for mothers, physical changes, newborn characteristics (stools, temperature, skin, sleep, eating, behavior), and suggested reading and sources of help in the community. For breast-feeding mothers there might be a page on breast and nipple care, and for bottle-feeding mothers, one on engorgement and formula preparation. Each mother could also receive a page with concerns requiring notification of the health care provider and the name and number to call. If the postpartum unit offers telephone consultation, that number could be provided. Developing written materials for different cultures and languages can be accomplished using nurses and lay people in the community. Materials from other communities may be adapted to fit the needs in a local area.

A library containing various helpful lay literature may be maintained by prenatal and in-hospital nurses for perusal by client families. Nurses might find it helpful to use the article by Meier and Mead (1978) for suggestions of resource books for the library as well as for recommending to parents who wish to purchase books of their own. The early months of the *Growing Child* series, a few books on breast feeding, and parenting magazines and books comprise a good beginning library. A more complete list of books and magazines is included in the supplementary bibliography.

Car Seats. It has long been a practice when discharging a mother and infant to help the mother into the car and place the infant in her arms. Thus, health care professionals give tacit dismissal to the importance of car seat use. If infants are properly restrained approximately 90 percent of the deaths and 70 percent of the injuries due to automobile accidents could be avoided. Additionally, car restraints keep the child still and thus less distracting to the driver, reduce injury from noncrash events, and reduce motion sickness. Some states now mandate the use of infant car seats.

A study by Goebel, Copps, and Sulayman (1984) found that a postpartum car seat education program did not significantly increase the procurement or use of infant car seats. A prenatal program may be of more use in this regard. Parents may need assistance in choosing and obtaining a car seat prior to hospitalization (see supplemental bibliography). Local communities may have infant car seat loan programs through the health department or voluntary service organizations. Physicians may write a prescription for a car seat prior to discharge so that the cost of the seat may be deducted. A return program may be initiated whereby the seat is donated when no longer needed and a charitable deduction may be taken.

As reported in *Physicians Journal Update* (Dec. 28, 1983), the Verdugo Hills Hospital in Southern California has begun a program to help parents use car seats while offering positive reinforcement for their use. Each mother on a day prior to discharge is shown how to place her infant in the car seat. On the day of discharge the mother buckles her baby into the car seat and then carries baby and seat on her lap to the car. The nurse then shows the family how to properly secure the seat in the car. Since the advent of the program, 98 percent of infants are discharged in a car seat.

THE POST-HOSPITAL PERIOD

Postpartum concerns at 1 week (Bull, 1981) and at 1 month (Gruis, 1977) have been studied. Women asked about themselves, return of their figures, and their emotional needs, particularly fatigue. They had questions about infant behavior patterns. Multiparas wondered how they could meet the needs of their families and how to incorporate the infant into the family. Some anticipatory guidance can be given in the hospital. The new mother who says to her postpartum nurse "I wish I could take you home with me" is expressing her wish for an experienced guide to help her master what she needs to know as unfamiliar situations arise in her new role. She needs someone she can feel comfortable calling on to validate her knowledge or help her see alternate solutions to problems. She is motivated and in a state of readiness for the health teaching described in Chapter 2.

Postpartum Telephone Calls. The most appropriate help for the postpartum mother following discharge would be several home visits; because, however, this is not usually practicable, alternatives need to be found. Far too often postpartum families are abandoned until the pediatric or obstetric office visit. This is unfortunate for these 2 to 4 weeks are often the time of greatest need (Sumner & Fritsch, 1977). Postpartum telephone calls (Haight, 1977) fill this need well when provided through a carefully planned program and by a person familiar to the family, for instance the hospital postpartum nurse. This is optimal if available 24 hours a day with appropriate support. To provide this care, staff in-services are needed, to insure staff confidence and consistency of information as well as to validate competency to medical colleagues. In-service content includes routine newborn care (Vanderzanden, 1979), normal postpartum obstetrical care, and breast-feeding, as well as skills for eliciting and recognizing problems that might require immediate assistance, and familiarity with community resources and the care programs of local care providers. Two helpful guides are described by Marecki (1979) and Donaldson (1981). An evaluation of such a program is described by Rhode and Groenjes-Finke (1980).

Most parents will use such a service a great deal at first and will taper off rapidly as questions are answered and anxieties are allayed and as they establish a relationship with their infant's care providers. Telephone support often leads to the initial asking of a greater number of questions that benefits the family and encourages participation in their health care.

Each new family will receive a great deal of advice about caring for the mother and the baby. Some of it will be excellent and practical, some will not. New families need help in sorting out this advice and bearing up under the onslaught of well-meaning but sometimes conflicting advice. It may be helpful for a new mother to discuss the matter with her health care professional.

Post-hospital Groups. Post-discharge parenting groups are not generally successful unless community-based. It is difficult for a new mother to get herself and her infant out to a group when there are so many demands on her time and energy. Evening groups to include fathers are sometimes difficult to time to fit around meal times. The press of economics and the desire of many women to return promptly to work further reduces the usefulness of this tool. Many churches and community groups offer some type of parenting support groups. Nursing involvement in such groups is important. Balik and Foley (1981) offer a theoretical basis for such groups and reiterate the importance of meeting the needs of the parents rather than nursing or general objectives, however well-intentioned. Nurses can organize lay groups of experienced mothers and fathers who can provide telephone support to new parents much as La Leche League provides support for breast-feeding mothers. Cooksey and Goetting (1982) reported the development of a successful neighborhood lay group in St. Louis. In addition to support groups, this organization also published a newsletter that provided information about programs and community resources. Such support has proved effective in relieving anxiety and promoting successful parenting.

The Working Mother. Encourage the mother who plans to return to work soon after childbirth to anticipate how she will manage a dual role. Sharing her feelings about motherhood and work with other working mothers rather than with relatives, neighbors, and friends who disapprove of combining these roles, can lessen her vulnerability to negative opinions (Hardin & Sherrett, 1981).

Ash (1980) recommends strategies to help working parents become more effective and confident. Some women may be able to plan with their employers a work schedule that allows them to continue breast-feeding or to pump their breasts during the work day.

EVALUATION

Evaluating an educational program for postpartum parents presents an equal challenge to the one of developing and teaching the program. Postpartum mothers in the hospital present the most convenient population for evaluation techniques. This may prove a good time to evaluate prenatal programs in terms of satisfaction and competency of birth preparation. It is, however, not a good time to examine the effectiveness of postpartum teaching. There are two reasons. First, much of the teaching is not completed at this time. Second, the family experiences, which can help to indicate whether or not the program is successful, have not yet occurred. In-hospital examination can only provide information on the short-term retention of material provided and patient reaction to teaching methods.

There are several ways of evaluating a postpartum program. Sophisticated evaluation of the program can be accomplished by looking at outcomes. For example, breast-feeding programs might be evaluated by looking at the success (length of time breast-feeding, etc.) of breast-feeding pairs. Infant care might be looked at by examining the appropriateness of calls to the care provider and/or the appropriateness of emergency room use during the first 6 weeks postpartum. Infant interaction can be evaluated by looking at maternal–infant interactions 3 or 6 weeks postpartum. These are the most helpful evaluations but the most difficult to accomplish.

Formal questionnaires may be useful. Filshie and colleagues (1981) have described such an evaluation. The timing of the questionnaires might be 2, 4, and 6 weeks postpartum. They could be mailed to the families or proffered during an office visit or done as part of a home visit. Such a questionnaire should evaluate both the recall of information and the usefulness of that information to the family. Specific questions need to be asked. A family may report themselves as eminently satisfied with the care they received, but actually be enduring great postpartum difficulties in some areas because they did not expect their care providers to assist them in those areas. Additional open ended questions can be very enlightening but are of limited usefulness. To be helpful, responses require either precision timing, asking the question right in the midst of a specific difficulty, or a very astute and articulate respondent. Formulating such questionnaires and getting an adequate response is not easy. It may prove easier to periodically evaluate small portions of the program.

A less precise but nevertheless useful method of evaluation is the use of logs of postpartum telephone calls (and/or home visits). Monthly tallies of questions asked, problems raised, and so on, give everyone an idea of whether the program is effective and underscore areas for further work. Frequent discussions among care providers and community parenting resource groups can also aid in evaluating an educational program. An open and vibrant communication may be the most economical way to discover how the program is doing and what needs to be adjusted.

CONCLUSION

Client education in the unique situation of the postpartum period offers you a challenge. Ideally a program should begin during pregnancy and continue through the new family's first year. The health care provider's skill can help a new family pull together the vast amount of information they need to take on new roles and responsibilities and cope with rapid physical and emotional change. We are still searching for the ideal coordinated, creative response to the educational needs of the developing family in the months of the postpartum period. By assessment and planning, professionals can provide an environment and identify resources to support new mothers and their families.

BIBLIOGRAPHY

Affonso, D. Missing pieces—A study of postpartum feelings. *Birth and the Family Journal,* 1977, *4*(4), 159–164.

Affonso, D. The newborn's potential for interaction. *JOGN–Nursing,* 1976, *5*(6), 9–14.

Als, J., Tronick, E., Adamson, L., & Brazelton, T. The behavior of the full-term but underweight newborn infant. *Developmental Medicine and Child Neurology,* 1976, *18*, 590–602.

Ash, M. J. Working and parenting: Can we do both? *Issues in Health Care of Women,* 1980, *2*, 15–23.

Avery, M. D., Fournier, L. C., Jones, P. L., & Sipovic, C. P. An early postpartum hospital discharge program. *JOGN–Nursing,* 1982, *11*, 233–235.

Balik, B., & Foley, M. K. Developing a community-based parent education support group. *JOGN–Nursing,* 1981, *10*, 197–199.

Banton, M. *Maternal–infant attachment: Evaluation of an early postpartum nursing intervention.* Unpublished Master's thesis, University of Rochester, 1980.

Bills, B. J. Enhancement of paternal–newborn affectional bonds. *Journal of Nurse-Midwifery,* 1980, *25*(5), 21–26.

Brazelton, T. B. Neonatal behavioral assessment scale. *Clinics in Development Medicine,* 1973, *50*.

Brown, B. Maternity–patient teaching—A nursing priority. *JOGN–Nursing,* 1982, *11*, 11–14.

Brown, M. S., O'Meara, C., & Krowley, S. The maternal–child nurse practitioner. *American Journal of Nursing,* 1975, *75*, 1298–1299.

Buckner, E. Use of Brazelton neonatal behavioral assessment in planning care for parents and newborns. *JOGN–Nursing,* 1983, *12*, 26–30.

Bull, M. J. Change in concerns of first-time mothers after one week at home. *JOGN–Nursing,* 1981, *10*, 391–394.

Carr, K., & Walton, V. Early postpartum discharge. *JOGN–Nursing,* 1982, *11*, 29–30.

Chao, Y. M. Cognitive operations during maternal role enactment. *Maternal–Child Nursing Journal,* 1979, *8*, 211–274.

Cooksey, N., & Goetting, T. An open school for parents. *JOGN–Nursing,* 1982, *11*, 117–120.

Croog, E. H., & Zigrossi, S. T. Parenting luncheons on the postpartum unit. *MCN,* 1983, *8*, 277–279.

Dean, P. G., Morgan, P., & Towle, J. M. Making baby's acquaintance: A unique attachment strategy. *MCN,* 1982, *7*, 37–41.

deChateau, P., & Wilberg, B. Longterm effect on mother–infant behavior of extra contact during the first hour postpartum. *Acta Paediatric Scandanavia,* 1977, *66*, 145–149.

Dickson, M. Community hospital-based obstetrical primary nursing. *JOGN–Nursing,* 1982, *11*, 292–295.

Donaldson, N. E. The postpartum follow-up nurse clinician. *JOGN–Nursing,* 1981, *10*, 249–254.

Dunn, D. M., & White, D. G. Interactions of mothers with their newborns in the first half-hour of life. *Journal of Advanced Nursing,* 1981, *6*, 271–275.

Family centered care for mothers and newborns at home. Rochester, New York: Home Care Association, 1981. (Pamphlet.)

Filshie, S., Williams, J., Osbourn, M., Senior, D., Symonds, E., & Backett, E. Post-natal care in hospital—Time for change. *International Journal of Nursing Studies,* 1981, *18*(2), 89–95.

Fomon, S. J., Filer, L. J., Anderson, T. A., & Ziegler, E. E. Recommendations for feeding normal infants. *Pediatrics,* 1979, *63*(1), 52–59.

Gates, S. Children's literature: It can help children cope with sibling rivalry. *MCN,* 1980, *5*, 351–352.

Giefer, M. A., & Nelson, C. A method of help new fathers develop parenting skills. *JOGN–Nursing*, 1981, *10*, 455–458.

Goebel, J. B., Copps, T. J., & Sulayman, F. Infant car seat usage: Effectiveness of a postpartum program. *JOGN–Nursing*, 1984, *13*, 33–35.

Gottlieb, L. Maternal attachment in primiparas. *JOGN–Nursing*, 1978, *7*(1), 39–45.

Growing child. Dunn and Hargitt, Inc., 22 N. Second Street, Lafayette, IN 47902.

Gruis, M. Beyond maternity: Post-partum concerns of mothers. *MCN*, 1977, *2*, 182–188.

Grubb, C. A. Perception of time by multiparous women in relation to themselves and others during the first postpartal month. *Maternal–Child Nursing Journal Monograph 10*, 1980, 225–320.

Haight, J. Steadying parents as they go—by phone. *MCN*, 1977, *2*(5), 182–185.

Hall, L. A. Effect of teaching on primiparas' perceptions of their newborn. *Nursing Research*, 1980, *29*(5), 317–321.

Hames, C. T. Sexual needs and interests of postpartum couples. *JOGN–Nursing*, 1980, *9*, 313–315.

Hardin, B., & Sherrett, K. Counseling working mothers. *Journal of Nurse-Midwifery*, 1981, *26*(4), 19–25.

Health Sciences Communication Center. *The amazing newborn*. Cleveland: Case Western Reserve University, 1976. (Film).

Howley, C. The older primipara. *JOGN–Nursing*, 1981, *10*, 182–185.

Inglis, T. Postpartum sexuality. *JOGN–Nursing*, 1980, *9*, 298–300.

Jennings, B., & Edmundson, M. The postpartum period: After confinement, the fourth trimester. *Clinical Obstetrics and Gynecology*, 1980, *23*, 1093–1103.

Jordan, A. Evaluation of a family-centered maternity care program, Part II: Ancillary findings and parents' comments. *JOGN–Nursing*, 1973, *2*(2), 15–27.

Kilker, R., & Wilkerson, B. Assessment. *Nursing '73*, 1973, *3*(5), 56.

Klaus, M. H., & Kennell, J. H. *Maternal infant bonding*. St. Louis, Mo.: C. V. Mosby, 1976.

Kraus, N. Postpartum hospital visits for children. *Issues in Health Care of Women*, 1979, *1*(4), 29–39.

LeMasters, E. Parenthood as crisis. In H. J. Parad (Ed.), *Crisis intervention: Selected readings*. New York: Family Service Associations of America, 1965.

Martell, L. K., & Mitchell, S. K. Rubin's "Puerperal change" reconsidered. *JOGN–Nursing*, 1984, *13*, 145–149.

Marecki, M. P. Postpartum follow-up goals and assessment. *JOGN–Nursing*, 1979, *8*, 214–218.

Meier, P. P., & Mead, L. P. A nurse's guide to "how to parent" manuals. *JOGN–Nursing*, 1978, *7*, 46–52.

Mercer, R. T. The nurse and maternal tasks of early postpartum. *MCN*, 1981, *8*, 341–345.

Mercer, R. T. She's a multip . . . she knows the ropes. MCN, 1979, *4*, 301–304.

Moss, J. R. Concerns of multiparas on the third postpartum day. *JOGN–Nursing*, 1981, *10*, 421–424.

Osofsky, J. D. Neonatal characteristics and mother–infant interaction in two observational situations. *Child Development*, 1976, *47*, 1138–1147.

Overton, B. *Pediatric phone call study*. Project done while R.W.J. Faculty Fellow, University of Rochester, 1981–82.

Parenting Pictures. *Are you ready for the post partum experience?* RD1, Box 355 B, Columbia, NJ, 07832. (Film).

Petrick, J. M. Postpartum depression. *JOGN–Nursing*, 1984, *13*, 37–40.

Prechtl, H. The directed head turning response and allied movements of the newborn. *Behavior*, 1958, *13*, 212–242.

Rhode, M. A., & Groenjes-Finke, J. M. Evaluation of nurse-initated telephone calls to postpartum women. *Issues in Health Care of Women*, 1980, *2*(2), 23–41.

Reisch, S. Enhancement of mother–infant social interaction. *JOGN–Nursing*, 1979, *8*, 242–246.

Rossi, A. S. Transition to parenthood. In A. Skolnick & J. H. Skolnick (Eds.), *Family in transition*. Boston: Little, Brown, 1980.

Rubin, R. *Maternal identity and the maternal experience*. New York: Springer, 1984.

Rubin, R. Binding-in in the postpartum period. *Maternal–Child Nursing Journal*, 1977, *6*, 67–75.

Rubin, R. Basic maternal behavior. *Nursing Outlook*, 1961a, *9*(11), 683–686.

Rubin, R. Puerperal change. *Nursing Outlook*, 1961b, *9*(12), 753–755.

Scupholme, A. Postpartum early discharge: An inner city experience. *Journal of Nurse–Midwifery*, 1981, *26*(6), 19–22.

Shaffer, H. R. Early interactive development. In H. R. Shaffer (Ed.), *Studies in mother–infant interaction*. London: Academic Press, 1977.

Shea, N., Klatskin, E., & Jackson, E. Home adjustment of rooming-in mothers and non-rooming-in mothers. *American Journal of Nursing*, 1952, *52*, 65–72.

Snyder, C., Eyres, S. J., & Barnard, K. New findings about mothers' antenatal expectations and their relationship to infant development. *MCN*, 1979, *4*, 354–357.

Sumner, G., & Fritsch, J. Postnatal parental concerns: The first 6 weeks of life. *JOGN–Nursing*, 1977, *6*(3), 182–185.

Sweet, P. T. Prenatal classes especially for children. *MCN*, 1979, *4*, 82.

Taubenheim, A. M. Paternal–infant bonding in the first-time father. *JOGN–Nursing*, 1981, *10*, 261–264.

Trause, M. A. A birth in the hospital: The effect on the sibling. *Birth and the Family Journal*, 1978, *5*(4), 207–210.

Vanderzanden, E. C. Anticipatory guidance for the first two months of life. *Journal of Nurse–Midwifery*, 1979, *24*(5), 28–34.

Vestal, K. W. Siblings: Adapting to accommodate the neonate. *Issues in Health Care of Women*, 1979, *1*(4), 15–25.

SUPPLEMENTAL BIBLIOGRAPHY

Adolescents

Mercer, R. T. Teenage motherhood: The first year. *JOGN–Nursing*, 1980, *9*, 16–27.

Tankson, E. A. The adolescent parent: One approach to teaching child care and giving support. *JOGN–Nursing*, 1976, *5*, 9–15.

Audiovisual Sources

American College of Obstetricians and Gynecologists Film and Video Service. P.O. Box 299, Wheaton, IL 60187.

Martin, E. J. Annotated film bibliography. *Journal of Nurse–Midwifery*, 1979, *24*(6), 9–17.

Multimedia Programs for Health Care and Nursing Education. Career Aids, Inc., 8950 Lurline Ave., Dept. N9, Chatsworth, CA 91311.

NAACOG Continuing Education Catalog Patient Information Booklets, One East Wacker Drive, Suite 2700, Chicago, IL 60601.

National Foundation of the March of Dimes. Box 2000, White Plains, NY 10602.

NLN Publications Catalogue. 10 Columbus Circle, New York, NY 10019.

Polymorph Films. 118 South St., Boston, MA 02111.

Publications and Teaching Aids. Maternity Center Association, 48 East 92nd St., New York, NY 10028.

Pyle, M. M. Life Circle. 2378 Cornell Drive, Costa Mesa, CA 92626.

Breast–feeding

Cadwell, K. Improving nipple graspability for success at breastfeeding. *JOGN–Nursing*, 1981, *10*, 277–279.

Eiger, M. S., & Olds, S. W. *The complete book of breastfeeding*. New York: Bantam Books, 1972.

Hervada, A. R., Feit, E., & Sagraves, R. Drugs in breastmilk. *Prenatal Care*, 1978, *2*(8), 19–25.

La Leche League International. *The womanly art of breastfeeding*. Franklin Park, Ill.: Interstate Printers and Publishers, 1977.

Lawrence, R. A. *Breastfeeding—A guide for the medical profession*. St. Louis, Mo.: C. V. Mosby, 1980.

Nichols, M. G. Effective help for the nursing mother. *JOGN–Nursing*, 1978, *7*(2), 22–30.

Pryor, K. *Nursing your baby*. New York: Pocket Books, 1973.

Riordan, J., & Countryman, B. A. Basics of breastfeeding. *JOGN–Nursing*, 1980, *9*, 207–210, 210–213, 273–277, 277–283, 357–361, 361–366.

Tibbetts, E., & Cadwell, K. Selecting the right breast pump. *MCN*, 1980, *5*, 262–264.

Whitley, N. Preparation for breastfeeding. *JOGN–Nursing*, 1978, *7*, 44–48.

Car Seats

Child safety seats. *Consumer Reports*, 1982, *47*, 171–176.

Krozy, R. E., & McColgan, J. J. Auto safety, pregnancy and the newborn. *JOGN–Nursing*, 1985, *14*(1), 11–15.

Culture

Bampton, B., Jones, J., & Mancini, J. Initial mothering patterns of low-income black primiparas. *JOGN–Nursing*, 1981, *10*, 174–178.

Bush, D. M. Jewish religious practices related to childbearing. *Journal of Nurse–Midwifery*, 1980, *25*, 5, 39–42.

Dempsey, P. A., & Geese, T. The childbearing Haitian refugees—Cultural applications to clinical nursing. *Public Health Report*, 1983, *98*, 261–267.

Grosso, C., Barden, M., Henry, C., & Vieau, M. G. The Vietnamese American family . . . and grandma makes three. *MCN*, 1981, *6*, 177–180.

Hautman, M. A. Folk health and illness beliefs. *Nurse Practitioner*, 1979, *4*, 23–34.

Meleis, A. I., & Sorrell, L. Arab American women and their birth experiences. *MCN*, 1981, *6*, 171–176.

Satz, K. Integrating tradition into maternal–child nursing. *Image*, 1982, *14*(3), 89–91.

Slevin, K. F. Motherhood, culture, and change. *Pediatric Nursing*, 1982, *8*, 403, 405–409.

Stern, P. N., Tilden, V. P., & Maxwell, E. K. Culturally-induced stress during childbearing: The Philipino-American experience. *Issues in Health Care of Women*, 1980, *2*, 67–81.

Thomas, R. G., & Tumminia, P. A. Maternity care for Vietnamese in America. *Birth*, 1982, *9*(3), 187–190.

Wadd, L. Vietnamese postpartum practices. *JOGN–Nursing*, 1983, *12*(4), 252–258.

Zepeda, M. Selected maternal–infant care practices of Spanish-speaking women. *JOGN–Nursing*, 1982, *11*(6), 371–374.

Reinhard, S. C. Nursing responsibility in infant car safety. *The American Journal of Maternal–Child Nursing*, 1980, *5*, 64–66.

Evaluation

Adom, D., & Wright, A. S. Dissonance in nurse and patient evaluations of the effectiveness of a patient-teaching program. *Nursing Outlook*, 1982, *29*, 132–136.

Gardner, S. L. Mothering the unconscious conflict between nurses and new mothers. *Keeping Abreast Journal of Human Nurturing*, July-September 1978, *3*, 193–200.

Fathering

Becoming a father. Cincinnati, Ohio: Procter & Gamble, 1979.

Hangsleben, K. L. Transition to fatherhood: Literature review. *Issues in Health Care of Women*, 1980, *2*, 81–97.

High Risk Families

Baker, M. H. When the Down's syndrome baby is yours. *RN*, 1977, *40*(7), 67–70.

Cordell, A. S., & Apolito, R. Family support in infant death. *JOGN–Nursing*, 1981, *10*, 281–285.

Devaney, S. W., & Lavery, S. F. Nursing care for the relinquishing mother. *JOGN–Nursing*, 1980, *9*, 375–378.

Iyer, P. My baby was premature. *JOGN–Nursing*, 1981, *10*, 304–307.

Varner, B., Ossenkop, D., & Lyon, J. Prematures, too, need rooming in and care-by-parent programs. *American Journal of Maternal Child Nursing*, 1980, *5*, 431–432.

Wong, D. L. Bereavement: The empty-mother syndrome. *MCN*, 1980, *5*, 385–390.

Wooten, B. Death of an infant. *MCN*, 1981, *6*, 257–260.

Parenting

Brazelton, T. B. *Infants and mothers*. New York: Dell, 1979.

Caplan, F. (Ed.). *The first twelve months of life*. New York: Grosset & Dunlap, 1981.

Consumer Guide. *The complete baby book*. New York: Simon & Schuster, 1979.

Fraiberg, S. *The magic years*. New York: Charles Scribner's Sons, 1959.

Korner, A. J. The effect of the infant on the caregiver. In M. Lewis & L. A. Rosenbloom (Eds.), *The effect of the infant on its caregiver*. New York: John Wiley & Sons, 1974.

Shereshefsky, P. M., & Yarrow, L. J. *Psychological aspects of a first pregnancy and early postnatal adaptations*. New York: Raven Press, 1973.

Stern, D. N. Mother and infant at play. In M. Lewis & L. A. Rosenbloom (Eds.), *The effect of the infant on its caregiver*. New York: John Wiley & Sons, 1974.

Spock, B. *Baby and child care* (rev.). New York: Pocket Books, 1976.

The Middle Years Woman: Education for Health Promotion and Maintenance

14

Barbara N. Adams

Change of life, the common term used for menopause, provides an apt description of the middle years woman. Historically, it has not necessarily been seen as a positive change for women in our culture. For example, the nineteenth century, upper class, middle years woman was seen as one who had used up her "energy stores" with childbearing and childrearing and was "put out to pasture" so to speak. She was often considered to be an invalid without a vital role in family and community functioning. A stereotype of the middle years woman as a bedraggled, irritable, ineffective person evolved and is still portrayed in media advertisements and, unfortunately, held as true by many women and men alike.

A changing life can be a positive, rewarding experience for women in their middle years. Although there are a multitude of physical, psychosocial, developmental, and environmental alterations that occur during this period, it can also be seen as a time of freedom from the burden of the maternal role, an opportunity for personal growth and pursuit of a professional career, and the chance to do "all those things there was never time to do before."

It is the premise of many health care professionals that anticipatory guidance for the middle years can prevent a "mid-life crisis" and prepare women for health maintenance, illness prevention, and coping with problems as they occur (Gelein & Heiple, 1981). With increased knowledge middle years women will be able to make informed choices about their health and their attitude toward the aging process itself may be enhanced. Women will be better able to maintain or gain self-determination and control over their lives.

Hence, the reason for this chapter, to provide the health care professional with the tools to prepare women for their middle years experiences. Included are sections on assessment of learning needs, content areas, methodologies, and evaluation.

Assessment of Learning Needs

When should anticipatory guidance begin for the middle years woman? This author suggests the age range of 35 to 40 as being most appropriate. However, as health care providers we must be alert to discreet signals, questions, and comments made by a woman of any age that are indicative of her readiness to learn about her future aging process.

Given this age guideline, how does one begin? General variables affecting learning such as age, sex, culture, health–illness values, and health status have been discussed by Littlefield in Chapter 2 and should be considered first in making an assessment of learning needs. Other areas needing assessment that were addressed in the same chapter are readiness for learning, anxiety, and resources available to the client and the family. These, as well as several other factors particular to the middle years, are important to evaluate before information is given or discussion begun. Table 14–1 lists assessment areas with sample questions that the interviewer may use to obtain needed information.

Content Areas

As with each developmental stage the learning needs of the middle years woman are great if the woman is to be viewed in a holistic sense. Ideally, teaching–learning would include all the physiological, psychosocial, and developmental changes included in this section to promote total health, adaptation, and growth. However, it must be remembered that the scope and depth of education provided for each middle years woman must be based on the assessment already made. The individual woman's needs are those that are to be met.

Definitions. Traditionally, the word climacteric (from the Greek word meaning "rung of the ladder") has been used to define the middle years. It refers to the physiological changes that occur for women generally between the ages of 40 and 60 and includes that period of time from the occurrence of the first menstrual irregularities until after cessation of menses. It is often divided into three phases: premenopausal, menopausal, and postmenopausal. Menopause itself, or the end of menses, is considered complete when there has been an absence of menstruation for 1 year. The average age of menopause for women in the United States is 51 years (Gelein & Heiple, 1981).

The middle years is a relatively new term developmentally encompassing those adult years when childbearing is usually completed and continuing until the aging phase, generally coinciding with the climacteric and the ages of 40 to 60. It describes this age as a stage of transition, certainly including the menstrual changes that occur, but also considering that period of time when other physiological and psychosocial changes take place. It describes a life stage unto its own.

Physiology of Menopause. In menopause, a decrease in follicular maturation and formation of the corpus luteum in the ovary occurs causing ovulation to become irregular, less frequent, and finally ceasing. This results first in a disturbance of the cyclic estrogen and progesterone production from the ovary and finally in the cessation of menses due to lack of sufficient estrogen to stimulate endometrial growth. The ovaries, in many women, continue to produce estrogen in small amounts for several years, but the main source of estrogen after menopause is the conversion of circulating androstenedione from the adrenals into estrone (Green 1977; Martin, 1978).

At the same time, the pituitary loses the "braking effect" of estrogens, becomes overactive, and produces high levels of follicle stimulating hormone (FSH) and luteinizing hormone (LH) (FSH is maintained at a higher level than LH). This increase in gonadotropins remains into old age, when the body eventually adjusts to the new levels.

Physical Changes. Numerous symptoms experienced by women in their middle years as well as signs of aging have been attributed to estrogen decline. It is well recognized that this decline can have systemic effects and a direct relationship has been found to exist

TABLE 14–1. LEARNING NEEDS ASSESSMENT

	Sample Questions
Assessment Area	
Knowledge	Have you heard about a life stage called menopause or middle years? Tell me what you know about it.
Learning style	Where have you obtained this information you've been telling me about?
Readiness	Some people like to be prepared for things that will be happening to them, such as childbirth or parenting; others do not. How do you feel about this?
Attitude	What do you think it will be like for you to enter your forties and fifties? What have you heard or read that concerns you? What things do you see for yourself and family as you enter your middle years related to your physical, emotional, environmental relationship with others?
Prior experience	What has middle years been like for others you know?
Sense of control	Are you a person who likes to take charge of your life or do you like others to do this for you? What differences do you see your middle years making in this?
Goals for self	Where do you see yourself 10 years from now and what will you be doing?
Coping strategies	What things have happened in your life that have been stressful? When you feel stressed what do you do?
Support systems	With whom do you like to share your happiness, your sadness, your pleasures and problems?
Possible deterrents	
Stereotypes	When you have seen women in their forties and fifties on TV or in pictures in magazines, how have they looked to you? How do you think you will look and act compared to them?
Culture	What has menopause been like for members of your family? As a member of (name of culture), menopause and the middle years may have special meaning for you. Can you tell me things I should know about this?
Time and financial constrictions	You seem like a busy woman. Can you tell me what time you would like to give to learn more about your middle years? Discuss cost of individual or group sessions with adjustments that can be made within constraints of agency or practice.

between a decrease in estrogen and two common problems associated with the middle years: vasomotor instability and vaginal atrophy. Osteoporosis in the aging woman has also been attributed to decreasing estrogens but this has not been proven conclusively in light of other factors involved. The physical changes of the middle years and their relationship to the signs and symptoms reported by many women are discussed here.

Vasomotor Instability. The most commonly noted change related to the vasomotor system is the "hot flash" phenomenon. It is caused by the disequilibrium of the hypothalamic–pituitary–ovarian axis that affects the autonomic nervous system causing dilation of the cutaneous blood vessels (McCarter, 1982). Hot flashes are experienced as a sensation of warmth usually beginning at the waist and spreading to the neck, face, and arms, are associated with flushing and perspiring, and sometimes are followed by chills. Because they often occur at night, sleep disturbances are common. Not only is the woman awakened by hot flashes but she may need to change drenched pajamas and bedding and has difficulty returning to sleep. Hot flashes last from a few seconds to a minute and may occur a few times a day or several times an hour. They tend to be provoked by emotional stress, exercise, heavy clothing, sexual excitement, illness, alcohol, and eating, in other words by heat-generating activities. It is estimated that between two-thirds and three-quarters of all women experience hot flashes, which often begin a year or so before menopause and usually continue from 1 to 5 years thereafter. They end when the woman's body adjusts to its new levels of estrogen and gonadotropins.

Women's response to this vasomotor symptom is variable. Although 10 to 20 percent of women have symptoms severe enough to seek treatment, many are able to cope when they understand the normalcy of the changes and the nature of their spontaneous cessation (McCarter, 1982).

Menstrual Changes and the Genital Tract. As the hormonal relationships within the hypothalamic–pituitary–ovarian axis begin to fluctuate, menstrual patterns change. Menses become irregular with their pattern often changing from month to month as the levels of estrogen and progesterone vary. When estrogen levels are low, ovulation does not occur, progesterone levels remain low, the endometrium is thin, and a scantier period results. At other times the endometrium is hyperstimulated with prolonged estrogen, no ovulation occurs without the peaks of estrogen and pituitary LH, low progesterone levels are maintained, and women experience heavier, longer periods. At times regular periods will occur because of normal ovarian function. Eventually, sometimes 5 years or more after irregular menses begins, ovarian function diminishes to the point where in each cycle estrogen levels are low and menstrual periods are scant and infrequent. When ovarian function ceases, menses end and the menopausal period has begun.

Excessive bleeding or intermenstrual spotting must be watched carefully throughout the middle years because of the increased risk of endometrial cancer in this age group. Careful recording of bleeding patterns by women themselves can help health care providers determine the need for further investigation.

Structural, as well as functional, changes in the genital tract begin in the premenopausal period. There is a gradual decrease in size as well as function of the ovaries. Major changes in the entire reproductive system, however, occur when menopause is complete and estrogen levels are permanently low.

Within the vulva, the labia majora and the labia minora become flatter as subcutaneous fat decreases. Pubic hair thins. The vagina has several changes. The loss of estrogen causes the epithelium to thin and become less elastic while the rugae disappear. Less cervical secretion and a decrease in vascularity leads to an increase in dryness of the vagina. The pH of the vaginal secretions becomes more alkaline. Atrophic vaginitis (irritation of the vagina, susceptibility to infection and dysparunia) is often a concern to postmenopausal women because of these changes (Gelein & Heiple, 1981).

The supporting tissue of the pelvis also loses tone or atrophies. The organs of the pelvis, uterus, bladder, and rectum can then be displaced, leading to a cystocele, a rectocele, or a uterine prolapse. The uterus as well as the ovaries diminish in size after menopause.

Breast and Skin. With the wide fluctuations in hormonal levels there are times when the premenopausal woman experiences high peaks of estrogen. This can result in engorged and painful breasts. She may also note an increase in breast size because of the increase in subcutaneous fat. The postmenopausal woman, however, will find that her breasts tend to sag or become pendulous as the subcutaneous fat atrophies and loses elasticity (Gelein & Heiple, 1981).

The decrease in estrogen has an overall effect on skin and muscle contributing to a loss of elasticity and diminished muscle strength. In particular, women note more wrinkles and lines in facial skin and sagging of tissue in the upper arms.

Musculoskeletal. Osteoporosis is a serious disorder in part attributed to estrogen decline. Twenty-five percent of those women within 10 years past menopause will experience fractures as a result of osteoporosis. The most common sites are the vertebrae, with hip or wrist fractures often occurring after falls. The role estrogen plays with bone is to stabilize bone formation and resorption; with estrogen decline there is increased resorption of bone resulting in decreased mass (Martin, 1978).

Calcium deficiency has been identified as a contributing factor in the development of osteoporosis (Heaney et al., 1982). Many older women have a lower intake of calcium and they are less able to absorb it from the intestine. It was also thought that the high intake of phosphorus common in the American diet (processed foods, excessive bread, meat, soft drinks) negatively influenced calcium balance (Gelein & Heiple, 1981). Recent research, however, shows no direct evidence of deterioration in calcium balance of bone loss when high phosphorus diets are ingested (Heaney et al., 1982; Spencer, Kramer, & Osis, 1982). It appears that bone loss can be retarded with an intake of 1000 mg of calcium per day for all adult women and 1500 mg per day for postmenopausal women (Heaney et al., 1982). This intake can be achieved through dietary sources and/or supplements. Calcium supplementation risks are low. Soft tissue calcification is rare and renal stone formation can be avoided with adequate fluid intake (Whedon, 1981).

The high protein American diet contributes to the loss of calcium from the bone because calcium is needed to buffer the increased acid the kidneys must excrete. Fluoride and vitamin D are also important in the maintenance of bone density.

Exercise is the final factor that needs to be considered in the development of osteoporosis. Those individuals who exercise regularly throughout their lives are known to have a decreased incidence of this disorder. The rationale for this is the fact that the more bone is used the more calcium is deposited and density increased. Regular exercise may also increase muscle and ligament strength relieving some of the aches and stiffness noted by postmenopausal women. Improvement of circulation, weight maintenance, and an increase in self-esteem are other benefits of exercise (Gelein & Heiple, 1981). A sedentary life for the middle years woman is ill advised.

Diet and Exercise Changes. Obesity is not caused by menopause but is a problem seen frequently for the middle years woman. Because metabolic rates are lowered, and often exercise decreased, fewer calories are needed for weight maintenance as women grow older. Excess weight increases the middle years woman's risk for coronary heart disease, hypertension, arteriosclerosis, high cholesterol, and late-onset diabetes.

Table 14–2 lists the recommended daily allowance (RDA) for middle years women. As can be seen from this table, changes are needed in the diet as women move out of their childbearing years. Iron needs as well as caloric requirements are decreased. Care must be taken that daily intake includes all of the essential nutrients while reducing the amount of cholesterol and saturated fats. Good nutritional status can be maintained with a diet high in vitamins and minerals selected from natural foods as much as possible and with calories adjusted for age, body build, size, and activity level.

Exercise patterns that were established in adolescence or young adulthood have often gone by the wayside by the middle years. Even with the increased emphasis on physical fitness in this country, most athletes and exercise participants fall in younger age groups. The pace at which women work both as homemakers and in employment outside the home often leaves little time for organized exercise programs. It is unfortunate that this happens for lack of exercise may predispose women to weight gain, muscle atrophy, stress, and insomnia. Exercise promotes relaxation, improves muscle tone, increases work performance, reduces chronic fatigue, and enhances the efficiency of the cardiovascular system. Because exercise has a positive effect on total health it should be considered as a means of health promotion as well as maintenance and encouraged for middle years women.

Medical Problems of Middle Years Women. The mortality table (Table 14–3) shows that black women die in greater numbers than white women in their middle years. The most frequent cause of death for black women is cardiovascular disease, followed closely by

TABLE 14–2. RECOMMENDED DAILY ALLOWANCES

Women (Age)	Weight (lb)	Height (in)	Energy (kcal)	Protein (g)	Fat-soluble Vitamins		
					Vitamin A (g R.E.)	Vitamin D (g)	Vitamin E (mg T.E.)
23–50	120	64	2000	44	800	5	8
51–75	120	64	1800	44	800	5	8

Women (Age)	Water-soluble Vitamins						
	Ascorbic Acid (mg)	Folacin (g)	Niacin (mg)	Riboflavin (mg)	Thiamin (mg)	Vitamin B₆ (mg)	Vitamin B₁₂ (g)
23–50	60	400	13	1.2	1.0	2.0	3.0
51–75	60	400	13	1.2	1.0	2.0	3.0

Women (Age)	Minerals					
	Calcium (mg)	Phosphorus (mg)	Iodine (g)	Iron (mg)	Magnesium (mg)	Zinc (mg)
23–50	800	800	150	18	300	15
51–75	800	800	150	10	300	15

(Source: Adapted from *Recommended Dietary Allowances, revised 1980. Dairy Council Digest, 1980, 51, 7–10.*)

TABLE 14–3. LEADING CAUSES OF DEATH PER 100,000 POPULATION

White Female, Age 40–44		Black Female, Age 40–44	
Cause	*Number*	*Cause*	*Number*
Malignant neoplasms	71.5	Cardiovascular	105.9
Cardiovascular	35.8	Malignant neoplasms	97.3
Suicide	12.2	Cirrhosis	30.4
Motor vehicle accidents	9.6	Homicide	14.7
Cirrhosis	9.4	Motor vehicle accidents	12.2

White Female, Age 45–49		Black Female, Age 45–49	
Cause	*Number*	*Cause*	*Number*
Malignant neoplasms	131.5	Cardiovascular	187.1
Cardiovascular	68.7	Malignant neoplasms	161.2
Cirrhosis	15.8	Cirrhosis	38.7
Suicide	12.2	Diabetes mellitus	16.1
Motor vehicle accidents	9.3	Influenza and pneumonia	12.9

White Female, Age 50–54		Black Female, Age 50–54	
Cause	*Number*	*Cause*	*Number*
Malignant neoplasms	211.2	Cardiovascular	326.3
Cardiovascular	125.2	Malignant neoplasms	260.7
Cirrhosis	22.4	Cirrhosis	41.6
Suicide	12.1	Diabetes mellitus	31.3
Motor vehicle accidents	9.8	Influenza and pneumonia	16.3

White Female, Age 55–59		Black Female, Age 55–59	
Cause	*Number*	*Cause*	*Number*
Malignant neoplasms	303.9	Cardiovascular	535.7
Cardiovascular	225.6	Malignant neoplasms	365.1
Cirrhosis	23.9	Diabetes mellitus	51.2
Diabetes mellitus	16.1	Cirrhosis	37.8
Suicide	11.6	Influenza and pneumonia	23.2

(*Source: U.S. Department of Health and Human Services. Vital Statistics of the U.S. 1978, Vol. II Mortality, Part A. Hyattsville, Md., 1982.*)

malignancies. Breast cancer takes the highest toll throughout this period whereas lung and genital tract cancers are not far behind for women in their forties. Digestive tract cancers are higher for women in their fifties than those of the genital tract. Of significance as well is the number of older black women who die from diabetes mellitus. White middle years women die most frequently from cancer with the pattern following that of black women. Cardiovascular disease is the second leading cause of death. The high rate of cirrhosis throughout the middle years signifies the alcohol abuse problem that exists for both white and black women.

Women can identify for themselves whether or not they are at high risk for these disorders. Heart disease risk factors include hypertension, stress, elevated serum cholesterol, diabetes, lack of exercise, family history, heavy smoking, and obesity. The same risks apply to vascular lesions with the exception of obesity. Excessive alcohol consumption puts a woman at risk for cirrhosis. Polyps, rectal bleeding of unknown cause, history of ulcerative colitis, and a low roughage and fiber diet are predictive factors for cancer of the rectum and intestine, whereas smoking places a woman at risk for lung cancer (Martin, 1978). The malignant neoplasms can often be detected early with the health maintenance techniques discussed later in this chapter.

Contraceptive Needs. A variety of emotions will be evoked for middle years women as health care providers raise the issue of contraception. For some women who have not given birth to the children they wanted, menopause and the end of the childbearing period can be unwelcome. For those whose families are complete, a sense of relief will be evident that soon fertility and contraceptive needs will be over. At a time when it is important to avoid pregnancy because of increased medical risks, however, these women learn that the risks of some of the most effective methods of contraception also increase with age, making contraceptive planning challenging for client and provider.

Although ovulation becomes less frequent in the premenopausal years, the potential for pregnancy exists until the completion of menopause, that is, when there has been an absence of menses for 1 year. Contraception should be continued throughout this year (Millette & Hawkins, 1983).

The family planning options available to the middle years woman are somewhat limited. Oral contraceptives should be discontinued at age 30 to 35 if a woman smokes, and between the ages of 35 and 40 if she does not, because of the increased risk of thromboembolic disorders. Table 14–4 illustrates this risk very clearly.

Intrauterine devices are not absolutely contraindicated but must be used with caution because they often cause irregular bleeding that could be confused with bleeding indicative of endometrial cancer. Natural family planning is difficult because of the irregularity of cycles, but can be managed by the woman who makes a dedicated effort in following her cervical mucous changes.

The diaphragm is often the method of choice for many women who do not have severe relaxation of the supporting structures of the pelvis. The cervical cap would be preferable for these women. Foam and condoms used together also provide an effective method of preventing conception for motivated couples. This method has a distinct advantage in terms of adding lubrication to the vagina from the foam and a lubricated condom.

As the new vaginal sponge is marketed an additional contraceptive option for the middle years woman will be available. Studies thus far demonstrate effectiveness in the same range as other vaginal contraceptives. However, clinical trials have not yet been

---

TABLE 14–4. SMOKING AND THE PILL: AGE IS THE KEY

- The real key to increased risk of heart attack, stroke or death in women who smoke heavily *and* use the pill is *age*
- Women over 30 take a big risk if they smoke and take the Pill
- Smoking and use of the Pill are associated with heart attack (myocardial infarction) and stroke (subarachnoid hemorrhage)
- Age underscores every risk
  - Risk of heart attack doubles every decade of life
  - Risk of death in women over 30 is 3 to 4 times higher in smokers than in nonsmokers

---

(Source: Adapted from Hatcher, R.A., Stewart, G.K., Stewart, F., Guest, F., Josephs, N., & Dale, J. Contraceptive Technology. 1982–1983, New York: Irvington, 1982.)

large enough to assess the risk of developing toxic shock syndrome. Research on effectiveness and toxicity continues (Vorhauer et al., 1983).

In recent years sterilization has become the most common method of fertility control for married couples over 30 (Hatcher et al., 1982). It is an appropriate choice for couples whose families are complete, and is a safe procedure for either the man or the woman.

Sexual Response. The four stages of the sexual response cycle remain the same throughout the middle years as they were for women in their younger years. However, the intensity and duration of response are lessened. In the excitement phase, vaginal lubrication is produced more slowly and is lesser in amount. Clitoral sensitivity and response remain the same. The erectile tissue of the breast may be less responsive. Although there is an increase in muscle tension it now may be lessened. In the plateau phase the sex flush occurs less often. The expansion of the vagina is less pronounced and the degree of muscular tension is decreased. Orgasm is similar in younger and older women except that contractions are often fewer in number. Some women experience painful contractions of the uterus with orgasm. Following orgasm, in the resolution phase, there is a rapid return of all tissues to the preexcitement stage (Masters & Johnson, 1966). Postmenopausal women are also psychologically as well as physiologically capable of remaining sexually active. However, sexual activity decreases significantly for women in their fifties and sixties compared to men (Brecher, 1984). This phenomenon is attributed to the decline in health, or absence or death of husband or viable partner rather than to physiological changes (Bachmann, 1983).

Paralleling the changes in the sexual response cycle for women are those for men in that the duration of each of the phases is altered. After age 50, men experience a longer resolution period and after age 60 find that it takes longer to achieve an erection and more stimulation to achieve orgasm (Brecher, 1984; Gress, 1978). Both men and women report a decline in sexual desire with aging (Brecher, 1984).

Much of the sexual decline with aging is concerned with the frequency of sexual activities rather than enjoyment. Many men and women find the pleasure with their sexual relationships is as great or even more satisfying than when they were younger. Others find techniques for maintaining or enhancing their sexual expression despite physiological or physical changes that make sexual activity in later life an enjoyable experience (Brecher, 1984).

Emotional Changes. Women report other symptoms during their middle years that are sometimes called "other vasomotor disturbances" and are sometimes called psychological or emotional changes. The conflict in identification occurs because it is not clear whether or not hormonal changes have a relationship with these symptoms. Indeed, they may be precipitated by a hormonal imbalance but the effect of the aging process on an individual woman as well as her adjustment to a different life-style, role changes, and the sociocultural implications of growing older also need to be considered.

Emotional lability, palpitations, and anxiety are among those problems middle years women may verbalize. Mood swings and palpitations are noted in pregnancy where hormonal fluctuations also occur and may have the same basis during the menopausal years. "Going crazy" is not a result of menopause as some women fear; education about the normalcy of these symptoms may allay this concern.

Insomnia, fatigue, and irritability are also common concerns. It is reasonable to expect that the woman who experiences hot flashes at night with her resultant sleep disturbance would experience fatigue during the day and appear irritable to family and friends. The headaches noted by some women may be related to fluid retention or the combination of hormonal and psychosocial changes described earlier. Depression in the middle years, often attributed to grief over loss of one's youth, children, or role changes, may also have a physiological basis. It is known that natural estrogen increases the level of free tryptophan (a precursor of serotonin that may be related to depression) in the plasma. When estrogen decreases, as occurs in the perimenopausal years, the amount of tryptophan also decreases, leading to the possibility of depression (Gelein & Heiple, 1981). Again, a combination of factors needs to be examined when considering the etiology of this symptom.

Developmental Tasks and Role Changes. Each phase of life brings with it new tasks to be accomplished and an adjustment in roles. Stevenson (1977) has written about developmental tasks based on the work of Maslow, Erikson, and Pikunas that provide us with a current examination of the continuing process of growth that takes place throughout the life span. She has divided the tasks for the middle period of life into two divisions: middlescence I—ages 30 to 50 and middlescence II—ages 50 to 70 (Table 14–5).

In the early middle years individuals are expected to be independent of parents, to be socially and economically responsible for self and possibly a significant other, to help

TABLE 14–5. DEVELOPMENTAL TASKS FOR THE MIDDLE PERIOD OF LIFE

Developmental Tasks of Middlescence I, the Core of the Middle Years

The major objective is to assume responsibility for growth and development of self and of organizational enterprises. Another objective is to provide help to younger and older generations without trying to control them.

1. Developing socioeconomic consolidation
2. Evaluating one's occupation or career in light of a personal value system
3. Helping younger persons (e.g., biological offspring) to become integrated human beings
4. Enhancing or redeveloping intimacy with spouse or most significant other
5. Developing a few deep friendships
6. Helping aging persons (e.g., parents or in-laws) progress through the later years of life
7. Assuming responsible positions in occupational, social, and civic activities, organizations, and communities
8. Maintaining and improving the home or other forms of property
9. Using leisure time in satisfying and creative ways
10. Adjusting to biological or personal system changes that occur

Developmental Tasks of the New Middle Years, Middlescence II

The major objective here is to assume primary responsibility for the continued survival and enhancement of the nation.

1. Maintaining flexible views in occupational, civic, political, religious, and social positions
2. Keeping current on relevant scientific, political, and cultural changes
3. Developing mutually supportive (interdependent) relationships with grown offspring and other members of the younger generation
4. Reevaluating and enhancing the relationship with spouse or most significant other or adjusting to their loss
5. Helping aged parents or other relatives progress through the last stage of life
6. Deriving satisfaction from increased availability of leisure time
7. Preparing for retirement and planning another career when feasible
8. Adapting self and behavior to signals of accelerated aging processes

(*Source: Stevenson, J.S. Issues and crises during middlescence. New York: Appleton-Century-Crofts, 1977, by permission.*)

those in younger and older generations become (or continue to be) independent human beings, and to make significant contributions to the community, country, and society. One is also to "come to grips" with changes in self, family, work, and social relationships that occur in the middle years. Continued physical and mental health and well-being are also the responsibilties of the individual.

In the late middlescent years the tasks of the 30- to 50-year-old continue, with an even greater expectation for contributions at the societal level. Energy is more intensely spent on preparations for and acceptance of one's aging. Relationships with children change so that neither is parenting the other, but each provides respect, understanding, and assistance when needed by the other. Helping the older generation successfully move into the last stage of life is also a major task of the older middle years person.

Caution must be taken in expecting these tasks to be undertaken solely during the ages of 30 to 70. Some individuals may still be working on young adult tasks at 35, whereas others at the other end of the spectrum may be accomplishing tasks of middle years and aging at the same time. Individual variations must also be considered for the single person, married couple, and those in differing socioeconomic classes and cultures.

Both women and men need to accomplish the developmental tasks as defined by Stevenson (1977). Certain role changes, however, can be more outstanding for women. These include changes in relationships with partners, children, and parents as well as role changes in the world of work. Divorce, widowhood, early death of friends, or having close friends move away can be experienced by women in their middle years. Continuing supportive friendships are important to middle years women whereas the establishment of new relationships can be a renewing and rewarding experience.

For those women whose adult life was devoted to childbearing and childrearing, the "launching" of children can bring a feeling of loss, sometimes called the "empty nest syndrome." Other women feel a sense of pride and accomplishment when their children leave home to begin their own lives, and enjoy the freedom from maternal responsibilities. The changing relationship with one's children from parent–child to adult–adult can be disturbing for some, and a joy to others who enjoy the new friendships that can evolve.

Often the middle years are a time when women feel they are able to continue their education or enter the work force or both. For those who may be experiencing a lowered self-image as they face the physical and psychosocial changes of the middle years, work can increase positive feelings about self and provide a new means of finding satisfaction in life. For the woman who has been working throughout adulthood, the middle years bring the same need for reevaluation as they do for men. Both may be peaking in their current careers and need to make decisions about career changes or accepting the end of their careers in the not too distant future. Retirement planning is also a necessity for these women.

Role reversal is common for middle years women and their mothers and fathers. They may find they must parent their parents as they become more frail in mind and body. This can be a role they had not considered, and that most find difficult, for it is not easy seeing one's parents moving toward death. It may also be the first time the middle years woman has been forced to face her own mortality. Parenting issues may even be more difficult for women in the future. Many are now postponing their childbearing until their thirties and will find they still have responsibilities to teenagers and young children at a time when their parents are also becoming more dependent on them. The drain on time and energy sources could be overwhelming unless careful planning within families is done.

Management

The Estrogen Replacement Therapy (ERT) Controversy. The use of ERT to relieve symptoms of menopause has been under scrutiny since reports of a relationship between the administration of exogenous estrogen and endometrial cancer were reported in the mid 1970s (Smith et al., 1975; Ziel & Finkle, 1975). These studies were done on women who were using high doses of estrogen over long periods of time. All variables were also not considered when the studies were done. Objective criticism of these studies can be found in Martin (1978, p. 215). Whether or not present day ERT therapy causes endometrial cancer is uncertain, but concern exists and current thinking is that ERT therapy is appropriate for women with severe vasomotor symptoms and atrophic vaginitis not relieved by other means. The lowest effective dose of estrogen should be used cyclically with 3 weeks on estrogen and 1 week per month without medication. Most clinicians include a progestogen for 1 week with the estrogen to allow shedding of the endometrium thereby preventing hyperplasia. ERT is contraindicated for women with breast or reproductive system malignancies, kidney or liver disease, or thromboembolic disorders. Before beginning therapy women themselves must be fully informed about the potential risk of endometrial cancer and that ERT can contribute to hypertension, gallbladder disease, decreased glucose tolerance, change in lipid metabolism (Gelein & Heiple, 1981), thrombophlebitis and embolism, and aggravation of fibrocystic breast disease, endometriosis, and fibroids (Martin, 1978). They must be screened for risk status and be provided with close follow-up with breast and pelvic examinations every 3 to 6 months and Pap smears every 6 months (Martin, 1978).

ERT is also now considered an appropriate treatment or preventive measure for osteoporosis by some health care providers. It must be started within 3 years of estrogen deficiency and continued throughout the life span (Martin, 1978). In light of the effects of estrogen on all body systems this is a serious step to take but may be appropriate for high-risk women or those with early osteoporosis. As a result of osteoporosis, 25 percent of the women over 60 will have spinal compression fractures and many will have hip fractures. Half the older women with hip fractures will die from complications such as pneumonia within 1 year of their accident (Swartz, 1981). For some women with severe problems, ERT is the only alternative. Preventive measures, including nutritional supplementation and exercise, need to be offered to women early in their adult years.

Self-help. In increasing numbers, women are choosing to use less medication and more natural remedies for middle years problems. Table 14–6 provides a review of the self-help measures commonly used by women. Where vitamins are suggested, dosages are given in the therapeutic range and where contradictions are known, they are noted. No megavitamins should be suggested to women because vitamins in high dosages can alter the body's chemistry and lead to serious side effects. The alternative vitamin preparations are not as yet supported by valid research findings. Unless otherwise noted, vitamin and herbal information is taken from Seaman and Seaman (1977).

Methodologies

Resources for anticipatory guidance are currently not easily found by the middle years woman. Society, community, and health care professionals are only touching the surface in meeting their obligation to provide services. The well-educated and financially secure woman is now beginning to seek information and service from physicians, nurses, and counselors and to attend workshops and conferences, where she can learn more about this stage of life. For the less-educated, poorer woman there is little available. Her questions are often not well received in prenatal, well-child, and traditional gynecological clinics where she usually receives care and no specialized services have been set up for her. We have the obligation, then, as health care providers to find a mechanism to offer both anticipatory guidance and support to all women during their middle years. The following are some alternative ways that can be used to help women better understand and appreciate their middle years experiences.

One-to-one Education. Women are known to be more frequent users of the health care system than men. Why not use the woman's visit for a Pap smear, sore throat, or urinary tract infection to assess readiness for learning about the middle years? This "captive audience" approach can work well. Often the woman is only waiting to be asked about that period of life and may not be comfortable discussing it with her partner or a friend. A statement can be made such as, "Often women your age who come to see us have noticed changes in their bodies and their periods. Which changes have you noticed? What questions can I answer for you today?" Depending on the direction of response, the health care provider can begin her assessment and anticipatory guidance. With limited time, appropriate booklets and reference lists should be available. If books can be loaned and returned they are an even more valuable resource. During follow-up visits discussion can continue. Partners or other family members can be included as the woman wishes.

Groups. Two kinds of groups are appropriate to consider: self-help and facilitator-led.

Self-help. Self-help groups are those where women come together as equals to obtain knowledge and share the experiences of their middle years. They have the advantage of everyone having equal status, often allowing for a very free flow of ideas, and can rapidly move into a working group. (See Chapter 3 for a discussion of groups as a method of learning, group process, and the developmental sequence of groups.) There is a disadvantage in that groups without a facilitator can wander aimlessly, with the women not having their needs met. In addition, expert knowledge must be sought from outside the group. This can be problematic for some groups, for new people entering and leaving the group from week to week can disrupt the group's continuity and have a stifling effect on the sharing of thoughts and ideas.

Self-help groups may initially focus on physiological changes, physical symptoms, and treatments of menopausal problems, but can quickly turn into discussions of feelings about the middle years and aging. Some groups can go even further, with sessions on societal views of menopause and political action planning (MacPherson, 1981).

Health care providers can take a leadership role in organizing self-help groups or can be members. As members, care must be taken by professionals that they do not become a focal point or monopolize the group. This can easily happen if they have a greater knowledge of the subject matter or group process than other group members.

Facilitator-led. Groups with a leader or facilitator can also be useful to middle years women. A variety of health care providers are appropriate to assume a leadership role with the important consideration being that the group leader is knowledgeable about the middle years, has group leadership abilities, and has a genuine interest in middle years women. (See Chapter 3 for information on leadership and Chapter 16 for a discussion of co-leadership and a resource list for group leaders.) A female leader for women's groups is suggested. A male health care provider would be more appropriate for comparable

TABLE 14–6. SELF-HELP MEASURES FOR MIDDLE YEARS WOMEN

Need	Remedy
Knowledge of middle years	Preparation and support by knowledgeable health providers
Health maintenance	Monthly breast self-examination Appropriate nutrition and exercise Yearly Pap smears and breast examinations by a health care provider Regular stool guiac tests Eliminate smoking and use alcohol moderately
Hot flashes	Wear layered clothing *Vitamin E* Action: Prevents excessive FSH and LH production Dietary sources: Wheat germ, whole grains, vegetable oils, soybeans, peanuts, spinach Dose: Varies with individual's nutritional status. Usually begin with 100 IU increasing over weeks or a month or two, to 600 IU until relief of symptoms Note: Ingest after meals with fat or take with lecithin (contains phosphorus) to aid absorption. Medical supervision needed for those with hypertension, heart disease, and diabetes. Sometimes used in combination with Ginseng. Takes 2–6 weeks to be effective *Ginseng (herb)* Action: Unknown. Said to increase feelings of well-being, and changes in body metabolism Dose: Varies with body weight Note: Take on empty stomach before or between meals. Should not be taken with vitamin C. Difficult to be sure of purchasing pure ginseng. Contains small amounts of estrogen, has a component closely resembling digitoxin, and appears to affect blood levels of glucose and glycogen levels in liver and muscle. Use questionable by diabetics and those taking cardiac glycosides (Dukes, 1978). May be packaged with mandrake root (contains scopolamine) and snakeroot (contains reserpine) (Siegel, 1977) *Vitamin B Complex* Action: Aids in detoxification and elimination of FSH and LH by liver Dietary sources: Whole grains, wheat germ, yogurt, brewer's yeast, milk Dose: One to two daily after meals
Vaginal dryness	Continued intercourse and/or masturbation aids circulation and helps keep tissues flexible. *Lubrication:* water soluble jelly, vegetable oil, or if necessary, estrogen cream
Osteoporosis prevention	Exercise: Any that puts traction on long bones as walking, tennis, dancing, bicycle riding Increase calcium intake Dietary sources: Milk, cheese, yogurt, green vegetables, sesame seeds, maple syrup, turnip greens, seaweed Supplements available as calcium lactate, carbonate or gluconate Dose: Sufficient (with dietary sources) to equal 1 g/day beginning age 25, 1.5 g/day postmenopausal years
Nervousness, irritability, "feeling blue"	Vitamin B_6, 5–25 mg daily (Do not exceed 100 mg) Dietary sources: Brewers' yeast, bran, wheat germ, organ meats, molasses, walnuts, peanuts, brown rice

TABLE 14–6. (cont.)

Need	Remedy
Insomnia	Warm milk at bedtime (contains tryptophan). Calcium at bedtime. Tryptophan tablets, 2–3 g at bedtime. No coffee, tea, chocolate or cola after evening meal Chamomile tea. *Caution:* can cause hypersensitivity for people allergic to ragweed, asters, chrysanthemums (Benner & Lee, 1973) Valerian tea (strong odor). Both teas slow digestion if used daily
Pelvic relaxation	Weight loss if overweight. Kegal exercises to increase muscle tone
Muscle cramps	Calcium tablets or calcium–magnesium products such as dolomite
Prevention of urinary tract infection	Increase fluids, void frequently, urinate after intercourse, maintain good hygiene, wear cotton underwear

men's groups. Couples are also expressing interest in learning more about middle years. Couple leaders for these groups should be considered.

A semi-structured format will allow for giving of information, raising of issues, and expression of feelings. A group of 10 to 12 women in the middle years age group is small enough for everyone to be comfortable with one another and yet large enough so that no one individual stands out. A closed group (one that stays together without new members joining as the weeks progress) allows for more rapid development of the group than an open one. A series of four to six meetings, perhaps one-and-a-half to two hours in length, is manageable. At the end of the series the group can choose to stay together, continue as a self-help support group, or disband.

A series of four group sessions with objectives for each session follows. Exercises and teaching tools are included. The reader is referred to Chapter 2 for a review of teaching–learning principles and instructions in writing objectives before beginning this section.

Group Session 1

Objectives: Assist individuals to come together as a group. Determine the group's goals.

Plan:

1. Ask each member to introduce herself, tell a little about herself, and explain the reason she joined a middle years group. Encourage group interaction to avoid stilted introductions.
   Example: A woman says she's come because she has hot flashes and doesn't know what they are. Ask the group if anyone else is experiencing them. Stay with the subject until several women have participated. This technique also helps the facilitator determine the level of group knowledge.
2. Contract with the group for time, place, number of weeks the group will run, roles of facilitator and members, refreshments, and so on. Announce those things that are not negotiable. The group should decide anything that is.
3. Have each woman share her menstrual experiences. This can include her preparation and feelings about menarche and menopause, the menstrual changes occurring now, and their significance for her.
4. Provide information about middle years as questions arise. Use group members as resources as much as possible. If myths and misconceptions are raised, handle

with care to prevent "put downs." For example, a woman may say she's heard that women feel like they're "going crazy" during menopause. Rather than saying, "That's an old wives' tale," ask what that means to her and ask others the same. After discussion, explain the emotional changes some women feel, the rationale for them, and provide reassurance. Self-help measures for the changes can be incorporated into the discussion.

5. Close with having the group indicate the information they'd like to have provided and issues needing discussion. These can be written down and the group can decide priorities for the following week.

Group Session 2

Objectives: Further group development. Move members into a working group if possible. Provide information group has requested and yet maintain a balance between education and discussion.

Plan:

1. Show a film or slide-tape program such as "My Menopause" (see resource list at end of chapter for source). Lead discussion in fashion similar to that suggested by manual accompanying tape that includes:

   • Menopause: what is it, from whom do we receive information, with whom do we discuss it?
   • Change of life: stereotypes, role changes and their impact on women (and men).
   • Physiology and physical changes.
   • Sexuality.

   Other audiovisual programs could be used with equal effectiveness if they provide a format that allows the leaders to easily move the group through the major topics of importance to the group.

2. Check with group members to see if the group is progressing as they had hoped. If not, have group members make suggestions for changes.

3. Tell the group that they should come prepared to get down on the floor and exercise the following week.

Group Session 3

Objectives: Actively engage group members in group work. Discuss medical and self-help therapy for middle years problems.

Plan:

1. Have group members come to the blackboard and list all the middle years problems they knew about before they came, and those they have learned about in the group. Encourage more than one member to come up at one time. Have them write all over the board, not make tidy columns. As leader, collapse the list as appropriate. Taking the problems one at a time, have group members offer medical and self-help remedies for each. Provide information as necessary, dispel myths, and give guidance if unsafe measures are suggested.

2. Save preventive measures for osteoporosis until last. After discussing dietary needs, show the group some easy exercises appropriate for putting traction on long bones. Have the group practice. If the leaders do not feel prepared to teach these, have a qualified person join the group for this part of the session.

3. End the group with a demonstration and some practice of relaxation techniques useful in reducing stress and promoting rest and sleep. Kegal exercises could also be introduced here.
4. Ask each member to bring a snack that is especially appropriate for middle years women's nutritional needs to the final group session. Suggestions might be fresh fruit with a yogurt dip, sesame seeds, whole wheat bread, chamomile tea.

Group Session 4
Objectives: Help women plan for future aging. Terminate group.

Plan:

1. Mingle with group members while munching on snacks they have brought. Share other ideas about nutrition, meal planning, etc.
2. Draw a "time line" such as this on the blackboard.

   0 ——— 15 ——— 25 ——— 45 ——— 65 ——— 85

   Have group members draw a similar line on their own paper and write or draw in those things that have been important to them during their lives. They need to predict for those years not yet experienced. The leader(s) can do this exercise with the group. When completed, have the group relate what they have learned from their time lines. Usually the lines will be very full for the younger years and sparse from middle years on. Talk about why this happens, what goals women can have for their aging years, and circumstances that must be considered, such as widowhood. Have the group help one another with future planning. Leaders need to be aware that these discussions about selves, families, and women's issues can be intense for some groups. Other groups might move into topics related to societal issues or political action, less personal, but of equal importance.
3. Allow time for any final questions, issues, and concerns members want to raise.
4. Termination, a difficult task for some groups, must be addressed. If it is possible for the group to stay together as a support or self-help group and they wish to do so, arrangements for continuing can be made. If the group is a short-term group and is ending, the following questions can be used for closure:

   - How do you feel about what we did in the group? Were your needs met?
   - How do you now feel about your middle years?
   - How do you feel about one another?

   If leaders wish to end on an "upbeat" note, the following short exercise is suggested. The leader begins a sentence as indicated and group members all offer endings.

   - One thing I learned about in the group was . . .
   - I'm glad that . . .
   - I wish that . . .
   - In the future, I . . .

Community Workshops. Workshops provide a way to share knowledge with large groups of women in a short period of time. They can evolve from smaller support groups when women decide they want to share information and feelings with more women. Organiza-

TABLE 14–7. MENOPAUSE WORKSHOP

1. Pick a date that is far enough in advance to do publicity
2. Find a place to hold the workshop
   A. Community center
   B. Church
   C. School
   D. Clinic
3. Do the publicity for the workshop
   A. Make posters and distribute around the town
   B. Prepare radio announcements
   C. Put an announcement in the local papers
   D. Send out invitations
   E. Go to various club meetings to invite the members
4. Gather and prepare materials
   A. Bibliography (use locally obtainable books)
   B. Outline of the workshop
   C. Diagrams
   D. Definitions
   E. Printed materials
5. Be flexible: During the workshops women need to talk. Allow for this in your time plan.

(Source: Menopause: A self-care manual. Santa Fe, N.M.: Santa Fe Health Education Project, 1980, by permission.)

tions, such as women's groups, churches, businesses, and professional organizations, can sometimes be even more effective in offering workshops because of easy access to numbers of women. Health care providers can take a leadership role in their professional and community organizations to initiate workshops for middle years women.

Members of the Santa Fe Health Education Project (1980) have outlined the steps in setting up workshops in their booklet *Menopause: A Self Care Manual* (Table 14–7).

An effective model for conducting a one-day workshop on middle years has been designed by the Women's Center for Theological Education in Rochester, New York. An adaptation of one of their workshop programs can be found in Table 14–8.

Adjunct Teaching Materials. Numerous books, pamphlets, and some films are now being produced to aid individual women in understanding their middle years. They can be used successfully in conjunction with individual and group teaching. An annotated list of these resources can be found at the end of this chapter.

Evaluation
The general activities for evaluation, including understanding, specifying, describing, comparing, judging, valuing, and influencing, are reviewed in Chapter 2. Following are a few techniques used by this author to evaluate her own work in one-to-one teaching, group work, and community workshops on the middle years.

One-to-one. Evaluation will be illustrated by a case study.

Mrs. M. is a 48-year-old woman who came to the office for her annual gynecological examination. Her history and physical examination were normal except for a continuing intermittent discharge from one breast, and being 20 pounds overweight. She runs 3 miles, three to four times a week, is active in coaching athletics and community activities, does regular breast self-examinations and is comfortable with her sexuality and premenopausal changes. She has no contraceptive needs since a bilateral tubal ligation was done 8 years ago. She and her husband are enjoying the freedom of their middle years.

Teaching and counseling at this visit includes:
- Reinforcement of breast self-examination
- Need for follow-up mammogram for breast discharge
- Guidance for weight loss
- Need for yearly gynecological examinations

Two years later the client returned for another gynecological appointment. She was continuing her monthly breast examinations, had obtained a mammogram, and had purposely and sensibly lost 20 pounds.

An evaluation of the teaching based on these outcomes indicates:
- Breast self-examination was appropriately reinforced because client continued to perform them.
- Teaching was effective for weight loss and the mammogram.
- Teaching was unsuccessful around appointment timing. This client had not had gynecological care in 2 years.

This case study illustrates that through evaluation, the provider is given clear direction for where emphasis should be placed in the teaching and counseling activities for the current visit. Evaluation of one's assessment and intervention strategies should be done before proceeding.

Group. One way of measuring group effectiveness is by the regularity of attendance by members and their participation in the group. From the closing discussion of the group, the leaders can subjectively evaluate the degree of learning that took place as well as

TABLE 14–8. COMMUNITY WORKSHOP ON MIDDLE YEARS

Morning Session

1. Welcome
2. Get acquainted exercise. Divide large group into smaller groups. Use the "time line" or "menstrual history" exercise described earlier in the section on small groups. Bring the group together and ask for representatives from the small groups to tell about some of their group's findings.
3. Speaker: "Women in History, Myth, Religion and the Current Media"
   Question and answer session to follow.
4. Speaker: "Tasks and Transitional Events of the Middle Years"
   Question and answer session to follow.
5. Speaker: "Physiology of Menopause, Physical Changes and Common Discomforts"
   Question and answer session to follow.

Afternoon Session

(Each person chooses three small groups which are run simultaneously)
   Diet and exercise for the middle years
   Medical therapy and self-help measures
   Depression
   Understanding the aging process
   Psychology of middle age
   Mid-life career changes
   Sexuality and contraception in the middle years
   Planning for retirement
6. Closing and Evaluation

Source: Adaptation of Middle Years Workshop Agenda. Rochester, N.Y.: Women's Center for Theological Education, 1980.

TABLE 14–9. EVALUATION OF MIDDLE YEARS WORKSHOP

1. What did you hope would happen today?
2. Were your expectations met?

not at all   so-so   totally
1   2   3   4   5

Explain:

3. What was most helpful to you in the morning? In the afternoon?
4. What was the least helpful to you in the morning? In the afternoon?
5. What would you like in a future workshop?
6. Additional comments

(Source: Adaptation of Middle Years Workshop Evaluation Tool. Rochester, N.Y.: Women's Center for Theological Education, 1980.)

evaluate the comfort of the women toward their own middle years. Wanting to continue the group or planning for a reunion could be considered a measure of group success. Objective evaluation can be done with pre- and posttests and will show knowledge gain. Attitude change can be determined through the use of a questionnaire. These concrete tools are useful for agency reports and group research.

Workshops. Pre- and posttests measuring knowledge and attitude-change questionnaires are also appropriate for workshops. A general questionnaire can also be used (Table 14–9).

Workshop sponsors and participants will find this information helpful in planning future sessions.

CONCLUSION

This chapter provides health care professionals with guidelines for the education of women in their middle years. It is hoped that readers will be stimulated to become active in working with women in this age group, for it is through this mechanism that we will be able to assist women to reach their full potential, to cope successfully with the aging process, and to find their middle years a rewarding time of life.

ANNOTATED EDUCATIONAL RESOURCES

Books

Boston Women's Health Book Collective. *Our bodies, ourselves.* New York: Simon and Schuster, 1984. *(Chapter on "Women Growing Older" includes physical changes, psychological issues, medical and self-help measures. Many questions from middle years women.)*

Cherry, S. H. *The menopause myth.* New York: Ballantine Books, 1976. *(Questions and answers about menopause and the myths surrounding it.)*

Clay, V. S. *Women: Menopause and middle age.* Pittsburgh: Know, 1977. *(The social and psychological implications of the middle years.)*

Cutler, W., Garcia, C., & Edwards, D. *Menopause.* New York: Norton, 1983. *(Information and resources about menopause including consideration of hormone therapy and hysterectomy.)*

Israel, J., Poland, M., Reame, N., & Warner, D. *Surviving the change: A practical guide to menopause*. Detroit: Cinnabar, 1980. *(Basic information on menopause and ways to cope with changes based on a series of workshops the authors conducted.)*

Millette, B., & Hawkins, J. *The passage through menopause: Women's lives in transition.* Reston, Va.: Reston, 1983. *(Written to demythologize menopause, emphasize normalcy of the development stage, and provide information. Good film and literature resources.)*

Reitz, R. *Menopause: A positive approach.* New York: Penguin Books, 1977. *(A woman experiencing menopause writes about menopause and middle years changes based on interviews and workshops.)*

Rubin, L. B. *Women of a certain age.* New York: Harper & Row, 1979. *(Sociological study provides accounts of women experiencing the "mid-life crises.")*

Seaman, B., & Seaman, G. *Women and the crisis in sex hormones.* New York: Bantam Books, 1977. *(Includes a chapter on menopause and alternative therapies to hormonal treatment.)*

Sheehy, G. *Passages.* New York: Bantam Books, 1976. *(Adult developmental stages, crises, and methods for creative change.)*

Sheehy, G. *Pathfinders.* New York: Bantam Books, 1981. *(Report of men's and women's solutions to adult crises based on questionnaires and interviews.)*

Stewart, F., Guest, F., Stewart, G., & Hatcher, R. *My body, my health: A concerned woman's guide to gynecology.* New York: Wiley, 1979. *(Sensitive approach to a wide variety of reproductive and other women's health issues with one chapter devoted to menopause.)*

Weideger, P. *Menstruation and menopause.* New York: Delta Book, 1977. *(Biology and psychology of the menstrual cycle with special attention given to menopause.)*

Booklets

Menopause: A self care manual. Sante Fe, N.M.: Santa Fe Education Project, 1980. *(Tools and information needed for the organization of menopause groups.)*

Reimer, B. L. *The menopausal years.* Daly City, Calif.: Physicians Art Services, 1980. *(Physical and emotional changes of menopause described in text with color graphics—close to comic book format.)*

The menopause vs. the myth. New York: Ayerst Laboratories, 1980. *(Concise information pamphlet to be used as an office handout.)*

Other

Menopause resource guide. Washington, D.C.: National Women's Health Network, 1980. *(Listings of references and resources.)*

Dodds, J. *My menopause.* Rochester, N.Y.: Planned Parenthood of Rochester and Monroe County, 1982. *(A slide-tape program with accompanying manual that contains discussion questions. Useful for groups of middle years women.)*

American Cancer Society films, 777 Third Avenue, New York, NY 10017

> *Breast self-examination*—Demonstration of technique
> *For a wonderful life*—Pap tests
> *Women in the middle years*—Menopause and endometrial cancer

The invisible woman. Women Make Movies, 257 W. 19th Street, New York, NY 10011. *(Film examining society and aging, menopause, sexuality.)*

BIBLIOGRAPHY

Bachmann, G. A. Sexual response and hormone therapy. *Menopause Update*, 1983, *1*(2), 21.

Benner, M. H., & Lee, H. J. Anaphylactic reaction to chamomile tea. *Journal Allergy Clincal Immunology*, 1973, *52*, 307.

Brecher, E. M., and The Editors of Consumer Reports Books. *Love, sex and aging.* Mount Vernon, N.Y.: Consumers Union, 1984.

Dukes, M. N. G. Ginseng and mastalgia. *British Medical Journal*, 1978, *1*, 1621.

Gelein, J. L., & Heiple, P. Aging. In C. I. Fogel & N. F. Woods (Eds.), *Health care of women: A nursing perspective*. St. Louis, Mo.: Mosby, 1981.

Green, T. H. *Gynecology: Essentials of clinical practice*. Boston: Little, Brown, 1977.

Gress, L. Human sexuality and aging. In M. V. Barnard, B. J. Clancy, & K. E. Kranz (Eds.), *Human sexuality for health professionals*. Philadelphia: Saunders, 1978.

Hatcher, R. A., Steward, G. K., Steward, F., Guest, F., Josephs, N., & Dale, J. *Contraceptive technology 1982–1983*. New York: Irvington, 1982.

Heaney, R. P., Gallagher, J. C., Johnson, C. C., Neer, R., Parfitt, A. M., Behir, M. B., & Whedon, G. D. Calcium nutrition and bone health in the elderly. *American Journal of Clinical Nutrition*, 1982, *36*, 986.

MacPherson, K. I. Hot flash!! Women reclaim menopause. *Sojourner*, 1981, 11.

Martin, L. L. *Health care of women*. Philadelphia: Lippincott, 1978.

Masters, W., & Johnson, V. *Human sexual response*. Boston: Little, Brown, 1966.

McCarter, S. S. Physical changes related to aging. In S. L. Tyler & G. M. Woodhall (Eds.), *Female health and gynecology: Across the lifespan*. Bowie, Md.: Brady, 1982.

Menopause: A self care manual. Sante Fe, N.M.: Sante Fe Health Education Project, 1980.

Millette, B., & Hawkins, J. *The passage through menopause: Women's lives in transition*. Reston, Va.: Reston, 1983.

Recommended Dietary Allowances Revised 1980. *Dairy Council Digest*, 1980, *51*, 7–10.

Seaman, B., & Seaman, G. *Women and the crises in sex hormones*. New York: Bantam, 1977.

Siegel, R. K. Letter to the editor. Reply to: Kola, ginseng and mislabeled herbs. *Journal American Medical Association*, 1977, *237*, 25.

Smith, D. C., Prentice, R., Thompson, D. J., & Hermann, W. L. Association of exogenous estrogen and endometrial carcinoma. *New England Journal of Medicine*, 1975, *293*(23), 1164–1167.

Spencer, H., Kramer, L., & Osis, D. Factors contributing to calcium loss in aging. *American Journal of Clinical Nutrition*, 1982, *36*, 776.

Stevenson, J. S. *Issues and crises during middlescence*. New York: Appleton-Century-Crofts, 1977.

Swartz, D. P. *Women's health care lecture*. Rochester, N.Y.: University of Rochester School of Nursing, 1981.

U.S. Department of Health and Human Services. *Vital statistics of the U.S. 1978*, Vol II Mortality, Part A. Hyattsville, Md., 1982.

Vorhauer, B. W., Edelman, D. A., North, B., & Soderstrom, R. M. Today vaginal contraceptive sponge: A technical review. *VLI Corporation*, 1983.

Whedon, G. D. Osteoporosis. *New England Journal of Medicine*, 1981, *305*, 397.

Zeil, H. K., & Finkle, W. D. Increased risk of endometrial carcinoma among users of conjugated estrogens. *New England Journal of Medicine*, 1975, *293*(23), 1167–1170.

Women in Their Later Years: Special Educational Considerations

15

Ann Marie Dozier

The importance of patient education for women has been emphasized throughout this book. Until recently younger patients were the focus of research and descriptive studies. As the predicted demographic shifts take place, a larger percentage of our population will enter the elderly cohort (over age 65).* This trend will continue for several decades until the post-World War II babies reach old age. Another aspect of this demographic trend is the increasing number of older women. They outlive men particularly in the age 75 and older group. These two trends are responsible for the increasing number of elderly female clients in our health care system.

Some professionals do not fully understand how these changes can and will impact health care delivery. This is mainly due to a less than full appreciation of the unique and special needs an elderly woman has, distinct from those of the younger woman or, even, the elderly man.

This chapter examines why special consideration is required, what research has shown about teaching–learning in the elderly population, what content should be addressed, and what health care professionals can do to facilitate learning.

Why Special Considerations

In terms of patient education, special consideration is necessary on three fronts: (1) aging as different from illness, (2) health differences between older and younger women, and (3) aging changes that are normal versus those that are abnormal.

Aging Versus Illness. Many health care professionals inadequately understand that aging is not a disease. Age-related problems are approached and treated as if they were acute and reversible processes. Approaching aging as if it were an illness is unrealistic (Gelein, 1982). This does not imply that the elderly never have conditions requiring acute intervention, but that the acute reversible event and the chronic palliative event must be differentiated. This focus on aging as illness also creates provider frustration because some conditions may not be alleviated despite one's best efforts. Stereotypes also affect

---

*Elderly is used throughout this text to refer to individuals over age 65. Because there is no standard in the literature and the phrase older adult is less specific, the word elderly is employed. This term is not viewed with negative connotations by the author.

the diagnosis. Because the professional "knows" what the problem is, inadequate time may be taken in determining its true etiology. Treatment decisions are similarly affected. A simpler method such as prescribing medication might be chosen over spending the time and energy to counsel, teach, or do behavior modification. The complaint cycle is perpetuated because the patient's problem may not have received adequate evaluation or treatment. The client then may change providers or return still complaining. From this cycle the derogatory names such as "crock" are generated (Forbes & Fitzsimons, 1981).

Another circumstance that fosters this image is that health care providers usually come into contact with the *ill* elderly, who offer a biased picture of the population as a whole (Gelein, 1982). As a rule the impact of this image is negative and does not enhance the elderly woman's quality of health care.

Health Differences Between Older and Younger Women. The second reason why special consideration is crucial to the promotion of the elderly woman's health is that distinct differences exist between older (over age 65) and younger women. These differences relate to:

- Functional deficits or limitations, such as those created by normal age-related changes (Table 15–1).
- Self-concept, as it affects how the client perceives the problem or whether it is deemed a priority in her life.
- Makeup of local support systems that may contain many extrafamilial members. (The extended family system is likely to see the elderly woman as a support to them, not the reverse.)
- Changes in living situation, specifically financial resources, kind and location of residence, or co-habitants.
- Previous experiences with the health care system.
- Current acute and chronic illnesses that may affect function in addition to cognitive processing. They may also magnify the above differences.
- Impaired cognitive processing.

This list does not imply that every elderly woman will have a problem related to each of the above items. In fact, some women may not exhibit any. Nevertheless, these areas do clarify why the health care provider needs to view older women as a group separate from middle-aged and younger women. Later in this chapter the differences are discussed in more detail.

Aging Is Normal. The final reason requiring the health care professional to pay the elderly woman special attention is that no body system is unaffected by the aging process (Table 15–1). What differs among individuals is that one system may be affected to a greater extent than the same system in another individual. From a provider–educator standpoint, these differences mean alerting women to the normal changes that accompany aging. This may seem simplistic, but many women are unaware of the range of normal events that occur as one ages. Reversing this lack of knowledge can be useful to the woman from a preventive standpoint (e.g., maintaining an exercise regimen) or from an illness standpoint (e.g., seeking attention for postmenopausal bleeding).

In addition to clarifying what changes are normal and abnormal, health education can meet another need of elderly women: identifying conditions for which they are at risk and teaching prevention or early detection measures. This intervention is not unique to

TABLE 15–1. AGE-RELATED CHANGES BY BIOLOGICAL SYSTEM BASED ON OBSERVED BEHAVIORS AND RESPONSES

Nervous	Slower reaction time Lesser degree of overstimulation causing anxiety and tension Delayed return to base activity level after autonomic nervous system stimulation (e.g., drugs to change heart rate) Increased difficulty resolving new problems Decreased efficiency of short-term memory Longer latency time before falling asleep Less nocturnal sleep required
Cardiovascular	Increased blood pressure Reduced cardiac response to increased demand; lengthened return to normal heart rate Increased varicose veins Diminished mobility Decreased blood flow to extremities
Respiratory	Reduced vital capacity Increased residual volume Decreased oxygenation of blood Less effective cough
Gastrointestinal	Less effective chewing Dry mouth Decline in tastiness of foods Early satiety "Heartburn" sensation after eating Smaller bowel movements (if eats less) Decreased caloric needs
Endocrine	Slowed basal metabolic rate
Urinary	Impaired reabsorption of fluids in kidney Decline in concentration of urine Nocturia Reduced bladder capacity Inadequate bladder emptying
Genital	Decreased vaginal mucous secretion Relaxation of perineal floor muscles
Musculoskeletal	Reduced range of motion and skeletal flexibility Reduced hand grip strength Shortened stature and postural changes Increased fragility of bones
Integumentary	Normal body temperature reduced Decreased skin turgor and elasticity Diminished perspiration Decreased quantity and quality of hair Decreased body fat Loss of subcutaneous fat
Sensory	Decreased visual activity and peripheral vision Decreased reaction and accommodation of pupils Hearing loss of high tones increased Progressive loss of smell Decreased response to pain

(Source: Adapted from Birchenall, J. M., & Streight, M. E. Care of the older adult. *Philadelphia: J. B. Lippincott, 1982. Forbes, E. J., & Fitzsimons, V. M.* The older adult. *St. Louis, Mo.: C. V. Mosby, 1981.)*

elderly clients but the conditions for which this group is at risk are different than those of younger women (e.g., osteoporosis or cancer versus sexually transmitted diseases).

The final aspect of health education to be explored is teaching related to treatments for pathological conditions. This may include, but is not limited to, medications, diet, mobility, or self-care. It is at this level that the majority of providers have had experience working with the elderly.

Summary

The elderly female client deserves special consideration from the health care professional because of (1) the need to distinguish aging changes from acute events, (2) the differences between elderly women and middle-age or younger women and men, and (3) the lack of knowledge about normal changes and the preventive or treatment regimens as they relate to the maintenance of health. The following sections examine the assessment of learning needs, research about learning, and some recommendations and teaching strategies for their practical application.

ASSESSMENT OF LEARNING NEEDS

The identification of learning needs is a complex process in which the provider must assess the client's objective and subjective data as well as the situational and environmental variables. Using the topics presented in the introduction to this chapter, the assessment process as it relates to patient education is highlighted.

Assessment Tools or Guidelines

Nearly every publication about the elderly discusses assessment. Each varies slightly in its focus (wellness versus illness) and its audience. The following are recommended resources for additional reading (the full citations are at the end of this chapter).

- *Care of the Older Adult* by J.M. Birchenall, & M. E. Streight. Focus on elderly in institution. Much information. Readable.
- *Gerontological Nursing* by C. Eliopoulos. Focus on well and ill elderly. Thorough. Incorporates the nursing process.
- *Health Assessment of the Older Individual* by M. D. Mezey, L. R. Rauckhorst, & S. A. Stokes. Excellent assessment tool. Focus on function.
- *Nursing Management for the Elderly* by D. D. Carnevali, & M. Patrick. Organized around functional assessment. See outline in Tables 15–2 and 15–3.
- *The Aged Person and the Nursing Process* by A. Yurik, S. Robb, B. Spier, & N. Ebert. Exhaustive assessment by system deals with psychosocial aspects of deficits/changes. Excellent.
- *The Older Adult* by E. J. Forbes, & V. M Fitzsimons. Focus on nursing approach to elderly. Separates physical from psychosocial. Applicable to ill and well.

Reliability and Realism. The majority of elderly individuals provide reliable and accurate assessments of their health. Their idea of health, however, may differ from that of the provider. One assessment tool (Mezey, Rauckhorst, & Stokes, 1980) described the health optimist and the health pessimist. The former is described as someone who minimizes symptoms, carrying out normal activities to her satisfaction. The pessimist, in contrast, is preoccupied with her body, exaggerating and dwelling on the age-related changes. It is likely that this person has not yet completed the developmental tasks of aging (Mezey, Rauckhorst, & Stokes, 1980).

Functional Deficits. Functional deficits are probably the most frequently completed part of the assessment. Evaluation of range of motion and use of corrective lenses typifies these data. However, it is necessary to emphasize the word *functional* (Mezey, Rauckhorst, & Stokes, 1980; Lawton, 1971). The typical assessment or workup does not routinely include functional capacities. Knowing whether someone wears glasses does not yield information about whether the corrective lenses help or whether the individual is even using them. Similarly knowing joint range of motion or strength does not necessarily reflect whether the person can climb stairs or walk without assistance. The information about function can be elicited by having the client describe her daily activities (Table 15–2). Some providers may see this information as too detailed, but the detail is likely to help the client work with the provider to schedule exercise, determine why she is having bowel difficulties, or develop a medication schedule that would be adhered to (see Mezey, Rauckhorst, & Stokes, 1980, for additional discussion).

Sensory Deficits. Similarly querying a woman about sensory deficits can elicit useful data. Ask whether she has difficulty digesting or chewing certain foods or if the taste of food has changed. Vision should be evaluated using examples such as the ability to read a newspaper or drive a car. An eye chart test can also be used. Remember also that there are five senses. Often times the tactile one is taken for granted as is taste and the ability to distinguish colors.

TABLE 15–2. CATEGORIES OF FUNCTIONAL STATUS AREAS IN TERMS OF IMPACT ON DAILY LIVING

Breathing	Shortness of breath, pain on coughing, wheezing, bloody sputum
Circulation	Heart: Pain-nature, heaviness, episodes of rapid heart beat, skipped beats, dizziness, blackouts Vessels: Varicose veins, cold hands or feet, charley horses, leg pains walking and at rest
Eating	Appetite, enjoyment of food, diet or dieting, weight, chewing problems Cooking: Skill, enjoyment, resources Shopping: Transportation, skill, frequency, finances Eating patterns: Meals/day, typical foods Locale: Home/restaurant, alone/with others
Elimination	Bowels: Frequency, time, concerns, associated problems, medications Urine: Frequency, urgency, pain, leaking, up at night
Grooming	Importance to them, capabilities, frustrations
Mobility/safety	Patterns and location of activities, gait, accidents, balance, weakness, dizziness, stiffness, pain, status of feet/shoes, appropriate clothing available
Senses	Vision, hearing, tactile, sensory stimulation—desired/available—use of glasses/hearing aid
Sleep	Sleep patterns: night/naps, number of pillows, medications, times up at night
Social/emotional/cognitive	Memory problems, satisfaction with social life, barriers, use of time, difficult times

(Source: Carnevali, D. L., & Patrick, M. Nursing management for the elderly. Philadelphia: J. B. Lippincott, 1979, p. 29, by permission.)

Cognitive Functioning. Other functions such as the ability to speak, follow directions, or recall something relate more to cognitive processing. A deficit in this area is as serious as it is difficult to quantify or evaluate. Data concerning cognitive deficits can be collected during an assessment by varying the type of question.

- Use an example:
  Some women find they have difficulty remembering a recipe they had previously known by heart, have you experienced this?
- Offer choices:
  Do you think your memory is better, worse, or the same as it was 5 years ago?
- Request a description:
  Tell me (or describe) what you do to relax.
- Request an opinion:
  What do you think of our waiting room (or hospital)?
- Request an evaluation:
  Did you have to wait long?

Not only should the health care provider be attentive to the answer itself, but also whether the question asked was the question answered. Also note the ease with which the different formats were responded to. While this will not tell you whether the person has cognitive processing difficulties, it may give you an indication of possible problems. (See Mezey, Rauckhorst, & Stokes, 1980, for additional details. Also see Yurik et al., 1980, p. 271–273.)

Self-concept. Self-concept can also affect patient education outcomes. Three areas will be discussed to exemplify this relationship: locus of control, client perception of the problem, and client's perception of her body.

Locus of Control. The concept of locus of control (Rotter, 1966) is based on client perception of control over events in her life. The theory states that an internally controlled person would perceive her behavior as responsible for the events in her life. An externally controlled person sees *not* her own behavior, but an agent such as chance, luck, or powerful others as responsible. Belief in the supernatural falls into this category. Rotter (1966) notes that a person in the external group would be more amenable to guidance and suggestion. In addition she may view illness as punishment. Because her outcome or fate is controlled by others, she would question the usefulness of doing preventive tasks or early detection measures. The crisis of illness may make an externally controlled person sense helplessness, guilt, or even anger. In contrast, the internally controlled person would likely take a more active stance related to illness, seeking information and validation. However, this person would want to make an independent decision and would be less easily persuaded. Both of these extremes can reduce or enhance the effectiveness of a teaching intervention.

Certainly clients will not fall into one of the theoretical extremes described above. Incorporating the locus of control concept into an assessment, however, can provide added insight to a client's learning abilities. Attending to the client's comments about illness or beliefs in her ability to rectify a circumstance may decrease the number of questions the health care provider needs to ask. This information can then help direct teaching efforts.

Client's Perception of the Problem. The second aspect of self-concept that may affect patient education is the client's perception of the problem or need (Dodge, 1969). Should the client not view preventive activities as useful or if she does not think she will have a problem maintaining mobility, efforts to teach her may be heard but are not likely to be heeded. The first recourse, then, is to determine what the client sees as a problem or need. In some cases the perception and the assessment are similar. In this case the provider and client can jointly agree on a solution to the problem and their respective responsibilities in achieving the goal.

In cases where the assessment and the perception are quite different it may be necessary to compromise the health care provider's goal(s) to meet those of the client. This andragogical approach fosters the development of rapport and trust. Subsequently, the provider and client can work toward seeing the situation from each other's perspective. This may not be timely, nor can one convince every client to learn to apply what is taught; however, over time inroads can often be made.

Client perception can affect learning in another way. Should the woman find what is being taught either unacceptable or repulsive, she is not likely to listen or to practice what has been taught. For example, breast self-examination involves touching an organ with implicit and explicit meanings. To feel one's breasts may signify something more than mere examination. This can be a barrier to the client's learning or doing this screening technique. The health care provider might ask the client if she feels comfortable touching her breasts. When asked in a nonthreatening manner, the client may share her concerns or distaste at doing this activity. Caring for a colostomy or the perineum may be equally distasteful. It is important to be aware of what the client is being asked to do.

Client's Perception of Her Body. The final area in self-concept that deserves attention is the woman's perception of her body. Just as generational differences exist about rearing children and sexual practices, so too are there differences in how women perceive their bodies. This is directly related to the value of the body or organ to the woman. Some women may not have taken care of their bodies, may not see themselves as a priority, or may have led a life that offered them few choices and many burdens. These situations have had a dramatic effect on how a woman perceives her body. This also relates to how she sees herself as a woman, mother, friend, and so forth. As a provider it is critical to assess how this woman views herself. When a woman is a patient in a health care system she is likely to be in a dependent role or be the center of attention (of her family and/or providers). If she does not see herself as deserving or important, she is not likely to agree with the goals of treatment or follow-up. Involving the family, usually the children, can help reduce some of these problems. The best solution, however, is to work with the woman so that she understands the goals whether they be related to treatment or prevention.

Environmental and Situational Factors. Environmental or situational factors that affect client learning include support systems and living situations (Gelein, 1980). They are presented together because of their interrelatedness. Assessment must include the above information. This entails logistical data such as who her main supports are, where they live, and what familial relationships exist both within and outside the household. Extrafamilial relationships should be identified also. Information about the client's place of residence, dependents, and resources, financial and otherwise, is also useful (Table 15–3). Recent losses or changes in relationships should be noted. Although these details will not have a direct effect on teaching they may be utilized in an overall plan to help this client meet an

TABLE 15–3. NURSING DATA BASE ON SUPPORT SYSTEMS

Housing	Type: Single family dwelling, yard, apartment, hotel room, retirement center, lighting, risk factors (wires, loose rugs, etc.)
	Neighborhood: Risk, hills, location of stores, transportation, churches, health services, other services.
Personal network	Living alone or with spouse/children/housemate/commune. Relationship and distance from siblings, children, relatives, friends, neighbors.
	Club/church contacts, types of contacts (letters, phone, visits)
Communication responses	Phone? Emergency contacts, intercom systems
Transportation	Public transportation availability, personal rides, senior citizen passes
	Barriers to getting in and out of vehicles
	Own car, status of driver's license
Finances	Adequacy, problem areas, resources, concerns
Need for support	Nature of desired support, usable support, available support
	Ability to maintain support systems (mechanical, personal)

(Source: Carnevali, D. L., & Patrick, M. Nursing management for the elderly. New York: J. B. Lippincott, 1979, p. 31, by permission.)

identified need. For example, the health care provider may recommend that someone else learn the client's treatment regimen or help remind her to take medications. If no one is available who could serve in this role then it is inappropriate to make this recommendation. Alternatives are available, however, and these should be discussed with the client. Similarly, resources may be scarce. Costs of food, medication, or dressings must be compared to available resources as plans are devised to meet identified needs. Use of generic brands, identifying alternative, nontraditional food sources, and reviewing the plan for what is minimally required versus what is ideal may help reduce expenditures.

Previous Experience. The client's previous experiences with the health care system will affect how much she will allow the health care provider to do with or for her. Asking her about past experiences can offer insight into her concerns and perceptions. Note what she identifies as useless or negative experiences. Understanding this allows the health care provider to learn from the mistakes others have made. Asking how she thinks a similar situation could be avoided gives the health care provider a place to start. Reversing bad experiences is not simple. Being aware of the past can help health care providers know what a specific client prefers.

Current Health Status. The current health or illness state of the client was listed last because it affects all of the above items. During an assessment this information is acquired throughout the interview as different systems are examined. It is mentioned here as a separate entity to emphasize its deleterious effect on learning abilities.

Illness can be categorized as short- or long-term on the basis of length of required hospitalization (less than or greater than 30 days). In addition some long-term illnesses become chronic. It is reported that 86 percent of the population over age 65 has one or more chronic conditions. However, few of these individuals classify their health as anything but good or excellent (Birchenall & Streight, 1982). This is supported by the fact that 95 percent of the elderly are not institutionalized. From a teaching–learning standpoint it is important to be knowledgeable of the ways in which illness, both chronic and acute, impact learning. Similarly the teaching content would differ. This is explained in more detail later in this chapter.

TABLE 15–4. SUMMARY OF BURNSIDE'S ASSESSMENT CONTENT

Detailed description of problem(s)
> Duration; onset; characteristics; frequency of occurrences/treatments; factors which relieve/aggravate; self-treatment method; impact on ADLs

Description of associated symptom/problems

Symptoms commonly associated with psychosocial problems
> Sleep disturbance; change in bodily function; change in mental state; memory impairment; appearance of hallucinations or delusional thinking

Past health history

Drug history
> Prescribed medications; OTC medications; ETOH intake; caffeine intake

Family history

Social history

Present activities

Other topics
(pertinent to the aged)
> Loss/separation experiences, e.g., loss of spouse; loss of purpose; loss of material goods/ownership; food intake; significant others—spouse, children, siblings, friends, social groups; finances; need to feel useful; concern with death and dying

Objective data
> Personal appearance; affect; mentation—speech, orientation, memory/recall, unusual ideation; vital signs; review of systems

(Source: Adapted from Burnside, I. M. Psychosocial nursing care of the aged. *New York: McGraw-Hill, 1980.)*

Psychosocial Assessment

This component was added to draw attention to the fact that some of the elderly client's complaints may be due to psychosocial problems. Chaisson (1981) comments that depression is the most often overlooked diagnosis in the elderly population. Burnside (1980) identifies that clients seeking attention for symptoms are not just identifying physical problems but psychosocial ones as well. Table 15–4 summarizes Burnside's assessment content. These are shared to highlight the scope of difficulties that may present as physical problems but whose etiology is in the psychosocial realm.

Summary

These areas are, in many cases, already a part of health care assessment. Consider them as learning needs are identified, and a plan is developed, implemented, and evaluated. Determine how any adjustments worked or failed. It is only through clinical application and experimentation that our knowledge base about effective strategies can be expanded. The next section explores what research has shown regarding the elderly learner.

THE ELDERLY LEARNER

Insights from the research of other disciplines lend an understanding to the complex problem of the elderly learner. Research generated by gerontologists and developmental psychologists has examined the process of learning as it applies to the older person. The process includes inputs, outputs, and transactions occurring within the brain, referred to as central or cognitive processing. Performance on a posttest, for example, is determined by adequate integration of these transactions (storage, retention, retrieval, and recall). A deficit in any one of these four areas would affect performance. However, no measurement tool has been or is available to identify the specific area of deficit and indirect measures are considered to be far from accurate (Hulicka, 1977).

Because the area of actual deficit cannot be identified, any attempt to improve learning has been aimed at all four areas. Thus in the following research, general learning principles were employed in hopes that the area of actual deficit would be compensated for. The principles used to facilitate learning in the elderly were separated into those examining the kind of content and format of the information to be learned, those analyzing the format or method of the learning, and those involving memory.

Kind and Format of Information

The kind of information to be learned affects outcomes. Researchers discovered that elderly patients demonstrated a poorer performance on postlearning tests when the learning consisted of memorization of meaningless word–pairs or syllables (Hulicka, 1967; Hultsch, 1974; Wittels, 1972). However, when the material presented had some relevance attached to it, the posttest results improved dramatically. For example, the learner in the study was told to pretend that he was in a new city and had to learn the names of a doctor or grocer, thus the word–pair was "grocer–Knox," for example. The researchers believed that this would increase the motivation of the elderly learner. Given more time to study the pairs and increasing the pairs' relevance, elderly subjects' scores improved to the point of equaling younger adults' scores (Hulicka, 1967). Thus to facilitate learning, the purpose or relevance of the material should be made explicit to the elderly learner.

Another aspect of motivation is arousal. According to Burnside (1976), there seems to be an optimal level of arousal necessary for good performance. The individual who is over- or under-aroused will not perform well. Although research supports the optimal level idea, it is not clear whether the elderly are over- or under-aroused (Botwinick, 1973), nor what conditions might contribute to this (e.g., inadequate sleep, disinterest, or disuse).

Several researchers examined the impact format had on learning by, again, measuring word–pair memorization (Canestrari, 1963; Hulicka & Grossman, 1967; Hulicka & Weiss, 1966). The experimenters used both concrete and imaginary relationships to help the elderly learn. (The issue of relevance, discussed above, was not addressed by these experimenters.) For example, for the pair "glass–noodle" the concrete relationship described a noodle on a glass dish or with a glass of milk. An imaginary relationship described a glass made out of noodles or noodles turning into glass. Regardless of which relationship was used, performance improved in all age groups when compared with a group memorizing the pairs without any descriptions (Hulicka & Grossman, 1967; Murrell, 1970; Rowe & Schnore, 1971; Winograd, Smith, & Simon, 1982). When comparing just the elderly subjects, an interesting dimension was noted: better performance occurred when concrete rather than imaginary relationships were employed (Rowe & Schnore, 1971). This finding implies that use of visual or other sensory aids can therefore facilitate learning.

Perlmutter (1979) examined whether recall could be improved if learners generated their own relationships for the word–pairs. Compared to younger learners, the elderly learner utilized self-generated relationships less frequently and had poorer recall. Therefore, the elderly person's learning was not impeded when the teacher generated visual or other sensory aids.

Researchers also manipulated the learning phase (Hulicka & Weiss, 1966; Moenster, 1972; Schonfield, 1969). Usually the number of times a subject could review the word–pair list prior to the performance test was limited. In these studies each participant was allowed to review the list until a certain standard or performance criterion was met, for example, two errorless reviews. This allowed each subject to attain the same performance level prior to testing, assuring equal competency at the time of testing. This was called learning to criterion. The results of studies using this method demonstrated that even though the elderly took more trials to attain the criterion, their postlearning performance was equal and sometimes better than that of younger subjects (Hulicka & Weiss, 1966). To facilitate learning in the elderly, then, the format should allow enough time for learning to take place and provide a mechanism to measure learning.

Another format evaluated was self-pacing. This means learning the information at a rate set by the learner and not the teacher. Interestingly, people of all ages performed equally well using this method (Arenberg, 1965; Canestrari, 1963; Goodrow, 1975; Hulicka, Sterns, & Grossman, 1967; Sieman, 1974). However, when self-paced learning was used with self-instruction, limitations were found. The use of sophisticated equipment or complex directions led to elderly clients' poorer performances and refusals to participate (Dozier, 1978, 1980). This finding was supported by Kim and Grier (1981). Their evaluation of self-paced medication instruction indicated that patients were cautious about the material initially. After repeated exposure, however, they were able to absorb the content. These researchers found the visual material hepful, a finding not supported in preoperative teaching modules (Dozier, 1980). The differences encountered may be due to the fact that Kim and Grier had multiple opportunities to teach patients. This is contrasted with the preoperative situation where a deadline is set. They also discussed concerns about self-pacing and the elderly. These included instructional variables such as expected pace, relevance, and difficulty of the task(s). Before self-instruction is automatically used for teaching the elderly, these areas deserve attention. Because both studies were with hospitalized elderly, caution must be taken before generalizing to the elderly population as a whole.

Memory. Memory is the key to all the aforementioned manipulations. However, researchers have yet to explain what actually caused the improved test performance. Again, cognitive processing, the sum of storage, retention, retrieval, and recall, cannot be directly measured. Several studies have shown improved posttest scores when mediators were used (Craik, 1977; Hulicka, 1967; Moenster, 1972; Poon et al., 1980; Schonfield, 1969; Schonfield & Robertson, 1966). These were memory aids that placed the word to be learned within a frame of reference. Using the word in a sentence, drawing a picture, or explaining a concrete relationship are three examples of mediator use. This apparently assisted the subject to mentally visualize the word he or she was learning. Although the exact mechanism of their effect remains obscure, mediators do have a role in promoting learning in the elderly.

The ability to ignore irrelevant information has also been studied (Hoyer, Rebok, & Sved, 1979; Kausler & Kleim, 1978). Each study found that the elderly subject had difficulty ignoring irrelevant stimuli. This reduced their ability to learn, caused more errors to be made, and increased reaction time.

Although these studies about the elderly seem impressive, their results and conclusions must be noted with a degree of caution. All participants were volunteers and no random selection process was used. Furthermore the nonelderly adults were college students. Thus, neither the elderly nor the nonelderly adult subjects were truly representative of their respective populations. Even though these considerations detract from the findings, they are not invalidated.

It is obvious from these studies that the elderly person's learning can be potentiated. Methods that accomplish this would need to include statements that (1) clarified the purpose of the learning, (2) provided the learner with time for review and a frame of reference, and (3) avoided inclusion of irrelevant information and distractions. The value of mediators and repetitions was also pointed out.

Strategies for Teaching the Elderly Woman

As the teaching plan is set up, first set goals with the client. These can be short- and long-term. Use measurable outcomes so the client and health care provider can identify progress. Discuss with her how she learns best, by reading, doing, or listening. She is likely to offer some useful suggestions.

In preparing the content, include only information relevant to the client's need. If she needs to learn about a medication it is not usually necessary for her to understand the pathology causing the problem or the pharmacology of the drug (see Chapter 2 for a discussion of teaching doses). Be concise and avoid excessive detail. Anticipate questions and have simple answers prepared. Identify the key points. Anecdotal information is not usually helpful and can detract from the message. Incorporate examples or parallels to promote learning. The use of mediators or associations can be useful. Names of drugs or conditions can be rhymed or a catch phrase developed. Perhaps the client can devise her own mnemonic. Remember to be consistent. Use the same word or phrase each time. Similarly, avoid jargon or abbreviations as you speak.

The actual content that these strategies will be applied to is determined by the situation in which the elderly woman is encountered and the health needs identified. Table 15–5 lists suggested content areas, broken down into maintenance of wellness and adaptation to illness. Unfortunately information in the literature about maintenance is somewhat lacking and is usually anecdotal. The information presented is a compilation from numerous sources, presentations, and clinical experiences. The information about adaptation to illness is better developed to the point that the depth of content cannot be thoroughly represented. To supplement the items mentioned, see the references by Perdue and colleagues (1981) and Carnevali and Patrick (1979). Both provide detailed intervention strategies.

Use of Multimedia Aids. Consider supplementing the oral presentation with stimuli from the other senses (see Chapter 2 for criteria and description of use). Visual aids can include pictures, drawings or diagrams, or contact with the actual equipment (e.g., crutches or medication bottles). Visual experiences may also include an on-site visit. Although using another sensory mode facilitates learning, use only one mode at a time. For example, when using pictures or diagrams, do not show the picture until oral information has been given. Then allow the client a minute of uninterrupted silence to examine the visual stimuli and ask questions. It may help to ask the client a question about what was just said to determine if the key point has been grasped. If diagrams are being used make sure they are not too schematic, but have enough detail to be recognizable. Test these out with similar age patients before hand. With pictures take care that the photograph is not of an offensive or distasteful area. These may be better represented by drawings or diagrams.

Hands-on experience uses visual and tactile senses. This level of teaching is effective once the content has been taught and generally understood. Do not teach and do hands-on experience simultaneously. This uses more than one sensory mode. Experience with the equipment must also be done in a quiet environment, free of distractions. Avoid communicating haste to the patient. The easiest way to prevent learning is to tell someone to hurry. This emphasizes the outcome rather than the process.

Use of Written Instructions. Written instructions should only be used in concert with other teaching. It is preferable to develop them ahead of time so they may be reviewed by other professionals and selected clients. Before writing up anything, clearly state your goals and agree on how the written information would meet the goals. Then agree on the content. Take care to highlight the ideas you want the woman to remember. Also be sure the printing is large and diagrams clearly labeled. Conduct a readability test (see Chapter 2) to determine the grade level of the material. You may also want to consider developing it in a language other than English.

The timing of distribution of written information varies. It may be helpful to have the client review the written material and then be instructed. In other situations the written information can be introduced at the conclusion of the teaching. If it is something the client can keep, it is helpful to have it at hand while teaching. The client can put her notes right on the instruction sheets. Similarly, if you use a diagram that is in the instructions your notes or arrows will be there for her to review at a later date. Include a name and telephone number for the client to contact for clarification once she leaves the teaching setting.

The Teaching Environment. During the actual teaching find a quiet area away from distracting sounds, interruptions, or activity. This may be difficult. The public address systems in many institutions often invade even the most secluded area. It may be necessary to identify a room for patient education or negotiate to be uninterrupted in order that teaching and learning take place. At the beginning explain to the client how the teaching is to be organized, whether she should wait until the end for questions, and how long it will take. Allow her ample opportunity to ask questions. During the teaching, ask her to repeat the idea in her own words, or ask her a question about it. This will give the health care provider an indication of whether the concepts are being learned. If the amount of information required is lengthy, it is recommended that it be broken down into sections of no longer than 15 to 20 minutes. As each section is begun take a few minutes to confirm with the client what has been taught previously.

The elderly woman can become frustrated if she does not learn something the first time. Clarify for her that perfection is not expected. Help her understand that it will take time for her to incorporate a new activity into her daily routine. Express understanding of how in the beginning she may be less consistent. Talk with her about ways she can remind herself. Find out how she remembers other things.

Determining whether the client has learned and can apply the learning to her daily life is as complex a task as preparing and carrying out the teaching plan. Testing her or having her demonstrate what to do is a beginning step toward incorporating learning into practice. Make sure she talks about how she will incorporate it into her daily routine. The true evaluation comes when the client is able to complete the regimen in her normal environment.

TABLE 15–5. POTENTIAL TEACHING CONTENT FOR THE ELDERLY WOMAN

	Maintenance of Wellness	Adaptation to Illness
Personal hygiene	Facial care including daily washing with tepid water; moisturizer recommended even if makeup being applied; remove makeup daily; reapply moisturizer at bedtime. Avoid glycerin-containing products. Hair care, including daily brushing; washing may be necessary only every other week; use of permanent and hair coloring should be done only with recommendation from beautician knowledgeable of elderly hair care. Restrict soap use to axilla and genital areas. Fully bathe once or twice a week only. Apply nonperfumed emollient. Blot skin dry, do not rub.	Energy for this may be reduced. Pacing or assistance with care is recommended until energy level returns. Even when ill, good hygiene and grooming can contribute to a sense of well-being.
Clothing	Base dressing on weather report, not how cold/hot it feels. Recommend layered clothing so it can be removed/added as necessary. If living in climate not previously accustomed to, may be intolerant of extremes in humidity and temperature. Clothing from undergarments out should be nonrestrictive. Avoid 100% polyester clothing. Wear protective clothing to prevent trauma, i.e., gloves for chores, wash new garments before wearing and pad body surfaces subjected to trauma (e.g., knees when gardening).	See guidelines to left
Mobility	Focus on activities that develop skill and coordination (as opposed to speed, strength, and skill). Undergo a warm up and cool down activity before and after exercise. Use of firm mattress. Build on client's normal pattern of activity (e.g., gardening or walking). Avoid pressure, cold and smoking. See Resource A for specific exercises. Avoid heavy lifting.	Pacing of activities critical, schedule rest periods. Spread time-consuming tasks over several days. Do not stay in bed; do usual self-care activities. Avoid focusing on length of time to complete normal activity. Guidance about way to move from lying to standing position. Identify positions that reduce discomfort. Utilize relaxation techniques. Identify compensating mobility aids active and/or passive ROM.

Sexuality/ sexual functioning	Review human sexual response phases. Validate the normalcy of client concerns. Suggest water soluble lubricants or use of estrogen for vaginal dryness. Encourage regular sexual activity (masturbation, intercourse, etc.). Timing after a full night of sleep is recommended. Explore client perceptions of health/illness impact on sexual functioning. Identify position changes that may increase comfort.	Identify the importance of intimacy as a part of healing/feeling better. Involve partner in discussion. Identify actual limitations. Identify importance of maintaining previous patterns of sexual expession.
Sleep/ rest patterns	Rest or relaxation period (not sleep) in early afternoon recommended. For sleep suggest bathing or eating protein (e.g., milk). Avoid night time medications, especially OTCs hypnotics, which suppress REM sleep. Maintain activity patterns and stimulation during waking hours. If awakened during night, engage in a diversion such as reading, listening to music. Do not sleep in chair (causes hyperextension of neck).	Disturbances related to illnesses and hospitalization common. Apply concepts presented under maintenance of wellness. Avoid scheduling night time disruptions: medications, treatments. Attend to environment (which previously may have not influenced sleep): heat of room; noise/light; number of pillows; weight/warmth of blankets/sheets. Follow guidelines at left.
Nutrition/ fluid and electrolytes	Balance meals combining basic food group (see Young, 1974). Maintain protein intake at 1 g/kg body weight. Include fats in diet. Avoid utilizing convenience foods for primary carbohydrate source (substitute whole grain cereals or breads). Achieve vitamin and mineral intake by consuming fruits (canned or fresh). Vegetable intake should be either from fresh or frozen not canned sources. Maintain fluid intake of 2500–3000 cc daily. Encourage social contact around mealtimes. Maintain exercise level. Cutting cost while maintaining nutritional value (See Carnevali & Patrick, 1979, p. 163).	Increase protein intake to 1.5 g/kg body weight if weight loss or muscle atrophy has occurred. Increase calorie content of foods consumed; drink fruit juices not water or coffee, drink whole milk not skim; plan six meals a day. Exercise to stimulate appetite and efficient use of calories/protein. Follow guidelines at left. Check weight every 3 days or weekly.

(continued)

TABLE 15–5. (cont.)

	Maintenance of Wellness	Adaptation to Illness
Bladder function	Teach perineal floor exercises, should do several hundred per day. Practice stopping urinary stream mid-void. Respond to urge to urinate. Nocturnal frequency can be reduced by reducing fluid intake and caffeinated beverages in evening; also avoid salty or spicy foods before retiring. Thorough cleansing after voiding.	Bladder retraining to simulate normal filling and emptying. Prevent accidents, e.g., time excursions after diuretic has had effect; know where bathrooms are; void every 2–3 hours even if urge is absent; void before leaving home. Avoid caffeinated beverages. Time fluid intake for when bathroom is accessible. Review methods to stimulate voiding. If indwelling catheter required, aseptic technique must be implemented. See section to left. See also section under Adaptation to Illness, sexuality/sexual functioning.
Bowel function	Avoid irritating laxatives. Increase bulk in diet or use of non-irritating laxative. Maintain exercise level. Wiping front to back.	If client has colostomy, teaching about care must be undertaken (see Resource A in Chapter 22 for additional content). Reestablish bowel reflex by an every other day regimen of suppository use to stimulate filling and evacuation of bowel. Protect skin with ointments to prevent excoriation. Change soiled undergarments as soon as possible.
Sensory changes visual	Reduce glare (change lighting, avoid shiny objects). Provide adequate lighting (e.g., stairwells). Use protective eyewear. Undergo annual vision screening. Provide information about conditions associated with aging (e.g., cataracts, glaucoma).	Identify low-vision aids (e.g., lighted magnifying lens). Use contrasting colors. Survey room if peripheral vision affected. Instruct on eyedrop adminstration. Do not rearrange objects in environment. Incorporate tactile sensations whenever possible. Reduce glare.
Taste	Identify nonsalt based spices to enhance flavor.	Use other senses—visual, olfactory to enhance food appearance/smell and thereby taste.

Hearing	Protective wear if environmental noise of long duration or intensity. Regular hearing screening, especially if on ototoxic medication. Prompt treatment for inflammatory processes. Do not probe ears with cotton swabs, fingers or other objects.	Identify alternatives for communication: hearing aids, auditory training, speech reading. Environmental alterations focusing on other senses, e.g., flashing lights. Reduce background noise.
Smell	Enhance odors in environment, pleasant and familiar.	Enhance odors that client identifies as pleasant.
Touch		Use rough textures and heavy or weighted objects.
Cognitive	Identify importance of sensory stimulation; variation in type, intensity, pattern. Identify importance of changing/expanding one's environment (e.g., outside home, new stores, parks). Identify importance of forming new social relationships. Avoid overstimulation, i.e., stimuli from multiple sources using several senses (e.g., driving with radio on and conversation occurring).	Teach only one step at a time. Avoid irrelevant stimuli/distractions in environment. Use notes/cards with concisely written information. Use terms/objects familiar to client. Provide variable stimuli (e.g., colors, environment). Teach when client well rested.
Self-esteem	Increase awareness of present and past achievements through review/discussion. Identify positive attributes. Encourage reminiscence. Help client set realistic goals. Provide for client self-determination. Identify importance of privacy. Encourage independence. Identify ways in which client can or is making a contribution to society. Identify support persons in environment who care about client. Involve family as needed to provide recognition, respect, etc.	Recognize that stages of grieving or loss are normal expected steps for dealing with change. Involve family and significant others in discussion to provide ongoing support. Initiate behavior modification if needed. Provide time for decision-making, acceptance, adaptation. Ensure that other areas are not neglected (e.g., environment or health).

SUMMARY

Health education is a complex process, entailing variables that can and cannot be manipulated. The provider who does health education with the elderly woman must be aware of the variables specific to that age group and the range of normal problems that can occur. Preventive content should not be overlooked while resolving client problems. Teaching strategies or approaches should closely examine the content and use supplemental instruction or reinforcing experiences. By incorporating the suggestions presented here the health care provider can improve the outcome of teaching elderly clients.

Life Is Movement

Committee on Physical Fitness of Elders*

BASIC SITTING POSITION (GOOD POSTURE)

1. Find a chair low enough to allow both feet to be firmly placed on the floor.
2. The seat should be flat or slightly raised in front.
3. The back should be straight.
4. Place hands in lap. Sit with weight evenly divided between both legs.
5. Imagine that your spine is an accordian held vertically. One handle is at the top of your head, the other at the base of your spine. Lengthen your spine by stretching the handles away from one another. Make sure your shoulders and chest stay down and that your chin stays parallel to the floor.
6. Your abdominal muscles press back toward your elongated spine.
7. Allow your breath to flow in and out easily.
8. To relax and rest, slowly curve your back allowing your head to bend towards chest. Let your shoulders, arms and hands hang loosely at your sides or on your lap.

FLEXIBILITY EXERCISES—SITTING

All these exercises should be done slowly. Remember to stop if discomfort appears. Try these exercises five times each to start, gradually increasing the number of repetitions.

Warmup

Sitting in chair with good posture, raise arms over head, hugging ears, try to reach for ceiling! Then stretch your right side up, then stretch your left side up. Relax, bringing arms down. Try to inhale as you lift arms and exhale when dropping them.

Abdominal breathing. Breathe in and out slowly, expanding abdomen as you inhale. Slowly exhale, pulling abdomen in.

Exercises for Each Part of the Body

Eyes

Flirting. Good for your eye muscles. Look to the left—look to the right—up, down, and all around, without moving your head.

Neck

Head Roll. To relieve stiff and tense neck and shoulder muscles: In comfortable sitting posture, close eyes and *slowly* allow head to come forward, resting chin on chest if possible. Slowly lift head, stretching chin to ceiling. Return head to normal position. Turn head slowly from one side to the other. Also, try moving your head so one ear drops toward your shoulder. Now do the other side. Keep shoulders down throughout the exercise (Fig. 15A–1A).

Arms

Six-count movement. Start with hands in lap. When doing the exercise, keep arms straight (Fig. 15A–1B). On the count of:

1— Raise your arms in front of chest
2— Slowly move arms to the sides of your body, shoulder height
3— Raise arms over head
4— Return arms to sides of your body, shoulder height

---

*Reprinted with permission from: Connecticut State Department on Aging, 1979. *Authors' note:* Illustrations have been added to clarify some of the exercises.

5—Bring arms to front of chest
6—Return hands to lap

Then pretend you are swimming! Use your arms to do the crawl or the breaststroke.

Arm Circling. Extend arms out to side, keeping them straight. Circle them moving first in one direction then the opposite. Make large circles, then make small ones (Fig. 15A–1C).
   Rest and breathe deeply.

Shoulders
Do the Shrug. Raise your shoulders up toward your ears (Fig. 15A–1D). Lower away from the ears as much as you can.

Roll Your Shoulders. Slowly move your shoulders forward, up, back and down. Repeat going back first, then up, forward, and down.

Fingers
Wrist and Finger Stretcher. Clasp hands in front of chest. Turn palms away and stretch arms forward keeping hands clasped. Return to beginning position. Place arms out in front of chest, keeping arms straight. Open and close palms with fingers. Try palms up, then palms down. Try squeezing a soft, crocheted or foam rubber ball. Loosen your fingers and play an imaginary keyboard; from left to right, right to left.

Wrist
Circles. Extend arms forward to a comfortable position. Rotate hands downward, sideward, upward, sideward. Do motion clockwise, then counterclockwise.

Shake. Loosen hands and shake from the wrists. Sure helps get the old stiffness out!

Back
Beginning with your hands on your lap, bend forward, dropping hands toward the front of your body, trying to reach the floor (Fig. 15A–1E). As you return to your sitting position, slowly bring arms up over your head. (Try to touch the ceiling!) Return to original position. (If you have high blood pressure, do not drop head down when bending.)

Waist
Sit straight in chair. Raise right arm. Reach toward ceiling. Continue reaching (arm stays near ear) leaning head and torso toward the left side. Make sure right hip stays down in chair. Do the opposite side.

Stomach and Legs
Knee Lifts. Slowly raise bent knee—return and then raise the other. Raise bent knee, straighten leg forward, bend knee, return to place. Repeat other side.
   Raise bent knee, place hands under thigh, draw knee toward chest. Simultaneously bend head and torso forward. Straighten and return to original position. Relax.

Foot and Ankles
Ankle Flex. Extend leg forward. Flex ankle. Stretch toes up toward ceiling, down toward floor. Now roll your ankles in circles—clockwise then counterclockwise.
   The ol' rockin' chair is good for you! Rock back and forth—to Lawrence Welk or to your favorite radio music. Great for the circulation and the back: remember President Kennedy and his rocker?
   Rest and breathe deeply.

FLEXIBILITY EXERCISES—STANDING

Warmup
March in Place. How high can you lift those knees? Now slow your march, purposely balancing one leg at a time.
   All the sitting exercises can be done in a standing position.

Some Additional Standing Exercises
Trunk Bend. With hands on hips, slowly bend forward as far as comfortable, straighten up, relax. Then try sideways too. Can you bend a little toward the back?

Be a Tall Man. Stand erect. Slowly raise up on toes and down again. You can hold on to a chair if you need to.

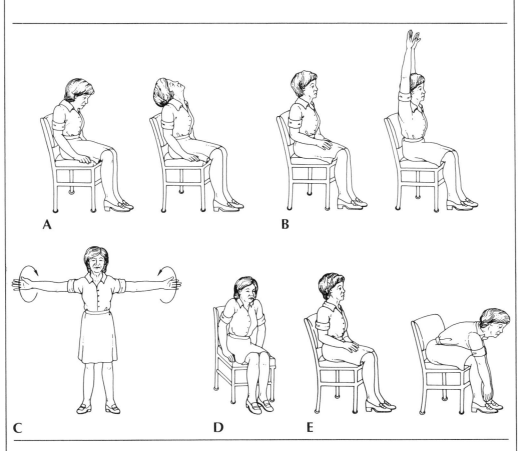

Figure 15A–1. A. Head roll. **B.** Six-count arm movement. **C.** Arm circling. **D.** Shoulder shrug. **E.** Back exercise. *(cont.)*

Crazy Walking. Walk on your toes, forward and backward.

Cross left leg in front of right, tapping your toe to the side. Return leg to original position, and then cross your right leg in front of your left. Move forward as you are doing this.

Walk with toes pointed toward each other. Walk with toes pointed away from each other.

Warm-down

March in place, moving quickly at first, then slowing down the pace.

Rest and breathe deeply.

FLEXIBILITY EXERCISES—LYING ON FLOOR OR ON BED

All exercises from sitting position can be done lying down. Also try these exercises:

Stretching. Start every day by stretching and relaxing, just like a cat. Stretch, relax, change position, stretch, relax. Repeat, changing positions, until the whole body has been treated to a flexing. (Sometimes good for relaxing before sleeping too.)

Liver Stretcher (Knee-chest). Lying on back, both knees bent, place hands under one thigh and pull your knee toward chest (Fig. 15A–1F). Hold position as long as it is comfortable. Return to original position. Relax. Now try the other knee.

Leg Lift. Slowly raise leg, return, and then raise the other. Always keep one leg bent as you raise the other (Fig. 15A–1G).

Modified Sit-up. Lying on back with both knees bent, raise head, moving chin to chest, hold to count. On next try, if comfortable, slowly lift head and shoulders; hold to count. Relax—lift head, shoulders, and upper body (Fig. 15A–1H). Then maybe you'll feel good enough to try this next exercise.

Full Sit-up. Strengthens abdominal muscles. With arms over head, raise head, moving chin to chest. Start to move shoulders and torso toward knees, slowly bringing arms between the bent knees (Fig. 15A–1I). Slowly roll back with the end of the spine first until lying flat on back again. The more slowly, the better—it is in the slowness that the muscles are strengthened.

    Rest and breathe deeply.

Canes: Canes or walking sticks can also be used as an exerciser, standing or sitting. They should have a rubber tip at the end for safety.

- Hold cane in front of your chest, squeeze the cane with your fingers, release, then squeeze again, relax.
- Hold cane in front of your chest, arms straight, bend your wrists, pushing cane up and down.
- Hold the cane with the palms of your hands facing upward, resting the cane across your knees. Bring the cane toward your chest. Return to starting position.
- Reverse your hand position so that palms are facing downward. Raise the cane toward your chest. Return to starting position.
- Hold cane across your knees. Bend down with the cane toward the floor. Return to original starting position. Slowly lift the cane up over your head. Return to starting position. Now try bending down with the cane on your left side, then your right side.
- Try rowing with your cane!

HOW TO EXTEND THESE EXERCISES CREATIVELY

Stretch your mind and your imagination along with your muscles. Adapt these suggestions to your capabilities:

To Loosen Up When You Are Feeling Tense or in Need of Extra Energy
Yawn. Take a breath, exhale, rounding your back while sitting in the chair. Let your arms fold across your chest. Start to unfold, stretching your back and your arms out as much as possible. Make a loud oooh sound. Return to original position. Repeat three times.

To Get Your Circulation Going
Seated, with one hand pat briskly up and down the opposite arm. Extend that patting to the whole opposite side. Go from arm downward to toes, upward to top of head, patting briskly. Stop, close your eyes, feel that side of you, compare it with your other side. Then do the other side. Feel yourself tingle.

    Vary this by gently massaging with the whole hand. Take a dry shower.

Sideways
Be aware of action lines in your body.

Feeling Your Width. Stretch outward to both sides with your arms as if you could touch both walls with your fingertips; then

Feel Yourself Narrow. Bring your arms together, press them momentarily against your sides, then release. Repeat these two.

Up/down
Elongating Your Spine. Feel yourself growing tall, pulled up by an imaginary string attached to the top of your head (crown); then

    Give in to gravity, sink down, rounding your back, chin lowered toward chest, feel your weight. Repeat these two.

    Open your arms out to sides, stretch, then close arms around you, give yourself a hug. You deserve it!

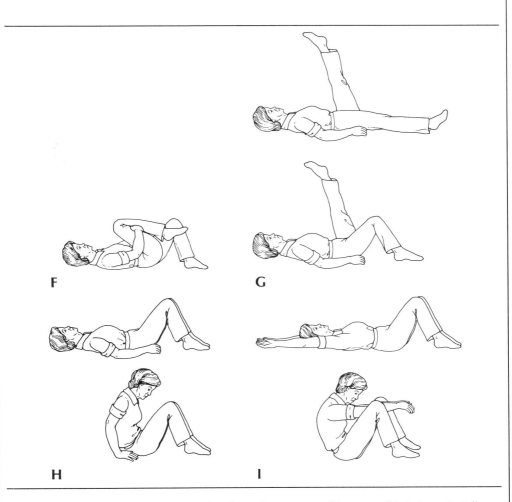

Figure 15A–1. (cont.) F. Liver stretcher (knee-chest). **G.** Leg lift. **H.** Modified sit-up. **I.** Full sit-up.

Walking Variations

Walk slowly, eight steps in one direction, stop, change direction, walk eight steps, stop, change direction. Then pick up the speed. Repeat several times. A variation: Somewhere in the sequence, add a pause for eight counts. Hold very still. Try standing in different positions on the hold.

Sidewise Walk. Holding table or kitchen counter if you need to, walk sideward crossing one foot in front of the other. Then

Return to the other side, this time crossing one foot in back of the other.

Walk sideward again, this time cross once in back, once in front (the grapevine walk). (You can practice feet crossovers beforehand while seated in your chair. Move left foot over right, return to place. Move right foot over left, return to place.)

More Loosening Up

Shake hands, then add arms, shoulders, then stop.

Shake legs, add voice and head, and arms again—as if using a jack hammer.

Then stop and relax and breathe deeply.

KINESPHERE

Find *your* kinesphere . . . all the space you can reach with your fingertips from where you are, sitting or standing—above you, below you, in front of you, behind you. Imagine standing or sitting inside a globe of which you are the center. Now stretch to reach all around the confines of that globe. With an imaginary paintbrush in your hand, "paint" the whole inside of your kinesphere. Use one hand, then the other.

Try varying the feeling of the above exercise by actually holding in your hand

1. A thin scarf
2. A leaf
3. A tube from a roll of paper towels
4. A pencil

Open your arms out to sides, stretch, then close arms around you. Give yourself another big hug!

CARDIORESPIRATORY EXERCISES

Walk! Walk around the table, up and down the hall, during commercials on TV—get up and get a glass of water—it cleans the pipes and gets blood moving again. Walk outside when weather is nice . . . around the block . . . to the store . . . to the mailbox . . . in the park, enjoy nature! Walk to see a friend . . . ask your friend to come for a walk. Above all walk a little briskly—enough to cause you to breathe a little deeper! *Excellent* for cardiorespiratory toning.

Note: Jogging is for the experts—don't attempt unless you are a regular daily jogger. If you wish to try it, consult your doctor first and then join a physical fitness program, and then attempt only when the trained director feels you are expertly fit and ready!

Brisk walking may be the ticket for you.

Dancing. If you like ballroom dancing and have continued to do it over the years, keep it up. If dancing never was your cup of tea, especially the couples variety, why not try folk dancing. If you are interested, ask your senior center director to organize a group—or get together with a few of your friends, invite someone who knows some folk dances, get a few records and learn. If 20 people get together and request a teacher from your local Adult Education Director, the teacher will be provided at the time and place you indicate. It doesn't have to be evenings—try an afternoon!

Swimming. A great way to exercise too, the water is not only an aid in buoyancy, but can be a great resister. Try moving your arms about under water and feel the resistance on your muscles. Walk or march in water up over your knees.

- Water exercises: Learn with a qualified leader from the local "Y" or Red Cross or recreation program.
- Floating: On your stomach or back for starters. Add a flutter or frog kick, then a breast stroke until you're
- Swimming: Breast stroke with frog kick—a good breathing exercise to increase cardiorespiratory endurance. You may want to try other swimming techniques, one side and then the other. *Don't overdo!* Relax at water's edge when winded; try again if you're feeling up to it.

Social Games. Shuffleboard—hand or with pusher, ring toss, beanbag toss, darts, shooting pool or billiards, and croquet.

MUSCULAR ENDURANCE (REPETITIVE ACTIVITY)

All of aforementioned activities, if repeated, could increase muscular endurance. *Do* start slowly with the bending and stretching flexibility exercises. *Don't* do more than you are comfortable doing. *Do* build up to repeating the exercises and adding new ones. Pace yourself. Exercise and activity should be enjoyable. *Don't* force yourself beyond endurance or try for medals!

RELAXATION TECHNIQUES

Too much stress and anxiety is harmful and wasteful of human energy. Below are a few techniques that should help you to relax, for *relaxation is a skill that must be learned and practiced*.

Setting

Practice these techniques in as near a perfect setting as possible.

1. Wear comfortable clothing.
2. Lie on floor that is well padded or sit in a comfortable chair.
3. Place a small pillow under the knees.
4. Have room semidarkened.
5. Use either a metronome or neutral record (bells, ocean, etc.) in order to dull out disturbing sounds.

Procedure

Diaphragmatic Breathing. It will give you a more complete exchange of air and is the most important technique, for it can be easily employed at any time once it is mastered.

1. Lie flat.
2. Place hands on stomach, fingertips barely touching.
3. When you inhale, push stomach out (fingertips will separate).
4. Exhale, stomach goes in (fingertips will come together). All of this will feel awkward at first but in a few days you will recognize and feel the results of diaphragmatic breathing.

Passive Scene. With eyes closed, picture a pleasant passive scene. See yourself in this scene happy and relaxed—spend a few minutes enjoying this scene. This procedure should rest your mind, for it is impossible to be worrying or unhappy if your mind is concentrating on something enjoyable.

Progressive Relaxation. (Developed by Dr. Edmond Jacobson) Brief contraction of a muscle (feeling of tension) followed by feelings of relaxation. *Important: anyone over 40 should not hold the contraction for longer than 3 seconds.*

1. Feet and legs: Curl toes downward, tensing until you feel a slight discomfort (no longer than 3 seconds), then slowly and passively let your whole body relax. Wait a few seconds then proceed with all the following in this same manner. Flex foot so toes point to your head. Push heels into floor. Pull legs together and press.
2. Arms and hands: Make a fist. Press palms into floor. Press back of hands into floor. Press arms against body.
3. Shoulders and head: Lift shoulders up to ears. Close eyes tightly. Close jaws.

(Source: Forbes, E. J., & Fitzsimons, V. M. The older adult: A process for wellness. St. Louis, Mo.: C. V. Mosby, 1981.)

BIBLIOGRAPHY

Arenberg, D. Anticipation interval and age differences in verbal learning. *Journal of Abnormal Psychology,* 1965, *70*(6), 419–424.

Birchenall, J. M., & Streight, M. E. *Care of the older adult.* Philadelphia: J. B. Lippincott, 1982.

Botwinick, J. *Aging and behavior.* New York: Springer, 1973.

Burnside, I. M. *Psychosocial nursing care of the aged.* New York: McGraw-Hill, 1980.

Burnside, I. M. (Ed.). *Nursing and the aged.* New York: McGraw-Hill, 1976.

Burnside, I. M. (Ed.). *Psychosocial care of the aged.* New York: McGraw-Hill, 1973.

Canestrari, R. E. Paced and self-paced learning in young and elderly adults. *Journal of Gerontology,* 1963, *18*(2), 165–168.

Carnevali, D. D., & Patrick, M. (Eds.). *Nursing management for the elderly.* New York: J. B. Lippincott, 1979.

Chaisson, G. M. *Depression in the elderly.* In S. V. Anderson and E. E. Bavwens (Eds.), *Chronic health problems.* New York: C. V. Mosby, 1981, pp. 262–273.

Craik, F. I. M. Age differences in human memory. In J. E. Birren & K. W. Schaie (Eds.), *Handbook of the psychology of aging.* New York: Van Nostrand Reinhold, 1977.

Dodge, J. S. Factors related to patients' perceptions of their cognitive needs. *Nursing Research,* 1969, *18*(6), 502–513.

Dozier, A. M. *Preoperative preparation by nurses to improve the elderly's postoperative recuperation.* Unpublished master's thesis, University of Rochester, 1980.

Dozier, A. M. *Preoperative teaching with the older learner.* Research report, University of Rochester, 1978.

Ebersole, P., & Hess, P. *Toward healthy aging.* St. Louis, Mo.: C. V. Mosby, 1981.

Eliopoulos, C. *Gerontological nursing.* New York: Harper & Row, 1979.

Fillenbaum, G. G. Social context and self-assessments of health among the elderly. *Journal of Health and Social Behavior,* 1979, *20*(1), 45–51.

Forbes, E. J., & Fitzsimons, V. M. *The older adult.* St. Louis, Mo.: C. V. Mosby, 1981.

Gelein, J. L. Aged women and health. *Nursing Clinics of North America,* 1982, *17*(1), 179–185.

Gelein, J. L. The aged American female: Relationships between social support and health. *Journal of Gerontological Nursing,* 1980, *6*(2), 69–73.

Goodrow, B. A. Limiting factors in reducing participation in older adult learning opportunities. *The Gerontologist,* 1975, *15*(5), Pt. I, 418–422.

Harris, D. M., & Associates, Inc. *The myth and reality of aging in America.* Washington, D.C.: National Council on Aging, 1975.

Harris, D. M., & Guten, S. Health-protective behavior: An exploratory study. *Journal of Health and Social Behavior,* 1979, *20*(1), 17–29.

Hoyer, W. J., Rebok, G. W., & Sved, S. M. Effects of varying irrelevant information on adult age differences in problem solving. *Journal of Gerontology,* 1979, *34*(4), 553–560.

Hulicka, I. M. *Psychology and sociology of aging.* New York: Thomas Y. Crowell, 1977.

Hulicka, I. M. Age differences in retention as a function of interference. *Journal of Gerontology,* 1967, *22*(1), 180–184.

Hulicka, I. M., & Grossman, J. L. Age-group comparisons for the use of mediators in paired-associate learning. *Journal of Gerontology,* 1967, *22*, 46–51.

Hulicka, I. M., & Weiss, R. L. Age differences in retention as a function of learning. *Canadian Journal of Consulting Psychology,* 1966, *29*, 125–129.

Hulicka, I. M., Sterns, J., & Grossman, J. Age group comparisons of paired associate learning as a function of paced and self-paced association and response times. *Journal of Gerontology,* 1967, *22*(3), 274–280.

Hultsch, D. F. Learning to learn in adulthood. *Journal of Gerontology,* 1974, *29*(3), 302–308.

Kausler, D. H., & Kleim, D. M. Age differences in processing relevant versus irrelevant stimuli in multiple-item recognition learning. *Journal of Gerontology,* 1978, *33*(1), 87–93.

Kim, K., & Grier, M. Pacing effects of medication instruction for the elderly. *Journal of Gerontological Nursing,* 1981, *8*, 464–468.

Lawton, M. P. The impact of the environment on aging and behavior. In J. E. Birren & K. W. Schaie (Eds.), *Handbook of the psychology of aging*. New York: Van Nostrand Reinhold, 1977, pp. 276–301.

Lawton, M. P. The functional assessment of elderly people. *Journal of the American Geriatrics Society*, 1971, *19*(6), 465–481.

Lindeman, C. A. Nursing intervention with the presurgical patient: Effectiveness and efficiency of group and individual preoperative teaching—phase two. *Nursing Research*, 1972, *21*(3), 196–209.

Lindeman, C. A., & Van Aernam, B. Nursing intervention with the presurgical patient—The effects of structured and unstructured preoperative teaching. *Nursing Research*, 1971, *20*(4), 319–332.

Long, J. M. (Ed.). Caring for and caring about elderly people: A guide to the rehabilitative approach. Rochester, N.Y.: Rochester Regional Medical Program and the University of Rochester School of Nursing, 1972.

Mezey, M. D., Rauckhorst, L. H., & Stokes, S. A. *Health assessment of the older individual*. New York: Springer, 1980.

Moenster, P. A. Learning and memory in relation to age. *Journal of Gerontology*, 1972, *27*(3), 361–363.

Murrell, F. H. The effect of extensive practice on age differences in reaction time. *Journal of Gerontology*, 1970, *25*(3), 268–274.

Norton, D., McLaren, R., & Exton-Smith, A. N. *An investigation of geriatric nursing problems in hospitals*. Edinburgh: Churchill Livingstone, 1975.

Pearson, L. J., & Kotthoff, M. E. *Geriatric clinical protocols*. New York: J. B. Lippincott, 1979.

Perdue, B., Mahon, N., Hawes, S., & Frik, S. (Eds.). *Chronic care nursing*. New York: Springer, 1981.

Perlmutter, M. Age differences in adults' free recall, cued recall, and recognition. *Journal of Gerontology*, 1979, *34*(4), 533–539.

Poon, L. W., Fozard, J. L., Cermalk, L. S., Arenberg, D., & Thompson, L. W. *New directions in memory and aging: Proceedings of the George A. Talland Memorial conference*. Hillsdale, N. J.: Lawrence Erlbaum Assoc., 1980.

Rebuk, G., & Hoyer, W. The functional context of elderly behavior. *The Gerontologist*, 1977, *17*(1), 27–34.

Rotter, J. B. Generalized expectancies for internal versus external control of reinforcement. *Psychological Monographs*, 1966, *80*, 1–28.

Rowe, E. J., & Schnore, M. M. Item concreteness and reported strategies in paired associate learning as a function of age. *Journal of Gerontology*, 1971, *26*, 470–475.

Schonfield, D. In search of early memories. *International Congress of Gerontology*, 1969, 295–301.

Schonfield, D., & Robertson, B. A. Memory storage and aging. *Canadian Journal of Psychology*, 1966, *20*(2), 228–236.

Sieman, J. R. Learning from programmed material as a function of age. *Gerontological Society 27th Annual Scientific Meeting*, 1974, *2*, 67.

Winograd, E., Smith, A. D., & Simon, E. W. Aging and the picture superiority effect in recall. *Journal of Gerontology*, 1982, *37*(1), 70–75.

Wittels, I. Age and stimulus meaningfulness in paired-associate learning. *Journal of Gerontology*, 1972, *27*(3), 372–375.

Young, C. M. Nutritional counseling for better health. *Geriatrics*, 1974, *29*(83).

Yurik, A., Robb, S., Speir, B., & Ebert, N. *The aged person and the nursing process*. New York: Appleton-Century-Crofts, 1980.

Health Education When There Are Special Reproductive Needs

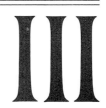

Reproduction when there are medical or social problems brings complications and difficulties for women and their families. Special efforts to provide information and support become necessary. Part III focuses on several major reproductive complications. For example, Chapter 16 discusses group methodologies to use with pregnant adolescents, and Chapter 17 describes methodologies to assist women in making decisions about an unintentional pregnancy. Chapter 18 details content for women and their significant other where cesarean birth is anticipated or occurs. The last chapter in this section describes one medical complication, diabetes, and the content needed for educating women about this condition. Appendix B provides detailed guidelines for educating the woman who is both pregnant and diabetic. The description and guidelines for diabetic women who are pregnant is presented as a model so health care providers can develop guidelines for other medical conditions.

Adolescent Pregnancy: Use of Prenatal Groups

16

Barbara N. Adams

Nearly one million young women under the age of 20 become pregnant each year. Of this number, approximately 600,000 carry their pregnancies to term. Although the number of births has declined somewhat since 1973, the costs associated with adolescent pregnancy for both the teenager and her baby remain a national concern (ACOG,1979). An overview of the medical and psychosocial risks surrounding adolescent pregnancy follows. This chapter, however, focuses on other important needs of the pregnant teenager: preparation for labor, delivery and initial parenting, and assistance with the developmental tasks of pregnancy and adolescence. Use of the group modality is described and sample prenatal group sessions are included.

Risks of Adolescent Pregnancy

Investigations during the last decade have shown that obstetrical complications for the primigravid teenager age 15 and older are no greater than for the woman in her twenties if she receives early and consistent prenatal care and adequate nutrition (Phipps-Yonas, 1980). Age alone is also not the critical factor in increased medical risk for babies when their mothers are older adolescents (Merritt, Lawrence, & Naeye, 1980). Agreement has not been reached on the question of risk for younger adolescents. Some studies indicate higher rates of pregnancy-induced hypertension and cephalopelvic disproportion for these young women (Dunhoelter, Jimenez, & Baumann, 1975). Low birth weight babies, however, have been shown to be a significant problem in this lower age group (Elster & McAnarney, 1980) and are a major cause of infant mortality and neurological defects (Guttmacher Institute, 1980).

Even though teenagers (particularly aged 15 and older) may not be at a higher risk by virtue of age alone, other factors contribute to their reproductive disadvantage. Low socioeconomic status, inadequate nutrition, poor health habits, inadequate prenatal care, substance abuse, and a high incidence of sexually transmitted diseases can adversely affect pregnancy outcome (ACOG, 1979).

The greater risk for morbidity lies in the psychosocial area. Developmental tasks are interrupted and the psychological tasks of pregnancy are difficult for the teenager to complete. Socially, pregnant adolescents often experience educational dysfunction and face future vocational and financial disadvantages. The outcome for those who choose to marry is guarded because nearly three-fourths of the teenagers who marry between the ages of 14 and 17 will be divorced (Mercer, 1979).

Adolescent parenting has been under close scrutiny in recent years. Although it has not been shown that adolescents abuse their children more than adults (Sahler, 1980), the ineffective or inconsistent parenting behavior that professionals have observed in this population is cause for concern. Repeat pregnancy during the adolescent years is a major problem. The medical outcome is grave for second and third babies born to teenage mothers because they are at considerably higher risk of prematurity and perinatal death than the first born babies (Jekel et al., 1975). The psychosocial outcome is equally bleak. The teenager with more than one child is even more likely to be trapped in the familiar cycle of pregnancy followed by educational, emotional, developmental, and social instability and further repetition of pregnancy.

Comprehensive Programs for Pregnant Teenagers

To effectively meet the multiple needs of pregnant adolescents, comprehensive programs have been developed throughout the country. Each program offers services designed to meet the medical, psychosocial, and educational needs of pregnant teenagers through the use of a multidisciplinary staff. One such program is the Rochester Adolescent Maternity Project (RAMP) in Rochester, New York. Individual care is provided to young women, families, and boyfriends throughout the prenatal, labor and delivery, and postpartum periods (see McAnarney & Adams, 1977, for a complete description of RAMP services). In addition, a group experience is offered to each adolescent while she is receiving prenatal care in the program.

The RAMP group experience provides the basis for the remainder of this chapter.

Rationale for Prenatal Groups

Groups are advocated as a mode of therapy and teaching for teenagers because of the importance of the peer group to adolescents. It is also believed that the level of satisfaction during the labor and delivery process can be enhanced for women of all ages when they are prepared for childbirth. (Adams et al., 1976, p. 467)

Consideration of both these factors led to the development of the RAMP prenatal groups with the objectives of helping the teenagers work through the developmental tasks of adolescence and the psychological tasks of pregnancy, along with preparing them for labor, delivery, and initial parenthood. The theory behind these objectives as well as the theory of groups provides the framework for the prenatal groups.

Issues and content related to childbirth education can be found in Chapters 11, 12, 13, 18, and 19 and Appendix A and B in this book. A discussion of adolescent tasks, psychological tasks of pregnancy, and group process as they relate to groups for pregnant adolescents follows.

Developmental Tasks of Adolescence. The developmental tasks of adolescence include:

1. Striving for independence
2　Achieving comfort with a new body
3. Becoming comfortable with relationships with the opposite sex
4. Learning to verbalize conceptually
5. Developing a value system (Adams et al., 1976)

Pregnancy often causes a teenager who is making strides toward independence to regress and become more dependent because of her increased needs for physical, emotional, and financial support from her family. Conflicts can arise within families as the teenager struggles with her now ambiguous place in the family. Within the group setting, the common conflicts in families with a pregnant daughter such as attending school versus staying home, rest versus exercise, household responsibilities versus going out with friends, or curfew time can be discussed. The group leaders can guide the group in problem solving. Alternative solutions can be considered by the teenager and tried out in her own situation, allowing her to keep her own goal of independence while maintaining the care and nurturing of significant others that pregnancy requires.

It is difficult for a teenager to accept a changing pregnant body at a time when she may not have resolved feelings about her new adolescent contours. Having an opportunity within a group situation to discuss feelings about the changing self can be helpful. Some pregnant teenagers feel that only others experiencing a similar situation can truly understand their problems.

Peer support in the group is also valued if the pregnant teenager is abandoned by her boyfriend or female friends when they learn of her pregnancy. For some, the adult world places a "bad girl" image on the pregnant teenager and, again, it is within a supportive group atmosphere that feelings can be shared, values of teenagers and adults can be explored, and self-worth restored.

Finally, groups provide adolescents who are learning to put their thoughts into words an opportunity to try out new thoughts and ideas in a safe atmosphere. Some may be able to leave the group with enhanced verbal skills.

Psychological Tasks of Pregnancy. Bibring and colleagues (1961) have described the psychological tasks of pregnancy. Early on, a woman must accept the fetus as part of herself. Gradually, she recognizes the fetus as a separate person, and prepares emotionally and physically for its birth. Finally, each woman must make the transition to motherhood. Rubin (1975) expanded the work of Bibring with her maternal tasks in pregnancy. Described as pregnancy work, they include seeking safe passage for herself and child, ensuring the baby's acceptance by her family, binding-in to her child, and giving of herself to the baby.

Some teenagers do not fulfill the first tasks until well into their pregnancies because of denial of the pregnancy. This often means delayed prenatal care as well. The group provides a place where feelings about being pregnant can be explored, the reactions the teenager is receiving from others can be discussed, pregnancy options presented, and consistent prenatal care encouraged. A teenager who is not able to face her pregnancy may be helped to move through these early tasks when she sees she is not alone with her feelings, has the opportunity to explore both the negative and positive sides of pregnancy, and can test her values and choices in an atmosphere of acceptance and support. She will then be able to move on to the process of binding-in with her child, having accepted the idea of the pregnancy itself.

Acceptance of the pregnancy and the new baby are not automatic when there is conflict between the teenager and her parents or she and the baby's father as is often the case for pregnant adolescents. A reordering of relationships with boyfriend or young husband and family is necessary and is modeled as the teenager establishes new relationships with other group members and the leaders. It is also difficult for an adolescent to give of herself as a mother when she has not yet resolved the dependent–independent nature of her relationship with her own mother. Often a group leader is tested by the teenagers as a mother figure providing the opportunity to discuss mother-daughter conflicts and explore alternative ways of dealing with them. The adolescents can incorporate such problem-solving experiences into their lives to be used in an ongoing basis after their baby's birth. The concrete nature of learning breathing techniques to help oneself in labor, and the planning and purchasing of baby equipment and supplies, offers the teenager additional ways to prepare for the baby's birth.

Group Process. Because pregnant teenagers are experiencing both a developmental and a situational crisis, a unique group experience is required, that is, one that meets both their learning objectives and their interaction needs. This can be accomplished by incorporating the techniques described by Littlefield and Siebert in their group method of learning (Table 3–5). Using their suggested methodology, content is given by the leaders only after members share their knowledge of the subject being discussed. Group members are helped to find their own answers to questions and to develop their own coping mechanisms.

Goals of the group process and the developmental tasks of groups, necessary for leaders to understand before beginning group work, are also discussed in Chapter 3.

Group Co-leadership. Co-leadership has been found to enhance the group experience for teenagers and leaders alike. The adolescents are able to observe the leaders as role models as they demonstrate adult behaviors, communication patterns, and simulated family interaction. They can see first hand a relationship based on trust, respect, and shared responsibility, a healthy model of interpersonal relationships (Marram, 1978).

The egalitarian approach to co-leadership in which leaders accept one another as equals and share responsibility for the group's development is suggested. They decide on goals and interventions jointly and have equal opportunity to participate in the group. Often they will alternate behaviors in the group such as being active or passive, directive or nondirective, observer or participant. The leaders also profit from peer involvement because they can validate or challenge one another's perceptions of the group and the activities that are carried out (Marram, 1978). The sex and professional background of the leaders is not important as long as they complement one another with their knowledge of adolescence, labor, delivery, and parenting, their philosophy of group leadership and process, and their willingness to work on their own relationship within the group.

Setting and Structure of Groups. Opportunity for a group experience can be explained to all teenagers upon entry into their prenatal program. Health care providers should reinforce this during individual visits. At approximately 26 to 28 weeks' gestation each teenager should be sent an invitation by mail with a follow-up telephone call from her group leaders informing her that her own group is beginning. Some of the group activities should be described. Ten to 12 teenagers can be assigned to each group, because six to eight will probably attend regularly. Because not all adolescents are developmentally ready for a group experience, it is expected that some group members would drop out. Eight to 10 weekly meetings of one to one-and-one-half hours in length are usually needed. These should be scheduled at the end of a clinic session, making them as convenient as possible for the teenagers. A large quiet conference room away from the busy clinic is an appropriate setting for the group meetings.

The leaders can choose whether their group will be available for only pregnant teenagers, or whether boyfriends, mothers, or labor coaches will be included. Some leaders will want these significant others to be included to promote family-centered care and to provide opportunity in the group for the teenager to work on the task of changing family relationships. Other leaders may want to focus on the teenagers themselves, and feel that the young women will raise concerns more readily and express themselves more freely without others present. Leaders with this preference may choose to have two additional group sessions for those teenagers who wish to include boyfriends or labor coaches. A short course on the labor and delivery process, breathing techniques, and role of the coach can be given. If time allows, a delivery film or tour of the labor and delivery area can be included. Separate "grandmothers" groups have been shown to be a way to give mothers of pregnant adolescents an opportunity to share their feelings, problem solve with other mothers, and be updated on the labor and delivery experience (Dohr, 1979). A developmental and situational crisis can develop for these women as they are confronted with the role changes and new stresses on the family that occur when a daughter becomes pregnant. The group approach may be helpful in resolving the crisis and may contribute to growth in the mothers' ego development and a strengthening of the family system (Dohr, 1979).

Leaders may wish to have open groups for the first 3 weeks, during which time outreach needs to be done to encourage the teenagers to participate. This is necessary because the adolescents usually have not been asked to participate in a group before, and approach it with some timidity. The present orientation of teenagers also does not lend itself to planning ahead for a series of group sessions. Thereafter, meetings can be closed, allowing for group cohesion to develop.

A semistructured format is appropriate for all sessions. This allows the leaders to present some of the essentials of childbirth education or to raise issues the group members may have been skirting for an in-depth discussion. At the same time it provides for extended interaction by group members when they raise a subject or issue of interest. Leaders should keep lengthy didactic presentations to a minimum and not feel impelled to complete any specific amount of educational material in one session.

Common Problems in Adolescent Groups

Inconsistent Attendance. As previously mentioned, with the teenagers' present rather than future orientation group attendance is often sporadic. Outreach by mail, by phone, and in person during prenatal visits is often necessary when a group is initiated. Thereafter, contact must be continued after each session with anyone who has not attended to keep the group viable. This is a time consuming role for leaders but should be considered a usual function for those leading adolescent groups.

Polarized Emotional Leadership. An individual group member may assume either a negative or positive emotional leadership role as the group moves into the working stage (Adams et al., 1976). Negative emotional leadership can be attempted by a member as she competes for attention in the group. She can be identified as the member who embellishes a personal experience such as a visit to the emergency room for a vaginal infection. She describes her visit in such a way as to have the group believe that she was experiencing a miscarriage and found health care providers inattentive to her needs. A technique that can be used with this group member is to help her focus on the situation and response she received rather than her interpretations of the experience. Questions about why she went to the emergency room, who took care of her, what she was told, and the results of her examination and tests will help her relate the incident more accurately and help to reassure other group members.

The positive counterpart in the group can be equally problematic. She may be so positive about everything related to her pregnancy that she may not permit the expression of fears or a discussion of problems by other members. She often is the person who changes the subject to a lighter vein. The leaders must not allow this to happen if they sense that other group members are ready to explore an issue in depth.

Although these polarized members are important in the development of the group's emotional process and their activities recognized as part of the adolescents' need for independence, the group needs to be pulled out of these experiences by a neutral member. She is the person who relates a problem about her pregnancy, expresses her initial concern, and describes realistically the information and reassurances she received from others. If a neutral member is not present the leaders can take on this role, using a typical situation as an example for the group.

A Monopolizing Member. When one person in a group monopolizes the conversation, others are deprived of their share of participation. This tends to create bad feelings within the group with resultant anger and frustration. It also prevents others from offering their viewpoints on the topic being discussed, a primary goal of the groups being suggested here (Sampson & Marthas, 1981).

Excessive talking can reflect anxiety or a need for attention. The goal of intervention should not be to examine these dynamics but to effect a change in behavior. If this behavior is caught early on, interrupting the individual in a supportive manner may suffice: "That's a really good idea Sue. Let's see if others have some suggestions." If it is repetitive and an effort is to be made to help the individual see her behavior and its effect on others, different strategies are needed. Leaders can reflect on the individual's behavior, interpret it for the individual and the group (example: mentioning anxiety as a cause), or reflecting the group's feelings such as pointing out the boredom or anger of the group. Confronting the individual or the group can be done by skilled leaders who will take care that this is done in a supportive fashion (Sampson & Marthas, 1981).

The Silent Group. Silence, the most common problem in groups, can mean many things: punishment of the leader, escape from conflict, fear of the reactions of others, inability to formulate responses, ambivalence, or in a positive vein, may indicate that members are silently problem solving (Hinkley & Herman, 1951). Leaders also can cause silence by making unilateral decisions, dominating the discussion, or cutting off members' participation (Sampson & Marthas, 1981).

The first task of the leaders of a silent group is to examine their leadership and to intervene on themselves if leadership style is adversely affecting the group. At times, silence could be related to a specific topic that members feel is irrelevant. The group can be asked if they would prefer to be talking about something else or if there is an activity they would rather be doing. If the silence seems based on an interpersonal issue, such as fear or anger, a statement such as, "I wonder if you are angry about what I've said?" can be made. An equally worthy approach is to let the issue pass if the group has otherwise been moving along well. Sporadic silence can be handled by nonintervention but continued silence and apathy of a group must be dealt with or the important work of the group will not be carried out by the members, the very people who are expected to do this (Sampson & Marthas, 1981).

Development of Prenatal Groups. In group work, as in individual teaching and counseling, a knowledge of teaching–learning principles is needed. The reader should refer to Chapter 2 for a review of these as well as instructions for writing objectives. The following assessment, objectives, methodology, and evaluation are based on these principles and provide added information specific to adolescent prenatal groups.

Assessment of Learning Needs. Because the determination of learning needs of teenage group members is difficult, several alternative methods of assessment can be tried. A very structured approach can be used with paper and pencil pretests. The other extreme, a very unstructured approach, can also be utilized in which the teenagers are asked their needs and expectations at the first group meeting. The first method is probably too rigid, too much like school, for a group of adolescents who in general have not had good educational experiences (a highly pedagogical approach). The latter may be too free flowing. Having no frame of reference, they may be unable to say what they want and need. In addition, they are being asked to respond to an abstract concept when developmentally their thinking is still concrete (a highly andragogical approach).

A dual method of assessment can be devised that is more satisfactory for group members and leaders alike. At the initial meeting a list of possible discussion topics can be listed on the blackboard (see initial group meeting outline that follows for a sample list). Additions are requested from the group. Each member then chooses six topics and lists them in order of importance to her. The lists are placed in a bowl; each teenager chooses one and reads from that list as a group leader tabulates the results on the blackboard. Those topics with the highest rankings will be the discussion items for the next few weeks. Once topics are chosen, group members will expect that they will be raised in subsequent weeks. This appropriately gives them some independence and control over their situation. However, members will also shift the agenda of an individual group session around to meet their own immediate needs. Leaders need to be flexible enough to allow for this. A lively discussion can follow that often includes both information giving and expression of feelings.

Learning needs around individual topics can be assessed as subjects are raised. For example, at a session where signs of labor are to be introduced, a leader might ask, "What have you heard about the ways labor begins?" Usually some correct and some incorrect responses are given. The leaders can build on the knowledge the group already has as well as dispel myths and misconceptions.

Objectives. Objectives for each session should be written with the overall group objectives clearly in mind. Each group meeting then will have goals pertaining to preparation for the childbirth experience as well as helping the teenagers progress with their tasks of adolescence and pregnancy. Group process objectives should also be included. It must be clear from the objectives that both a cognitive and an affective dimension exist in each group. This will promote the philosophy that is key to the adolescent groups, that is, every subject raised is approached as having a need for information giving and expression of feelings.

Methodology. Four sample prenatal group sessions follow with objectives for childbirth education content, promotion of developmental tasks, and group process. Content and interaction techniques are provided.

Initial Group Session

Objectives
1. Orient members to the group.
2. Determine the group's goals for childbirth education.
3. Promote independence and decision making.

Process

1. As teenagers enter the room have a nutritious snack such as milk and granola or juice and nuts ready on a table. Encourage members to pour for one another and pass the snack plate.

2. A leader explains the need for name tags. Have one group member pass out the tags and pens. Have a limited number of pens, making the teenagers share with one another.

3. The second leader presents an introductory game. A member passes around a box with pictures that are cut in half (choose pictures appealing to pregnant teenagers). Explain that each member is to find the person who has the other half of her picture and then talk with that person for a few minutes to learn a little about her. Come back and sit down, and everyone will take turns introducing the person she just met. The teenagers always ask one another when their babies are due, and usually whether they would like a boy or a girl. While the introductions are taking place, one leader can begin a chart with each teenager's name, EDC, and sex of the child she would like. Space is left for the actual EDC and sex. These can be filled in as deliveries occur by the teenager herself if she is on the postpartum unit over a group session and is able to come to the group, or by a leader who keeps track of deliveries. Comments about the information on the chart by leaders and members can conclude this exercise.

4. Group contract is explained around meeting time, place, length of session, and attendance. Emphasis is placed on starting time. The open and closed nature of the group is explained. A decision about refreshments can be left to members.

5. One leader asks the group, "Why have you come to the group?" Leaders interact nonsystematically to follow up on

Rationale

Sets the scene for a semistructured group.

Encourages member interaction.

Encourages member interaction.

Demonstrates equal status of leaders. Helps group members recognize commonalities with one another and encourages social development of the group.

Provides initial orientation to group members, gives structure and parameters to the group appropriate for guidance of teenage behavior.
Recognizes adolescents' present rather than future orientation.
Promotes independence and decision making.
Promotes initial group development (leaders should expect stilted interaction and inability to directly express feelings).

responses, encourage discussion, and give brief answers to direct questions.

6. As a follow-up to prior discussion, a leader might state, "While we've been talking you've mentioned several things you'd like to discuss in the groups. Let me list those on the board." She then asks for other suggestions, adding items from her own list. A sample of a final list may look like the following:

tour of labor and delivery area
newborns
bottle feeding
how labor begins
legal rights of teenagers
pain relief in labor and delivery
different ways to give birth
breast-feeding
movie of labor and delivery
birth control
how babies are born
relaxation
being home with the baby
breathing techniques for labor and delivery
pregnancy options
circumcision
school alternatives
role of labor coach
pediatric care
my body after delivery

The process of choosing the topics of importance to the group from this list has previously been described. Often the topics can be combined for subsequent weeks, allowing for all essential information and discussion to take place.

7. Conclude the group with a review of activities that have taken place. Positive reinforcement should be given for the initial progress of the group. The expectation for meeting time and place for the following week should again be mentioned. Urge members to call leaders if they know they must be absent from a group meeting.

Demonstrates adult communication patterns. Provides initial childbirth education.

Promotes independence and decision making.
Identifies the teenagers' objectives for the group. Promotes initial group development.

Acknowledges concrete nature of adolescent thinking and present rather than future orientation.

Second Group Session

Usually topics related to labor and delivery head the list of each group. To understand the process of labor and delivery, the adolescents need to have a good understanding of their reproductive system. Often teenagers have fairly good knowledge of their anatomy, but their understanding of physiology is limited. Knowledge of the teenagers' educational strengths and deficits provides the basis for the organization of the second group meeting.

Objectives

1. Promote continued group development.
2. Provide initial preparation for childbirth.
3. Increase the teenagers' acceptance of body changes and functions.

Process	Rationale
1. Review attendance status. Inform group members about those who called to say they would be absent. Ask if members know about anyone else who is absent. Introduce new members. Add names, sex choices and EDC's to chart. Explore choice of sex and thoughts and feelings of teenagers about delivering a baby of the opposite sex from the one desired.	Encourages group commitment. Helps integrate new members into group. Continues recognition of commonalities among members. Begins an examination of the adolescent's self image and relationship with others.
2. Review group contract.	Integrates new members into group. Reinforces structure of group for old members.
3. The topic list from the previous week (copied from the blackboard to poster board by the leaders) is shown to the group, indicating the high priority given to labor and delivery topics. A leader explains the need to understand the reproductive system before moving to the labor and delivery process.	Provides visual reminder of group decisions reinforcing the teenagers' control and independence within the group. Equalizes the learning level among members.
Through the use of a flannel board and cutouts for the various organs of the reproductive system, ova, sperm, menstrual flow, fertilized egg, embryo, and various stages of development of the fetus, the menstrual cycle, fertilization, and fetal growth and development can be explained.	Demonstrates use of concrete audiovisual materials appropriate for the adolescent stage of development. Reinforces learning when both audio and visual stimulation are provided.
When fetal development is raised, group members will choose their own direction for discussion. Some possibilities include: comparison of the stages of fetal development among members, sex determination, tests for fetal well-being during pregnancy, or	Continues prenatal education and identification of group commonalities. Demonstrates cognitive and affective dimensions of the group. Equalizes the roles of the leaders. Helps move the group from leader to member orientation.

activities of a fetus in utero. One leader can facilitate discussion while the other uses the flannel board. Help from the teenagers can be requested throughout the demonstration.

4. The group is now ready for labor and delivery information and discussion. If they have asked to learn "how a baby is born," this group session can easily be moved into a discussion of the mechanism of labor, contractions of the uterus, and effacement and dilatation of the cervix.

Responds to group's identified need for prenatal education.

A pelvis and doll should be available for a demonstration of the mechanism of labor. A leader can show the group a pelvis and have them feel the pelvic landmarks on themselves. Members, in pairs, can try to move the doll through the pelvis. Because it is always difficult for the teenagers, they are reassured when the smooth process is demonstrated. They might like to try again once they have seen the demonstration. A knitted uterus with doll inside or posters can be used for a demonstration of contractions, dilatation and effacement. Using the flannel board or commercial posters, the relationship between these two facets of labor and delivery can be shown.

Capitalizes on the activity orientation of teenagers.

While this activity is taking place, some groups will move the discussion to bodily changes taking place in pregnancy or to fears of labor and delivery (as examples). Leaders can promote the discussion by asking indirectly for feelings, such as, "What is that (or will that be) like for you?" A projective technique is also valuable. For example:

a. What have you heard about labor and delivery?
b. What has happened to friends or relatives in labor and delivery?
c. What do you think labor and delivery will be like for you?

Acknowledges the teenagers' inability to apply abstract labels to their feelings.

5. Recap briefly the group's movement through its second meeting. Positive reinforcement (as appropriate) should be given for members' attendance and participation. Give general plan for the following week.

Increases group cohesiveness.

Eighth Group Session

Objectives
1. Promote trust and emotional expression among group members.
2. Provide information about infant feeding methods and the newborn.
3. Prepare teenagers for the transition from pregnancy to motherhood.
4. Begin group termination.

Process
1. Group members and leaders discuss absences and deliveries. Deliveries are added to the chart and member comments are invited.
2. Have a newly delivered group member return to the group to demonstrate breast-feeding. (A bottle-feeding demonstration could also be included but most teenagers seem familiar with at least the basics of this method.) The invited teenager can talk about breast-feeding in any way she chooses, that is, describing what she is doing at present, how someone begins breast-feeding, what help she received in the hospital, etc. The teenagers will ask her questions regardless of where she begins. Leaders may facilitate the interaction in areas difficult for adolescents to talk about. These may include the decision-making process, breasts as functional rather than sexual parts of the body, sensations of breast-feeding, feeding in public, and the response of others to breast-feeding. At the conclusion of the feeding, leaders can give information not already covered, giving the breast-feeding teenager opportunity to participate. Comparing and contrasting bottle- and breast-feeding can be done at this time. Gaps in information about bottle feeding can be filled and feelings about this feeding method explored.

Rationale
Continues promotion of group cohesion.

Promotes member rather than leader orientation of the group.

Provides opportunity for intimate, personal sharing among members.

Promotes independence for adolescents.

Demonstrates the decision-making process.

Helps to form and build on relationships within the group that may be transferred to an individual's situation.

The infant can be depended upon to have a crying episode, spit up, need a diaper change, etc., which offers an opportunity for the leaders to begin a discussion of initial motherhood, common problems, and changing relationships and to give information on the newborn.

Orients the teenagers to the reality of motherhood.

Encourages the adolescents' affective response to mothering.

Provides a real life situation consistent with adolescent concrete thinking.

3. Remind teenagers that the group will end in 2 weeks. Time should be saved for comments. Prepare the group for further discussion of termination at the next group session. Present the overall plan for the following week.

Begins the termination process.

Ninth Group Session

Objectives
1. Promote problem solving to prepare the teenagers for independent decision making as mothers.
2. Provide a framework for the adolescent to use in making family planning decisions.
3. Provide information about contraceptive methods.
4. Address termination of the group.

Process
1. Group members and leaders discuss absences and deliveries. Deliveries are added to the chart and member comments are invited.

2. While one leader is placing contraceptive materials on the table, the other can introduce the subject of family planning. Saying something such as, "Several of you have mentioned that you would like to wait a while before having more children," is a good beginning. "Let's look at methods of birth control available for you and how you can decide what to use" can be a follow-up statement.

The leaders should have multiples of each method on the table to enable the adolescent to look at and feel each as she wishes. Questions, answers, myths and past experiences will come out of this method exploration. Leaders can encourage information seeking among members, and can be available to

Rationale
Continues promotion of group cohesion.

Allows the teenagers control over their future reproduction.

Provides accurate contraceptive information.
Demonstrates equal status of leaders and member orientation of the group.
Demonstrates adult communication.

dispel misconceptions, discuss concerns, and give added facts when necessary. All necessary information can be provided within this unstructured format. It can be facilitated by having one leader interact with the group while the other keeps track of information given. Roles can switch back and forth easily throughout the group session.

3. Decision-making process

A. At some point the group will raise a concern that will ease the discussion into decision making. It may be, "My boyfriend won't use condoms" or "I can't decide" as examples. With careful listening, the leaders will know when to guide the group into this process.

Provides a problem-solving activity. For teenagers, decision making should be based on concepts including teaching–learning, role modeling, and adolescent development. The process includes identification of the goal to be attained, consideration of alternatives and the consequences of each course of action, and selection of the alternative that will most likely lead to goal attainment (Taylor, 1976).

B. Present an exercise that includes a familiar example such as buying a pair of jeans to teach the decision-making process. Help members examine motivating and inhibiting factors, alternatives, and consequences of their actions (see Taylor, 1976, for a complete description of this exercise).

Illustrates a process that the adolescents can use in the future for themselves and their babies.
Promotes participatory learning.
Promotes formation of self-identity.
Promotes understanding of others' communications and judgment.
Accounts for differences in culture, customs, and personalities, and their relationship to the use of contraception.

4. Values clarification process

A. Introduce an exercise such as "Strongly Agree–Strongly Disagree" (Taylor, 1979). Each group member is given a list of statements about contraception and responds with strongly agree, agree somewhat, disagree somewhat, strongly disagree. Share and discuss responses in the group.

Allows examination of future goals, self-image, parental expectations, beliefs and attitudes all having an influence on contraceptive usage.

B. Use a second exercise, "Values Choice," that builds on the first (see Morrison & Price, 1974, for a complete description of this exercise). A list of four or five statements is read to the members and

Unifies teenagers' thoughts, feelings, and actions consistent with the development of an adolescent's own value system.

they quickly answer each by themselves. An example from the first list might be:

> The method of birth control I would choose would be:
> no sex
> the pill
> diaphragm
> loop (IUD)
> foam and rubbers
> vaginal sponge (when marketed)
> other

Encourage the group to share responses after each set of statements. The group can try to answer questions as, "What made me choose this statement?" "Why not another?" "What does this tell me about myself?"

Two to four sets of statements can be used depending on time available.

5. Summarize group session. Address termination with question such as "What will it be like next week when we don't all meet at 4:00 p.m. on Mondays?" Leaders and members alike should have opportunity to express their loss in both concrete and emotional terms. Some groups will want to make special plans for their final week together. Give members major responsibility for this.

Confronts members with the task of termination.
Acknowledges leader and members' loss.
Acknowledges adolescents' ability to make independent decisions and the importance of members rather than leaders in the group.

Following is a list of additional and alternative methodologies for various prenatal topics. The format for presentation should be similar to the four sample sessions just presented.

Additional and Alternative Methodologies

Learning Need

Birth alternatives

Methodology

Tour labor and delivery rooms. Describe and show alternatives. Follow-up with discussion. Leaders should be alert to the teenagers' signals indicative of their fear of death that often can be noted when labor and delivery is discussed. Ventilation of feelings should be encouraged.

Newborn

Take group to newborn nursery and show them a newborn, its features, activities and developmental status. Demonstrate diapering or feeding if requested by the group.

or

"Play the Pregnancy Game" (see Mercer, 1979, for complete description). The adolescents, in pairs, examine a question written on a card that has been drawn from those provided by the leaders. The questions might include, "You're breast-feeding your baby and the doorbell rings. What will you do?" or "What will be fun to do with your baby when he/she is 1 month old?" Each pair can read their questions and answer(s) to the group. Have others suggest alternatives.

Breast-feeding

Show a breast-feeding film followed by discussion.

Relaxation

Discuss stress and group members' means of handling their own stressful situations.

Teach and have group practice relaxation techniques.

Apply these to labor.

Breathing techniques for labor and delivery

Demonstrate and have teenagers practice in pairs.

Keep the number of techniques to a minimum.

Practice several weeks in a row.

Contraception

Information

Show film "A Matter of Choice" (see Resource List) followed by discussion.

Decision making

As previously described.

Values clarification

Introduce a series of exercises (see Taylor, 1979; Simon, Howe, and Kirschenbaum, 1972; and Morrison and Price, 1974).

Legal rights of minors

Distribute cards with a vignette of a common legal problem of pregnant teenagers to each group member. Lead a discussion that includes information giv-

TABLE 16–1. GROUP QUESTIONNAIRE

	Check if This Happened in the Group	Helpful	Some-what Helpful	Very Helpful
Instructions: Please read each statement carefully and check the response that explains best how you feel.				
Altruism	1. Listening to others talk about their concerns.			
	2. Offering suggestions or help to others.			
	3. Talking with others about my concerns and feelings.			
Group cohesiveness	4. Being part of a group that has similar concerns.			
	5. Belonging to a group that understands and accepts me.			
	6. Not feeling so alone with my problem.			
Universality	7. Learning I'm not the only one with my type of problem; "we're in the same boat."			
	8. Learning that others have some of the same thoughts and feelings as I do.			
	9. Seeing that I'm no worse off than others.			
Imparting information	10. Seeing the labor and delivery area.			
	11. Seeing the film on birth of a baby.			
	12. Film and discussion on birth control.			
	13. Learning about breathing exercises.			
Catharsis	14. Being able to say what's bothering me instead of holding it in.			
	15. Getting things off my chest.			
Instillation of hope	16. Realizing there are ways to solve some of my problems.			
	17. Learning how others have solved problems similar to mine.			
Family reenactment	18. Being in the group was, in a sense, like being in a family, only this time a more accepting and understanding family.			
	19. Being in the group somehow helped me to understand old hang-ups that I had in the past with my family.			
Existential factors	20. Recognizing that life is at times unfair.			
	21. Learning that I must take final responsibility for my life no matter how much guidance and support I get from others.			

Note: The curative factors would not be listed on the questionnaire for patients, but are illustrated here for identification of what each question is designed to test.
(Source: Adapted from Yalom, I. D. The theory and practice of group psychotherapy (2nd ed.). New York: Basic Books, 1975, pp. 78–81; Dohr, M. S. An experimental study of a group intervention and its effects on mothers' ego development and empathetic identification with their pregnant daughters. Unpublished master's thesis, University of Rochester, 1979, pp. 135–137.)

	ing, dispelling of myths, and exploration of concerns after each issue is read.
	or
	Have a legal expert make a videotape that addresses the common legal concerns of pregnant teenagers with information consistent with their own state laws. A discussion should follow the showing of the tape.
Postpartum changes	Show film "Are You Ready for The Postpartum Experience" (see Resource List) followed by discussion
	or
	Have a delivered teenager return to the group and describe her postpartum experiences. Leaders should facilitate the discussion to ensure inclusion of physical, emotional, and relationship changes.
Labor and delivery	Show a film (see Resource List) followed by discussion. Expect a stilted discussion to follow because teenagers find the reality of these films difficult to handle. Use of a projective technique may help. Leaders should again be alert to signals from the adolescents about fear of death.

Evaluation. Evaluation must be integrated into these prenatal group sessions, as with any teaching–learning strategy. Each session must be evaluated by the leaders for them to make changes as the group sessions progress. This process of evaluation should be based on the weekly objectives and could include members' attendance, participation, comprehension of information as demonstrated in the discussion portions of the group sessions, adherence to regimens suggested by health care providers, or ability to correctly perform relaxation and breathing techniques.

Outcome evaluation is also appropriate, and could include satisfaction with the labor and delivery experience, positive bonding with infants, selection of feeding method before delivery with good rationale, appropriate use of contraception, and demonstration of good decision making with pediatric calls and visits. The group process goals can be measured through the use of a questionnaire based on Yalom's (1975) curative factors (Table 16–1). A description of the curative factors can be found in Chapter 3.

Summary

This chapter has reviewed the process and content of prenatal groups based on those held in the Rochester Adolescent Maternity Project. Using this model, health care providers can provide pregnant teenagers with appropriate childbirth education, can give them opportunity for support from their peer group, and can enhance their decision-making skills and confidence as they assume their new roles as mothers. The groups can aid in making pregnancy a positive experience for pregnant adolescents, one that they leave with a good self-image, more independence, and having made strides toward the development of their own self-identity and value system.

RESOURCES

Books and Articles for Health Professionals

Groups

Bonavich, L. Participation: The key to learning for patients in antepartal clinics. *Journal of Obstetric, Gynecologic, and Neonatal Nursing*, 1981, *10*(2), 75–79.

Janosik, E. H., & Phipps, L. B. *Life cycle group work in nursing*. Monterey, Calif.: Wadsworth Health Services Division, 1982.

Kagey, J. R., Vivace, J., & Lutz, W. Mental health primary prevention: The role of parent mutual help groups. *American Journal of Public Health*, 1981, *71*, 166–167.

Loomis, M. E. *Group process for nurses*. St. Louis, Mo.: Mosby, 1979.

Adolescent Pregnancy

Baldwin, W., & Cain, V. S. The children of teenage parents. *Family Planning Perspectives*, 1980, *12*, 34–43.

Barr, L., Monserrat, C., & Gaston, F. *Working with childbearing adolescents*. Albuquerque, N.M.: New Futures, 1980.

Card, J., & Wise, L. Teenage mothers and teenage fathers: The impact of early childbearing on the parents' personal and professional lives. *Family Planning Perspectives*, 1978, *10*, 199–205.

Furstenberg, F. F. Jr. *Unplanned parenthood: The social consequences of teenage childbearing*. New York: Macmillan, 1976.

Furstenberg, F. F. Jr., & Crawford, A. G. Family support: Helping teenage mothers to cope. *Family Planning Perspectives*, 1978, *10*, 322–333.

Heald, F. P., & Jacobson, M. S. Nutritional needs of the pregnant adolescent. *Pediatric Annals*, 1980, 9, 21–31.

McAnarney, E. R. (Ed.). *Premature adolescent pregnancy and parenthood*. New York: Grune and Stratton, 1983.

McAnarney, E. R., & Stickle, G. (Eds.). *Pregnancy and childbearing during adolescence: Research priorities for the 1980's*. March of Dimes Birth Defects Foundation, Birth Defects: Original Article Series. New York: Liss, 1981, 17(3).

McAnarney, E. R., & Thiede, H. A. Adolescent pregnancy and childbearing: What we have learned in a decade and what remains to be learned. *Seminars in Perinatology*, 1981, 5(1), 91–103.

Zelnick, M., Kantnor, J. F., & Ford, K. *Sex and pregnancy in adolescence*. Beverly Hills, Calif.: Sage, 1981.

Books and Booklets for Pregnant Teenagers

Barr, L., Monserrat, C., & Gaston, F. *Teenager pregnancy: A new beginning*. Albuquerque, N.M.: New Futures, 1980.

Berg, G. L. *The 1st gifts*. Tuckerton, N.J.: Caring Mothers Cooperative, 1978.

Edwards, M. *Childbirth: A teenager guide*. Seattle: The Pennypress, 1979.

Pregnancy in anatomical illustrations. Los Angeles: Carnation Co., 1962.

You and your baby: A guide for teenaged mothers. Fremont, Mich.: Gerber Products Co., 1981.

Films

Labor and Delivery

Bernita's film. Centre Films, Inc., 1103 N. El Centro Ave., Hollywood, CA 90038 (*This is the story of one inner city teenager as she attends her prenatal visits and childbirth education classes. It also traces her experiences in labor and delivery and her first 6 weeks postpartum with her new baby.*)

Have a healthy baby: Labor and delivery. A Churchill Film, 622 N. Robertson Blvd., Los Angeles,

CA 90069 *(Two couples are followed through labor and birth. One has a normal delivery whereas the other is difficult. Physiology and the process of birth are explained with animation. The feelings, expectations, and experiences of the two couples are also explored.)*

The teenager pregnancy experience. Parenting Pictures, 121 N.W. Crystal Street, Crystal River, FL 32629 *(Realistic situations are presented in an effort to prepare expectant teenage parents for birth and parenthood. Options for the pregnant adolescent are addressed and discussion is promoted on pregnancy, labor and delivery, sexuality, birth control and parenting.)*

Contraception

A matter of choice. Department of OB/GYN, Albany Medical Center, Albany, NY 12208 *(A straightforward presentation of all contraceptive methods by health providers interspersed with client comments and concerns.)*

Postpartum

Are you ready for the postpartum experience. Parenting Pictures, 121 N.W. Crystal Street, Crystal River, FL 32629 *(The first 6 weeks postpartum for a couple with their new baby are realistically portrayed. Good discussion takes place as the couple seeks solutions for managing their problematic child.)*

Other

Childbirth Graphics, P.O. Box 17025, Irondequoit Post Office, Rochester, NY 14617 *(Company producing teaching supplements that include color slides, illustrations and models on pregnancy, physiology, labor, birth, breast-feeding, exercise, sibling at birth materials and the newborn. Maternity Center Association Materials are included. Catalogue available.)*

Inside my mom. March of Dimes Local Office or Box 2000, White Plains, NY 10602 *(A slide series or film strip focusing on good nutrition in pregnancy.)*

Omni Health Communicator, Division of Ortho Pharmaceutical Corp., Somerville, NY 08876 *(Separate self-teaching inserts for hand-held device showing pelvic exams, breast self-exam, IUDs, diaphragms, vaginal applicators.)*

Sunny. Under the Cabbage Leaf, 3830 S.W. 19th Street, Gainsville, FL 32601 *(A 7-pound doll for demonstration and practice of skills for the newborn. Placenta, cord and pouch for vaginal and cesarean deliveries are available.)*

REFERENCES

Adams, B. N., Brownstein, C. A., Rennals, I. M., & Schmitt, M. H. The pregnant adolescent, a group approach. *Adolescence,* 1976, *11*(44), 467–458.

Adolescent perinatal health. Chicago: The American College of Obstetricians and Gynecologists, 1979.

Bibring, G., Dwyer, T., Huntington, D., & Valenstein, A. A study of the psychological processes in pregnancy and the earliest mother–child relationship. I. Some propositions and comments. *The Psychoanalytic Study of the Child,* 1961, *16*, 9–71.

Dohr, M. S. *An experimental study of a group intervention and its effect on mothers' ego development and empathetic identification with their pregnant adolescent daughters.* Unpublished master's thesis, University of Rochester, 1979.

Dunhoelter, J., Jimenez, J., & Baumann, G. Pregnancy performance of patients under 15 years of age. *Obstetrics and Gynecology,* 1975, *46*, 49–52.

Elster, A. B., & McAnarney, E. R. Medical and psychosocial risks of pregnancy and childbearing during adolescence. *Pediatric Annals,* 1980, *9*(3), 89–94.

Hinkley, R. G., & Herman, L. *Group treatment in psychotherapy.* Minneapolis: University of Minnesota Press, 1951.

Informing social change. New York: The Alan Guttmacher Institute, 1980.

Jekel, J., Harrison, J. T., Bancroft, D. R. E., Tyler, N. C., & Klerman, L. V. A comparison of the health of index and subsequent babies born to school age mothers. *American Journal of Public Health*, 1975, *65*, 370–374.

Littlefield, V., & Seibert, G. The group approach to problem solving for pregnant diabetic women. *American Journal of Maternal Child Nursing*, 1978, *3*(5), 274–280.

Marram, G. D. *The group approach in nursing practice* (2nd ed.). St. Louis, Mo.: Mosby, 1978.

McAnarney, E. R., & Adams, B. N. Development of an adolescent maternity project in Rochester, New York. *Public Health Reports*, 1977, *92*, 154–159.

Mercer, R. T. The pregnant adolescent. In R. T. Mercer (Ed.), *Perspectives on adolescent health care*. Philadelphia: Lippincott, 1979.

Mercer, R. T. Prenatal care. In R. T. Mercer (Ed.), *Perspectives on adolescent health care*. Philadelphia: Lippincott, 1979.

Merritt, T. A., Lawrence, R. A., & Naeye, R. L. The infants of adolescent mothers. *Pediatric Annals*, 1980, *9*(3) 100–110.

Morrison, E. S., & Price, M. U. *Values in sexuality: A new approach to sex education*. New York: Hart, 1974.

Phipps-Yonas, S. Teenage pregnancy and motherhood: A review of the literature. *American Journal of Orthopsychiatry*, 1980, *50*, 403–431.

Rubin, R. Maternal tasks in pregnancy. *Maternal–Child Nursing Journal*, 1975, *4*(3), 143–153.

Sahler, O. J. Z. Adolescent parenting: Potential for child abuse and neglect? *Pediatric Annals*, 1980, *9*(3), 120–125.

Sampson, E. E., & Marthas, M. *Group process for the health professions* (2nd ed.). New York: Wiley and Sons, 1981.

Simon, S. B., Howe, L. W., & Kirschenbaum, A. *Values clarification: A practical handbook of practical strategies for teachers and students*. New York: Hart, 1972.

Taylor, D. A new way to teach teens about contraceptives. *American Journal of Maternal Child Nursing*, 1976, *6*, 378–383.

Taylor, D. Contraceptive counseling and care. In R.T. Mercer (Ed.), *Perspectives on adolescent health care*. Philadelphia: Lippincott, 1979.

Yalom, I. D. *The theory and practice of group psychotherapy*. New York: Basic Books, 1975.

Unintentional Pregnancy: Education for Choice

17

Colleen Keenan

Approximately one-half of all pregnancies occurring in the United States are unintentional (Dryfoos, 1982; Henshaw et al., 1982). Many factors contribute to the incidence of unplanned pregnancies such as lack of understanding about contraceptive use, contraceptive method failure, degree of fertility, and contraceptive risk taking. Millions of women in the United States face an unplanned pregnancy each year. Three options are available: (1) motherhood; (2) adoption; (3) abortion.

Figure 17–1 depicts the decision outcomes of the unintentional pregnancy. Since the advent of legally available abortion, few women elect to give up their child for adoption. This trend may be due in part to the increasing acceptance of single parenthood in addition to the increasing acceptance of abortion as a pregnancy choice (Leynes, 1980).

The most common choices for the woman or a couple with an unintentional pregnancy are abortion and motherhood. According to current estimations, approximately one-quarter of all pregnancies (or one-half of unplanned pregnancies) end in abortion, with the balance ending in live births or miscarriages (Henshaw et al., 1982).

Regardless of the ultimate outcome, however, pregnancy often creates a crisis in a woman's life. Developmentally, it is a time of potential growth. The unintentional pregnancy may even heighten this potential. A woman may find that many of her beliefs and perceptions about her role identity, body image, sexuality, fertility, and contraception are all challenged. Conflicts regarding the above issues frequently emerge and create ambiguities and complexities in the decision-making process. These factors may result in a reassessment of the importance or appropriateness of previously held values, and may lead to growth producing change.

In this chapter, we focus on the pregnancy decision-making process and the methods health care providers can use to assist women who have an unintentional pregnancy. Education and counseling strategies, which can enhance or reinforce decision-making skills and self-determination, are presented.

PREGNANCY DECISION MAKING

Pregnancy decision making is a complex process in which the woman must examine multiple conflicting alternatives, assess the potential costs and benefits of each, and ultimately choose the option most congruent with the demands and resources of her

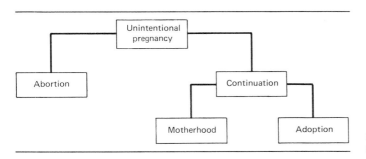

Figure 17–1. Decision outcomes of unintentional pregnancy.

current life situation. Chapter 3 presents the general theory and process of decision making as it relates to the health care of women. In this section, we examine the specific process of pregnancy decision making.

Even if a woman and her partner have consciously decided to avoid pregnancy and faithfully contracept, pregnancy is still a possibility; contraceptive methods can fail and isolated risk taking occurs. Regardless of the reason for the pregnancy, a choice must be made whether or not to continue. A decision *not* to decide ultimately ends up as a choice to continue the pregnancy once the time limits for termination have been exceeded.

Stages of Decision Making. Bracken, Klerman, and Bracken (1978) described the stages of unintentional pregnancy decision making. They are: (1) acknowledgment of the pregnancy, (2) formulation of alternatives, (3) assessment of the relative merit of each choice, (4) commitment to one choice over others, and (5) adherence to the choice.

Acknowledgment of Pregnancy. The first state usually occurs gradually, the length of time varying for each individual woman. Frequently, the first missed menses and symptoms of early pregnancy are concrete signs confirming conception. However, factors such as irregular periods and absence of pregnancy symptoms may prolong this stage. Denial of existing pregnancy signs is another factor that may delay the ackowledgment of pregnancy. This stage may last several weeks and in rare instances a few months.

Formulation of Alternatives. The second stage occurs as the woman examines the three options available to her—abortion, adoption, and motherhood. In some cases, the woman may immediately exclude a particular choice.

Assessment of the Relative Merit of Each Choice. The third stage occurs as the result of hypothesizing potential circumstances that would occur if the woman chose one of the options over the others. For example, she might envision herself as the mother of an infant while trying to manage a new marriage and a demanding career. Or she might imagine the response of her own mother if she were to have an abortion. Potential events are played out in her mind and the benefits and costs of each are weighed. Many women experience intense conflict during this stage and ambivalence is not uncommon. Significant others are frequently consulted for their advice and reactions to the pregnancy. And multiple factors such as personal resources, readiness for parenthood, career goals, and moral values and beliefs must be considered. Ultimately the woman must assign value to these factors in terms of their importance to her in the present situation and assess their impact on her alternatives.

Commitment to One Choice Over Others. The fourth stage represents the beginning resolution of the conflict experienced in the previous stage. The woman may actively seek out additional data that confirm her choice and avoid information or input from significant others that might provoke conflict.

Adherence to the Choice. The last stage occurs as "the decision is adhered to even in the face of new negative information concerning the choice" (Bracken, Klerman, & Bracken, 1978, p. 322). For example, a woman may remain firm about her decision to continue the pregnancy despite the fact that her partner has threatened to break off the relationship because of her plans.

These stages provide a general overview for the process of pregnancy decision making. Although many women move through the stages with relative ease, others encounter difficulties with potential barriers to decision making. Table 17–1 summarizes the stages developed by Bracken and colleagues (1978) and the facilitators and barriers to this process.

Developmental Considerations. From a developmental perspective, certain unique issues may affect decision making for women in particular age groups.

Adolescence. The establishment of intimate relationships outside of the family is a hallmark task of adolescence. When the need for intimacy is expressed sexually, the adolescent frequently is unprepared for the practice of contraception, if pregnancy is not desired. Many adolescents feel that contraception takes away from the spontaneity of sex, that it is not "natural" or that it connotes a planned sexual encounter. Peers take on an

TABLE 17–1. PREGNANCY DECISION MAKING

Stage	Task	Influencing Factors	Barriers	Facilitators
1	Acknowledgement of pregnancy	Pregnancy symptoms	Denial	Regular menstrual cycle Presence of pregnancy symptoms
2	Identification of alternative outcomes	Availability of information	Passive problem solving	Active problem solving skills
3	Assessment of relative merit of each alternative	Problem-solving style, support network	Passive problem solving	Utilization of support network Active problem solving skills
4	Commitment to one choice over others	Conflict	Ambivalence	Strong support network Developed coping skills
5	Adherence to choice	Support network	Inadequate supports or resources	Utilization of supports and available resources

(Source: *Adapted from Bracken, M. B., Klerman, L. V., & Bracken, M. Coping with pregnancy resolution among never-married women.* American Journal of Orthopsychiatry, *1978, 42(2).*)

increasingly important role in the adolescent's life and pressure to engage in sexual activity and even to have a baby may be very strong among certain groups of adolescents. Independence from parents becomes a particularly acute issue as well and can be actualized initially as a departure from family norms and values. Pregnancy is also seen by many adolescents as a desirable sign of adult womanhood. Finally, the physical sexual development during early adolescence and the necessary adjustment to a new female body image is followed closely by additional adjustments of body image changes during pregnancy. For some adolescents these changes are perceived negatively whereas for others they may be experienced as quite positive. All of the above factors may figure prominently in the adolescent's decision-making process about her pregnancy.

Young Adulthood. Issues arising in young adulthood concerning autonomy and intimacy are associated with questions about long-term commitment to the partner, the suitability of the partner, the woman herself as a parent, and the readiness for parenting. Many young adults plan to begin families at some point in the future rather than at the time of the unintentional pregnancy. Young adulthood is certainly the time when career training and development are paramount goals for many individuals. Women in particular may feel conflict concerning career and family.

Middle Adulthood. The transition to the thirties and beyond is frequently a "now or never" situation as the woman realizes that for her the traditional childbearing years are drawing to a close. This "time squeeze" may be accentuated by the typical life assessment common in the thirties. Middle adulthood may increase the underlying ambivalence a woman feels about pregnancy, particularly for the primigravida. This situation may also be compounded by the woman's awareness that fertility gradually declines in the third decade and another pregnancy at a later time may not be as easy to achieve. Many couples who delay parenting until their middle adult years find that infertility is a problem.

Pregnancies occurring in the perimenopausal period frequently present an unexpected dilemma. Women in this age group commonly have completed their family several years prior and a major consideration is whether the woman wants to begin the process of childbearing again. Perhaps even more importantly, the risks of genetic defects increase with advanced maternal age. A genetic amniocentesis can be performed at approximately 16 weeks of pregnancy, which will provide additional information about the fetus upon which to base a pregnancy decision. For some women, however, there is no advantage to obtaining the amniocentesis, because either they would not terminate a pregnancy in any case or not beyond the first trimester.

ROLE OF THE HEALTH CARE PROVIDER

The role of the health care provider is facilitative and can be expressed in the following counseling and educational behaviors:

1. Provide necessary data to make an informed choice after considering all potential alternatives.
2. Explore the potential impact of factors affecting the decision to continue or terminate the pregnancy.
3. Assist in mobilizing resources and enhancing coping skills.

4. Provide a secure environment in which the woman can determine the most reasonable alternative for her at this point in her life.
5. Enhance self-determination through deliberate decision making by the woman.

Each woman must ultimately make her own decision concerning the outcome of her pregnancy. The health care provider is available as a resource. In the process of helping the woman make a decision, it is essential that health care providers examine and resolve personal bias concerning pregnancy options. Many pregnancy choices carry strong negative sanctions and may be totally unacceptable in certain segments of our society. Abortion and single adolescent motherhood are examples of socially controversial decisions that nevertheless should not be eliminated or minimized as a pregnancy alternative if the woman herself is considering it. Nonjudgmental counseling is critical if the woman is to fully consider all available options and, therefore, maximize the base from which her decision is made. If the health care provider has a strong bias against a particular option, it is then appropriate to refer the client to another provider who can provide comprehensive counseling.

Assessment

Thorough assessment is required to provide a strong base for health education and promotion interventions. The health history, psychosocial assessment, decision-making status, and individual learning needs all determine the direction the counseling or teaching session will take. In many instances, assessment, counseling, and teaching occur during one interview and the woman is referred to another provider or setting based on the decision she makes. In other situations, more complex needs may arise and time may be available to develop and implement an intensive plan for teaching or counseling or both as the individual patient requires. Many other settings provide comprehensive women's health care in which the provider is consistently involved from the initial assessment (or before), throughout the decision-making process and the pregnancy outcome (and beyond). In this situation, other members of the health care team will be involved according to the woman's need and the health care provider's other areas of expertise. Regardless of the setting in which the initial encounter occurs, a thorough assessment and individualized plan of care is essential.

Health History. The health history yields important information regarding health status, risk factors, pregnancy dating, and previous health behaviors. The following are critical elements in the history related to pregnancy decision making and health education:

1. *Current history:* Pregnancy symptoms (fatigue, nausea, skipped menses, breast tenderness, urinary frequency, quickening)? Patterns of sexual activity? Use (regular or irregular) or nonuse of contraceptives?
2. *Last menstrual period:* Was it normal or abnormal? Previous menstrual period, normal or abnormal? Use of oral contraceptives within the past three months?
3. *Menstrual history:* Age of onset of menses, frequency, duration? Amount of flow? Premenstrual or menstrual symptoms?
4. *Obstetrical history:* Number of full-term births, premature births, spontaneous or induced abortions and number of living children? Any complications of pregnancy, labor, delivery or the postpartum period?
5. *Gynecological history:* Previous gynecological surgery? Difficulty becoming pregnant? Sexually transmitted diseases? PID? Other gynecological illnesses? Previous contraceptive use (with dates)? Breast disorders? Current symptoms of infection?

6. *Past medical history:* Any serious medical illness (past or present) or hospitalizations? Current medications? Allergies or drug sensitivities? Surgery? Thrombophlebitis? Rh type?
7. *Family history:* Diabetes? Cardiac disease or MI before the age of 50? Hypertension? Cancer? Genetic disorders?
8. *Health habits:* Usual sleep patterns? Bowel and bladder habits? Last Pap smear and health visit? Breast self-examination? Use of caffeine (coffee, tea, colas, chocolate)? Use of tobacco? Marijuana? Other street drugs? Alcohol?

The above data provide a useful base for an initial thorough evaluation of health risks and health behaviors that might have a direct impact on pregnancy decision making for an individual woman. In addition, the critical historical elements of early pregnancy dating have been included. Regardless of whether a woman chooses to continue or to terminate her pregnancy, the gestational age of the fetus must be clearly determined as early in pregnancy as possible. If the woman chooses to continue her pregnancy, early dating is much more reliable in determining fetal gestation and maturity, should an unanticipated complication and early delivery be required. If the woman chooses to terminate her pregnancy, precise dating is required to determine the type of procedure undertaken.

Psychosocial Assessment. The psychosocial component in the health assessment of women with an unintentional pregnancy is integrated into the health history interview. Because the psychosocial element in the assessment has many facets, however, a separate section in the chapter is devoted to this area.

General Coping Skills. Any pregnancy has the potential to create stress in a woman's life and the unintentional pregnancy may trigger a crisis situation. After an initial and often intense response comprising various feelings such as shock, anger, pleasure, sadness, or fear, the woman must begin to mobilize both internal and external resources to cope and adapt to her new situation. Conflicting emotions may occur with any pregnancy and may even be heightened with an unplanned pregnancy. Ambivalence is a common emotional response. How the woman copes with conflicting feelings regarding her pregnancy has a direct impact on how well she adapts to whatever pregnancy decision she ultimately makes. Resolution of ambivalence may never be complete. However, the high levels of ambivalence that can psychologically immobilize a woman and cause emotional sequelae are rarely encountered (Shusterman, 1979). Most women adjust to their pregnancy decision within a relatively short period of time and the crisis of pregnancy begins to resolve.

Women use various coping strategies to deal with the conflicting feelings so often encountered with the unintentional pregnancy. Previous patterns, whether adaptive or maladaptive, are incorporated into the woman's current problem-solving approach. The use of defense mechanisms on the unconscious or semiconscious level is also implemented to reduce the anxiety inherent in ambivalent or conflicted states. Certain defense mechanisms, such as the use of humor, sublimation, and suppression, are healthy ways to cope with stress by channeling negative feelings into positive or neutral behaviors (Garland & Bush, 1982). Other defense mechanisms, such as denial, projection, and displacement, are less adaptive and may actually impede effective coping. For example, denial of pregnancy despite obvious subjective symptoms such as amenorrhea, nausea, breast tenderness, and weight gain may occur if the pregnancy is too painful or threatening to acknowledge. This defense, while helping to avoid the immediate anxiety, creates an immobilized state that precludes active coping and decision making. Anger, another unpleasant emotion associated with unintentional pregnancy, may be projected (attributed to another person) or displaced (vented on an inappropriate person or situation). For example, a woman may feel angry with her partner for failing to use withdrawal during intercourse and for her subsequent pregnancy, but she might displace her anger on a friend who perhaps would be less likely to reject her. In another situation, an adolescent woman might project her own anger toward her parents, which is unacceptable, and refuse to disclose the pregnancy because "they would be furious" although they had been supportive in other situations.

Previous problem-solving styles also influence how the woman will cope with an unintentional pregnancy. Active problem solving involves the direct confrontation of the situation, careful examination of the contributing factors, and creative identification of possible solutions. Active problem solving implies mastery and a sense of control over the final outcome. The woman assumes responsibility for her decision and its outcome, but she is able to realistically assess and utilize the resources she has available, including support persons, her own coping abilities, current finances, and future career and family plans.

Another woman may assume a more passive stance when confronted with an unintentional pregnancy, based on her previous coping styles. In passive problem solving, confrontation is avoided with the expectation or hope that the problem will somehow resolve itself. Magical thinking is an example of passive problem solving. The problem, if one is recognized, remains amorphous and ill-defined. The situation takes control of the woman and she believes she cannot exert influence over the outcome. In the case of unintentional pregnancy, however, even passivity leads to an outcome. No decision is ultimately a decision to continue the pregnancy if delay persists beyond the gestational age for abortion. A woman also makes a decision if she allows influential others to coerce her into terminating the pregnancy. The style of problem solving the woman is most comfortable with has a direct impact upon how she will deal with her current pregnancy and also how satisfied she will be with her decision. In assessment of the general coping skills of a woman with an unintentional pregnancy, the following questions are useful:

1. What are the woman's previous coping patterns and problem-solving style? Her initial response to the pregnancy?
2. The reason for delay, if any, in seeking contact with a health care provider?

Social Supports. The quality of social support available to a woman may have a dramatic impact on her ability to deal effectively with the stressful events surrounding an unintentional pregnancy. In particular, the man involved in the pregnancy, female friends, and family members all play a potentially critical role. In the case of the male partner, his initial response to the pregnancy and subsequent validation or lack of validation of her decision-making process may have a major impact. Shusterman (1979) found that as intimacy in the partnership increased, the man was more likely to provide emotional support and validation of the pregnancy decision. In many instances, the decision may be joint and may reaffirm the stability of their relationship. In other instances, the crisis of pregnancy may prove disruptive and severely strain the relationship. Conflict between partners regarding the pregnancy options may estrange a woman from an important source of support. It is essential to remember that men are not solely biological participants in the pregnancy and often have strong emotional responses and needs regarding this event. Whenever possible, it is advantageous to involve the man in the assessment and counseling process.

Close female friends are often consulted and confided in when a woman experiences an unintentional pregnancy. The values and previous pregnancy experiences of the confidant can serve as a reality base upon which to validate and test the woman's own feelings and weighing of alternatives. Family members, particularly women, are also frequent sources of support. The continuity and intimacy of these relationships can be valuable in helping the woman gain a perspective on this crisis and in making her pregnancy decision a satisfactory one.

The assessment of social supports involves ascertaining not only the availability of persons, but also whom the woman actually seeks out for help. In many instances, a woman may have a very close relationship with an individual and frequently give and receive support in various circumstances, but elect not to divulge her unintentional pregnancy. For example, a woman may choose not to tell her mother of her decision to terminate a pregnancy because she knows that her mother would not support her seeking an abortion and would be angry or disappointed. Another woman might delay telling her partner of the pregnancy until it becomes too late for him to pressure her into having an abortion.

Important areas for assessment of social support are:

- Usual makeup of support network?
- Individuals consulted in pregnancy decision?
- Response of partner?
- Quality of supports related to current pregnancy?
- Degree of influence exerted by support persons on pregnancy decision?
- Potential for continued support after pregnancy decision is made?

Pregnancy Antecedents. The current life situation of the woman usually influences the decision she makes concerning her pregnancy. Variables such as career or school plans, age, financial resources, and marital status are all important considerations. Many women will hesitate to bring a child into the world unless they believe they can provide an optimum environment. It is important to assess the woman's perceived ideal circumstances for childrearing because there are wide variations. And although the woman may choose to continue the pregnancy in less than the ideal situation, she must acknowledge these factors as potential stressors and plan accordingly.

Contraceptive Behaviors. Assessment of previous patterns of contraceptive use can yield important information regarding plans for future pregnancy prevention. Because many women's contraceptive history is complex with mutliple methods implemented, development of a time line is often helpful to determine utilization patterns. In addition to obtaining dates of use, contraceptive risk-taking behavior, partner input, and method satisfaction should also be elicited. From this time line, contraceptive patterns can be more easily examined with the woman. Based on this information, an appropriate contraceptive method can be slected should the woman decide to terminate her pregnancy. Regardless of her decision, important insights can be gained that will help prevent future unintentional pregnancies.

Decision-making Status. Decision-making status is one of the most important areas requiring assessment. Many women reach the health care provider with a decision already in mind. Given the complexity of this process, however, thorough evaluation is indicated to ascertain if the woman has completely thought through her decision and to prevent dissatisfaction with her choice after the decision is irrevocable. The woman should be asked if she has made a choice concerning her pregnancy and if so, what the reasons are.

Alternative choices should be raised by the health care provider and explored with the woman. The role of significant others in the decision must also be examined to determine whether or not the woman has been unduly influenced in her choice. This is particularly true in the case of adolescents who are more likely to perceive their choice as externally determined (Lewis, 1980) and, therefore, may be at greater risk for experiencing a negative psychological outcome.

Educational Needs. "The success of our teaching is measured not by how much content you have imparted, but by how much the patient has learned" (Narrow, 1979). The range and depth of educational content related to pregnancy decision making is vast and must be tailored to the individual's own learning needs. The education needs assessment is based on the woman's current knowledge, previous pregnancy experiences, if any, and the woman's preferred learning style. In addition, decision-making status and the degree of anxiety or ambivalence the woman is experiencing must also be assessed before an appropriate teaching plan can be developed.

In many instances, the educational needs assessment occurs concurrently with the general assessment of the woman with an unintentional pregnancy. For example, while obtaining the menstrual cycle and contraception histories, the woman's familiarity with normal menstrual physiology and understanding of birth control methods can also be evaluated. After current level of knowledge (as well as level of language skills) has been assessed and the woman's learning style identified, decision-making status will determine the actual direction client education will take. The educational content for the woman deciding upon an abortion differs dramatically from the content appropriate for the woman who intends to continue her pregnancy. Thus, it becomes clear how important the role of assessment is in planning for quality health care for the individual woman. The generic process of assessment of learning needs is included in Chapter 2. The specific content for the woman with an unintentional pregnancy is outlined in later sections of this chapter and in other chapters of this book.

Counseling Strategies

Health care providers are frequently involved in counseling the woman with an unintentional pregnancy. In many cases, counseling occurs at the time the woman receives the result of her pregnancy test. Depending on the needs of the woman, follow-up sessions may be indicated. In other instances the woman may be referred for counseling. When the woman decides to terminate her pregnancy, there are frequently counselors available as part of the abortion service. Regardless of the initial setting for counseling, however, the purposes are to:

• Facilitate decision making
• Assure an informed choice
• Identify high-risk individuals and initiate intervention

An initial strategy is the exploration of the problem as the woman perceives it and the possible alternatives. The pros and cons of each choice are examined even if the woman has previously excluded a particular option. This process is often facilitated by writing the choices and listing the positive and negative aspects of each to determine more objectively the factors that enter into the decision. The roles of each member of the support system and their potential for support in decision making about the pregnancy are reviewed. If possible it is also beneficial to retrace the chain of sexual decision making from the beginning and examine the underlying rationales for those choices. Issues of contraception may also be raised at this time, if appropriate. During this phase of counseling, information exchange and reality validation are crucial elements in the decision-making process.

Another focus is on the decision itself. Many women have difficulty making a choice because previous values may conflict with the present set of circumstances in her life. In this situation it is helpful to emphasize the "best possible" choice given all the factors she must consider. The resolution of conflict regarding such important issues is very difficult indeed and this fact should be acknowledged by the counselor.

Decision making is fostered by engaging the woman in playing an active role. The insights that are gained by the woman can then be more easily incorporated into future coping and health behaviors. The role of the counselor is facilitative rather than advisory. The participation of the counselor includes information gathering and assessment, reflection on the content and process of the interview, and the use of summary and appropriate validation of the knowledge and insights of the woman.

In counseling the woman with an unintentional pregnancy, psychological risk factors should be screened and assessed, and referrals made where appropriate. Women with severe ambivalence are at risk for regretting their decision and for coping dysfunctionally. Both the very young teenager and the woman nearing the end of her reproductive years may also be at risk because of developmental issues and, of course, women with previous psychological difficulties may experience an increased sense of crisis and not be able to cope effectively with the demands of making a difficult decision (Shusterman, 1979). Women who choose abortion after a diagnostic amniocentesis may also be at risk for psychological problems. Generally speaking, however, most women are satisfied with the decision they have made. When a woman does regret her choice after a reasonable length of time and psychological functioning is affected, referral for more intensive psychotherapy is indicated.

CHOICES—ABORTION, ADOPTION, MOTHERHOOD: CLIENT EDUCATION

As has been seen, the decision is complex. Once the decision is made and counseling and assessment are undertaken the focus shifts to client education. The content and available time to impart the content differ for the woman who chooses to continue her pregnancy versus one who selects termination. In the former case, education is aimed toward maintenance of a healthy pregnancy and postpartum period over a time span of several months and frequent health care encounters. The latter, pregnancy termination, focuses on preparation for a surgical procedure and minimization of complications. The time frame is short term, usually with a maximum of two to three visits. Regardless of choice, comprehensive education will help facilitate acceptance and satisfaction with her choice. In the following sections, specific educational content is presented for abortion. Brief discussions follow related to pregnancy continuation (motherhood or adoption) as specific content on prenatal education is included in Appendix A.

ABORTION

Although induced abortion continues to be a controversial subject for certain groups in our society, the practice of termination of an unwanted pregnancy has a long-standing historical precedence. Attempts to end pregnancy through ingestion of toxic substances

TABLE 17–2. TYPES OF INDUCED ABORTION

Type of Procedure	Technique	Laminaria	Pain Management	Complications	Setting	Expense	Psychological Impact Woman	Psychological Impact Staff
1st Trimester (up to 12 weeks of pregnancy)								
ME (up to 6 weeks)	Suction curettage	No	Paracervical block; optional IV/po; sedation	Incomplete abortion; cervical laceration	Outpatient	Low; few or no lost work days	Low	Low
D & S (up to 12 weeks)	Cervical dilation and suction curettage	Yes	Paracervical block IV sedation; po analgesia prn	Uterine perforation; bleeding infection	Outpatient	Low; laminaria requires additional visit day before	Low–moderate	Low
2nd Trimester (13–24 weeks of pregnancy)								
D & E (13–20 weeks)	Cervical dilation and suction curettage; sharp curettage	Yes	Paracervical block and IV sedation or general anesthesia	Uterine perforation and increased bleeding with gestational age;? cervical incompetence	Generally inpatient	Moderate; may require overnight hospitalization	Low–moderate	Physician high
Intraamniotic saline instillation (16–20 weeks)	Injection of 20% saline; amount varies with gestation; labor and delivery of fetus		Local anesthetic at injection site limited amounts of analgesia during labor	Hypernatremia; coagulopathy bleeding; uterine rupture	Inpatient	High; unpredictable length of hospital stay	Moderate–high	Nurse high
Prostaglandin (13–20 weeks)	Intraamniotic injection or vaginal suppositories most common route; labor and delivery of fetus		Local anesthetic if intraamniotic; limited amounts of analgesia during labor	Retained placenta; frequent GI side effects; nausea, vomiting, diarrhea	Inpatient	High; unpredictable length of hospital stay	Moderate–high	Nurse high

or the use of crude, unsanitary instrumentation were associated with a very high incidence of maternal morbidity and mortality. With the advent of legal abortion by skilled providers, however, the incidence of complications declined dramatically in the United States and worldwide. Termination of first trimester or midtrimester pregnancy is acknowledged to have fewer relative risks and significantly lower mortality rates than delivering a full term pregnancy (vander Vlugt & Piotrow, 1973; Tietze, 1984). In addition to the growth of medical and surgical skills in the technical aspects of pregnancy termination, counseling and patient education interventions have been incorporated very effectively to assure that a woman receives the highest quality care available when she chooses abortion. Thorough preparation, anticipatory guidance, and close follow-up must all be individualized to meet the specific needs of the woman and her significant others.

Types of Procedures

Several medical and surgical techniques of pregnancy termination are available depending on gestational age, preference and skills of the physician and the health status of the woman. The important characteristics of each technique are summarized in Table 17–2.

First Trimester

Dilation and Suction (D & S). D & S is a surgical procedure in which the cervix is dilated and the products of conception are removed from the uterus by vacuum aspiration. The D & S procedure is used through the twelfth week of pregnancy. A paracervical block provides local anesthesia to reduce the pain associated with cervical dilation. In many instances and usually beyond 10 weeks of pregnancy, laminaria are used to provide a more gentle and gradual cervical dilation. Laminaria (Fig. 17–2) are dried, sterile pieces of seaweed that are inserted into the cervical os up to 24 hours before surgery. During that time, the laminaria absorb moisture, increase in diameter, and gradually dilate the cervix. Uterine contractions also occur because of the presence of these foreign bodies. The advantages of laminaria are decreased cervical lacerations and the elimination of

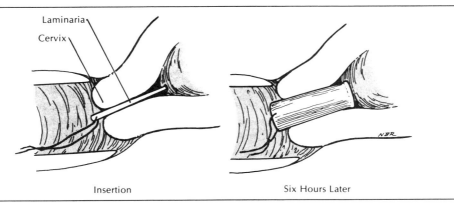

Laminaria
Cervix

Insertion   Six Hours Later

Figure 17–2. The physician may insert a laminaria rod in the cervical canal. The laminaria will absorb moisture, swell, and gradually widen the canal in about 6 hours. (Source: *Stewart, F., Guest, F., Stewart, G., & Hatcher, R.* My body, my health: The concerned woman's book of gynecology. *Toronto: Bantam Books, 1981. Reproduced with permission from Nelva B. Richardson and Bantam Books.)*

painful, rapid dilation of the cervix. One disadvantage of the laminaria is that an additional visit to the health care provider is required before the actual termination is performed. Occasionally mild analgesia is required for uterine cramping. The risk of infection is also slightly increased. On the day of the procedure, the woman may be given a mild intravenous sedative such as diazepam. Laminaria are then removed, the vagina is cleansed with an antiseptic solution, a tenaculum is applied to stabilize the cervix, and local anesthesia is administered to the paracervical area. The cervix is then further dilated if necessary (Fig. 17–3). At this point, the suction procedure begins. A flexible plastic curette attached to suction tubing and the source of vacuum is inserted into the uterine cavity and suction is applied at about 60 mm Hg. The suction curette is gently rotated and the products of conception are removed. The entire procedure lasts approximately 15 minutes.

The major risks of this procedure are uterine perforation, infection, and bleeding from incomplete removal of tissue. As mentioned above, cervical trauma is minimized with the use of laminaria.

Menstrual Extraction (ME). ME is virtually identical to the D & S procedure. But because this procedure terminates very early pregnancies (usually up to 6 weeks and not exceeding 8 weeks gestation) cervical dilation is usually not required and laminaria are rarely used. Following a paracervical block, a small lumen suction catheter is inserted into the uterus and the pregnancy is removed by suction. A decade ago, when tests detecting very early pregnancy were not available, a major disadvantage of the ME was that some women underwent the procedure needlessly because they were not in fact pregnant. With the advent of serum and urine assays for human chorionic gonadotropin

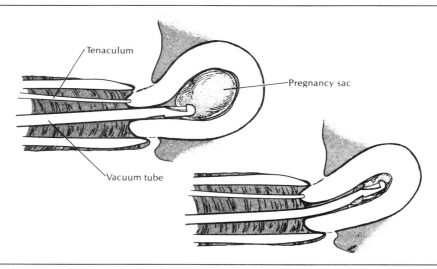

Figure 17–3. The vacuum tube draws the pregnancy sac out of the uterus. Near the end of the abortion procedure, the uterus begins to contract. (Source: *Stewart, F., Guest, F., Stewart, G., & Hatcher, R. My body, my health: The concerned woman's book of gynecology. Toronto: Bantam Books, 1981. Reproduced with permission from Nelva B. Richardson and Bantam Books.)*

(HCG), which are generally sensitive 10 to 14 days post-conception, a positive pregnancy test is indicated before a termination is undertaken. Another disadvantage of the ME is the potential for missing the pregnancy, necessitating a repeat procedure.

Second Trimester
Dilation and Evacuation (D & E). D & E is an appropriate pregnancy termination procedure for the second trimester (13 to 20 weeks' gestation). Similar to the D & S, the cervix is dilated with laminaria and with metal dilators if needed. A larger lumen suction curette is required because of the increased volume of tissue. Extraction instruments (ring forceps) are also used to remove the products of conception. Either a paracervical block or general anesthesia is used for pain management.

The complications associated with pregnancy termination, particularly uterine perforation, increase as gestational age increases. However, risks of surgical termination are still markedly lower than induced abortions using prostaglandins or saline instillation (Grimes & Cates, 1981). The D & E is used with increased frequency by experienced surgeons. This technique offers advantages to the woman seeking a midtrimester abortion because she does not have to experience the labor and delivery of the fetus as in saline or prostaglandin abortions. However, many physicians find the procedure emotionally stressful and elect not to perform it.

Saline Abortion. Saline abortion is a medical technique for pregnancy termination in which a hypertonic solution of saline is infused into the amniotic sac, causing death of the fetus and placenta. This procedure is generally performed between 16 and 24 weeks' gestation because earlier attempts to puncture the amniotic sac are usually unsuccessful. This can be a major disadvantage for the woman in the early midtrimester who must then wait up to 3 weeks between her decision to terminate and the time of the actual procedure.

For the procedure itself, the abdomen is cleansed, local anesthetic is injected, and a large gauge needle is inserted transabdominally into the amniotic sac. Amniotic fluid (100 to 250 cc) is withdrawn and replaced with 150 to 250 cc of 20 percent saline solution. Labor usually begins within several hours and the abortion is usually complete within 24 to 36 hours (Kerenyi, 1981).

Several major complications are associated with saline abortion. Hypernatremia is usually the result of injecting the sodium solution directly into the maternal vascular system. Coagulation defects resulting from fibrin depletion following hemorrhage or placental clot formation may also occur. In addition uterine rupture and cervical laceration from the rapid progression of labor are additional complications (Kerenyi, 1981).

Prostaglandin Abortion. This method of medically inducing an abortion is being used with increasing frequency for midtrimester terminations because of the lower associated risks. Prostaglandins stimulate uterine contractions and labor is usually complete within 24 hours (Neubardt & Schulman, 1977). Commonly used routes are intraamniotic injection and vaginal suppositories. Peripheral administration is associated with a higher incidence of gastrointestinal side effects such as nausea, vomiting, and diarrhea, although it is a less invasive procedure.

The major complication of prostaglandin abortion is an incomplete abortion with retention of the placenta or missed abortion. Infection and bleeding are also associated factors. In addition, advanced midtrimester procedures can make the delivery of a living but nonviable fetus possible.

Hysterotomy. Hysterotomy is no longer used as a primary technique for terminating a pregnancy. The procedure involves a uterine incision and manual extraction of the uterine contents. The surgery has been referred to as a mini-cesarean. Because of the morbidity and impact on future pregnancies from a uterine scar, this procedure is reserved for emergencies when other methods have been unsuccessful (Bolognese & Corson, 1975).

Summary and Discussion. Several methods of pregnancy termination are currently used. Although first trimester abortions have minimal risks, maternal morbidity and mortality increase significantly in the second trimester. In addition, long-term sequelae of late abortions have an unknown impact on future fertility although a number of factors such as cervical incompetence, uterine synechiae (Asherman's syndrome), and complications from infection have been identified. However, secondary infertility after induced abortion with appropriate surgical technique is very uncommon (Stubblefield et al., 1984).

Health Assessment for Induced Abortion
When the woman chooses to terminate her pregnancy, certain health data must be elicited from the general assessment described earlier in this chapter. In preparation for induced abortion, the following areas should be assessed: (1) pregnancy dating, (2) medical risk factors, and (3) psychosocial status.

Pregnancy Dating Based on Uterine Size and Date of Last Menstrual Period. Ultrasound may be used for more exact determination, particularly if there is a discrepancy between dates and uterine size or if the gestational age is borderline for a particular procedure. Dates of positive HCG tests may also be useful in retrospectively dating a pregnancy. History of quickening (first perceived fetal movement) and fetal heart tones are generally not used in pregnancy dating for a termination.

Medical Risk Factors. Preexisting medical problems such as diabetes, asthma, and cardiac or renal disease may preclude an outpatient procedure. Allergies to medications, particularly antibiotics, analgesics, and iodine must be noted, as well as adverse effects to anesthetics both general and local. History of bleeding disorders, anemia, thrombophlebitis, gastrointestinal disease, previous surgery (especially gynecological), and syncope or seizures should also be recorded (Neubardt & Schulman, 1977). Pre-existing reproductive tract infections should be ruled out.

If the woman is Rh negative, there is a risk that she may become sensitized if Rh positive fetal blood cells enter the maternal circulation at the time of the abortion. For this reason, immune globulin D (Rhogam for 12 weeks and above, Microgam for under 12 weeks) is administered to all Rh negative women at the time of the pregnancy termination unless it is known for certain that the father is also Rh negative.

In addition to the complete history and a phsyical examination, common laboratory work includes routine urinalysis, CBC, RPR (syphilis screen), Pap smear, cervical culture, and blood type.

Psychosocial Status. As described previously, coping skills, pregnancy antecedents, and social supports all have an impact upon the woman and her decision. In addition, what is her decision-making status? If she is ambivalent, is this conflict likely to be resolved? If not, the abortion may need to be delayed until the woman is able to choose a pregnancy option with less ambivalence.

Client Education. The general goals of client education for the woman seeking pregnancy termination are as follows:

1. Provide information and anticipatory guidance
2. Promote well-being before, during, and after the procedure, minimizing complication and emotional difficulties
3. Enhance client independence in self-care activities

To meet these goals, interventions must be client centered. Based on the education needs assessment described earlier, you can begin to develop a plan based on the individual client. An example of a teaching plan for a patient undergoing a dilation and suction procedure is presented in Table 17–3.

Emotional Status. The decision to terminate a pregnancy often is accompanied by emotional turmoil for the woman. Feelings of impending loss, anxiety about the pain associated with the procedure, and other unknowns may all contribute to this turmoil. This must be recognized and care taken not to unnecessarily overload the woman with volumes of information in brief periods of time. In addition, terminology such as "the baby" or "father of the baby" is not appropriate and should not be used. Terms such as "fetus," "pregnancy," and "partner" are less psychologically loaded and adequately convey the meanings.

Learning Style. Many women prefer to learn in one-to-one situations with their health care provider, particularly in the situation of pregnancy termination where privacy and confidentiality may be desired. In many instances, however, the woman may request that a significant other be present for all or part of the session. This is particularly true in the case of very young adolescents whose parent must sign the consent form for termination. However, the woman should also be given the opportunity for some time alone with the health care provider to discuss any topics she may not feel comfortable raising in the presence of others.

Another aspect of learning style is the degree to which the woman actively seeks out information. Some women come prepared with a list of extensive questions about the abortion and its risks, anesthesia, and postabortion contraception. Others prefer to be told only what the provider thinks is necessary. In either case, the woman should be encouraged to ask questions, think about the information given to her, and then follow up by telephone with any further questions.

Content Level. Obviously, the amount of content depends to a certain extent upon the woman's age, intelligence, and willingness to receive it. Minimally, the woman must have enough information to prevent complications and to cooperate with her care. The level of language should be tailored to the individual client and technical terminology limited in many cases. Additionally, graphic details of the surgical procedures are usually not indicated unless the woman requests it and may contribute unnecessarily to her feelings of guilt or anxiety.

PREGNANCY CONTINUATION

The initial crisis of the unintentional pregnancy may seem far away to the woman as she progresses through the second and third pregnancy trimesters. The decision making accomplished in a deliberate and self-determined way, however, will help make the

TABLE 17–3. TEACHING PLAN: DILATION AND SUCTION

Preprocedure objectives
1. To prepare the client for the termination procedure
2. To promote the opportunity for answering questions and providing necessary information

Content Area	Method	Evaluation	Plan
1. Basic anatomy and physiology of early pregnancy	Review signs and symptoms of early pregnancy: skipped menses nausea fatigue breast tenderness urinary frequency	States signs and symptoms Describes own experience	Review as needed at follow-up visit
	Discuss dating of pregnancy LMP Uterine size	Is aware of calculation of gestational age from LMP and exam	Review as needed at follow-up visit
2. Pregnancy decision making	Review alternatives	States desire for termination and reasons Able to verbalize feelings	Follow-up discussion at postabortion visit
3. Laminara	Describe laminaria and purpose Review written information Limited activity overnight May experience cramping Notify health care provider for: excessive bleeding, cramps or temperature elevation	States purpose of laminaria Is aware of warning signs	Review at time of laminaria insertion
4. Procedure	Describe anesthesia, paracervical block, general Describe cervical dilation Describes suction technique Use of visual aids	States preference for local or general anesthesia Understands procedures	Review at time of procedure

			Review at time of procedure
5.	Pain Management	Describe measures for reducing pain: relaxation techniques IV sedation, anesthesia Describe pain in familiar terminology, e.g., strong menstrual cramps	States preferences
6.	Laboratory work	Explain the following: routine urinalysis CBC PAP smear cervical culture RPR blood type Explain Rh factor Rhogam	States reason for receiving Rhogam if Rh negative
7.	Contraception	Discuss methods of contraception Identify previous problems with implementation of any of the methods	Client chooses best method for her needs States preferred method and specific details of method implementation	Follow-up postprocedure

During procedure objective
1. Provide anticipatory information to alleviate anxiety and insure client cooperation.

1.	Physical sensation	Prepare the client beforehand when she can expect the following: speculum insertion cleansing of the vagina paracervical block—often described as "stinging" cervical dilation pressure or cramping suction—noise of the machine sensation of pressure or strong cramping	Client remains relaxed Able to communicate level of discomfort

(continued)

TABLE 17–3. (cont.)

Postprocedure objective
1. To enhance self care practices to avoid complications of surgery.

Content Area	Method	Evaluation	Plan
1. Physical changes	Discuss: Bleeding—light moderate Bleeding for 7–10 days Avoid tampons Mild cramps Breast tenderness 48 hours postprocedure	States normal changes	
2. Activity	Discuss: No intercourse for 7 days Activity ad lib—normal to feel fatigue for a few days	States activity level plans for prn rest	
3. Contraception	Review plan for contraception Give pertinent instructions, written and verbal	States method of contraception, method of use	
4. Warning signs	Report to health care provider excessive bleeding, excessive cramping, temperature elevation	States warning signs Knows method of contacting health care provider	Follow-up prn
5. Emotional aspects	Discuss potential for feelings of sadness, loss, also relief All normal and usually self-limited		

Follow-up

Content Area	Method	Evaluation	Plan
1. Return visit 2–4 wks	Give appointment postprocedure At visit discuss plan for exam to check uterine size, repeat pregnancy test	Understands need for postprocedure check-up	
2. Contraception	Review contraceptive method	Provider assesses for appropriate use, any problems	

adjustment to pregnancy continuation possible. Another level of decision making, the choice between motherhood or adoption, must also be addressed.

Whether the woman decides on motherhood or adoption, comprehensive prenatal care is essential to maximize the health of both the mother and the fetus. In addition to client education, careful attention throughout the pregnancy must be directed toward the psychosocial adjustment and pregnancy bonding issues that may emerge.

Adoption

Adoption practices have changed radically in this country since the advent of legally available abortion. Before the early seventies when abortion was not a legal option, most young unmarried women with unintentional pregnancies faced two choices: motherhood or adoption. Single motherhood, particularly for the adolescent or young woman, was stigmatizing and resulted in strong negative social sanctions. As a result, many young unmarried women chose adoption as the most viable alternative. Changing social norms and the option of safe pregnancy termination have made the choices of abortion or single motherhood more acceptable. Many women feel that terminating an early pregnancy is preferable to giving up an infant after carrying a full term pregnancy. In many other cases, however, abortion is not an acceptable choice either because of personal (moral) reasons or because the gestational age of the fetus is too advanced.

The decision to relinquish a child after a lengthy pregnancy and the critical labor and delivery period is usually accompanied by grief and bereavement. As in the case of abortion, the woman usually experiences a sense of loss of what might have been, and of motherhood. In contrast to most women who opt for abortion, the relinquishing mother has had the additional experience of labor and delivery and in most cases, seeing her newborn. The reality of a viable infant often creates intense ambivalence for the relinquishing mother and, in fact, she may change her decision concerning the adoption.

With adequate assessment and counseling, anticipatory guidance, and appropriate interventions, the relinquishing mother can adjust to her choice with a positive outcome.

Assessment. The woman who relinquishes her child for adoption has special needs that must be assessed by the health care provider. Decision-making status, coping skills, and prenatal/postpartum educational needs are areas that must be considered.

As discussed earlier, ambivalence is common in pregnancy decision making. Despite this fact, the woman must complete the stages of decision making in order to become comfortable with her choice.

Previous coping skills and newly developing patterns should also be assessed. The use of an extensive support network is particularly important for the woman who will give up her child because of the complexities of her psychosocial situation. Involvement of parents and significant others should be encouraged if the relationships are supportive. Health care providers and social workers may also be an important resource for the woman. The use of defense mechanisms previously discussed in this chapter is also an important method of coping. In counseling the woman, the health care provider must be careful not to threaten fragile defense mechanisms (Berek, 1983). However, counseling should also be directed at assisting the woman to develop new and adaptive coping mechanisms.

Anticipatory Guidance. In addition to the prenatal and postpartum education included throughout this book, the woman relinquishing her pregnancy also requires anticipatory guidance specific to her situation.

The labor and delivery experience is particularly critical for the relinquishing mother (Devaney & Lavery, 1980). She must decide whether or not she wants to see and hold her infant. Although this experience will likely be a mixture of joy and sadness, it is usually recommended that the mother have contact with her baby after delivery and during the early postpartum period to make the experience real for her and to facilitate separation when she relinquishes her child (Berek, 1983).

The grief process is a normal response to loss and the young woman should be given the opportunity to ventilate her feelings in a supportive environmeent. Through verbalizing and expressing her responses to the loss of her biological child, she will begin to develop insights that will help her deal with the sorrow and move on to a new phase in her life.

SUMMARY

In this chapter, we have explored the complex area of unintentional pregnancy decision making. The health care provider is a pivotal person, providing counseling and client education. Thorough assessment is mandatory to facilitate the process of decision making. This period of crisis is potentially growth producing with adequate counseling and supportive interventions.

BIBLIOGRAPHY

Berek, J. Helping a patient surrender her child for adoption. *Contemporary OB/GYN*, 1983, *22*(6), 29–42.

Bracken, M. A causal model of psychosomatic reactions to vacuum aspiration abortion. *Social Psychiatry*. 1978, *13*, 135–145.

Bracken, M. B., Klerman, L. V., & Bracken, M. Coping with pregnancy resolution among never-married women. *American Journal of Orthopsychiatry*, 1978, *48*(2), 320–334.

Bolognese, R., & Corson, S. *Interruption of pregnancy: A total patient approach*. Baltimore: Williams & Wilkins, 1975.

Bygdeman, M. Prostaglandin procedures. In G. Burger, W. Brenner, & L. Keith (Eds.), *Second trimester abortion: Perspectives after a decade of experience*. Boston: John Wright, 1981.

Devaney, S., & Lavery, S. Nursing care for the relinquishing mother. *JOGN*, 1980, *9*(6), 375–378.

Dryfoos, J. Contraceptive use, pregnancy intentions and pregnancy outcomes among U.S. women. *Family Planning Perspectives*, 1982, *14*(2), 81–94.

Garland, L. M., & Bush, C. T. *Coping behaviors in nursing*. Reston, Va.: Reston, 1982.

Grimes, D., & Cates, W. Dilatation and evacuation. In G. Burger, W. Brenner, & L. Keith (Eds.), *Second trimester abortion: Perspectives after a decade of experience*. Boston: John Wright, 1981.

Henshaw, S., Forrest, J., Sullivan, E., & Tietze, C. Abortion services in the United States. *Family Planning Perspectives*, 1982, *14*(1), 5–14.

Kerenyi, T. D. Hypertonic saline instillation. In G. Burger, W. Brenner, & L. Keith (Eds.), *Second trimester abortion: Perspectives after a decade of experience*. Boston: John Wright, 1981.

Lewis, C. A comparison of minors' and adults' pregnancy decisions. *American Journal of Orthopsychiatry*, 1980, *50*(3), 446–453.

Leynes, C. Keep or adopt: A study of factors influencing pregnant adolescents' plans for their babies. *Child Psychiatry and Human Development*, 1980, *11*(2), 105–112.

Narrow, B. *Patient teaching in nursing practice*. New York: John Wiley & Sons, 1979.

Neubardt, S., & Schulman, H. *Techniques of abortion*. Boston: Little, Brown, 1977.

Shusterman, L. Predicting the psychological consequences of abortion. *Social Science and Medicine*, 1979, *13A*, 683–689.

Stubblefield, P., Monson, R., Schoenbaum, S., Wolfson, C., Cookson, D., & Ryan, K. Fertility after induced abortion: A prospective follow-up study. *Obstetrics and Gynecology*, 1984, *62*(2), 186–191.

Tietze, C. The public health effects of legal abortion in the United States. *Family Planning Perspectives*, 1984, *16*(1), 26–28.

vander Vlugt, T., & Piotrow, P. Uterine aspiration techniques. *Population Reports*, 1973, Series F, No. 3, F-25.

RESOURCES

Organizations

Adoption

Child Welfare League of America, 67 Irving Place, New York, NY 10003, (212) 254-7410, *(Information on adoption.)*

Birthright, 11055 S. St. Louis Avenue, Chicago, IL 60655, (312) 233-8000. *(Local chapters provide counseling oriented toward continuing pregnancy. Assists with pregnancy related matters.)*

Motherhood

Parents Without Partners, 7910 Woodmont Avenue, Washington, DC 20014, (301) 654-8850. *(Local chapters. Self-help groups.)*

Abortion

Abortion Information Hotline, 800-442-8178.

Publications

Adoption

Wishard, L., & Wishard W. *Adoption: The grafted tree*. New York: Avon Books, 1979.

Motherhood

Elvenstar, D. *Children: To have or have not?* San Francisco: Harbor Publishing, 1982.

Abortion

Stewart, F., Guest, F., Stewart, G., & Hatcher, R. *My body, my health: The concerned woman's book of gynecology*. Toronto: Bantam Books, 1981.

Health Education and Cesarean Childbirth

18

Diony Young and Jane Ahrens

The decade of the 1970s witnessed extraordinary technological developments in the practice of obstetrics, where the event of childbirth increasingly became transformed from a physiological process to a model of surgical intervention by cesarean section. It is necessary for health professionals and childbirth educators to have an understanding of the facts surrounding this procedure to know how to approach its multiple facets in an educational program. A unique feature of the cesarean delivery is that it involves both major abdominal surgery on one individual and the emerging life of another—a fact that requires an ongoing professional sensitivity to both the physiological and psychological aspects of the event.

From 5.5 percent of all births in 1970, the cesarean birth rate has risen to 17.9 percent in 1981—or 1 of every 6 births in the United States (Placek, Taffel, & Moien, 1983). The National Center for Health Statistics reports that from 1970 to 1978 this increase occurred within all regions, all age groups, all marital statuses, all hospital sizes, and all types of hospital ownership (Placek & Taffel, 1980). The trend continued in 1981, showing that the cesarean birth rate was highest in the Northeast (20.0 percent), followed by the South (18.8 percent), the West (17.1 percent), and the Northcentral states (15.9 percent).

Nationally, the rate is highest in hospitals of 500 beds or more, in proprietary hospitals, for Blue Cross as a source of payment, and for mothers aged 35 years and over (Placek, Taffel, & Moien, 1983).

Data from the National Natality Survey (1980) showed that nearly 40 percent of the cesarean deliveries were repeat procedures, and of the overall cesarean section rate of 17.1 percent, the primary rate comprised 11.2 percent (Placek, Taffel, & Keppel, 1983).

The Canadian cesarean birth rate has closely paralleled that in the United States, rising from 7.5 percent in 1972 to 1973 to 13.9 percent in 1979 (U.S. Dept. HHS, 1981). Although in Western European countries the rate is considerably lower, a trend toward an increase is reported in England, France, Norway, and the Netherlands (U.S. Dept. HHS, 1981).

The economic impact of a cesarean birth rate of almost 20 percent in the United States is enormous. For the 600,000 cesareans performed each year at an average of $4,000 each, a total of about $2.5 billion is spent of health dollars (Norwood, 1984).

In the United States a new policy of vaginal birth after a previous cesarean birth, described in The American College of Obstetricians and Gynecologists' *Guidelines for Vaginal Delivery after a Cesarean Childbirth* (1982a), has the potential for slowing the cesarean birth rate and improving the quality of the childbirth experience for American parents. It would also save a great deal of money. A 1979 University of Washington study calculated a savings of over $6 million for every 10,000 trial labors of women who had a previous cesarean section, even if some ended up having surgery again (Norwood, 1984). In 1984, this amounted to "a national saving of $100 to $120 million if even one half of today's 200,000 annual automatic repeat mothers were encouraged to labor" (Norwood, 1984).

Factors Contributing to the Increase in Cesarean Births

Two government reports have examined the subject of cesarean birth to determine the factors contributing to the increased rate and the characteristics of this trend. The Marieskind report, *An Evaluation of Caesarean Section in the United States* (1979), identifies multiple factors and notes that many of them may combine to increase the cesarean rate. Principal among the factors identified are: (1) physician fear of a malpractice suit and defensive obstetrical practices; (2) repeat cesarean sections; (3) lack of physician training and experience in uncomplicated obstetrics; (4) physician belief in superior outcome with cesarean section; (5) changing and expanding indications for cesareans (e.g., breech presentation); (6) shifts in childbearing patterns; (7) financial or economic factors; and (8) greater reliance on technological procedures for fetal assessment (e.g., electronic fetal monitoring).

The National Institutes of Health Consensus Development Conference on *Cesarean Childbirth* (U.S. Dept. HHS, 1981) found that four major factors had contributed to the increase in cesarean births between 1970 and 1978. They were dystocia (30 percent contribution to rise in rate), repeat cesareans (25 to 30 percent), breech presentation (10 to 15 percent), and fetal distress (10 to 15 percent). This does not mean to say, however, that "dystocia" is increasing. It is not. The diagnoses under this heading are simply being made more frequently in current clinical practice.

Psychological and Social Effects of Cesarean Birth

The psychological and social impact of a cesarean birth has been clearly documented (Affonso, 1981; Cohen & Estner, 1983; Marieskind, 1979; U. S. Dept. HHS, 1981). In comparison with a vaginal delivery, a cesarean delivery can evoke negative emotional reactions from parents that result from unmet expectations (Affonso & Stichler, 1980; Marut & Mercer, 1979). In addition, feelings of fear, frustration, anger, disappointment, helplessness, and failure are common. Often a woman's self-esteem suffers greatly because of loss of control over her body and failure for it to "work right" (Cohen, 1977; Cohen & Estner, 1983; Conner, 1977; Marut & Mercer, 1979). Fathers may also feel cheated and experience feelings of inadequacy, grief, and failure, which may carry over into the role of early fathering (Affonso & Stichler, 1980; Cohen, 1977).

The uterine scar may arouse feelings of mutilation and affect a woman's feelings of sexual attractiveness; the fear of rupture during sexual intercourse is often expressed (Cohen, 1977; Conner, 1977). One study reported that many cesarean mothers perceived the experience as abnormal and carrying a social stigma (Marut & Mercer, 1979).

Cesarean mothers express concerns and fears about their changing roles as wife and mother, and about changing family relationships and interactions, which can increase stress and cause conflict (Affonso & Stichler, 1980). Extreme disappointment may be felt by both mother and father if they cannot share the childbirth event as they had planned

(Cohen, 1977; Gainer & VanBonn, 1977). Cohen (1977) reports that "For a great many cesarean couples, the single most important factor influencing feelings about the birth is whether the father was present at the delivery."

Feelings of inadequacy and grief for the lost birth experience and immediate separation from the newborn may occur, and early mother–newborn interaction and attachment may be delayed because of maternal drowsiness, general anethesia, and removal of the baby to a nursery (Affonso, 1981; Cohen, 1977; Conner, 1977). In such situations, initiation of bonding with the father is essential (Affonso, 1981; Enkin, 1977). Some women may feel initial resentment toward the baby as being the "cause" of the cesarean (Lipson & Tilden, 1980).

Strong negative reactions and anger may be expressed toward the nursing and medical staff—that the "cesarean was unnecessary" or the "surgery was the doctor's fault" (Affonso & Stichler, 1980). Women mention feeling abandoned by the attending health professionals, a sense of powerlessness, disorientation, lack of information, perceptual distortions, and a loss of continuity (Affonso, 1981). Affonso and Stichler (1980) also report in their study that 30 percent of 105 women made positive comments about having a cesarean and were relieved that they had the operation, because they saw it as a way of ending the long hours of labor.

The process of psychological assimilation or integration of the cesarean birth has been examined by Lipson and Tilden (1980), who found that five general phases are manifested. Phase one, occurring in the immediate postpartum hours, is a period of shocked numbness and a sense of suspended animation. Phase two extends over the hospital stay of 5 to 7 days, and the "just coping" by the woman is replaced by feelings of intense disappointment at the loss of the anticipated vaginal birth. She may feel relief, guilt, anger, envy of other women, and detachment toward her baby. Phase three, from discharge to about 8 weeks postpartum, is an "emerging awareness" of the meaning of the cesarean to the individual. Self-image problems and dreams (nightmares) about the event may occur. Phase four, which seems to be from 2 months postpartum to the end of the first year, is a period of "intermediate resolution," when the woman struggles to understand and accept the experience, using various coping mechanisms. Support groups can help during this time. Phase five is the final resolution of the experience beginning about 1 year after the cesarean, in which the woman accepts and places it within the framework of the rest of her life. This phase is analogous to the resolution phase in grieving, where "a new and more realistic appraisal of the lost object becomes possible" (Lipson & Tilden, 1980). The recovery phase includes some positive evaluation of the cesarean birth by the mother that frequently refers to the baby's health and well-being. A new responsibility and assertiveness as a health care consumer combined with feelings of personal growth are other aspects of this last phase. A subsequent pregnancy can trigger maternal anxieties but also a new sense of active participation and decision making in childbirth (Lipson & Tilden, 1980).

Fairley emphasizes to pregnant women that "Having a cesarean does not mean that every goal is abandoned nor does it mean that you must relinquish control over the experience. . . . Maintaining understanding of oneself and of the event will result in feelings of satisfaction with the birth itself, whether the birth is vaginal or cesarean" (Fairley, in Cohen & Estner, 1983). Ways to minimize negative feelings about a cesarean section include prenatal knowledgeable participation in the birth, birth plan for vaginal cesarean birth and postpartum, and advance determination of family-centered cesarean birth options in the hospital. During labor and cesarean birth, the mother will feel more involved when she can receive loving support from her partner and have regional anesthesia. She should have maximum contact with her newborn and other family members, and be given as much help as possible at home after discharge to allow energies to be directed to "mothering and recovering" (Fairley, in Cohen & Estner, 1983). It also appears that the woman who has tried a variety of nonmedical measures to augment labor (e.g., position changes, standing, walking, warm water, relaxation techniques) feels more positive about herself and her experience, even if ultimately a cesarean section becomes necessary (Shearer, 1982a; Young & Mahan, 1980).

Additional measures that can enhance the cesarean birth are discussed later in this chapter.

Mortality and Morbidity

Although the risks of cesarean section have been greatly reduced with the advent of sterile technique, improvements in operating methods, and availability of blood and antibiotics, the procedure does involve an increased risk of maternal mortality, estimated to be two to four times that for vaginal delivery, although comparison of maternal mortality by method of delivery is difficult (U. S. Dept. HHS, 1981). In addition, maternal deaths during childbirth are underreported by perhaps as much as 50 percent, according to a recent analysis in Georgia (Rubin et al., 1981).

Cesarean section is a major surgical procedure for which maternal morbidity, including infections, hemorrhage, pulmonary emboli, venous thrombosis, and anesthesia-related morbidity, is substantially higher than that for vaginal delivery (U. S. Dept. HHS, 1981). In addition, significant maternal psychological disturbances, as described earlier, may occur.

Some authorities have attributed much of the decline in perinatal mortality to the increased use of neonatal intensive care and cesarean sections (Williams & Chen, 1982), but another recent report contradicts this suggestion and describes results that "do not support the contention that the expansion of cesarean birth rates has contributed significantly to reduced perinatal mortality in recent years" (O'Driscoll & Foley, 1983). In fact, at a large hospital in Dublin, Ireland, the perinatal mortality rates have dropped in parrallel with rates in the United States, but the hospital's cesarean rate remained unchanged at under 5 percent (O'Driscoll & Foley, 1983). Others have pointed out that improvements in prenatal care and nutrition, use of contraception, lowered fertility, availability of abortion, and socioeconomic factors have significantly affected perinatal mortality (Marieskind, 1979).

Frequently, a timely cesarean section has saved the life of a newborn. At the same time, this procedure, especially in the absence of labor, is associated with an increase in asphyxia and neonatal respiratory distress syndrome (Marieskind, 1979; U. S. Dept. HHS, 1981). Therefore, the necessity of avoiding iatrongenic premature birth has been stressed by the Consensus Development Conference on *Cesarean Childbirth* (U. S. Dept. HHS, 1981).

Indications for Cesarean Birth

Although the diagnosis and indications for performing a cesarean section cannot be discussed at length in this chapter, it is important to identify the more common indications, even though professional agreement about them varies considerably. Marieskind (1979) points out that there are no uniform definitions for what constitutes an indication for a cesarean. Also, during the 1970s the indications for the procedure changed and expanded. The most important conclusion that can be drawn is that the decision to do a cesarean section must be individualized according to each obstetrical situation and be based on the doctrine of informed consent (ICEA Position Statement, 1980; Young & Mahan, 1980).

When the data are examined by indication for cesarean, it has been found that dystocia (i.e., cephalopelvic disproportion, failure to progress, prolonged labor, and prolonged rupture of the membranes) is assoicated most prominently with the increase in the primary cesarean birth rate (Marieskind, 1979; U. S. Dept. HHS, 1981).

Previous cesarean delivery has been a major indication for cesarean section, but as already mentioned, professional opinion has recently changed, and in carefully selected cases, 50 to 60 percent of women can safely experience a vaginal delivery after a previous cesarean (Lavin et al., 1982; U. S. Dept. HHS, 1981).

The diagnosis of breech is another major indication for a cesarean section. Under specific conditions (discussed later), however, vaginal delivery for the term breech is considered to be acceptable (U. S. Dept. HHS, 1981).

Fetal distress is a common indication for cesarean section, and the use of electronic fetal monitoring (EFM) is associated with an increased frequency in this diagnosis. Questions of accuracy and interpretation of EFM need to be resolved before a reduction of the cesarean birth rate from this diagnosis can be achieved, because there is no evidence that the actual incidence of fetal distress has changed (U. S. Dept. HHS, 1981).

Other maternal conditions that are often an indication for cesarean section include maternal diabetes, placenta previa, severe toxemia, abruptio placentae, heart disease, and active genital herpes (U. S. Dept. HHS, 1981; Young & Mahan, 1980). A changing indication for cesarean section has been the presence of multiple pregnancy (U. S. Dept. HHS, 1981). The conditions of prolapsed cord and Rh disease (erythroblastosis fetalis) are two other indications for cesarean section, although the incidence of the latter condition is decreasing.

PRENATAL EDUCATION ABOUT CESAREAN BIRTH

The objectives and content for an educational program about cesarean birth need to be tailored to the participants in the childbirth education class. One group, the majority, anticipates and plans a spontaneous vaginal delivery, and for them, a contingency plan and preparation in the event of complications requiring an emergency cesarean section is necessary. A second group comprises expectant parents who have had a cesarean birth and are candidates for, and are planning, a vaginal birth this time. The third group, which is a minority, comprises those expectant parents who require an elective cesarean section, either elective repeat or elective because of a specific maternal or fetal condition for which cesarean section is the delivery of choice.

Irrespective of the group to which each pregnant woman and her partner belong, there are several general areas that need to be included in a comprehensive prenatal education program. The program itself can be conducted in one of three settings—the hospital, the community, and the private practice. Whichever setting is used, it is important that the educational courses be designed with consumer input and adapted to meet the needs of all educational, cultural, and socioeconomic groups (ICEA Position Paper, 1979). The expectant parents are the key members of the health care team, and they must be prepared so that they can actively participate in all aspects of the childbearing process.

The general objective of the prenatal education program described by the International Childbirth Education Association (ICEA) is "to prepare expectant parents emotionally and physically for a participating and individually satisfying pregnancy, labor, birth, and introduction to parenthood . . . and the right of the expectant parent to make informed choices based on knowledge of alternatives" (ICEA Teacher Certification, 1979). Similarly, the Nurses Association of the American College of Obstetricians and Gynecologists describes the health education objective as one that "should provide the patient and her family with pertinent information to enable them to participate in their own care, to make decisions, and to exercise choices" (NAACOG Standards, 1981).

The following curriculum for prenatal education for all childbearing parents, whether anticipating a vaginal or a cesarean birth, combines features from the *ICEA Position Paper on Planning Comprehensive Maternal and Newborn Services for the Childbearing Year* (1979), and from *NAACOG Guidelines for Childbirth Education* (1981).

- Normal reproduction, including anatomy, physiology, and psychology of labor, birth, and postpartum; signs of pregnancy; normal physical and psychological changes during pregnancy; health maintenance and care during pregnancy; fetal development; signs and stages of labor; postpartum health care.
- Danger signs in pregnancy; risks of alcohol, smoking, drugs, caffeine, communicable diseases, immunizations, radiation exposure, environmental hazards and contaminants.
- Basic nutritional needs and their relationship to fetal development.
- Self-help techniques and comfort measures for pregnancy, labor, birth, and postpartum, including posture, body mechanics, maintenance of muscle tone and physical fitness, tension–relaxation control; breathing techniques; childbirth and postpartum exercises.
- Labor support techniques for the companion; role of the companion in labor and birth.
- Social and psychological roles and relationships in the family; sexual roles.
- Roles of health care providers in the management of labor, birth, and postpartum.
- Options in labor and birth procedures; options in birth environment, including birthing rooms; options for rooming-in; early discharge; family visitation; home care follow-up.
- Rights of the expectant family; informed consent; responsibilities of the childbearing woman for self-involvement in care and decision making.
- High-risk birth, including discussions of procedures, indications, benefits, risks, and alternatives for prenatal tests for fetal growth and well-being, electronic fetal monitoring, intravenous fluids, induction and augmentation, analgesia, anesthesia, episiotomy, forceps, cesarean birth; parents' role and participation in the care of the sick newborn.
- Preparation for parenting, including roles of family members, infant care, infant feeding (breast and bottle), child growth and development; child safety; well-baby care; immunizations; family planning; sexual relations.
- Identification of community resource groups in breast-feeding, parenting, cesarean family support, nutritional programs such as WIC, physical fitness.
- Tour of the maternity–newborn unit.

As a supplement to the curriculum, *The Pregnant Patient's Bill of Rights, the Pregnant Patient's Responsibilities* (1977) is a helpful resource that can serve as a basis for class discussion.

The International Childbirth Education Association believes that all expectant parents should be educated about both vaginal and cesarean birth, with the primary focus on vaginal birth, and that "optimal birth outcome is directly related to an individualized rather than a routine approach to the management of each pregnancy, labor and birth" (ICEA Position Statement, 1980).

Cesarean Prevention

The current dependency on obstetrical intervention and technology and the high cesarean birth rate are realities that must be faced by all expectant parents and childbirth educators. At the same time, parents must be reminded that pregnancy and childbirth are healthy processes, not pathological conditions, and that with rare exceptions, a woman's body is fully capable of giving birth without medical or surgical assistance.

Concern about a trend of unquestioning acceptance for the rapid increase in cesarean birth by health professionals, childbirth educators, and parents in the 1970s has precipitated an emergence in the 1980s of a Cesarean Prevention Movement, with a growing number of chapters in the United States and Canada. Unnecessary obstetrical intervention and surgery have been critically examined in several recent books (Cohen & Estner, 1983; Harrison, 1982; Norwood, 1984; Young & Mahan, 1980). Articles in the medical literature also address the problem of how to reduce the cesarean birth rate (Dilts, 1981; O'Driscoll & Foley, 1983; Quilligan, 1983).

Reversing the long-established policy of repeat cesareans will be one key factor affecting the cesarean birth rate (ACOG Guidelines, 1982). A second factor involves changing labor management in ways that increase the likelihood of a spontaneous vaginal delivery. A third factor hinges on a prenatal educational approach that convinces women that their bodies are capable of giving birth without assistance. It needs to be pointed out that the very terminology associated with a woman's capabilities—inadequate pelvis, incompetent cervix, failure to progress, dysfunctional labor, lazy uterus—denote negative imagery that undermines a woman's faith in her body.

Not all childbirth educators are in agreement concerning what information, if any, should be given in a prenatal education program on the subject of complications and cesarean birth. For example, Young and Mahan (1980) suggest that "choices and facts relative to both avoiding and having a cesarean birth must be included." Peterson (1981), on the other hand, maintains that "in the educational setting, description of complications becomes preparation for complication for the pregnant woman. This preparation may become an expectation for the abnormal, precluding the ability to acquire healthy attitudes for normal delivery." It is obvious that the line between providing information and setting up an expectation is a fine and difficult one for the childbirth educator. Yet, if the right information is given and if an attitude of healthy skepticism toward unnecessary intervention in labor is conveyed, parents will be better equipped to cope with complications should they arise (Young & Mahan, 1980).

The cesarean birth component of a comprehensive prenatal education program should include the following information, according to the International Childbirth Education Association:*

1. Informed consent information, including advantages and side effects concerning the use of obstetrical procedures and technology, analgesics, sedatives, anesthetics, and drugs for labor induction and stimulation.
2. Maternal and fetal indications for cesarean birth.
3. Personal and medical choices in pregnancy and labor that may enhance the

---

*Source: ICEA position statement: Cesarean birth. ICEA News, 1980, *19*, 4–5, by permission.

likelihood of vaginal delivery and decrease the likelihood and necessity of cesarean section.

4. Information about antenatal tests to determine fetal maturity and well-being and to confirm the diagnosis indicating cesarean section.
5. Indications for, and advantages of, going into labor spontaneously and having a trial labor.
6. Possible links between cesarean section and the use of certain procedures, drugs, and intervention during labor (e.g., electronic fetal monitoring, recumbent position, epidural block, analgesics, induction) (Young & Mahan, 1980).
7. Brief review of obstetrical practices and procedures for cesarean section, including assessment of family-centered cesarean birth and postpartum programs in local hospitals.
8. Development of an optimal birth plan which includes personal and family-centered priorities for both vaginal and cesarean birth.

A woman's personal choices made when she is pregnant will increase or decrease the likelihood of a vaginal delivery (Young & Mahan, 1980). These choices include her birth practitioner (midwife or physician) and her birth environment (in-hospital or out-of-hospital birth settings). For an in-hospital birth, a birth practitioner and hospital with low cesarean section rates should be selected, and the pregnant woman should discuss with her practitioner all aspects of labor and birth management and family-centered choices for both vaginal and cesarean births.

The specific actions and steps during labor that will increase the likelihood of a vaginal delivery should receive major emphasis in the prenatal education program. These steps for the pregnant woman have been described as follows (Shearer, 1982b; Young & Mahan, 1980):

1. Stay home until active labor is well established.
2. Choose a supportive birth environment and atmosphere.
3. Be accompanied by a well-prepared labor partner plus a trained labor companion.
4. Use relaxation techniques without rapid breathing patterns.
5. Avoid surgical induction (rupture of membranes) and medical induction (Pitocin).
6. Use touching from a loving partner and verbal encouragement.
7. Urinate at least every hour.
8. Change position frequently; avoid flat-laying position; use standing, walking, sitting, side-lying, hands-and-knees positions; squat in second stage.
9. Eat and drink lightly to provide adequate calories and fluids.
10. If labor slows down, use nonmedical labor support techniques and insist on more time.
11. Use warm water (bath, shower, hot compresses).
12. In second stage, bear down as you feel the physiological need.
13. Avoid using sedatives, analgesics, and conduction anesthesia.
14. Avoid using electronic fetal monitor unless medically warranted; with fetal distress, request verification by a fetal scalp blood test.

Vaginal Birth After a Cesarean (VBAC)

The policy and practice initiated by Dr. Edwin Craigin in 1916 of "Once a cesarean, always a cesarean" has entered a new era as American childbearing parents enter the 1980s. Professional abandonment of this universally applied dictum has now been suggested by the National Institutes of Health (U. S. Dept. HHS, 1981) and the American College of Obstetricians and Gynecologists (1982a), who now recommend vaginal birth for a majority of women who have had a previous cesarean birth.

The validity of this option for expectant parents has been described by childbirth educators Cohen and Estner (1983), Keolker (1981), Shearer (1982a), Shulman (1978), Young and Mahan (1980), and others. In addition, during the 1970s and early 1980s the medical literature has abounded with studies confirming the safety of vaginal birth after a cesarean. A comprehensive review of these studies has been provided by Lavin and colleagues (1982) and also by O'Sullivan and colleagues (1981).

The primary reason physicians give for doing a repeat procedure has been the presence of a uterine scar from the previous cesarean surgery. The incidence of cesarean scar rupture in 28,742 pregnancies, and including prior classical and low vertical uterine incisions, is extremely low, however, varying from 0.6 to 1.2 percent (O'Sullivan et al., 1981). Perinatal mortality due to uterine rupture was 0.93 per 1000 births in the series of studies from 1950 to 1980, and during the same time period no maternal deaths occurred due to uterine rupture during labor among women with a prior cesarean scar (Lavin et al., 1982).

In January, 1982, *Guidelines for Vaginal Delivery After a Cesarean Childbirth* was published for physicians and hospitals. The *Guidelines* offer a welcome option for an increasing percentage of the childbearing population who would otherwise be committed to surgery for all pregnancies. The *Guidelines* read as follows (ACOG Guidelines, 1982a):

1. The woman and her physician should fully discuss the options of a trial labor early in the prenatal course to allow for appropriate planning.
2. The indication for the prior cesarean birth should be a nonrepeating condition, e.g., patients with previous cesarean birth for fetal distress or for failure to progress without documented fetopelvic disproportion.
3. The type of previous uterine incision should have been documented to be a low segment transverse type.
4. The pregnancy should be a singleton with a vertex presentation and a fetal weight estimated to be less than 4000 grams.
5. There should be no other obstetrical, medical, or surgical history of physical findings that contraindicates labor or vaginal delivery.
6. There should be capabilities for continuous fetal heart rate and uterine activity monitoring throughout labor.
7. The patient should understand that it may be necessary to terminate the trial of labor and proceed with cesarean section.
8. The anesthesiologist and pediatrician should be advised of the intent for a trial of labor and vaginal delivery.

Prenatal classes for vaginal birth following a cesarean (also called VBAC classes) were initiated around 1979 in Boston by Nancy Cohen; other childbirth educators soon followed suit. Cohen and Estner (1983) and Shearer (1982a) point out that the prenatal education program for parents who elect to have a vaginal birth after a cesarean section contains most of the same elements present in a traditional childbirth education program, described earlier in this chapter.

Shearer (1982a) describes four primary objectives in VBAC classes:

1. Replacing the "fear and mystery that surround birth in our culture with knowledge and confidence."
2. Providing sufficient information about the hospital—"its options, its restrictions,

the risk/benefit considerations of the various technologies"—to enable parents to make decisions about the childbirth.

3. Enabling women "to get in touch with their bodies, inner resources, and abilities."
4. Giving parents "specific tools with which to work in labor," that can be individualized to suit each woman's needs (discussed earlier).

There are two primary factors that make VBAC labor different from any other labor. First, the woman often brings with her negative feelings of fear, grief, and guilt about the previous experience, and both parents need to come to terms with that experience. Second, many obstetricians are nervous and tend to practice defensively with a VBAC labor and apply special restrictions (Shearer, 1982a). This management increases a woman's anxiety, limits her mobility, and increases the likelihood of a repeat cesarean. Such women should be encouraged to change physicians and find one who is experienced in doing vaginal births after previous cesareans (Cohen & Estner, 1983; Shearer, 1982a).

The following course outline for 12 VBAC classes of 2½ hours each is used by Cohen in teaching couples who are preparing for a vaginal birth (Cohen & Estner, 1983):

1. Welcome!

   - Introductions and group support
   - What do you need from these classes? Why are you here?
   - Why do you want to have your next child vaginally?
   - What are your expectations for your upcoming birth?
   - What are your concerns? Fears? Dreams?
   - How did you feel when the decision was made to perform the cesarean?
   - How do you feel right now?
   - Basic biology and brief discussion of labor and delivery physiologies
   - Instructor's philosophies about birth (upon which the rest of the course is based)
   - Uterine dependability

2. Increasing Your Chances for Vaginal Birth

   - Nutrition
   - Exercise
   - The consequences of medical and psychological interventions
   - Fetal/maternal/newborn interventions and risks
   - Tests during pregnancy—reliability and risks
   - Informed consent
   - Psychological aspects of childbearing
   - Seeing your cesarean as a learning and growing experience
   - Influence of body on mind and vice versa
   - Pain in childbirth—healthy and normal
   - Focus of control
   - Mother/daughter relationship, roles, and influences
   - Male energy at birth
   - Our own births
   - Birth as a sexual experience
   - Marital relationships
   - Spiritual aspects of childbirth

3. Planning Your Birth

   - Labor support
   - Choosing the place of birth
   - Interviewing doctors
   - Hospital "policies"
   - Designing a request list for your labor and birth
   - "Energies" at birth—self-confidence, loving support, strength, birth visualization, creativeness, trust
   - Children at birth
   - Consumer strength—regaining possession of childbirth, exercising options, making informed decisions, changing the way of birth

4. Films and slides (vaginal hospital births, home birth, cesarean birth) and discussion

   - When is a cesarean necessary?
   - Judicious uses of medical interventions
   - Remaining psychologically as well as physiologically conscious during a cesarean
   - Options for cesarean birth

5. Labor and Vaginal Delivery
6. Suggestions for Enjoying the Birth and Helping Yourself

   - For men: How to help your woman
   - Getting support from others during labor and birth
   - Psychological aids
   - Relaxation
   - Birth visualization exercise

7. Breast-feeding
8. Circumcision
9. Birth Control
10. Loving Your Newborn
11. The Family and Its Place in Today's World
12. Group party to share strength, love, and feelings

Cephalopelvic Disproportion and Dystocia

The diagnosis of cephalopelvic disproportion (CPD) or fetopelvic disproportion (FPD) generally means that the baby's head will not fit through the mother's pelvis, that labor is not progressing, or both. CPD is often included under the general term of dystocia, or dysfunctional labor, a condition that does not have a precise definition but that comprised the largest contribution to the increase in cesarean sections between 1970 and 1978 (30 percent) (U. S. Dept. HHS, 1981). In 1980, a cesarean section was done in 94 percent of the deliveries where the complication of maternal–fetal disproportion was noted (Taffel & Placek, 1983).

The Consensus Development Conference notes that the category of dystocia called "failure to progress" may, in fact, not be abnormal labor and the benefits of cesarean section for this diagnosis "are poorly supported in the literature." Thus further research clarifying the factors affecting the progress of labor is recommended (U. S. Dept. HHS, 1981). In addition, because many women who have had a previous cesarean section for CPD have subsequently given birth vaginally to larger babies, additional medical investigation should be undertaken in the event of a diagnosis of CPD (Young & Mahan, 1980).

It has also been recommended that in situations where fetal distress is absent, prior to considering a cesarean section, other measures to enhance labor progress should be tried, such as rest, ambulation, hydration, sedation, and use of oxytocin (U. S. Dept. HHS, 1981). Links between the more frequent use of lumbar epidural anesthesia through its effects on the forces of labor and the increase in cesarean birth have been suggested, and the debate about this issue continues (U. S. Dept. HHS, 1981).

In addition to following the steps outlined for increasing the likelihood of a vaginal delivery (discussed earlier), prenatal education about dystocia should emphasize the importance of tailoring labor management to an individual situation and may include these suggestions (Shearer, 1982b; Young & Mahan, 1980):

1. Seek second opinion if cesarean is recommended.
2. Discuss with your practitioner in advance: use, reliability, benefits, and risks of x-ray pelvimetry and ultrasound; trial of labor.
3. Request to begin labor spontaneously and have a trial of labor.
4. Stay at home until 5 cm dilation.
5. Emphasize birth as normal, physiological function to increase maternal self-confidence.
6. Use nonmedical support and relaxation measures (discussed earlier).

The guidelines for dystocia suggested by the American College of Obstetricians and Gynecologists recognize that slow progress in labor may be normal and cesarean section is not appropriate treatment for prolonged early labor (ACOG Guidelines, 1982b).

Breech Presentation

Breech presentation occurs in 3 to 4 percent of all deliveries. It is associated with an increase in both neonatal morbidity and mortality when compared with vertex presentation, irrespective of whether a vaginal or a cesarean delivery is done (U. S. Dept. HHS, 1981). The trend toward cesarean delivery of breech-presenting babies is continuing, and this complication accounted for 10 to 15 percent of the rise in the cesarean birth rate between 1970 and 1978 (U. S. Dept. HHS, 1981). In 1980, about 67.2 percent of breech presentations were delivered by cesarean section, compared with only 15 percent in 1970 (Taffel & Placek, 1983).

The Consensus Development Conference concludes that more data are needed to evaluate the best delivery method for breech-presenting babies. However, vaginal delivery of the term breech is considered to be an acceptable obstetrical choice under the following conditions (U. S. Dept. HHS, 1981):

1. Anticipated fetal weight of less than 8 pounds
2. Normal pelvic dimensions and architecture
3. Frank breech presentation without a hyperextended head
4. Delivery to be conducted by a physician experienced in vaginal breech delivery

In addition to following the steps described for increasing the likelihood of a vaginal delivery (discussed earlier), prenatal education about breech presentation may include these suggestions (Shearer, 1982b; Young & Mahan, 1980):

1. Discuss with your practitioner in advance: your desire and chances for vaginal birth; management of your labor and birth; risks of vaginal delivery to your baby and of cesarean delivery to you; trial of labor; use of postural exercise and external version, which might turn your baby.

2. If your practitioner routinely performs cesareans on all breeches or does not permit trial of labor or both, consider changing practitioners.
3. Have x-ray examination at labor onset and trial of labor.
4. Stay in bed if membranes rupture or with footling or full breech.
5. Use nonmedical and relaxation support measures (discussed earlier).
6. Be prepared for immediate cesarean.

Jordan, in an examination of external cephalic version for breech presentation, suggests that this procedure offers promise for transforming "some substantial proportion of the high-risk breech population into a low-risk cephalic population" (Jordan, 1983). It is important, therefore, that breech-presenting women discuss this option with their practitioner.

Multiple Pregnancy

Neonatal morbidity and mortality are higher for twins than they are for singleton babies, and the mortality appears to be higher for the second-born twin, especially when he or she is presenting as a breech (McCarthy et al., 1981). Lower birth weight among twins also increases the risk of neonatal death, and therefore special efforts must be made to enhance the likelihood of a term delivery. In an attempt to improve neonatal survival, cesarean delivery for multiple pregnancies has increased in recent years (U. S. Dept. HHS, 1981). In 1980, 32.8 percent of twin pregnancies were delivered by cesarean section (Taffel & Placek, 1983). Professional opinions differ on the appropriate management of multiple pregnancies, however, and Noble (1980) maintains that "Surgical delivery should be done only for special problems and not for multiple pregnancy itself."

The findings of McCarthy and colleagues (1981) do not support the contention that "a cesarean section will improve the neonatal survival rate of all twins" but there is "some evidence that cesarean sections will improve the survival rate of infants in breech presentations and other malpresentations (27 percent of all twins)."

In addition to following the steps for increasing the likelihood of a vaginal delivery (discussed earlier), prenatal education for the woman with a multiple pregnancy may include these suggestions:

1. Discuss with your practitioner: the possibilities for a vaginal birth; risks of vaginal birth to your babies and of cesarean birth to you; presentations of twins as determined by ultrasound examination and choices of labor and birth management for each twin; exercise and nutrition program and ways of reducing likelihood for premature birth.
2. If your obstetrician routinely performs a cesarean with all twin births, obtain a second opinion from an experienced obstetrician.
3. Maintain excellent nutrition, prenatal care, and sensible program of exercise, rest, and relaxation.
4. Request to begin labor spontaneously and have spontaneous delivery for *both* twins in absence of other complications.
5. Use nonmedical and relaxation support measures (discussed earlier).
6. If complications require anesthesia, regional anesthesia is preferable.
7. Be prepared for immediate cesarean section.

Elective Repeat Cesarean Birth

Repeat cesarean deliveries are the second most common reason for cesarean deliveries in the United States, according to the National Institute of Health Consensus Development Conference on *Cesarean Childbirth* (U. S. Dept. HHS, 1981). In 1980, more than 9 out of 10 women with a previous cesarean birth (96.6 percent) had a repeat cesarean procedure (Taffel & Placek, 1983). Most couples facing an elective repeat cesarean are unable to attain needed education about a cesarean birth with their first cesarean delivery because of the emergency nature of the situation. Couples anticipating the birth of their first child attend prenatal classes geared toward vaginal birth where little emphasis is placed upon complications that lead to cesarean deliveries. Even when exposed to information about cesarean birth, most couples choose to ignore this information, taking an "it can't happen to us" attitude. When facing an elective repeat cesarean birth, however, the opposite holds true. Couples need and seek information regarding events that take place during the preparation, delivery, and postpartum phases; types of anesthesias; sensations that may be experienced; and interaction with the newborn.

In the emergency atmosphere of their first birth experience, couples find that many questions are left unanswered due to the hurried nature of the delivery. This leads to fears and anxieties about the second birth. Cesarean birth classes are now offered in many parts of the country to help alleviate these fears and anxieties.

One such program was initiated in the 1970s by the Childbirth Education Association of Rochester, New York. Their consumer-oriented classes are entitled "Family-Centered Cesarean Birth." The following course outline for 4 classes of 2 hours each is used in their educational program. Each class consists of a lecture–discussion and an exercise portion as follows:

1. Introductions
   A. Instructor, assistants, couples
   B. Library (a lending library is available to couples)
   C. Handbook (*Family Centered Cesarean Birth*, a project by CEA of Rochester, 1985)
   D. Discussion of couples' previous cesarean delivery and current expectations or fears
   E. Goals:
      (1) Educational
      (2) Emotional
      (3) Physical conditioning
2. Anatomy and Physiology
   A. Reproductive organs and cesarean delivery diagrams (series of diagrams from Childbirth Graphics Ltd., Rochester, New York)
   B. Pelvic structures
   C. Tests to determine fetal maturity and health
      (1) Ultrasound
      (2) Amniocentesis, L/S ratio, and/or Pg test
      (3) Urinary estriol count
      (4) Nonstress test
      (5) Oxytocin challenge test
      (6) X-ray
3. Nutrition
4. Rationale for Cesarean Deliveries
   A. Safety
   B. Indications
   C. Emotional responses to unplanned cesareans

    D. Guidelines for discussion with obstetrician (Young & Mahan, 1980, p. 23):
       (1) Determine possibility of vaginal delivery.
       (2) Seek second opinion if warranted by your obstetrical status and practitioner's response to attempting vaginal delivery.
       (3) Attend cesarean or childbirth education classes.
       (4) Request to begin labor spontaneously to avoid premature birth.
       (5) Avoid surgical or medical induction of labor.
       (6) Discuss with your practitioner in advance: use, reliability, benefits, and risks of ultrasound and amniocentesis; benefits, risks, and types of incisions and anesthesia; family-centered cesarean birth.
       (7) Express desire for transverse uterine incision, Pfannenstiel skin incision, and conduction anesthesia, if possible.
       (8) Depending on responses to 6 and 7, consider changing practitioners.
       (9) Plan ahead for family-centered cesarean birth; have preferences written on your medical chart.
      (10) Discuss elective sterilization if you desire it after elective surgery.
  5. Hospital Admission for Cesarean Delivery
    A. Scheduling cesarean delivery
    B. Admission procedures
    C. Preoperative procedures
  6. Anesthesia
    A. General
    B. Spinal
    C. Epidural
    D. Cesarean delivery (slide series: *Family-Centered Cesarean Birth,* a project by CEA of Rochester, New York)
    E. Operating room
    F. Delivery
    G. Baby
    H. Recovery Room
  7. Postpartum Days
    A. Hospital
    B. At home
  8. Breast-feeding
  9. Parenting
    A. Adjustment to newborn
    B. Sibling concerns
    C. Emotions
    D. Paternal considerations
 10. Couples Presentation (couples returning from a previous class who have since delivered, discuss their labor and delivery experience)
 11. Exercises
    A. Posture and positioning
    B. Pelvic rock
    C. Touch relaxation
    D. Slow chest breathing
    E. Concentration–relaxation
    F. Kegels
    G. Abdominal tightening
    H. Arching position for spinal anesthesia

Throughout these classes, family-centered options for cesarean births are discussed. The primary goal is to make each individual birth experience one that is satisfying to each couple in the class. The following options are discussed in detail:

1. Father present at birth; in recovery room
2. Morning of surgery admission
3. Choice of anesthesia
4. Choice of incisions
5. Baby in recovery room; how soon can parents hold baby
6. Rooming-in
7. Minimal hospital stay
8. No preoperative tranquilizer
9. Insertion of Foley catheter after anesthesia given
10. Other arm free to touch baby after he or she is born
11. Anesthesia screen lowered at time of birth
12. Delivery room photography

One problem facing both childbirth educators and cesarean couples is the question of when these options may or may not be available. Many options that couples now request not only need the approval of the couple's practitioner but also the anesthesiologist assigned to their delivery. If it has been determined that a woman is physically and medically capable of beginning labor spontaneously and experiencing labor, only to have it end in another cesarean (which now becomes an emergency), she may find that the anesthesiologist on call will not allow her partner in the delivery room. She may also lose her choice of anesthesia, as well as many of the previously listed options. Therefore, in many parts of the United States, women who could be VBAC candidates are opting to be elective repeat cesarean candidates instead. By scheduling their surgery well in advance, they ensure for themselves the cooperation of the entire health care team in attaining the birth options they most desire.

For many of these women, having a family-centered cesarean birth experience is far more important than the possibility of delivering vaginally. Every woman who experiences labor ending in a cesarean delivery should have the right to the birth options she desires. The responsibility for resolving this conflict rests with the health professionals. The situation can only change as health professionals update hospital policies to meet changing consumer needs.

Cesarean Birth and Postpartum

The important needs, rights, and choices of families for whom a cesarean birth is necessary should be a major component of a prenatal education program for cesarean expectant parents. The humanistic, emotional, and social features that are integral to a program of family-centered maternity care should be available to all families anticipating a cesarean birth. No evidence of harm to mother, newborn, or father has been reported when family-centered care has been extended to the cesarean family (U. S. Dept. HHS, 1981).

The International Childbirth Education Association recommends that the following hospital options be available to cesarean families (ICEA Position Statement, 1980):

1. Family-centered cesarean childbirth in which cesarean mothers may share their labor, birth, and postpartum with their partner to enhance the emotional and social aspects of the experience.
2. Informed participation by expectant cesarean parents in decisions about preoperative sedation, anesthesia, incision, early breast-feeding, and early and extended parent–newborn contact.

3. Rooming-in for cesarean mothers and their babies, which provides the option for unrestricted access to the baby by the parents.
4. Twenty-four-hour visiting for the cesarean mother's partner and daily visiting on the postpartum floor for the other children in the family.
5. Participation by parents in the care of their newborn if he or she is premature or sick. If transport to a regional neonatal intensive care unit is necessary, transfer of the cesarean mother should occur as soon as possible.
6. Staffing patterns and protocols for cesarean mother–baby couples that provide supportive care and assistance and facilitate parent–baby interaction.

The presence of the cesarean mother's husband or partner at the birth is extremely important, as already mentioned. The Consensus Development Conference confirms that "The presence of fathers in the operating room and closer contact between mother and neonate appear to improve the postcesarean behavioral responses of the families" (U. S. Dept. HHS, 1981). Cesarean mothers experience more positive physical and emotional feelings if the father is present, and their perceptions of the birth are more satisfying (Gainer & VanBonn, 1977). In addition, fathers feel involved in the birth and a source of strength and emotional support to their wives/partners.

The family-centered program includes early contact between the cesarean parents and their newborn, and it is recommended that "the healthy neonate should not be separated routinely from mother and father following delivery" (U. S. Dept. HHS, 1981).

During their postpartum stay, the cesarean family should be offered the following options in the hospital (Young, 1982):

1. Extended parent–newborn contact and rooming-in.
2. Newborn admitted to the special care nursery only if required because of a medical problem.
3. Cesarean roommates in semiprivate rooms
4. Breast-feeding on demand.
5. Partner visitation on a 24-hour basis.
6. Daily sibling visitation of the postpartum floor.
7. Postpartum nursing support and comfort measures, education, and rehabilitation exercises.
8. Postbirth discussions with the birth practitioner concerning indications for cesarean birth, outlook for subsequent pregnancies, and family concerns.
9. Information about cesarean and breast-feeding support groups.
10. Home-help arrangements and follow-up, as necessary.
11. Early discharge, if appropriate.

It has been shown that when cesarean mothers received postpartum teaching about cesarean birth, uniformly and reliably positive effects on their physical and emotional responses to the birth were evident (Gainer & VanBonn, 1977). An important part of the postpartum program involves information about, and supervision of, special breathing, leg, abdominal, and rehabilitation exercises (Noble, 1982).

Several authors have described the value of cesarean support groups in helping cesarean mothers to share information, feelings, and concerns with peers and to resolve their experiences psychologically (Affonso, 1981; Lipson & Tilden, 1980; Young, 1982). Also incorporated in the cesarean support program should be a positive informational component about the prevention of unnecessary cesareans and the success and safety of vaginal birth after a previous cesarean birth (Cohen & Estner, 1983).

EDUCATIONAL PROCESS

Throughout this chapter, recommendations have been made to have the woman and her partner involved with their care provider in decisions about the cesarean birth experience and to challenge traditional, nonacceptable interventions. Even the decision to select the right physician or nurse midwife is important. These recommendations require expecting couples to feel in control, confident of their knowledge, and convinced that they can make good decisions regarding their care. Adult educational approaches have been recommended to assist learners to develop these characteristics. Thus if the overall goals of informed choice for a positive experience are to be met, the educational program must be designed toward this end.

The dilemma of whether to teach about all potential complications or limit information about complications could be resolved by enabling couples or groups to determine for themselves whether they wish to learn about all potential problems, some selected problems they are worried about, or few problems. Recognizing the ability of adults to determine what they need to know is important. An evaluation of whether parents make good decisions concerning what they need to know could be undertaken. Comparisons of couples who are taught about complications and those who are not could be made as to degree of anxiety, actual development of complications, and satisfaction with the birth experience.

Because vaginal birth after cesarean section requires decision making, it is important to discuss the decision-making process and how couples can use it to assist them in deciding whether vaginal delivery is a valid option in their situation.

THE HEALTH PROFESSIONAL AND THE CESAREAN FAMILY

It is clear that a cesarean birth has a profound physiological and psychological impact on a woman. The negative effects of the event, however, can be significantly alleviated with sensitive and supportive care from all hospital personnel who come in contact with the cesarean family.

Health care professionals need to critically examine the policies and the protocols in their institutions and determine whether the essential elements of family-centered maternity care are available to cesarean families. If they are not, immediate steps should be taken to implement a program for cesarean families that emphasizes parent participation in decision making about the labor and birth and family togetherness (Young, 1982). As Enkin (1977) points out, "Having a section is having a baby," and therefore, medical and nursing staff must find creative ways to enhance the emotional aspects of the birth. Every effort should be made to meet the expectations of the parents, irrespective of the manner of birth.

During the birth itself, a nurse, an anesthesiologist, or a monitrice can give a "running commentary" to allay fears and explain to the parents events as they occur (Cohen, 1977). Efforts should be made to maintain human contact and continuity. In the recovery area, simple explanations, information about the baby, and orientation as to time, place, and person will help to decrease distorted perceptions (Affonso & Stichler, 1980), and encouragement of parent–newborn interaction will enhance the initiation of family relationships (Enkin, 1977; Young, 1982).

During the postpartum hospital stay, the cesarean mother will experience major physical problems and pain as well as strong emotional reactions. Therefore, attention must be given to meeting both physical and psychological needs of the family. Especially important are physical comfort measures; reassuring explanations about procedures and care; listening to the parents' concerns; encouraging the father's involvement; promoting parent–infant bonding; supporting and advising the breast-feeding mother; and finding ways to help parents clarify, integrate, and understand the cesarean birth.

In addition to providing cesarean education programs for parents, there is a need for better preparation and training for nursing staff and other health care providers to enable them to better meet the needs of cesarean families (U. S. Dept., HHS, 1981). Sensitivity by health providers to the special needs of these parents and the implementation of family-centered practices and policies will go a long way toward increasing parental satisfaction about the birth and reinforcing the relationships of the cesarean family.

RESOURCES

Audiovisual Aids

Cesarean birth sequence and cesarean postpartum: 6 color illustrations ($20.00), 24 color slides ($24.00). *(From Childbirth Graphics Ltd., address below.)*

Cesarean childbirth, Cesarean birth incisions, Indications for cesarean, Reducing your chances for a cesarean birth, Vaginal birth after cesarean. *(These are available as a color illustration ($3.75 each) and slide ($2.00 each) from Childbirth Graphics Ltd., address below.)*

The cesarean birth experience (movie). *(25 min; 3-day rental $45.00; 16 mm, Super 8, or videotape From Parenting Pictures, 121 N.W. Crystal St., Crystal River, FL 32629.)*

Cesarean childbirth (movie). *(18 min. From Cinema Medica, 2335 W. Foster Ave., Chicago, IL 60625.)*

Cesarean bonding experience (80 slides/40 slides). *(From Tri-County Cesarean Parents Association, 1 St. James Road, Budd Lake, NY 07828.)*

Having a section is having a baby (138 slides, 30 min cassette). *(From Polymorph Films, 118 South Street, Boston, MA 02111.)*

Catalogs of Educational Books and Supplies

Childbirth Graphics Ltd., P.O. Box 17025 Irondequoit Div. 25, Rochester, NY 14671–0325. *Send for free catalog of excellent audiovisual and teaching aids.)*

Birth and Life Bookstore, P.O. Box 70625, Seattle, WA 98107. *(Send for free catalog of childbirth and parenting publications.)*

ICEA Bookcenter, P.O. Box 20048, Minneapolis, MN 55420. *Send for free catalog of ICEA publications and wide selection of childbirth and parenting publications.)*

The whole birth catalog: A source book for choice in childbirth, J. I. Ashford (Ed.). The Crossing Press, P.O. Box 640, Trumansburg, NY 14886. *(An encyclopedia and valuable resource and reference catalog of information about childbirth, including book reviews and descriptions of resources and organizations. Cost, $14.95, paperback.)*

Reading

Frankly speaking (rev. ed.). Framingham, Mass.: C/SEC, 1984.

Meyer, L. D. *The cesarean (r)evolution.* Edmonds, Wash.: Chas. Franklin Press, 1981.

Paul, R. H. (Ed.). Pregnancy management after prior cesarean section: An invitational symposium. *Journal of Reproductive Medicine,* 1984, 29(1), 1–44.

Royall, N. *You don't have to have a repeat cesarean.* New York: Frederick Fell, 1983.

Shearer, B. *Preventing unnecessary cesareans: A guide to labor management and detailed bibliography*. Framingham, Mass.: C/SEC, 1982.

Reading for Children

Allison, E. S. *Daniel's question: A cesarean birth story*. Willow Tree Press, 124 Willow Tree Road, Monsey, NY 10952, 1982. ($2.95 plus $1.00 postage.)
Baker, G. C., & Montey, V. M. *Special delivery: A book for kids about cesarean and vaginal birth*. Chas. Franklin Press, 18409 90th Ave., W. Edmonds, WA 98020, 1981. ($6.70 prepaid).

Resource Organizations

American Academy of Husband-Coached Childbirth, Box 5224, Sherman Oaks, CA 91413.
American Society for Psychoprophylaxis in Obstetrics (ASPO), 1411 K Steet, N.W., Washington, DC 20005.
Cesarean Birth Alliance, 39 Denton Avenue, East Rockway, NY 11518.
Cesarean Prevention Movement, Inc. (CPM), Box 152, Syracuse, NY 13210.
Council for Cesarean Awareness, 5520 S.W. 92nd Avenue, Miami, FL 33165.
Cesarean/Support, Education and Concern, Inc. (C/SEC, Inc.), 22 Forest Road, Framingham, MA 01701.
International Childbirth Education Association (ICEA), Box 20048, Minneapolis, MN 55420.
La Leche League International, 9615 Minneapolis Avenue, Franklin Park, IL 60131.
National Association of Parents and Professionals for Safe Alternatives in Childbirth (NAPSAC), Box 267, Marble Hill, MO 63764.

REFERENCES

Affonso, D. *Impact of cesarean childbirth*. Philadelphia: F. A. Davis, 1981.
Affonso, D., & Stichler, J. F. Cesarean birth: Women's reactions. *American Journal of Nursing*, 1980, *80*(3), 468–470.
American College of Obstetricians and Gynecologists. *Guidelines for vaginal delivery after a cesarean childbirth*. Washington, D.C.: ACOG, January 7, 1982.
American College of Obstetricians and Gynecologists. *Dystocia: Etiology, diagnosis, and management guidelines*. Washington, D.C.: ACOG, July, 1982.
Childbirth Education Association of Rochester. *Family-centered cesarean birth (rev. ed.)*. Rochester, N.Y.: Childbirth Education Association of Rochester, 1985.
Cohen, N. W. Minimizing the emotional sequelae of cesarean childbirth. *Birth and Family Journal*, 1977, *4*, 114–119.
Cohen, N. W., & Estner, L. J. *Silent knife: Cesarean prevention and vaginal birth after cesarean*. South Hadley, Mass.: Bergin & Garvey, 1983.
Conner, E. L. Teaching about cesarean birth in traditional childbirth classes. *Birth and Family Journal*, 1977, *4*, 107–113.
Dilts, P. V. How can we decrease the incidence of cesarean section? *Contemporary Obstetrics and Gynecology*, 1981, *18*, 19–28.
Enkin, M. W. Having a section is having a baby. *Birth and Family Journal*, 1977, *4*, 99–102.
Gainer, M., & VanBonn, P. *Two factors affecting the cesarean delivered mother: Father's presence at the delivery and postpartum teaching*. Ann Arbor: University of Michigan Press, 1977.
Harrison, M. *A woman in residence*. New York: Random House, 1982.
ICEA Position Paper on planning comprehensive maternal and newborn services for the childbearing year. Minneapolis: International Childbirth Education Association, 1979.
ICEA Position Statement: Cesarean birth. *ICEA News*, 1980, *19*, 4–5.

ICEA teacher certification philosophy. Minneapolis: International Childbirth Education Association, 1979.

Jordan, B. External cephalic version. In D. Young (Ed.), *Obstetrical intervention and technology in the 1980's*. New York: The Haworth Press, 1983.

Keolker, K. *Vaginal birth after cesarean*. Seattle: The Pennypress, 1981.

Lavin, J. P., Stephens, R. J., Miodovnik, M., & Barden, T. P. Vaginal delivery in patients with a prior cesarean section. *Obstetrics and Gynecology*, 1982, *59*(2), 135–148.

Lipson, J. G., & Tilden, V. P. Psychological integration of the cesarean birth experience. *American Journal of Orthopsychiatry*, 1980, *50*(4), 598–609.

Marieskind, H. I. *An evaluation of caesarean section in the United States*. Office of the Assistant Secretary for Planning and Evaluation of Health, Washington, D.C.: U.S. Government Printing Office, June 1979.

Marut, J., & Mercer, R. A comparison of primipara's perception of vaginal and cesarean births. *Nursing Research*, 1979, *28*(5), 260–269.

McCarthy, B. J., Sachs, B. P., Layde, P. M., Burton, A., Jerry, J. S., & Rochat, R. The epidemiology of neonatal death in twins. *American Journal of Obstetrics and Gynecology*, 1981, *141*(3), 252–256.

Noble, E. *Having twins*. Boston: Houghton Mifflin, 1980.

Noble, E. *Essential exercises for the childbearing years* (2nd ed.). Boston: Houghton Mifflin, 1982.

Norwood, C. *How to avoid a cesarean section*. New York: Simon and Schuster, 1984.

Nurses Association of the American College of Obstetricians and Gynecologists. *Guidelines for childbirth education*. Chicago: NAACOG, 1981.

Nurses Association of the American College of Obstetricians and Gynecologists. *Standards for obstetric, gynecologic, and neonatal nursing* (2nd ed.). Washington, D.C.: NAACOG, 1981.

O'Driscoll, K., & Foley, M. Correlation of decrease in perinatal mortality and increase in cesarean section rates. *Obstetrics and Gynecology*, 1983, *61*, 1–5.

O'Sullivan, M. J., Fumia, F., Holsinger, K., & McLeod, A. G. Vaginal delivery after cesarean section. *Clinics in Perinatology*, 1981, *8*(1), 131–143.

Peterson, G. H. *Birthing normally: A personal growth approach to childbirth*. Berkeley, Calif.: Mindbody Press, 1981.

Placek, P. J., & Taffel, S. M. Trends in cesarean section rates for the United States, 1970–1978. *Public Health Reports*, 1980, *95*, 540–548.

Placek, P. J., Taffel, S. M., & Moien, M. Cesarean section delivery rates: United States, 1981. *American Journal of Public Health*, 1983, *73*(8), 861–862.

Placek, P. J., Taffel, S. M., & Keppel, K. G. Maternal and infant characteristics associated with cesarean section delivery. In *Health: United States, 1983*. Hyattsville, Md.: U. S. Department of Health and Human Services, December 1983.

The pregnant patient's bill of rights, The pregnant patient's responsibilities. Prepared by Doris Haire and members of ICEA. Minneapolis: International Childbirth Education Association, 1977.

Quilligan, E. J. Making inroads against the C-section rate. *Contemporary Obstetics and Gynecology*, 1983, *22*(1), 221–225.

Rubin, G., McCarthy, B. M., Shelton, J., Rochat, B. W., & Terry, J. The risk of childbearing re-evaluated. *American Journal of Public Health*, 1981, *71*, 712–716.

Shearer, E. L. Education for vaginal birth after cesarean. *Birth*, 1982a, *9*, 31–34.

Shearer, E. L. Preventing unnecessary cesareans. Framingham, Mass.: C/SEC, Inc., 1982b.

Shulman, N. Labor and vaginal delivery after cesarean birth: A survey of contemporary opinion. In A. F. Cane & E. L. Shearer (Eds.), *Frankly speaking* (2nd ed.). Waltham, Mass: C/SEC., Inc., 1978.

Taffel, S. M., & Placek, P. J. Complications in cesarean and noncesarean deliveries: United States, 1980. *American Journal of Public Health*, 1983, *73*(8), 856–860.

United States Department of Health and Human Services. *Cesarean childbirth: Consensus development conference* (NIH Publication No. 82–2067). Washington, D.C.: National Institute of Health, October 1981.

Williams, R. L., & Chen, P. M. Identifying the sources of the recent decline in perinatal mortality rates in California. *New England Journal of Medicine*, 1982, *306*, 207–214.

Young, D. *Changing childbirth: Family birth in the hospital*. Rochester, N.Y.: Childbirth Graphics Ltd., 1982, chs. 14, 22.

Young, D., & Mahan, C. *Unnecessary cesareans. Ways to avoid them*. Minneapolis: International Childbirth Education Association, 1980.

Education When Pregnancy Is at Risk: The Woman Who Is Pregnant and Diabetic

19

Patricia M. Allen and Phyllis Sale

The high-risk pregnant client brings special challenges to the health care provider. The goal of assisting the client to enjoy the pregnancy and understand the numerous changes and preparations necessary is made more difficult because of the reality of a possible poor outcome and the added information a medical condition warrants. The health care provider must be friend, teacher, and counselor, as well as care provider. To meet the demands of each of these roles, the health care provider must have an in-depth knowledge of the pathophysiology of the medical problem, its course in pregnancy, the ability to interpret this information at a level appropriate for the client, and the technical skills necessary to care and teach the medically complicated obstetrical client. It is also important to remember the "normal" aspects of pregnancy because these aspects may get neglected for the high-risk client. Care providers have been accused of concentrating on the risks of pregnancy and excluding the overall aspects of childbearing (Snyder, 1979).

Caring for the pregnant diabetic may present a special challenge, because providing adequate and complete education for the pregnant diabetic is complex. Because of the necessity to maintain rigid blood glucose control for women who are diabetic and pregnant, they are often hospitalized on one or more occasions in the antepartum period. These admissions interrupt the teaching process in the ambulatory setting. There is rarely any mechanism designed for communicating information between the inpatient and the outpatient facilities and care providers. Continuity in the teaching–learning process is critical for the woman who is diabetic.

In addition, the treatment of diabetes has changed dramatically in recent years. With the availability of insulin, problems associated with diabetes in the female client improved; amenorrhea disappeared, fertility increased, and pregnancy became a possibility for more diabetic women. As a result, today, diabetes has gradually become a common complication of pregnancy. As more diabetic women experienced pregnancy, more was learned about medical management. As new information and improved technology became available medical management changed, frequently before changes were made known to care providers through published literature. Such rapid changes in the medical management of pregnant diabetic women require written protocols to be available to practicing physicians, nurses, and others who must teach clients and coordinate care between tertiary centers and primary physicians.

During the 1970s biophysical and biochemical monitoring became a routine part of "high-risk obstetrical" management. Ultrasound evaluation to confirm dating, evaluate fetal growth, predict macrosomia, and diagnose polyhydramnios has become a routine management protocol for managing the pregnancy of the diabetic. Urinary or serum estriol evaluation, maternal blood studies, and amniocentesis are additional examples of biochemical monitoring that provide information about the fetoplacental unit. Electronic fetal monitoring has also made possible early assessment of and intervention for fetal distress. These diagnostic evaluations require client cooperation and understanding, and confront the client and care provider with the reality of the status of the fetus. Pregnant, diabetic women need special assistance in understanding the rationale for these tests. They also need assistance in interpreting the results of these numerous tests. Such explanations place added responsibilities for education on care providers.

Consumer awareness including attitudes toward the delivery of health care has also changed drastically since the end of World War II. Butnarescu (1978, p. 246) describes three outcomes of this increased awareness: (1) "increased consumer interest in reproductive health care services, (2) emergence of preparation for childbirth programs, and (3) need for pre- and postconception sexual family life education and reproductive health maintenance programs." The women's movement has also supported women in their request for more information about health care.

Physicians now recommend preconceptual counseling for the overt diabetic. Because the outcome of diabetic pregnancies is directly related to the degree of control (Karlsson & Kjellmer, 1972), some authorities feel that it is desirable to achieve optimal control during the time a woman plans to conceive. This requires educational programs for women who are *contemplating* a pregnancy, not just those who *are* pregnant. For the overt diabetic whose pregnancy may be the fulfillment of a lifelong dream, it is imperative that she is given adequate information to be compliant with medical protocols. The gestational diabetic who unexpectedly finds herself in a "high-risk" pregnancy also deserves the opportunity to progress through pregnancy in as "normal" a manner as possible. This patient too needs the right "dosage" of education.

Regionalization of perinatal care is recommended for the gravid patient at risk. Because individual experience and expertise in the management of diabetic clients is limited, other than in perinatal centers, it is desirable to have these clients referred to a tertiary level institution for care and/or consultation. This fact frequently increases the number of individuals who provide care and education. It also necessitates agreement about what information is given and who gives it. Perinatal nurses, dieticians, physicians, social workers, laboratory personnel, community health nurses, and childbirth educators may all have a major role in educating and supporting the woman whose pregnancy is complicated by diabetes. Thus, communication between and among team members is vital to the productivity and effectiveness of the team, as is mutual respect for and understanding of individual roles within the team. This is best facilitated when there is agreement about what information is to be taught and how diabetes will be managed. If guidelines for teaching and management are in writing and available to all care providers, confusion for the client will be minimized. Another approach to facilitate coordination of care is to have one member of the team responsible for coordinating client care and education. In many centers, it is the perinatal nurse specialist who functions in this capacity.

Health care professionals in a perinatal center decided to propose a solution to this complex teaching problem for pregnant diabetic clients. Because no protocol for diabetic teaching existed, the initial undertaking was the development of teaching objectives, guidelines, and a form to facilitate routine recording of antepartum and postpartum teaching. This "tool" was patterned after the tool described in Chapter 12 and Appendix A. This chapter describes the tool designed to guide professionals in their teaching of the pregnant woman who is either an overt or gestational diabetic.

Assessment of Learning Needs

The Overt Diabetic. In the opinion of the authors, there does not appear to be any correlation between age of onset, length of time the patient has had diabetes, and her understanding of the disease process. With some overt diabetics, it is necessary to begin with basic information regarding the pathophysiology of diabetes and progress to the interaction of diabetes and pregnancy. Others will be extremely knowledgeable about their disease and its control and will be eager to have all available information about how pregnancy impacts their diabetes. For the overt pregnant diabetic, pregnancy may be the culmination of a dream fulfilled or just another problem compounding an already unacceptable situation. If an overt diabetic has never come to terms with her diabetes, pregnancy may or may not be the time she will. If the client has not accepted her diabetes, she is not apt to follow suggestions for maintaining diabetic control, presenting a challenge to the entire perinatal team. If the overt diabetic has been an active participant in her care prior to conception, and has been able to maintain diabetic control, pregnancy may create an emotionally charged situation for her. Insulin requirements vary from trimester to trimester, activity states may be altered, dietary needs may change, and frequent prenatal visits to the doctor along with the never-ending battery of tests of fetal well-being and tight diabetic control are required. The pregnant diabetic may have at least one and probably more hospital admissions in the antepartum period to establish diabetic control. Many adjustments to her life may be required. This frequently impacts the family as well.

Using White's (1978b) classification of diabetes it is possible to anticipate with some degree of accuracy pregnancy outcome. This is important information that should be given to the client early in pregnancy so that she will have an overview of what she can expect and what will be required of her. She must have the understanding that classification can change during pregnancy, requiring alternative management.

The client's financial and cultural status can impact her acceptance of diabetes and its treatment. The cost of a high-risk pregnancy can be excessive and nonreimbursable by third party payors. For the client with limited financial resources, the necessity of having to pay for numerous diagnostic tests or the need for repeated hospitalizations may create a problematic situation. In some cultures, childbearing is considered a natural function that does not require much medical intervention. It is indeed a challenge to convince clients who view pregnancy as normal to follow a strict medical regimen.

The Gestational Diabetic. The gestational diabetic also presents a challenge to the health care team. According to White's (1978b) classification, the gestational diabetic is one who has an abnormal glucose tolerance test but a normal fasting blood sugar during pregnancy and requires dietary or insulin management.

The need to identify the gestational diabetic has been well documented. In a study by Coustan and Lewis (1978), perinatal mortality among gestational diabetics treated as routine gravidas was between 4.9 and 19.8 percent, whereas it was between 0 and 6.4 percent in those patients treated as patients at risk (Coustan & Lewis, 1978). O'Sullivan also stresses the importance of managing the gestational diabetic in the high-risk environment (Felig, 1976). Once the gestational diabetic has been identified, she must be followed closely with fasting blood sugars and 2-hour postprandial blood tests because classification of diabetes may change during pregnancy and also in subsequent pregnancies. The life experience of the gestational diabetic greatly influences her reaction to diagnosis. If she has known diabetics who have had poor reproductive outcomes, she will be certain that hers will be equally as poor; if she has had negative information about insulin-dependent diabetics, she will react negatively or she may have virtually no information regarding diabetes and initially blame herself for causing her diabetic state. The approach of the team member giving the client the initial information relative to diagnosis is crucial. It must be a positive approach in an atmosphere of trust and caring where the client is encouraged to verbalize her concerns and feels comfortable in asking questions. The teaching–learning process will be enhanced and the client will be more motivated to take an active role in controlling her diabetes in this type of environment.

Teaching Tool Topics

The teaching guidelines and objectives are organized around selected topics (see Appendix B). The bibliography contains references to use with the guidelines. Instructions as to the use of the guidelines and the form for recording teaching–learning are included in Appendix B. Each topic is taught after an individual woman's needs are assessed. The exact amount of content taught varies depending on the woman's interest and needs and the preference of the care provider. Not all clients need, want, or can comprehend all the information presented in the guidelines. The health care provider needs to make a clinical and educational judgment as to what is critical for each woman. What is critical for each woman may vary due to the frequency of prenatal visits, the availability of health care providers to answer questions and monitor diabetic control, and the progress of pregnancy. The guidelines are complete; the actual objectives and content used need to be selected and planned for the specific situation. The next section provides suggestions concerning selected topics and the needs of pregnant diabetics.

General Information About Diabetes. To initiate teaching, the client's understanding of diabetes needs to be determined. If she has the basic information included in the first section of the guidelines (definition of diabetes, function of pancreas and insulin), it would be appropriate to omit what is known and proceed to other areas of instruction that either the health care provider or the client deems a priority. Most diabetic women need to understand the impact pregnancy has on their diabetic condition. There could be misinformation present, resulting in unnecessary fears. The guidelines were developed so that specific information could be given to the client at an appropriate time in her gestation. Thus the woman needing all the information about diabetes and the impact of pregnancy on diabetes would not be overwhelmed at any given time in pregnancy.

Predisposing Factors. The main predisposing factors to diabetes—pregnancy, heredity, and obesity—can be discussed if the client needs a clearer understanding of why she may have developed diabetes. A table describing the probability of developing diabetes is available in the guidelines to assist the health care provider in explaining the reasons and the probability of her offspring being affected. This is critical content for the client.

The guidelines describe the pathophysiology of diabetes in pregnancy. The health care provider needs a thorough understanding of this material; however, such specific information may not be needed by the client. Therefore, the objectives do not require the client to demonstrate her knowledge of this area. Some women may want more detail and a comprehensive understanding. This detail can then be provided.

Metabolism in Diabetes Mellitus. The diabetic woman may not fully comprehend how diabetes affects the metabolism of protein, fat, and carbohydrates. Having this information may allow the client to comprehend the consequences of having too much or too little insulin. By developing this information gradually, learning will be more effective because one learns better when a specific pattern is presented (Mort & Vincent, 1954). Factors that aggravate diabetes should be mentioned and the client cautioned to notify her care provider if complications occur.

Course of Diabetes in Pregnancy. Because insulin requirements vary in each trimester, the gravid diabetic must be prepared to accept the inevitable changes in treatment during the course of pregnancy. Knowing that insulin requirements vary in pregnancy will decrease the client's anxiety level. If the woman was informed that she was not responsible for these changes, guilt feelings will be minimized.

Because a diabetic pregnancy can be complicated by several problems, the client should be aware of symptoms that should be reported immediately to her care provider. This awareness will hopefully allow her to detect problems at an early stage and prepare her to cope with the additional stress created by the complications (Snyder, 1979).

Throughout the teaching guidelines, the health care provider is frequently reminded of the necessity of discussing the client's concerns and feelings about diabetes and pregnancy. This is extremely important because the high-risk mother is not only working through the normal tasks of pregnancy, but is also concerned with accepting herself as a high-risk mother. Included in this acceptance is the concern for her ability to maintain the pregnancy and the possibility of never being able to have another child (Galloway, 1976). The client does not look or feel sick; therefore it may be difficult for her to accept the restrictions of being a high-risk mother. This may interfere with her compliance (Galloway, 1976). The health care provider should encourage her client to express concerns. This will require an open, trusting relationship between client and care provider. It is also important that continuity of care be established so that concerns can be adequately dealt with throughout the pregnancy, the delivery, and the postpartum period.

Diet. Nutritional management is a major component of the pregnant diabetic's treatment plan. Her dietary habits and compliance can directly affect the course of the diabetes, as well as the outcome of the pregnancy. Although the dietician may assume primary responsibility for initial dietary instruction, other health care providers may contribute to learning about diet. The nurse's role will likely be one of coordinator of learning needs, assessor of patient understanding, and facilitator in making referrals to the community health nurse for home instruction and evaluation.

As in any pregnancy, weight gain must be monitored closely. If it is excessive or insufficient, or if a loss is noted, client and health care provider must work cooperatively to determine the cause. The public health nurse is a valuable resource to closely monitor the client's and the family's dietary habits and offer solutions that may be acceptable to the client. If the public health nurse and the dietician have copies of the teaching tool guidelines, the coordination and efficiency of teaching can be enhanced.

Effects of Diabetes on the Fetus. One of the major goals of the pregnant woman is to secure the safe passage of her infant (Galloway, 1976). She questions whether the baby will be normal and if not, will it be accepted by others. Therefore, it is extremely important that the diabetic client be aware of how diabetes may affect her fetus. When discussing this material it is important to create opportunities for the pregnant woman and significant other to verbalize their concerns.

Many tests are routinely performed to assess the well-being of the diabetic's fetus. The health care provider needs to stress: (1) the routine nature of the tests, (2) the preparation for the tests, and (3) what these tests tell her about her baby. The pregnant diabetic needs also to be aware of the possibility of an early delivery.

In many institutions the infant of the class B or greater diabetic is admitted to the special care nursery. To help the pregnant diabetic and her significant other better prepare for this experience a tour of the nursery should be offered prenatally.

Other Topics

Activity Levels. Although it is important for all pregnant women to maintain their normal activity state, it is of utmost importance for the diabetic who is pregnant. Activity levels directly influence insulin requirements, and therefore every effort must be made to provide consistent activity.

Insulin Injection Technique. Frequently, one of the most difficult tasks for the gestational diabetic to learn is to give self-injections. For the overt diabetic who has been insulin-dependent, there may be a change in requirements necessitating new learning. Because these are anxiety-provoking experiences, one must incorporate principles of learning when teaching this information. It is helpful to use a problem-solving approach: "What do you think would happen if you did not get all of the air bubbles out of the syringe?" For continuity, it is important to record the technique for insulin administration as taught to the client. The nurse must also address the special needs of the client, i.e., illiteracy, minimal level of reading and/or comprehension, visual impairment, or a physical handicap that may influence insulin administration.

Blood Glucose Monitoring and Urine Testing. Until recently the accepted method of monitoring glucose metabolism at home in the pregnant diabetic was by testing the urine for presence of glucose and ketones. This method provides only a rough guide to diabetic control. Pregnancy causes a rise in the glomerular filtration rate in the kidneys, and also causes a decreased tubular glucose reabsorption. Because of this the client may have glycosuria even though her blood glucose levels are normal. With the availability of chemical reagent strips for self-monitoring of blood glucose it is now possible to teach clients to perform this simple blood test at home.

Testing for Fetal Well-being. Assessment of fetal well-being is of prime importance throughout a diabetic pregnancy, and especially in the third trimester when it is important to determine the timing and mode of delivery. As stated earlier it is necessary for her to have a thorough understanding of each procedure, what is expected of her, why it is necessary, and what the implications are.

Written instructions for each of these tests are extremely helpful. After instruction, the patient should be given written guidelines as a reference for home use (see sample pamphlets in Appendix B). This practice is reassuring to the client and has helped to prevent problems associated with being improperly prepared for a given procedure.

Intrapartum. Clients also need to be prepared for the planned mode of delivery as well as an alternate mode. They are strongly encouraged to attend prenatal classes, especially designed for high-risk patients to prepare them for their labor and delivery experience.

This affords the pregnant diabetic an opportunity to discuss her problems with other mothers at risk in a positive setting, guided by the perinatal educator.

Labor, as any other form of intensive exercise, increases the energy needs of the body, thus increasing glucose requirements. This needs to be discussed with the client, assuring her that her insulin and glucose will be closely monitored throughout labor and delivery, and how that will be accomplished. She also needs to be aware that the fetus will be monitored during labor. Because she will be familiar with the fetal monitor from her repeated nonstress or contraction stress tests, this should not add to her anxiety during labor.

Postpartum Newborn. A thorough review of the diabetic's previous obstetrical history will provide a beginning data base upon which to develop teaching relative to the newborn. Included in the guidelines is a discussion of neonatal glucose metabolism. The pregnant diabetic will already be familiar with the terminology, which should facilitate her understanding of the need to monitor glucose levels in her infant.

Hopefully the diabetic mother will be familiar with the neonatal special care setting prior to delivery. She may, however, need encouragement to visit her infant, and needs information on the importance of doing so during her hospitalization as well as postdischarge. Special efforts to provide education for mothers who are discharged before their infants or without their infants is needed. This can be an important time for learning infant care.

Postpartum Maternal. Within 24 to 48 hours postdelivery, maternal insulin requirements diminish. The client needs to understand why this occurs and how it will be assessed and how it will change over the next few weeks.

Breast-feeding is encouraged for all women, including the diabetic, in many institutions. If the diabetic client chooses to breast-feed her newborn, she will need to be aware of the alteration in insulin and dietary needs during lactation, as well as information specific to breast-feeding required by all new mothers. Routine postpartum teaching, i.e., episiotomy care and danger signs, will also be needed.

Discussion of family planning should be initiated prior to delivery and continued in the postpartum period. The client needs to comprehend how specific factors impact her decision regarding contraceptive choice. For instance, her diabetic classification, her parity, her age, her proximity to a perinatal center, and the possible stresses involved in future pregnancies need to be discussed. It is helpful to the client if her partner can be included in these discussions to enable them to make a mutually acceptable decision.

Prior to discharge, the diabetic client should be given information relative to community resources. The guidelines list these resources. Local sources need to be added if the guidelines are adopted in other locales.

Method of Education

Throughout the guidelines, reference is made to several teaching aids used to facilitate the client's understanding of diabetes and pregnancy. The client is encouraged to use her senses of hearing and seeing while actually doing the task to be learned. Individuals learn more effectively if their learning is reinforced by the use of two or more senses (Mort & Vincent, 1954). Because learning is more effective when planned sequentially and not fragmented (Mort & Vincent, 1954), the guidelines are structured in that manner.

Also, when learning a new topic, learning takes place where the learner is and not from an imaginary starting point (Mort & Vincent, 1954). The learner can set her own pace of learning most information. The only area the health care provider must emphasize is the learning of critical content necessary for survival and to assure safety for the fetus. It is in these critical content areas that a more direct, pedagogical approach is needed.

When planning the teaching orientation, the current life experience of the client is important. Pregnant diabetics have to be extremely involved in their care. Use of adult learning strategies that respect the knowledge and experience of the learner seems especially relevant because many women have managed their diabetes for years. They may have insights and knowledge to share with the care provider.

Legitimate concerns and anxiety may prevent new learning; thus timing and reinforcement may become important. Asking the client about her comfort level and amount of knowledge needed is essential with these clients (see Chapter 3 for more details).

There is no problem in perinatal care in which the client requires the in-depth education to actively participate in self-management as pregnancy complicated by diabetes. If the client is highly motivated and eager to carry the pregnancy in spite of the demands it will place upon her, she will be anxious to learn all there is to know. In this situation an andragogical approach will be effective. However, the care provider must be cautious not to assume that every diabetic client is eager to learn. She may want the pregnancy but because of information previously learned about the chronic illness, may be fearful of her ability to have a healthy baby and remain healthy herself. This increased anxiety may cause her to be noncompliant with her care. It has been the authors' experience that pregnancy often reawakens unresolved anger in women with juvenile onset diabetes. For some, the restrictions of pregnancy and their attitude toward health care providers imposing those restrictions represent the same dilemma, confusion, and frustration as experienced at the time of the original diagnosis of diabetes mellitus. It may be helpful to involve this type of client in a group where she can share her feelings, frustrations, and fears with others who have similar experiences (Littlefield & Siebert, 1978). This can be very reassuring to the juvenile onset diabetic who must "relearn" control of her chronic illness because of the influence pregnancy has on diabetes. It was helpful to diabetic women contemplating pregnancy to join a group of women who were diabetic and pregnant (Littlefield & Siebert, 1978). Thus, recognizing that the stresses and strains of pregnancy can be confronted, the information about pregnancy's impact on diabetes and current medical management for mother and newborn can be discussed. This alleviates some anxiety and allows the pregnant woman to make a decision for or against being pregnant. Also the recently diagnosed diabetic may benefit from a discussion group because she must not only incorporate her pregnant self into her body image but also come to terms with an illness that may compromise her fetus and create an additional stress during pregnancy.

The client who appears resistant to recommendations of the health care team, refuses to become involved in self-management, and interferes with the teaching–learning process may be labeled as noncompliant. Her behavior may in fact be due to religious or cultural beliefs about illness and the positive or negative force they have on her life. For example, the client who views illness as a punishment for previous behavior may think she deserves the diabetes and should not do anything to interfere with the process of diabetic control through insulin and dietary management. The reverse may also be true. If the clients' life has markedly improved and this is attributed to her religious belief, she may feel that no other intervention is necessary to control illness or evil in her life. The health care provider will accomplish very little by demanding that the client perform certain tasks. If anything, such behavior would only serve to foster noncompliance in that type of patient. It would be far more effective to find out the client's reasons for not becoming involved in her care or doing various activities that allow diabetic control. Once reasons are identified, then together the care provider and the client can set mutual goals and expectations. Utilizing the client's strengths, previous positive experiences, and accomplishments as a basis for intervention will make the client feel more in control. The health care provider may need to accept the client's standards and goals. These may not be the ideal health standards and goals the health provider would wish, but they may allow the client to maintain her diabetes in enough control to not compromise the fetus. Clients may have alternate strategies to accomplish goals, especially those they have identified or agreed upon. Writing a contract offering "benefits" of the client's choice may be helpful (Steckel & Swain, 1977).

Evaluation of Client-centered Objectives. The major premise upon which these guidelines and objectives were written is that effective control of diabetes occurs most often in an informed client (Tribble & Hollenberg, 1977). Evaluation of the learning is facilitated because the objectives are client-centered and behavioral. Evaluation can be accomplished by asking the learner to restate what was taught, e.g., "What would be the signs you would notice if you were going into ketoacidosis?" A return demonstration of skills is also effective in evaluating learning. Another method of evaluation is to note how the client is adhering to her regimen by monitoring weight, blood sugar levels, and her compliance in reporting to her care provider when instructed to do so.

The effectiveness of the diabetic teaching tool will be evaluated in the near future. This evaluation, although not fully planned, should collect data to determine if the original goals of continuity and consistency are being met. In addition chart reviews to determine the degree of use and staff's perception of whether the tool saves time and simplifies documentation will be done. A chart review of the general guidelines revealed a need for more in-service on completing the form and more detailed written guidelines.

The complexity of teaching multiple providers how to use the new tool has taken time. It is just beginning to be used. It was decided that the general teaching tool discussed in Chapter 12 should be implemented first. This implementation has taken some time because many staff members needed to know how to assess learning needs and plan for teaching prior to using the tool. Numerous in-services have been held on principles of teaching–learning. Content knowledge was also needed prior to the use of the tool. Now that the staff is familiar with a similar tool (general teaching guidelines), it should be easy to use the new diabetic teaching tool. Currently, exploration of the use of a nursing Kardex is being devised that will incorporate client objectives for learning.

Management strategies for these clients change rapidly and vary; thus these guidelines may need to be adapted to specific and newly emerging protocol used in various perinatal centers. The guidelines do include critical content for these clients.

Other guidelines for high-risk clients need to be developed because of the difficulty in providing adequate, up-to-date information in the medically compromised patient. These guidelines represent one example of guidelines for high-risk clients. Other guidelines, once developed, can facilitate continuity and consistency in teaching for other high-risk obstetrical populations.

BIBLIOGRAPHY

Butnarescu, G. F. *Perinatal nursing. Reproductive health*. New York: John Wiley & Sons, 1978.

Coustan, D. R., & Lewis, S. B. Insulin therapy for gestational diabetes. *Obstetrics and Gynecology*, 1978, *51*(3), 306–310.

Felig, P. Diabetes mellitus. In G. Burrow & F. F. Ferris (Eds.), *Medical complications during pregnancy*. Philadelphia: W. B. Saunders, 1975.

Gabbe, S. G., Mestman, J. H., Freeman, R. K., Goebelsmann, U. T., & Lowensohn, R. I. Management and outcome of pregnancy in diabetes mellitus, Classes B to R. *American Journal of Obstetrics and Gynecology*, 1977, *129*(7), 723–732.

Gabbe, S. G., Lowensohn, R. I., Mestman, J. H., Freeman, R. K., & Goebelsmann, U. T. Lecithin sphingomyelin ratio in pregnancies complicated by diabetes mellitus. *American Journal of Obstetrics and Gynecology*, 1977, *128*(7), 757–760.

Galloway, K. G. The uncertainty and stress of high-risk pregnancy. *The American Journal of Maternal Child Nursing*, 1976, *1*, 294–299.

Good-Anderson, B. Home blood glucose monitoring in the pregnant diabetic. *JOGN-Nursing*, 1983, *12*(2), 89–92.

Gugliucci, C. L., O'Sullivan, M. J., Opperman, W., Gordon, M., & Stone, M. L. Intensive care of the pregnant diabetic. *American Journal of Obstetrics and Gynecology*, 1976, *125*(4), 435–441.

Gyves, M. T., Rodman, H. M., Little, A. B., Fanaroff, M. B., & Merkatz, I. R. A modern approach to management of pregnant diabetics: A two-year analysis of perinatal outcomes. *American Journal of Obstetrics and Gynecology*, 1977, *128*(6), 606–616.

Jovanovic, L. *Your guide to healthy, happy pregnancy*, Indianapolis: Bio-Dynamics, 1982.

Karlsson, K., & Kjellmer, I. The outcome of diabetic pregnancies in relation to the mother's blood sugar level. *American Journal of Obstetrics and Gynecology*, 1972, *112*(2), 213–220.

Kitzmiller, J. L., Cloherty, J. P., Younger, M. D., Tabatabail, A., Rothchild, S. B., Sosenko, I., Epstein, M. F., Singh, S., & Neff, R. K. Diabetic pregnancy and perinatal morbidity. *American Journal of Obstetrics and Gynecology*, 1978, *131*(5), 560–580.

Kitzmiller, J. L. Sweet success: Teaching diabetes and pregnancy management. *The Diabetes Educator*, 1983, *9*(2), 15–465.

Miller, N. R. Nutritional management of diabetes in pregnancy. *Perinatology–Neonatology*, 1983, *7*(1), 37–42.

Littlefield, V., & Seibert, G. The group approach to problem-solving for pregnant diabetic women. *Maternal Child Nursing*, 1978, *3*(5), 247–280.

Mort, P. R., & Vincent, W. S. *Introduction to American education*. New York: McGraw-Hill, 1954.

Olds, S. B., London, M. L., Ladewig, P. A., & Davidson, S. V. *Obstetric nursing*. Reading, Mass.: Addison-Wesley, 1980.

Queenan, J. T., & Hobbins, J. C. *Protocols for high-risk pregnancies*, Oradell, N.J.: Medical Economics Co., 1983.

Riblett, B. Insuring a safe pregnancy for your diabetic patient. *RN*, 1983, *46*(2), 50–55.

Roberts, J. E. Priorities in prenatal education. *JOGN-Nursing*, 1976, *5*(3), 17–20.

Snyder, D. J. The high-risk mother viewed in relation to a holistic model of the childbearing experience. *JOGN-Nursing*, 1979, *8*(3), 164–170.

Stekel, S., & Swain, M. Contracting with patients to improve compliance. *Journal of the American Hospital Association*, 1977, *51*(23), 81–88.

Surr, C. W. Teaching patients to use the new blood glucose monitoring products. *Nursing 83*, 1983, *13*(2), 58–62.

Tribble, N. M., & Hollenberg, E. E. The impact of a quality assurance program on diabetic education. *Nursing Clinics of North America*, 1977, *12*(3), 365–373.

White, P. Childhood diabetes, its course and influence on second and third generations. *Diabetes*, 1960, *9*, 345–355.

White, P. Pregnancy complicating diabetes. *American Journal of Obstetrics and Gynecology*, 1978a, *130*(2), 227.

White, P. Classification of obstetric diabetes. *American Journal of Obstetrics and Gynecology*, 1978b, *130*(2), 228–230.

Health Education When There Are Gynecological Problems

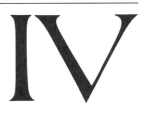

Part IV focuses on gynecological problems. Both minor (infections) and major (cancer) health problems are discussed. Chapter 21 presents a framework for teaching women how to prevent vaginal infections. Guidelines for teaching women specific content around such vaginal health problems as trichomoniasis, gonorrhea, herpes, toxic shock syndrome, amenorrhea, and dysmenorrhea are provided. Chapter 20 discusses the psychosocial needs of women who are infertile, as well as the content needed to understand various medical technologies to diagnose and correct infertility. Chapters 22 and 23 describe the knowledge needed for women who have cancer and must cope with the disease process and extensive medical and surgical intervention.

Infertility: Education for Understanding, Well-being, and Alternatives

20

Patricia Camillo

Infertility is not a modern phenomenon. It is a condition that has existed probably since the beginning of reproductive creation. Regardless of its long history, however, many individuals who are infertile continue to be very much alone, helpless, and misunderstood. Education regarding this condition is essential not only for those whom it directly affects, but also for the health care providers, families, and friends who play an intimate part in promoting positive (or negative) adaptation to this crisis.

With this in mind, the content areas explored in this chapter reflect the learning needs of not just infertile persons, but also all those who constitute the fertile world. We need to understand what it means to be infertile and how this condition affects an individual's life. With this heightened awareness, an assessment can be developed that incorporates not only the physiological, but the psychological, the sociocultural, and the developmental needs of the infertile person or couple, as well. Utilizing this holistic approach, intervention, in terms of education and counseling, encourages acceptance of meaningful alternatives by both the client and those around her.

Definition of Infertility

Traditionally, the medical profession has defined infertility as the inability of a couple to conceive after being sexually active for 1 year without using contraception. Some authorities have modified this length of time to 6 months if the woman is 30 to 35 years of age or older. This definition is sometimes extended to include those women who are unable to carry pregnancy to a live birth. The origin of the above definition of infertility is not clear, but it is generally accepted by most members of the medical profession.

As health professionals, we must address several questions if this standard definition is to remain appropriate in the clinical setting. First of all, it is important to recognize that there are many women who are "at risk" for being infertile (Table 20–1). If a woman falls into this category, does she have the right to a medical investigation that would evaluate her fertility status regardless of whether or not she has attempted to conceive? Is it essential that pregnancy be the immediate goal? Does the woman have to be married for her concerns to be legitimized? Does she have to be heterosexual?

The traditional definition of infertility does not consider these issues. It is defined, rather, on the concept of the nuclear family and the role of the woman as primarily housewife and mother. The single woman who seeks medical assistance to evaluate her

453

TABLE 20–1. RISK FACTORS FOR INFERTILITY (Not listed by degree of importance)

1. Advancing age, particularly over 35 years
2. Multiple abortions or dilatation and curettages (D & C)
3. Use of intrauterine device (IUD)
4. Pelvic infections, presently or in the past
5. Abdominal surgery or possibility of intraabdominal scar tissue
6. Prolonged birth control pill use
7. Endometriosis
8. Polycystic ovaries
9. Obesity
10. Endocrine imbalance
11. Malnutrition
12. Emotional stress
13. Exposure to DES in utero or exposure to occupational and/or environmental hazards.

fertility status is too often told not to worry until she is ready to settle down and have a family. Many women who are just beginning to establish their careers are haunted by the possibility that if they eventually decide to have a baby, they will not be able to. Lesbian women who are attempting artificial insemination without success rarely feel comfortable in seeking medical assistance to evaluate their fertility status. The traditional definition of infertility can no longer meet the health needs of these women.

In an attempt to redefine infertility, two basic questions emerge. First, "What does it mean to be infertile?" and, second, "When does a woman become infertile?" In response to the first question we must recognize the difference between infertility and sterility. The latter is a condition that absolutely prohibits an individual from participating in procreation. A blatant example of this would be the woman who has had a hysterectomy. Infertility, however, does not impose an absolute condition. The individual who experiences infertility is essentially disabled in terms of his or her reproductive function. In other words, these individuals are not as fertile as they or others have anticipated. In fact, they may never be fertile, but this is not actually known. Perhaps a better word to describe infertility would be "subfecundity."

In response to the second question "When does a woman become infertile?" let us examine two situations. Woman A seeks medical assistance because she and her husband have not used birth control for 1½ years and she did not get pregnant. They begin an infertility investigation and 3 months later, through no consequence of the medical workup, the woman is pregnant. Woman B, who has had two episodes of pelvic inflammatory disease (PID) in the past, seeks medical assistance to evaluate her fertility status. She is encouraged to actively try to conceive for at least 1 year before starting an expansive and costly medical evaluation. The woman returns 1 year later and it is found that her tubes are irreparably damaged. Three years later she has still not conceived.

Woman A was considered infertile when she was unable to conceive after 1 year. Woman B was probably infertile as a consequence of having PID, and yet recognition of her infertility was dependent on a fertility trial run! There is nothing magical that occurs either at 6 months, 9 months, or 12 months after an individual fails to conceive. One woman remarked "I have two more months to get pregnant before I become infertile."

This is clearly ridiculous when represented in this manner, but unfortunately the traditional definition of infertility encourages a very rigid standard before intervention can be planned.

As an alternative definition for infertility, the following statement is proposed. Infertility is a disability in terms of one's reproductive function that exists for an indefinite period of time and for which there is an indefinite outcome in respect to achieving a pregnancy. It is recognized in those women who are either at serious risk for reproductive failure or in those women who have failed to conceive over a variable period of time. The latter is collaboratively determined by both the woman and her health care provider, taking into consideration the woman's past history, family history, risk factors, and perception of her own personal fertility status. When considering the emotional impact of infertility, a woman is infertile from the time she begins to *feel* that her fertility is questionable. The subjective experience of being infertile is not dependent on any other variable, although it could certainly be influenced by other factors.

Incidence of Infertility. The 1978 United States Census Report states that there are 66 million (30 percent) Americans between the usual childbearing ages of 22 and 40 years. Using this information, Menning (1980) applied the generally accepted rate of infertility, 15 percent, and determined that 10 million people are currently affected by infertility in America.

When focusing on infertile couples, it is estimated that male factors account for approximately 40 percent of the problem, female factors for approximately 40 to 50 percent, and for the remaining 10 to 20 percent of the couples there will be no known cause for infertility (Speroff, Glass, & Kase, 1978).

At the present time, there is no organized system for collecting data on the incidence and prevalence of infertility. We can only make estimates based on the information that is known. Rosenfeld and Mitchell (1979) report that infertility data registries are being considered that would allow evaluation of the techniques used for management of infertility. Such registries would also provide more statistical information in terms of causative factors and outcomes.

Rationale for Education. Although infertility is not a phenomenon restricted to modern times, it is only within the past 5 to 10 years that there has been recognition of its consequences in terms of both physiological and psychological sequelae. As we move toward a more appropriate definition of infertility, there is a need to increase the awareness of women who are perhaps "at risk" of being infertile. As these and other women begin to explore their infertility status, issues related to role, sexuality, and life-style emerge. A perspective that incorporates the past, present, and future is necessary to examine the options and promote well-being.

Women who desire pregnancy and have been unable to conceive need to explore alternatives to biological parenthood. As health professionals, we need to anticipate this need and plan for appropriate guidance before the woman loses contact with the health care system. At the present time, there are very few resources that permit an infertile woman to reenter the system once an infertility investigation has been completed.

Fertility and the Female Role

Motherhood is central to a woman's identity and is characterized as a mandate that is built into our social institutions as well as our psyches (Russo, 1979). The media are particularly powerful in presenting motherhood in idealized and unrealistic terms. The "soap opera" frequently depicts pregnancy as a woman's way to compete for men, resolve conflicts, and become the center of attention. Although the process is often subtle, we can also find the seeds of this socialization growing in the school system, the job market, commercial industries, and the fine arts. The media may be different, but the message is the same: a woman's value and status in society is enhanced and often dependent on her ability to reproduce. Consequently, the woman who fails to become pregnant tends to see herself, and is often seen by others, as somewhat unnatural, shameful, and a failure as a woman.

The infertile woman has a disability that cannot be seen by others. She appears "normal" and yet is unable to fulfill the valued role of being a biological mother. Her competence as a woman is constantly being challenged. Family and friends repeatedly ask, "When are you going to start a family?" Her environment abounds in audio and visual displays of the joys of motherhood. There are an increasing number of books on natural childbirth, breast-feeding, and the working mother. Baby showers and traditional holidays for children such as Easter and Christmas are also constant reminders that this woman is ineffective in fulfilling her role.

Reproductive freedom is a concept that involves choice, and there are certainly women today who are choosing the alternative of being "child-free." However, the infertile woman is denied this decision-making process and is essentially "childless" as a consequence. She may begin to wonder what kind of woman she can be without children or whether or not she will be a "complete" woman in this society.

An exploration should be made of both past and present concepts of the female role as understood by the infertile woman. As health care providers, we should be prepared to assist women in identifying those factors that emphasize this role in their environment. It is not often possible or even desirable to negate or escape such environmental factors, but a recognition of their impact can lay the groundwork for seeking an alternative consciousness in terms of defining what is female.

INFERTILITY—A LIFE CRISIS

For most people, the question of having a child is a matter of choice. Fertility is assumed and, in fact, contraception is often of primary importance for several years before this decision becomes an issue. It is unexpected and often shocking when this option is no longer easily available to them.

Menning (1980) states that it is common for an infertile person to experience a state of crisis. In an attempt to further define this condition, Menning describes four common elements to any state of crisis:

1. *"A stressful event occurs that poses a threat which is insoluble in the immediate future."* The etiology and treatment of infertility is often entangled in a time-consuming investigation that seldom produces a solution in the immediate future. The individuals are dependent on the health care system for diagnosis, treatment, and supportive care. If pregnancy is not the desired outcome at that time, this threat hovers over the individual until attempts to conceive fail or until advancing age dictates the end of reproductive ability.

2. *"The problem overtaxes the existing resources of the persons involved because it is beyond traditional problem-solving methods."* Woods (1981, p. 264) discusses "the family planning mentality" as not only affecting infertile couples, but also pervad-

ing most of their social network. "It is assumed by others that not being a parent is a decision made voluntarily. As a result, most people are not sensitive to the feelings of the infertile individual or couple, particularly when they are unaware of their infertility." This lack of friends or family support or both, combined with the helplessness of the infertile person to create a change in the situation, greatly limits resources that are traditionally available for problem solving.

3. *"The problem is perceived as a threat to important life goals of the persons involved."* If raising a family is part of the life plan for a couple, then indeed infertility presents a threat to that plan and necessitates a reorientation of goals. The single woman is not excluded from this crisis if her life orientation has also centered around similar plans (Williams & Power, 1977).

4. *"The crisis situation may reawaken unsolved key problems from both near and distant past."* Wright (1960) discussed the phenomenon of spread in which feelings about a specific disability spread to encompass the individual's sense of self-worth and body image. As a crisis situation, infertility affects not only the ability to have children, but also the subsequent problems that arise from that disability such as alterations in self-esteem, sexuality, and body image (Mazor, 1978). It is conceivable that some of these problems have roots in the past as well as the present and are exacerbated by the stress of this crisis.

Burgess and Baldwin describe the resolution of a crisis as occurring in two phases—immediate and past crisis. Adaptive resolution during the crisis phase almost always dictates intervention by caring professionals. The individual needs assistance in defining issues, dealing with feelings, and learning how to cope in an effective manner.

Problems particular to infertility during this phase include:

1. Lack of knowledgeable professionals who are prepared to assist the individual;
2. Lack of experience on the part of the individual in dealing with this particular type of crisis;
3. Limited resources and support systems available for assistance in resolving the crisis.

In addition to the above, there is a dilemma in terms of "when" the individual initially experiences this crisis. Again, because of problems evoked by the traditional definition of infertility, this crisis is often not identified in its early stages and maladaptive resolution is the consequence. As part of this maladaptive response, the individual inadequately reduces the discomforts and returns to a level of functioning that is less adaptive than the precrisis period.

It is difficult to describe the postcrisis characteristics of infertility because, by its very nature, it is a condition that remains indefinite. It is not an event that occurs within a given space of time. Two women describe their perception of this crisis as being endless—"like having a miscarriage every month when I get my period" or "failing my law boards repeatedly every month." These women remain vulnerable to reactivations of this crisis because the conflicts associated with being infertile have never been resolved. An assessment of these individuals will reveal maladaptive behavior mechanisms and a general level of functioning that is less adaptive than their precrisis period. Of particular concern are those women who remain in this state for many years.

In an effort to promote adaptive resolution, the individual must first establish that there is a postcrisis period. Her reproductive status may never be totally defined until the physiological processes of menopause dictate an end to the possibility of conceiving a child. It is this indefiniteness that delays postcrisis adaptation. Acceptance of these uncertainties is paramount in moving toward a healthy resolution of this crisis.

Sexual Behaviors and Dysfunctions. In the past, the sexual difficulties of the infertile person or couple were frequently overlooked or knowingly neglected by practitioners who had very little awareness of these problems (Walker, 1978). Although this is gradually changing today, there is still a lack of anticipatory guidance and many individuals and couples do not seek assistance until a dysfunctional pattern has been set.

Concerns about sexuality and sexual function are universal no matter which partner has the infertility problem (Mazor, 1980). Some women may experience a loss of libido and even be nonorgasmic. Although they can still have intercourse, their relationships are likely to be compromised (Woods & Luke, 1979).

Menning (1977, p. 126) states that a major source of sexual difficulty is the temperature chart that must be kept as a record of ovulation patterns. She states that "a man, a woman, and a thermometer make strange bedfellows." Even when this type of charting is no longer necessary, a mental chart is kept of the woman's cycle, which creates demands for performance and removes spontaneity from the sexual relationship (Woods & Luke, 1979).

Some suggestions for minimizing this stress are:

1. The basal body temperature (BBT) chart should not be kept for more than 3 months at a given time. For the purposes of obtaining the type of information that this method provides, 3 months is an adequate amount of time.
2. The client should *not* be encouraged to synchronize sexual activity with the time of ovulation for at least the first month. Evidence of ovulation exists only in retrospect using the basal body thermometer, and cervical mucous must be observed for at least one cycle in order to recognize the fertile/infertile pattern.
3. The client's partner (if present) should take some responsibility for charting the information obtained. Too often, it is left entirely to the woman to take her temperature, record her findings, and encourage sexual activity at the right time. When this is a shared activity, each partner can take turns in being responsible for initiating sexual activity.

Following a final diagnosis of infertility, Menning (1977) indicates that some persons may call a moratorium on sex, whereas others may respond in the opposite way, by overcompensating. The single woman who has not entered into a sexual relationship may withdraw completely from contacts with men. There is a conscious or subconscious fear among many infertile women that their partners may abandon them for a fertile one (Williams & Power, 1977). The woman's feelings revolve around her loss of sexual desirability, which makes her overly sensitive to any sign of decline in sexual interest conveyed by her partner.

The Infertility Investigation

As women enter into and participate in an infertility investigation, there is a tremendous need for education regarding female anatomy and physiology as well as understanding the various tests and procedures that will be performed. Traditionally, these tests and procedures followed each other as, one by one, they proved to be negative. This could extend the investigation to a year and often longer. Concomitantly, there are increased anxiety levels in those individuals who are desperately waiting for answers.

Unless there is evidence to suggest preexisting psychogenic variables, it is certainly possible that a woman's reproductive status could be significantly compromised as a consequence of the stress associated with the length of time involved in this type of medical investigation. Although there are no data to support this at the present time, we do know that anxiety can interfere with ovulation as well as other body functions. It would be interesting to study the fertility outcome of those women for whom a deliberate attempt was made to reduce anxiety with those women for whom such efforts were not exercised.

The clinical/teaching plan presented in Table 20–2 was designed to expedite this investigational process while preserving as much client control as possible. Ideally, the physician (especially if she is a reproductive endocrinologist) would employ the services

TABLE 20–2. SUGGESTED TIME FRAME FOR INFERTILITY INVESTIGATION

Suggested Time Sequence	Clinical Goal	Education and Counseling
1st visit	1. History and physical 2. Assessment of risk factors 3. Interpret findings as they may or may not be pertinent to fertility status 4. Semen analysis arranged	1. Client establishes a beginning relationship with health care provider 2. Collaborative development of a plan for how the infertility investigation will be organized
2nd visit (preferably 1 week later)		1. Education regarding basic anatomy and physiology related to reproduction 2. Instruction on how to use the sympto-thermal method of detecting ovulation 3. Client advised *not* to try and schedule intercourse for this first month.
3rd visit	1. Examination of the cervix and cervical mucous (mid-cycle)	1. Problems associated with sympto-thermal method discussed 2. Psychosocial impact of infertility explored 3. Written and verbal information provided on postcoital test and endometrial biopsy
4th visit (mid-cycle)	1. Postcoital test performed	Explanation of results of postcoital test
5th visit (1 week later)	1. Endometrial biopsy performed	Explanation and preparation for hysterosalpingogram
6th visit		Summary of results and findings Plan for subsequent assessment and intervention

of a nurse clinician or other qualified health care professionals who are knowledgeable in fertility awareness as well as the emotional consequences imposed by infertility. Her expertise should include counseling skills and an appreciation of the grieving process. If such a person is not a member of the team, then a consultant should be secured who can provide these services.

The teaching plan incorporates the particular clinical aspects of the investigation with the learning and counseling needs that the client has or anticipates. At the initial visit, the client is given the opportunity to get to know her caretakers and to work collaboratively with them in organizing her particular needs for an infertility investigation. The order of the tests and procedures in Table 20–2 is only one example of how such an investigation can proceed. For instance, a woman may be particularly concerned about the patency of her tubes because of a past pelvic infection. In this case it would be more beneficial to proceed earlier with a hysterosalpingogram. All reasonable requests to alleviate anxiety in the infertile woman should be appreciated.

An explanation of the sympto-thermal method for detecting ovulation is reserved for the second visit. This is to ensure that an adequate amount of time is allotted for understanding the changes that occur throughout the cycle and the impact that all of this has on a woman's fertility. Traditionally, the client is quickly instructed at the first visit to take her temperature daily and to record it on a special graph. The mucous method is not usually included in this instruction. Many women do not understand the rationale for graphing their temperatures, yet try to figure out when they are ovulating. The anxiety associated with trying to schedule intercourse at the appropriate time is therefore intensified as a consequence of poor preparation and misunderstandings.

An alternative approach emphasizes instruction regarding basic physiology or reproduction and assisting the client in learning to investigate her particular body using the basal body thermometer and the mucous method of detecting ovulation. Any attempts to plan intercourse are not encouraged during this first month.

When one cycle is completed, the woman returns (preferably during mid-cycle) to review her findings and to compare her assessment of her mucous pattern with the findings of the examiner. This collaborative examination will add validity to the information being collected and correct any misunderstandings the client might have in using this method. Also at this visit, some of the emotional consequences of infertility are discussed with particular emphasis on sexuality and attempts to coordinate sexual intercourse with ovulation. Helping the client to understand some of the difficulties and providing suggestions for anticipated concerns will alleviate much of the turmoil that these individuals or couples experience. Also during this visit, verbal and written information should be provided that explains the postcoital test and the endometrial biopsy. The client should be encouraged to call if she has any further questions.

At the fourth visit, which should also be arranged during mid-cycle, a postcoital test is taken. The results of this test are thoroughly explained. One week later, the client returns for an endometrial biopsy. During this fifth visit, the hysterosalpingogram is explained. This test is particularly worrisome for many women. They often express their fears of cramping pain, which is sometimes experienced. Perhaps even more frightening is the amount of information that this single test provides. Tubal blockage is one of the leading causes of infertility in women. If her tubes prove to be patent and all other investigative procedures have been negative, the client moves closer to the possibility of never understanding why she cannot conceive. If her tubes prove to be blocked, the client might then face surgery, which may or may not restore her fertility. Consequently, the woman who is preparing for a hysterosalpingogram should be given ample time to express her feelings in an atmosphere that is clearly supportive of her emotional needs.

The hysterosalpingogram is done immediately postmenses. This is to ensure that ovulation and possible conception has not occurred. There are some physicians who believe that the actions of the dye pushing through the tubes can actually enhance the possibility of conception if done just prior to ovulation. It is certainly possible, but this has not been substantiated by current research data. It is also possible that the client could have a reaction to the dye and increase the inflammation that may or may not already be present.

The hysterosalpingogram is an invasive procedure with both benefits and risks. The client should be well informed of both.

The laparoscopy is a surgical procedure that is reserved as one of the final steps in the infertility investigation. This, too, is an invasive procedure and when general anesthesia is employed, there is a combined risk to the client that she should be fully aware of. The counseling that is involved in preparing for this procedure should emphasize that although the reproductive organs are usually visualized, the cause of the infertility may remain unknown.

Berger (1980) discusses the implications of an infertility workup in which the outcome did not pinpoint a definite cause for the infertility. He suggests psychiatric consultation, which would serve two functions:

1. To reassess in detail the sexual behavior and conflicts about pregnancy that may have been overlooked
2. To share and discuss the couple's uncertainty and to help plan a course of action for the future (1980, p. 556)

At the present time, there are very few health care settings that provide follow-up counseling for those individuals or couples who have been unable to conceive or for whom no known cause for being infertile has been found.

The Grieving Process. Mazor (1978, p. 148) states that regardless of the cause of infertility, the infertile woman "experiences a profound depression over the loss of her reproductive function, and feels herself to be damaged or defective." The disability thus incurred triggers a pattern of response that is characteristic of stressors involving loss, and is classically referred to as the "grieving process." Williams and Power (1977) outline this process in terms of the infertile individual as follows:

surprise $\rightarrow$ grief $\rightarrow$ anger $\rightarrow$ isolation $\rightarrow$ denial $\rightarrow$ acceptance

The element of surprise is especially significant in those women who have delayed parenthood and have been contracepting for years (Woods & Luke, 1979). Without having tried to conceive, surprise is profound in the single woman, who may have had no previous clues that anything was wrong.

The experience of grief may be deterred by individuals for several reasons (Woods & Luke, 1979, p. 240).

1. Their loss may be a potential rather than concrete one
2. They may have difficulty in discussing this loss
3. They may feel that their fertility is still uncertain so they do not grieve for its loss
4. Others may minimize or negate the loss
5. There may be no supportive persons available to comfort them in their grief

This loss is described by Williams and Power (1977, p. 328) as "the death of all one's potential children" as well as the loss of the experience of pregnancy, childbearing, and nursing. They discuss the mourning process associated with infertility as similar to that seen in the loss of wish fulfillment. There is grief for something that can never be.

Feelings of inadequacy may be associated with a period of anger and bitterness. Some women feel that they are unable to produce anything of worth because they are unable to produce a baby (Mazor, 1978). This anger can be internalized and result in a depression that often accompanies the stage of isolation. Infertility is a difficult subject for many people to discuss due to its very personal and inherently sexual nature. Denial then becomes the coping mechanism in responding to an overwhelming situation. Menning (1980, p. 315) describes chronically depressed men and women who "staunchly maintain that they never *really* wanted a family" or who refuse to apply the label "infertile" to themselves despite many years of involuntary childlessness.

Williams and Power (1977) state that for most women, acceptance is characterized by minimization of the loss. The process of resolution does not imply that the feelings associated with this loss will be forgotten, or that special reminders will not create new and different crises (Menning, 1980). However, the response is usually brief and not as overwhelming or difficult as the original crisis. Menning (1980, p. 317) describes the state of resolution as:

1. A return of energy
2. A surge of zest and well-being
3. An emerging perspective that puts infertility in its proper place in life
4. The return of a sense of optimism and faith
5. The return of a sense of humor
6. A disconnection of childbearing from sexuality, self-image, and self-esteem
7. A readiness to act on alternatives such as adoption
8. A willingness to go on with life planning for the future without the obstacle of infertility

Consideration of Alternatives

There are basically two options for those individuals and couples who have been unable to biologically create a child. These are adoption and child-free living. In any discussion of either of these options there must be a conscious realization of the fact that they are not primary choices. The fertile woman who voluntarily chooses child-free living is in many ways very different from the woman who must accept this life-style as an alternative due to infertility. The most important issue that separates the two is that of choice. We can best understand this difference in the use of the words "childless" and "child-free." The former describes the woman who *wants* a child but is infertile and the latter describes a woman who has freely chosen to live without children. The gap between these two life-styles can be bridged but only through holistic assessment and intervention that identifies the differences and moves toward maximizing the potential in each individual.

As a second option, adoption is becoming increasingly difficult. Whether this is a consequence of more liberal abortion laws or better use of contraceptive technology is not entirely clear. For the individual or couple who wants to adopt a child, the process is complex, time consuming, and emotionally painful. The complexity stems from a scarcity of resources that could assist the individual or couple in beginning an adoption procedure. As health care providers, many of us would have no idea where to send someone if they were considering adoption. We would know even less about international adoption.

When the information is finally obtained and the process is started, adoption can take between 3 and 8 years. A routine part of this process involves what is known as the "home study." In its most basic form, this is a home visit by a caseworker who then evaluates the adequacy of the environment and the life-style of the proposed family. Depending on which agency is handling the case, the individual or couple could be rejected based on lack of religious affiliation or full-time employment status of the woman. International adoption is also handled through home studies. Although adoption is often accomplished sooner, the process of applying for a non-American child can be much more intricate and detailed. The lengthy applications must be translated into the language of the country and in some instances, the new parents must spend a few weeks in that country before they are permitted to finalize the adoption. Depending on the current political atmosphere a country may suddenly close its doors and protect the child from leaving regardless of how far the adoption procedure has progressed.

The emotional implications of the adoption process can be overwhelming. Consider the fact that an individual or couple has already failed in being able to biologically create a family. They must then prove, through the present adoption process, that they are worthy of being parents and that they will provide a good home for a child. If they are fortunate enough to pass all the criteria of acceptability, they must then wait for several years before actually becoming parents. One woman described this waiting as "more intense than waiting for your period when you think you might be pregnant. . . . At least when my period comes, I know I'm not pregnant, with an adoption you never know. . . . I used to worry that they lost my papers or that my application would be passed aside for someone who had more influence."

Without question, the adoption process is another crisis in the life of an infertile person. Unfortunately, it is also at this time that individuals have very little contact with health care professionals who could provide supportive care. Anticipatory guidance should be provided as part of the infertility investigation. When all the tests have been completed and there is nothing more that can be done, time should be allotted to discuss alternatives and how these options will affect the individual's or the couple's life. Ideally, a system could be designed whereby the individual may return to her health care provider for counseling and supportive care if this becomes necessary in the future.

Assessment Variables. With an understanding of the content areas involved with infertility, we can now assess the individual or couple in terms of *their* learning and counseling needs. Table 20–3 outlines four major variables that comprise this assessment.

Physiological Factors. There are various known causes for infertility and when one such cause is identified, the client will exhibit learning needs particular to that diagnosis. For instance, the woman who has endometriosis is often placed on several months of drug therapy that may have side effects and that often places a financial stress on her situation. On the other hand, a woman with a tubal obstruction may have major surgery that might or might not affect her fertility status. Finally, a woman may not have a known cause for her infertility.

Length of time of known infertility is another important factor. A woman who has just started an infertility investigation will have learning needs that are obviously distinct from the woman who has seen several physicians over the past 8 to 10 years regarding her inability to conceive. The learning needs of the woman in the latter instance will focus on alternatives whereas the woman in the first example must learn about the often complex procedures involved in an infertility investigation.

TABLE 20–3. HOLISTIC ASSESSMENT OF HEALTH EDUCATION AND COUNSELING NEEDS FOR THE INFERTILE WOMAN

Physiological factors

1. Is the cause of infertility known?
2. How long has she considered herself to be infertile?
3. Is she presently trying to conceive?
4. Has she seen a physician regarding her infertility?
5. What has been done in terms of a medical investigation for the cause of infertility?
6. What risk factors are present that might suggest or complicate infertility?

Developmental factors

1. How old is the client?
2. What is her marital status?
3. What is her employment or career status?

Psychologic factors

1. Is infertility seen as a problem in her life now?
2. How important is it for her to be pregnant?
3. How important is it for her or her partner to have a baby?
4. Has she ever received individual or couple counseling?
5. Has she ever been a member of a support group?
6. Can she compare being infertile to any other experience she has had in the past?
7. How much emotional support does she receive from family and friends?
8. Has her sexual activity changed since she has been infertile?

Sociocultural factors

1. What is the client's concept of "being female"?
2. To what extent does her environment emphasize this role?
3. Has this changed since she has been infertile?
4. Who knows about her infertility?
5. Does she belong to any organizations for persons who are infertile (such as Resolve)?
6. Is adoption considered an acceptable alternative to self and partner?
7. If the client never has biological or adopted children, how does she perceive her life-style in the years to come?
8. What is her sexual preference?

If a woman is not presently trying to conceive, her learning needs will focus on an evaluation of her fertility status through a thorough consideration of risk factors while giving consideration to the possible alternatives that are available. This woman is not in a position to validate her infertility through failed attempts to conceive and therefore has increased counseling needs in terms of adapting to the uncertain and making appropriate plans for the future.

Developmental Factors. A woman who has postponed pregnancy and is now over 30 or 35 years of age will have learning and counseling needs that reflect a fear that perhaps she has waited too long and now it is too late. A younger woman will more often have to deal with issues that involve her plans for the immediate future. Will she stay home and hope that someday she will have a child or should she get involved in a career? The woman who is not married will need assistance in communicating her threatened fertility status to potential providers while considering possible alternatives to biological parenthood.

Psychological Factors. First of all, it is important to ascertain whether or not the client perceives infertility as a problem in her life now and to what extent. The woman who has an overwhelming need to be pregnant will have different needs than the woman who is focusing on having a baby, regardless of where it comes from.

Past experience with a similar crisis could provide the client with some possible adaptive mechanisms for dealing with the crisis of infertility. However, data from recent unpublished research (Camillo, 1982) suggest that this experience is limited. In this study, 104 women with primary infertility completed a questionnaire in which they listed numerous concerns, life-style changes, and coping behaviors that they perceived as being associated with infertility. Infertility could not be associated with anything that they had previously experienced in 41.3 percent of the women. The closest parallel that was identified involved the death of a close family member or friend. If the client cannot draw from past experience with a similar crisis then it becomes paramount to assess the social support systems that are currently available. It is often assumed by nurses and other health care providers that the family serves as the primary support network for individuals who are experiencing a crisis or are in the process of adoption. Camillo (1982) showed that although some family members knew about the subject's infertility, it did not necessarily follow that they provided emotional support (Table 20–4). With the exception of the husband, over 40 percent of those family members who knew about the infertility were perceived by the subject as not being supportive.

The client's past experience with seeking supportive care from individual or couple counseling or support groups must also be assessed. Are there resources which she can utilize in the community that specifically address the problems associated with infertility? One potential problem that should be carefully defined involves sexual fulfillment. Has infertility interfered with sexual pleasure? Has the client ever experienced problems with her sexuality in the past? Finally, in what way has infertility affected her relationship with her partner? For some individuals, the crisis acts as a very powerful positive force, whereas for others, it can evoke an entirely opposite effect. We must assess the situation very carefully to provide the most appropriate educational and counseling experience for the client.

TABLE 20–4. A COMPARISON OF FAMILY MEMBERS WHO KNOW ABOUT THE SUBJECT'S INFERTILITY AS COMPARED WITH THOSE FAMILY MEMBERS WHO OFFER EMOTIONAL SUPPORT

Family Members	% Who Know	Perceived Supportive	% Perceived Not Supportive
Mother	86.5	56.6	43.3
Mother-in-law	81.7	21.1	78.9
Father	75.0	30.7	69.3
Father-in-law	61.5	14.0	86.0
Husband	99.0	89.4	10.6

Note: % perceived supportive and % perceived not supportive are based on the number of family members who knew about the infertility.

Similarly, a comparison was made of the number of friends who knew about the subject's infertility with those who were perceived as offering emotional support. The findings show that although 8.7% of the subjects reported that at least five or more of their friends knew, only 31.7% reported that five or more of their friends were supportive.

(Source: Camillo, P. Psycho-social impact of infertility as perceived by women who are infertile. Unpublished thesis, University of Rochester, 1982.)

Sociocultural Factors. "Being female" has a long history of identification with successful mothering. It becomes necessary therefore to understand the client's concept of "being female" and to what extent this must be modified as a consequence of infertility. Can she see herself as a *complete* woman if she is unable to biologically have a child? How much does her environment emphasize the value of being a mother? Many women live in suburban communities where the female role is exemplified by the full-time housewife and mother. City living, on the other hand, offers a variety of life-styles with a more heterogenous population. It is important that the client become aware of how her present environment influences her ability to cope with infertility.

The consideration of adoption as a possible alternative requires careful assessment and intervention. Is this an acceptable alternative for the client, her partner, her family, her community? There is a tremendous need for information and education regarding the adoption process. Where does one go? Who does one contact? How long will it take? There are numerous other questions and details that must also be answered. Is there an organization in the community, such as Resolve, that can assist the client in this complex process?

If adoption is not an acceptable alternative, then the client must consider what her life will be like if she is never able to biologically have a child. Will her partner find child-free living an acceptable alternative? How does she envision her life as she grows older? For many women child-free living is not an acceptable alternative that has been decided upon but rather a consequence of finding adoption as unacceptable. Education and counseling regarding this life-style is long overdue. (See Resource list at end of chapter.)

Finally, in any assessment of sociocultural variables, it should never be assumed that an individual is heterosexual, regardless of the existence or nonexistence of a partner of the opposite sex. It is certainly possible that a homosexual individual would marry for the sole purpose of having a child. Infertility would then create specific needs that would be unique to this style of cohabitation.

In conclusion, a holistic assessment, based on the four major variables—physiological, psychological, sociocultural, and developmental—provides a tool whereby a woman's unique needs for education and counseling can be recognized.

Intervention for Well-being. A needs assessment is meaningless if we, as health care providers, cannot intervene in a manner that promotes the health and well-being of the clients who are served. Table 20–5 is an outline for wellness intervention that was adapted from Betty Neuman's "Total Person Approach to Patient Problems." The framework presented is specific to the infertile individual or couple but could certainly be used as an approach to other health related situations.

Primary intervention has a preventive focus that aims at reducing a woman's chance of becoming infertile while strengthening her ability to cope with the situation, should it occur. This mode of intervention is seldom offered because obstetrical and gynecological services in this country are provided primarily by physicians whose practice mode is disease-oriented. Alternative care providers, such as nurse practitioners, are becoming increasingly visible and available to provide the kind of health education and counseling that could meet the goals of primary intervention. This can be done with individuals or groups. Community education programs in local hospitals and health centers can serve as excellent vehicles for offering these kinds of service.

Secondary intervention becomes important once the stressor, in this case infertility, breaks through the client's "lines of defense." These are defined by Neuman as the

TABLE 20–5. APPROACHES TO PROVIDING HEALTH EDUCATION AND COUNSELING

Level of Intervention	Goals	Approaches	
		Individual	*Group*
Primary	1. Reduce possibility of encounter with infertility 2 Strengthen ability to cope with infertility should it occur	1. Provide for careful and competent OB/GYN health care services 2. Increase knowledge level of possible risk factors	1. Provide continuing education 2. Promote perception of women as people, not not necessarily mothers
Secondary	1. Early case-finding 2. Treatment of symptoms	1. Use of holistic assessment 2. Evaluation of present risk factors 3. Counseling for sexual dysfunctions 4. Crisis intervention 5. Supportive counseling during grieving process	1. Formation of support groups
Tertiary	1. Readaptation 2. Reeducation to prevent future stressors 3. Maintenance of stability	1. Education & counseling, re: alternatives 2. Education, re: stress associated with fertility 3. Counseling, re: individual adaptive ways of coping 4. Follow-up education and counseling	1. Encourage growth of of reliable social support network (e.g., Resolve, Inc.)

(Source: Adapted from Neuman, B. The Betty Neuman health-care systems model: A total person approach to patient problems. In J. P. Riehl & Sr. C. Roy (Eds.), Conceptual models for nursing problems *(2nd ed.). New York: Appleton-Century-Crofts, 1974, by permission.)*

individual's "usual coping pattern" or "steady state" (Neuman & Young, 1972, p. 265). Use of the holistic assessment tool presented in Table 20–5 is the first step toward intervention on an individual basis. Risk factors are evaluated and secondary stressors are identified. Counseling is provided with the goals of identifying those stressors with the client as early as possible and reducing the negative impacts that are likely to occur without this type of intervention. For example, the grieving process, when identified in its early stages, can be a growing experience for the individual or couple, whereas grieving which is prolonged or delayed can have serious and destructive consequences.

Tertiary intervention is particularly important when dealing with infertility. If pregnancy does not result, this is a crisis that often remains unresolved until menopause or sterility (as occurs with hysterectomy). Education and counseling regarding alternatives should be initiated by a competent professional before the infertility investigation ends. For many women, the search for answers continues for years. They may seek out specialist after specialist in a constant crisis over their fertility status. We do these women a grave disservice when we send them back into a fertile world unaware of the stressors they will experience as a consequence of their infertility and ill-equipped with positive ways for coping. Follow-up is essential so there can be legitimate access back into the health care system for emotional support, as needed. As a national organization for infertile persons, Resolve has done a wonderful service in meeting some of those needs.

The Educational Process. In determining an educational approach to be used with a client who is infertile, it is first necessary to assess the client's crisis state or stage in the grieving process. From that point, the health care provider can assess the psychological climate that will undoubtedly influence the client's ability to learn. For instance, during a client's initial appointment with an infertility specialist, there is usually a significant level of anxiety in the woman. She and possibly her partner have in a realistic and concrete manner identified that there is an infertility problem. This blatant recognition of infertility increases anxiety and, as such, is not a time to instruct the client on use of a basal body temperature graph. She will probably hear only half of what is being said. This type of learning requires a pedagogical approach that would evaluate the client's prior knowledge, provide explicit information, and perform some measure of testing that would evaluate the client's understanding of the information taught.

On the other hand, the initial visit is better conducted using an andragogical approach. Time is needed to listen to the client, identify her learning needs, and provide a supportive trusting environment. This approach would serve to decrease anxiety as well as prepare the client for what she and her partner could expect.

Throughout the infertility investigation and thereafter this type of assessment is necessary before deciding on a specific educational approach. Due to the highly emotional nature of an infertility crisis, this approach will probably fluctuate, perhaps from visit to visit, depending largely on the psychological climate and the client's individualized needs.

APPROACHES TO SPECIAL SITUATIONS

Women with Infertility of Unknown Cause

The findings presented in Table 20–6 (Camillo, 1982) compare women who had a known cause for their infertility with those who had no known cause. In terms of support networks, approximately twice as many women who did not have a known cause for their

TABLE 20–6. SELECTED PSYCHOSOCIAL VARIABLES COMPARING THOSE WOMEN WHO HAD A CAUSE FOR INFERTILITY WITH THOSE WOMEN WHO HAD NO KNOWN CAUSE

Variable	Cause Known[a] (%)	Cause Unknown[b] (%)
Presently trying to get pregnant	73.7	64.3
Visit to health care provider within past year specifically for infertility	82.9	67.9
Employed full-time	44.7	50.0
Perceives no support from friends	11.8	21.4
Perceives no support from family	5.3	10.7
Participation in support group	40.8	39.3
Received couple counseling	15.8	14.3
Received individual counseling	25.0	39.3
Adoption not acceptable to self	5.3	10.7
Adoption not acceptable to partner	6.6	21.4

[a]N—76
[b]N—28

infertility received no support from family and friends, than did those women who had a known cause. Although the percentage of those participating in support groups and those in couple counseling were almost identical, 14.3 percent more women who did not have a known cause received individual counseling. The reasons for these differences are not known. It can be hypothesized that perhaps the family and friends of those women who had no known cause found it difficult to feel empathy when the reason for being infertile could not be explained. Although it was not demonstrated in the study, it is also possible that these infertile women hesitated more before informing others of something they could not explain and subsequently did not receive support.

These results have special implications for assessment and intervention by health care providers. There is an obviously greater need for supportive care, and yet women who did not have a known cause for their infertility were less likely to have seen a health care provider within the past year. It is not certain whether this decision was made by the individual or her care provider, but for whatever reason, these women had less contact with a system that could have served as a potential resource for them.

In terms of adoption as a possible alternative, twice as many women who did not have a known cause for their infertility than those who had a known cause, found adoption to be an unacceptable alternative for themselves and more than three times as many stated that adoption was unacceptable to their partners. Although the reasons behind these responses were not explored in Camillo's (1982) study, it is clear that women without a known cause for being infertile have distinct educational and counseling needs, particularly in terms of tertiary prevention. Careful and systematic follow-up by specially trained care providers is essential.

Infertility and the Single Woman. Although single women are briefly mentioned throughout this chapter, they are a group who, when infertile, have very special needs that are rarely identified. The reason for this is probably related to our primary cultural norms that encourage childbirth only within the traditional family structure. In a very gradual way, these norms are changing, but it will be quite some time before this change impacts the situation of a single woman experiencing infertility.

Many may feel that the incidence of known infertility in single women is not significant enough to warrant special consideration. Often absolute sterility must be demonstrated before counseling is even considered for these women. This is not the same criterion that is used in counseling infertile married women, and yet many of the same disease processes or malformations may be present in both. Examples include endometriosis, polycystic ovaries, Turner's syndrome, and untreated venereal disease. There is a definite correlation between infertility and the existence of such conditions. Although it is true that many of these disease states may or may not be curable or significantly alter fertility status, it should be remembered that infertility is not defined as a definite or incurable condition. In all instances, a woman's reproductive freedom is being threatened and at the same time, a disability imposed.

In developing ways of helping the single woman resolve this crisis, it is essential that we first abandon the concept that infertility counseling is *primarily* and *exclusively* an effort to assist the "infertile couple" through the rigorous process of an infertility investigation and thereby enhance their ability to produce a living child. Although these problems certainly cannot be denied, there are, however, other equally important functions of infertility counseling. The single woman must be assisted in adapting to this loss, especially in terms of the grieving process, projected life-style alternatives, and defining the female role.

Support groups for "infertile couples" should include single women. By participation in the group process, the single woman can become aware of what happens in a marriage when the wife is infertile. The development of a female role that is distinct from reproductive ability is facilitated in an atmosphere that integrates the life-styles of both married and single women. Life-styles may change but the sense of integrity and self-worth in being a female and a sexual being can be supportive throughout life.

Single infertile women represent a silent minority whose needs are not being met by the present medical care system. As professionals we can anticipate these needs and provide the necessary guidance. The silence of single women cannot be interpreted as the absence of crisis if one recognizes the impact that infertility has on *all* women.

The Pregnant Woman Who Was Infertile: A Case Study

Laura had pelvic inflammatory disease when she was 17 years old. At that time she was informed that her fallopian tubes might be blocked with scar tissue and that someday she might have difficulty getting pregnant. Although she worried about this now and then, it was difficult for her to believe that she would never be able to have children.

One year later, Laura was admitted to the hospital for an ovarian cyst, which, when surgically removed, was diagnosed as endometriosis. Again she was told that her fertility was probably threatened, and, in fact, she might need a hysterectomy someday. Over the next 3 years the reality of Laura's situation became more apparent to her as she struggled with chronic pelvic pain and various hormonal treatments. Also, during this time, Laura married an old high school sweetheart who understood her situation and was satisfied to live a child-free life. However, for Laura, the issue of having a baby became more intense. She sought counseling to deal with her feelings and felt after a period of several months that she could accept a hysterectomy and subsequent sterility. A large part of Laura's emotional difficulty stemmed from her husband's rejection of adoption as a possible alternative.

The surgery was scheduled but Laura never got her period. A pregnancy test was done which was positive. Of course the surgery was cancelled and everyone was happy. The nine months that followed were not what Laura and her husband expected they might be. Instead of carefree excitement and expectation, which so often typifies a welcomed pregnancy, there was a constant and daily sense of anxiety. Some of the thoughts that were shared by Laura were as follows:

- "I don't know if I'm ready for this. . . . "
- "I should be so excited, this is a miracle . . . but I'm so frightened. . . . "
- "What if something goes wrong. . . . what if I miscarry or the baby dies. . . . "
- "Maybe all the hormone treatments I took will affect the health of the baby."
- "When I don't feel the baby move, I'm sure he or she is dead."
- "What if I loose this baby and I can't get pregnant again."
- "This could be my only chance. I'm even afraid of having sex—it might cause the baby to come too early—I can't wait for this pregnancy to be over."

Laura's situation is an actual case study and her comments were actual responses during several months of counseling throughout her pregnancy. There are too few care providers who can truly appreciate the daily emotional anguish of these women and couples. We seldom allow them to complain or express their negative feelings because, after all, they should be happier than most couples who take pregnancy for granted.

The bottom line for intervention in these situations is to open Pandora's box and discuss common fears and anxieties experienced during pregnancy and particularly during pregnancies that are "miracles." Most women will not feel comfortable to express these negative feelings and thoughts for fear that they would be shocking or unacceptable. When there are no positive outlets for releasing these anxieties, the interpersonal relationship between husband and wife can be compromised. In fact, it is entirely possible that the health and well-being of the baby might also be at risk because toxic levels of substances, potentially harmful to the baby, accumulate during times of increased stress.

SUMMARY

In summary, we can never assume in any of these situations that women will respond in any particular way or fashion. We are beginning to realize the complex series of emotional responses that occur as a result of infertility. There is still a great deal to learn. Holistic assessment with individualized intervention will increase our awareness of the problems that exist, promote the well-being of our clients, and encourage the acceptance and utilization of alternatives in a healthful manner.

RESOURCES

Resolve Inc., P.O. Box 474, Belmont, MA 02178, (617) 484-2424

Resolve is a national non-profit organization for individuals and couples who are having difficulty or are unable to conceive. It offers information on causes and treatments of infertility as well as a listing of medical resources throughout the country.

The bimonthly newsletter, which is distributed to members, often addresses the emotional consequences of infertility as well as offering suggestions for managing with infertility on a daily basis.

Resolve has local chapters in many cities that often offer individual and group support as well.

BIBLIOGRAPHY

Berger, D. Infertility: A psychiatrist's perspective. *Canadian Journal of Psychiatry*, 1980, *25*(7), 553–558.

Burgess-Wolbert, A., & Baldwin, R. A. *Crisis intervention theory and practice*. Englewood Cliffs, N. J.: Prentice-Hall, 1981.

Camillo, P. Psycho-social impact of infertility as perceived by women who are infertile. Unpublished thesis, University of Rochester, 1982.

Mazor, M. Psychosexual problems of the infertile couple. *Human Sexuality*, 1980, *14*(12), 32–39.

Mazor, M. The problem of infertility. In T. Malkak & C. Nadelson (Eds.), *The women patient: Medical and psychological interfaces*. New York: Plenum Press, 1978.

Menning, B. *Infertility: A guide for the childless couple*. New Jersey: Prentice Hall, 1977.

Menning, B. The emotional needs of infertile couples. *Fertility and Sterility*, 1980, *34*(4), 313–319.

Neuman, B. The Betty Neuman health-care systems model: A total person approach to patient problems. In J. P. Riehl & Sr. C. Roy (Eds.), *Conceptual models for nursing practice* (2nd ed.). New York: Appleton-Century-Crofts, 1974, pp. 99–114.

Neuman, B. M., & Young, R. J. A model for teaching total person approach to patient problems. *Nursing Research*, 1972, *21*, 264–269.

Rosenfeld, D., & Mitchell, E. Treating the emotional aspects of infertility: Counseling services in an infertility clinic. *American Journal of Obstetrics and Gynecology*, 1979, *135*, 177–180.

Russo, N. Overview: Sex roles, fertility and the motherhood mandate. *Psychology of Women Quarterly*, 1979, *4*(1), 7–15.

Speroff, L., Glass, R., & Kase, N. *Clinical gynecology, endocrinology and infertility*. Baltimore: Williams & Wilkins, 1978.

Walker, H. Sexual problems and infertility. *Psychosomatic Medicine,* 1978, *19*(8), 477–484.

Williams, L., & Power, P. The emotional impact of infertility in single women: Some implications for counseling. *Journal of the American Medical Women's Association,* 1977, *32*(9), 327–333.

Wright, B. A. *Physical disability—A psychological approach.* New York: Harper & Row, 1960.

Woods, N. Infertility. In C. Fogel & N. Woods (Eds.), *Health care of women: A nursing perspective.* St. Louis: C. V. Mosby, 1981.

Woods, N., & Luke, C. Sexuality, fertility and infertility. In C. Kopp (Ed.), *Becoming female: Perspectives on development.* New York: Plenum Press, 1979.

Promotion of Vaginal and Menstrual Health: Education for Health Maintenance

21

Leslie Skillman

In the ambulatory setting women present with a unique array of concerns. Often these concerns are not acute in nature but rather are client identified as temporary and specific self-care deficits. The client presents with a set of symptoms, expects an answer for the existence of the health status change, and expects an efficient remedy so that homeostasis is renewed. For a health care provider to meet the requirements of the woman's expectations, she must have previously identified a conceptual framework, developed a knowledge base that is pertinent, and utilize a process that contributes to the assessment, planning, intervention, and evaluation of the client's needs.

Contributing factors as to how this process is implemented include the health care provider's presence and initial introduction to the woman client, the provider's schedule and time frame and their compatibility with the client's schedule and time frame, and the physical environment of the clinic. If the above criteria are met without care provider or client conflict, the assessment process may proceed without compromise or distraction. In the event that one of the three contributing criteria is in conflict, the care provider and client must first deal with this before proceeding to the woman's concerns that initiated the appointment.

Simultaneous with assessment of the woman's presenting concerns, it is vital to obtain the woman's definition of health. Health in its most universal sense has been conceptualized as a continuum (wellness to illness), as coexistent states, or as mutually exclusive (bipolar) states. A continuum implies quantitative differences between states, whereas bipolarity implies qualitative differences between wellness and illness (Thibodeau, 1983, p. 7).

When the health care provider is working from a continuum perspective she may view the woman with a minor gynecological alteration as healthy but in need of temporary treatment or education. This would be enhanced by further assessment of her general well-being coupled with information about additional resources or assistance. Clients with this perspective are often eager for self-help aids and information.

The health care provider utilizing the bipolar definition may only treat the presenting symptom. The assumption the health care provider makes is that the woman would use other resources for health and education. Clients foster this approach to health care by accepting this framework and expecting to receive the miracle cure in pill fashion. The idea of self-help is rarely client identified. Also, it appears that this situation does not encourage client health maintenance activities.

Once the client's frame of reference is established, the care provider's understanding of her role can be matched with the client's. The care provider can then proceed to the assessment of the presenting concern, keeping in mind the future need to support or educate the woman regarding her self-care responsibilities in the maintenance and promotion of wellness.

This chapter focuses on the health education necessary for women with minor alterations in their gynecological health by first presenting conceptual frameworks and how these can provide the organizational schemas from which abstract and concrete concepts can be used for clinical assessment and patient educational purposes. This approach to women's gynecological health care also differentiates the short-term and long-term planning goals for health maintenance and promotion. A conceptual framework that focuses on health and health promotion versus treatment of symptoms will allow the health care provider and individual woman to establish participatory, complementary roles and encourage broad health teaching and intervention versus alteration of problems on a short-term basis. Vaginal and menstrual problems are the reason many women seek health care and the only reason some otherwise healthy women seek care. Such health problems result, in part, because of the lack of information about body functioning and potential threats to vaginal and menstrual health. Without a specific framework, health care providers may not take a holistic approach and health prevention strategies may be lost. Thus, a framework is presented, followed by examples of how to incorporate this framework in the assessment and the management of specific problems. Details of assessment, management, and teaching objectives can be obtained in tables.

CONCEPTUAL FRAMEWORKS

As in all scientific disciplines, each practice is based on a relevant theoretical structure. The health care professions are no exception to this rational method approach to practice. Nursing, traditionally defined as a "doing" profession, has recently been developing its theoretical base for practice by defining concepts of health practice and schematizing these graphically. Nursing has contributed to overall assessment of holistic health care by creating several models that assist the health care provider in making a complete assessment of the individual's health and illness. The following section gives examples of two health care models, first the Bermosk and Porter model that conceptualizes an approach to women's health needs and second the Health Belief model that looks at patient education via methods of information giving and derived outcomes.

Theory Base. The Bermosk and Porter model and the Health Belief model have been described in a previous chapter (see Chapter 4). Clinical application of these models is discussed in this section.

If a conceptual model is an outline, a representation of reality, then we can look at the Bermosk and Porter model (B & P) and see how it reports the health needs of a woman throughout the continuum of life emphasizing the health promoting activities. To understand the clinical application of the B & P model, the following two diagrams are used and interpreted. First, the mandala in its geometric form depicts the relationship of key concepts underlying the philosophy that considers each woman as a vital participant to achieving healthy behaviors (Fig. 21–1).

> The mandala may be regarded as an engine of change, releasing energy to the extent of which the individual using it and concentrating upon it is capable of identifying himself

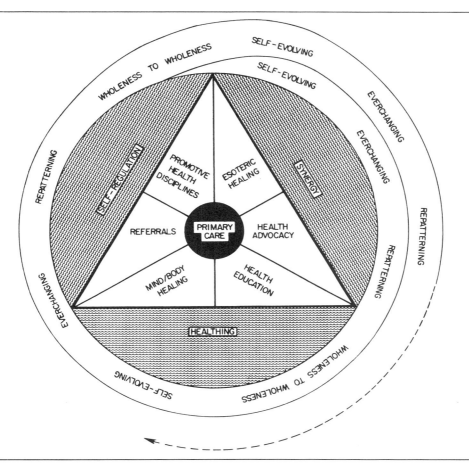

Figure 21–1. Mandala as logos for the women's healthing model. (Source: *Bermosk, L. S., & Porter, S. E.* Women's health and human wholeness. *New York: Appleton-Century-Crofts, 1979, p. 126, by permission.)*

with it. The principle of the mandala lies not in the external form, which is unique for each situation, but in the center, the source through which the form-creating energy flows. To be integrated, to be made whole, means to be able to maintain contact with one's center (Arguelles & Arguelles, 1972, p. 19–20).

The philosophy, a "holistic, cross-cultural approach directed toward the promotion, assessment, and maintenance of the health and human wholeness of women from birth to death" (Bermosk & Porter, 1979, p. 117), has seven components (primary health care, health educator consultation and referral, health advocacy, promotive health disciplines, mind–body healing, and esoteric healing). These components depict the means by which women clients and health care providers identify and communicate needs.

When the health care provider views the female client from this philosophical framework, it becomes evident that the approach to women with minor gynecological illnesses is not to treat the presenting complaint without also recognizing the long-range health care needs. To help the health care provider delineate aspects of the long-range health promoting activities the second of the Bermosk & Porter diagrams is useful (Fig. 21–2). This diagram shows the relationships between the seven service components within a health care system and also the routes by which women initiate contact with varying types of health care agencies and providers. Flow and direction of these relationships are noted by the arrows. An application of this model is provided in the following scenario.

In the case of M. S., a healthy 27-year-old nulligravida black female, who presents with the complaint of severe abdominal cramping on day 1 and 2 of her menstrual cycle and wanting relief, the health care provider would identify the mind–body healing component as the source in need of attention. Once the diagnosis of dysmenorrhea is made, several options or treatment modalities can be offered. Self-regulating activities may include biofeedback, massage or warmth to the abdomen, or prescribed medication to decrease the physical stress. Synergy is attained when appropriate information is given by the health care provider and understood by the patient. Once M. S. knows that the discomfort is self-limiting (only 2 days) and that it is a reminder that her endocrine glands are functioning normally she is better able to cope with the comfort alteration. Thirdly, healthing for M. S. is derived from the knowing what to do for the discomfort so she can begin to heal herself by doing something for herself. The perception of pain often diminishes with a decreasing state of anxiety promoted by understanding the circumstances.

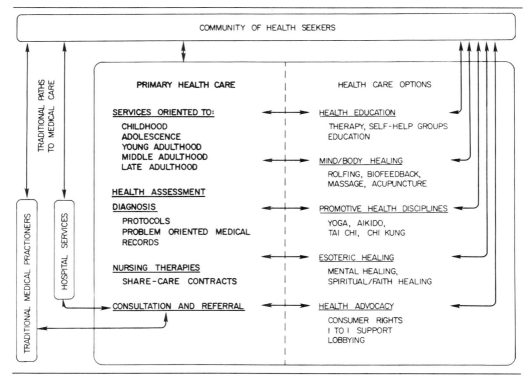

Figure 21–2. Women's healthing model. (Source: *Bermosk, L. S., & Porter, S. E. Women's health and human wholeness. New York: Appleton-Century-Crofts, 1979, p. 120, by permission.)*

The long-range implications are that M. S. will begin to realize that she has control in decision making regarding her health care needs. The hoped for outcome is that by identifying this control she will take on health promoting behaviors.

The Health Belief Model. Becker's Health Belief model (HBM) is a "partially developed theory" (1974, p. 143), geared toward developing a scientific base to serve in the education of educators. The focus is on behavior and motivation. The model "clearly specifies the motivational significance of its cognitive elements—the beliefs energize and direct behavior (or at least represent the existence of such forces in the person)" (Becker, 1974, p. 128).

The four elements to the model that conceptualize change and predict the outcomes from relationships between motivators and behavior are: (1) modifying factors that include demographical, sociopsychological, and structural variables; (2) the individual's perceived risk to disease susceptivity and severity; (3) the perceived threat of a disease; and (4) the likelihood of action derived from the benefits minus the perceived barriers. The diagram below of the HBM depicts these relationships (Fig. 21–3).

The idea of a cost to benefit ratio influencing health behaviors is not new. Becker utilizes this concept in his model. Identification of conflict that might block the actions toward health maintenance is a key point in his theory. The model's components help depict for the practitioner and the client the aspects blocking or promoting compliance. The model is also useful for identifying long-range health planning goals.

The following is a case study and diagram that uses the HBM for identifying the cost to benefit ratio motivating health promotion activity pertinent to the case.

T.J. is a 24-year-old white single female G_2P_{1011}. She is of low socioeconomic status and lives with her younger sister in a two-bedroom apartment. She works part time as a waitress and attends secretarial school. T.J.'s sister babysits her 3-year-old son. She comments that the sister seems to have a better relationship than she has with her son.

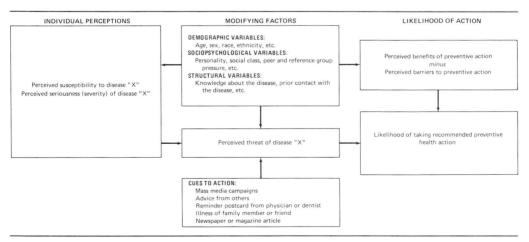

Figure 21–3. The "Health belief model" as predictor of preventive health behavior. (Source: *Becker, M. H. (Ed.). The health belief model and personal health behavior. Thorofare, N.J.: Slack, Inc., 1976, by permission.)*

T.J. has been sexually involved with one man for four months and is very happy about the relationship.

She was last seen by her health care provider (HCP) three months ago for an annual examination. At that time she was diagnosed with gonorrhea. She was successfully treated with IM penicillin 4.8 m.u. and probenecid 1 g po. Information regarding her partner was given to the local health department. Her partner states he saw his HCP who said he didn't need treatment.

Three months later T.J. returns with symptoms of pelvic discomfort and vaginal discharge. She suspects she has another gonorrheal infection. She continues to express happiness about her relationship and continued sexual involvement with the same partner. T.J. expresses concerns regarding her future fertility when she is told she definitely has gonorrhea again (Fig. 21–4).

Diagramming the aspects of this case study makes clear the struggle this woman has, perceived benefits minus perceived barriers, in attaining health promoting action. Because the major barrier is perceived loss of her male partner, an action that the health care provider can use to facilitate the likelihood of health promoting action is to invite the partner to be seen with the woman (T.J.) for health evaluation purposes.

In this section, theoretical models and concepts have been described to help aid the health care provider in organizing the way she would like to administer care. The next section examines the process by which the short-term and long-term health planning is achieved.

METHODOLOGIES

Separating these planning goals for health into two categories, short-term and long-term, helps the health care provider and the client focus on the immediate health deficits and the overall learning needs. Short-term health education goals for the woman presenting with a minor gynecological concern are usually dealt with through explanations of the diagnosis and consequential prescription. Long-term goals or the health promotion activi-

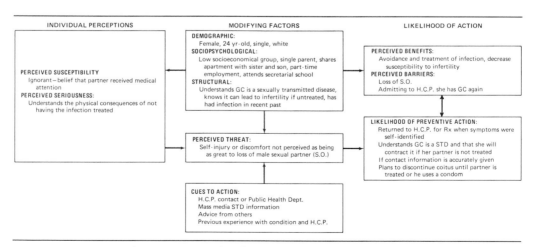

Figure 21–4. Specific adaptation of the health belief model.

ties vary depending on the philosophy and practice framework the health care provider uses, and the time and resources available the day of the visit. Rescheduling for additional health planning is certainly beneficial but often not immediately cost effective. Clients may not value this service depending on their orientation to how the health care delivery system benefits them. The outcome is, therefore, frustrating for both parties. The health care provider is disappointed by the poor compliance when the patient does not show for the appointment, and the client can be discouraged because she does not understand why she needs to see the health care provider when she feels fine. Health education for health promotion and self-care activities is neither sought nor valued by many women health consumers. The health care provider's goal then becomes one of enlightening women to health choices and participating in making informed self-help decisions.

If an adult learning orientation is used, the woman is encouraged to identify what she needs from the health care provider and what other resources are available to maintain her desired health status. A well-informed and motivated woman could be taught under these principles. Others may need a more pedagogical approach until they have enough information and experience to recognize the risks involved in poor health, for example repeated vaginal infections.

The next section focuses on the process for assessing client's needs. Later sections discuss the whys and hows of client education for short- and long-term planning.

ASSESSMENT OF LEARNING NEEDS

The Client's Agenda

When a woman comes to her health care provider with a concern, the most important thing her provider can ask is "What is your immediate concern?" This may be done either by providing space on the health history form which asks this question (Fig. 21–5) or by direct questioning during the interview. Appointments made by clients often contain hidden agendas. These agendas may be explicitly shared by the woman or withheld, anticipating that the health care provider will bring up the topics. When extensive hidden agendas are uncovered, the care provider's role is twofold. She will need to assist the client to take the responsibility for her concerns that will promote and maintain her health, and to learn to trust her provider so that her needs are met directly and efficiently. During the assessment of the client's ability to learn how to maintain her wellness health status, the care provider will not only determine the content appropriate for teaching but also the limits of the client's capacity to learn. Criteria such as age, developmental level, education level, and cultural influences determine whether or not adult learning processes are suitable.

Collecting health history data is a method that problem solves with the patient and identifies many potential health needs. Sandelowski supports this activity and adds:

> Promoting the health of women of all ages and developmental stages involves a "comprehensive ecological approach," designed to maintain their integrity as individuals living in a particular time and place. Because health is such an all-encompassing aspect of life, "prospective" health care is based upon the discovery of actual and the forecasting of potential health hazards and risks to the individual as s/he interacts with time and place. (Sandelowski, 1981, p. 258)

Inherent in this data collection process is the identification of support systems and how these work when the woman is experiencing stress or crisis; a review of the major life

Confidential Health History

University of Rochester Medical Center
Women's Health Care Clinic

Date _____ SMH Number _____

Name _____ Age _____ Birthdate _____

Occupation _____

Circle the highest year of school completed: 1 2 3 4 5 6 7 8 9 10 11 12 13 14 15 16 17 18

Circle your marital status: single married divorced widowed separated

Family History

Are you adopted? __ yes __ no

Brothers or Sisters

	Name	Age	Living/dead	Cause of death
Father				
Mother				

	Name	Age	Living/dead	Cause of death

Has anyone in your family had trouble with the following?
Include mother (M), father (F), brother (B), sister (S), grandfather (GF), grandmother (GM).

no yes who				no yes who				no yes who		
__ __ __	Diabetes			__ __ __	High blood pressure			__ __ __	Sickle cell disease
__ __ __	Heart attack (before 50)			__ __ __	Stroke			__ __ __	Birth defects/
__ __ __	Cancer			__ __ __	Breast disease				hereditary diseases

Medical History

Have you had any of the following?

no yes now			no yes now			no yes now	
__ __ __	Anemia		__ __ __	Cancer		__ __ __	Diabetes
__ __ __	Sickle cell		__ __ __	Breast disease		__ __ __	Thyroid problems
__ __ __	Sickle cell test			mass or discharge		__ __ __	Kidney problems
__ __ __	Heart disease		__ __ __	Severe depression		__ __ __	Bladder infection
__ __ __	Heart murmur		__ __ __	Numbness or tingling		__ __ __	Stomach/bowel problems
__ __ __	High blood pressure			of extremities		__ __ __	Gall bladder problems
__ __ __	Varicose veins		__ __ __	Epilepsy: seizures		__ __ __	Liver disease
__ __ __	Blood clots/		__ __ __	Stroke		__ __ __	Hepatitis
	bleeding disorders		__ __ __	Frequent headaches		__ __ __	Mononucleosis
__ __ __	Rheumatic fever		__ __ __	Migraine headaches		__ __ __	Jaundice
__ __ __	High cholesterol		__ __ __	Rubella titer		__ __ __	Contact lenses
			__ __ __	Rubella immunization		__ __ __	Asthma

Do you take any medications now? __ yes __ no
If yes, please list:

_____

_____

_____

Are you allergic to:

no yes	
__ __	copper
__ __	rubber
__ __	iodine
__ __	medications

Please list: _____

_____

Figure 21–5. Sample of a health history form. *(cont.)*

Menstrual History

Age period started _____

Periods come every _____ days. They last _____ days.

Periods are: __ regular __ irregular
__ light __ moderate __ heavy

Do you ever have period cramps? __ yes __ no
If yes, what do you do for the discomfort? _____

Do you bleed between periods? __ yes __ no

Do you ever use tampons? __ yes __ no

Do you ever use sponges? __ yes __ no

D.E.S. daughter? __ yes __ no

Pregnancy History

Age of first pregnancy _____

Number of:
___ pregnancies
___ living children
___ abortions
___ miscarriages

Have you ever had difficulty becoming pregnant? __

Gyn History

Age of first intercourse _____

Date of last PAP _____ LMP _____

Have you had any of the following?

no yes now
__ __ __ Vaginal discharge/infection
__ __ __ Unusual vaginal bleeding
__ __ __ Herpes
__ __ __ STD (eg, syphillis, gonorrhea, trichomonas)
__ __ __ Pelvic infection (PID)
__ __ __ Abnormalities of the uterus
__ __ __ Tumor/cysts of the ovaries
__ __ __ Pain/bleeding with intercourse
__ __ __ Abnormal PAP smear
__ __ __ Cervical lesions/biopsy/cryotherapy
__ __ __ Premenstrual symptoms (mood changes,
          water retention, headaches)
__ __ __ Toxic shock syndrome (T.S.S.)

Surgical History

List the date and type of surgery you have had:

Date   Type

_____   _____

_____   _____

_____   _____

Contraception

Have you ever used any form of birth control?
__ yes __ no

If yes, please list:

Method   Dates of use   Problems (yes/no)

_____   _____   _____

_____   _____   _____

_____   _____   _____

Present method: _____

Have you ever become pregnant while using a birth
control method? __ yes __ no _____ method

Health Habits

Average number of cups consumed per day.
__ coffee   __ tea   __ cola

Present weight is:
__ satisfactory __ unsatisfactory
__ less than   __ more than one year ago

Alcohol: How many drinks (beer, wine, hard liquor) per
week? ____

Cigarette smoking:
__ never   __ quit (when?)
How many per day? ___   How many years? ___

Marijuana use: __ yes __ no
Other street drugs: __ yes __ no

What do you do for exercise? _____

Sleep.
usually go to bed at ___, wake up at ___ Naps? ___

Breast self-examination:
__ no __ yes __ monthly __ occasionally

Sex: What questions do you have?

What concerns do you want your health care provider to
check out during your visit?

Figure 21–5. *(cont.)* Sample of a health history form. (Source: *University of Rochester, Strong Memorial Hospital, Rochester, NY, by permission.*)

events and what impact they have caused developmentally; and whether or not there has been positive adaptation to them.

The health history data can be acquired by an interview and a follow-up written summary or via a self-administered health history form. The latter is more efficient and allows for client participation. The health history is a tool that enhances communication not only between practitioner and client by helping the client to think through her particular health problems, but also as a means for practitioners to attain a comprehensive knowledge base efficiently and without repetition to the client. This tool also is a plan for future health education and health promotion by other providers and community resources. Figure 21–5 is a sample self-administered health history form used in a women's health clinic.

The form is organized so that family history, past medical history, and demographics are located on one side and the obstetrical, gynecological, contraceptive, and daily health habits are grouped together on the other side. A potential problem with self-administered forms is that they can not be used if the woman does not read or write in the language of the form.

The Teaching Process

The nursing diagnosis is differentiated from the medical diagnosis in that its primary focus is not cure, but rather care and advocacy for promoting the client's self-care goals. If health care providers have as one of their goals the promotion of self-health behaviors through education for their clients, then the care model of diagnosing alterations in a woman's health status is beneficial, especially when women are experiencing only a minor gynecological alteration. Techniques used by care providers to move in the direction of making a diagnosis are therapeutic communication and the teaching process.

Smitherman (1981) states that in therapeutic communication, a situation occurs in which one individual experiences attention on her concerns and needs so that she is helped by this interaction toward wellness. Social and formal communication methods may elicit some pertinent information; however, "it is through the use of therapeutic, individualized communications that a nurse has the greatest potential for influencing the health and well-being of patients" (Smitherman, 1981, p. 4).

The application of the first three phases of the teaching process, assessment, planning, and intervention (see Chapter 2), can be delineated by the following guide for the direction of information exchange between health care provider and client. This simplistic step by step diagnostic guide identifies the assessment and planning needs of the woman with a minor gynecological alteration and sets the stage for accomplishing the intervention needs.

1. Determine the facts (interview, history, and physical examination)
2. Diagnosis
3. Present the client with the facts
4. Determine what the diagnosis means to the client
5. Tailor education to the client's identified concerns and knowledge deficits

A pitfall that many inexperienced practitioners fall into is solely focusing on step 1, determining the facts so the correct diagnosis can be made. It is reassuring to the health care provider to make a right diagnosis. The consequence of focusing on this, however, is that the client may know what the alteration in health status is but leave without knowing its total ramifications. This picture needs to include immediate self-care promotion activities and an understanding of the diagnosis' relevance to future health maintenance. The process used to attain the scope of health promotion utilizes all five steps and does not allow the practitioner to be satisfied with just having made a diagnosis and sharing this with the client.

The following case study delineates this process.

Ms. Lake is a 26-year-old single white female who has been experiencing vulvar itching and a thin yellow-white discharge for 4 days. She has no previous history of vaginal infections. She is sexually active, uses oral contraceptives, and has a positive family history of diabetes. During the past month she has been under increased stress due to a job change. She also states that she uses tampons and has just finished her normal 5-day period.

Step 1. *Determine the facts.*
    A. History as per above (physical examination findings below)
        (1) Thyroid—nonpalpable
        (2) Breast—soft with no masses, does BSE
        (3) Abdomen—negative
        (4) Pelvic—B.U.S.—negative
            a. Vulvo/vagina—+ leukorrhea, + erythema
            b. Cervix—+ leukorrhea, NT, firm, mobile
            c. Uterus—Ant., NSSC, NT
            d. Adnexa—R and L are WNL
        (5) Extremities—WNL
        (6) Micro findings—budding yeast on KOH preparation
Step 2. *Diagnosis.*
    A. Medical diagnosis—candidiasis
    B. Nursing diagnosis—alteration in vaginal health
    C. Plan/Prescription—Rx nystatin, clotrimazole, or miconazole as per PDR
Step 3. *Present client with information.*
    A. A statement is made by the health care provider identifying the causative agent. "By symptoms, history and microscopic findings you have candidiasis often known as a yeast infection."
Step 4. *Determine what the diagnosis means to her.*
    A. The follow-up to stating the diagnosis is "What does this mean to you?" The client should be able to identify her familiarity with the diagnosis and ask for help in clarifying how the change in health status occurred and what she can do about it. If the woman is familiar with the diagnosis either by experience or having read about the subject, then the health care provider moves to step 5 and focuses on knowledge review and planning. If, however, the woman is unfamiliar with her health alteration, attention is focused on clarifying and logically providing information. The following is a sample dialogue.

Health Care Provider:	The clinical symptoms you have and the microscopic examination findings support the diagnosis of a candidiasis infection, sometimes known as a yeast infection. What does this mean to you?
Client:	I don't know. I've never had a vaginal infection before. Is this a contagious or venereal disease? How did I get it?
Health Care Provider:	(If the woman is anxious it is important to address the anxiety before proceeding with the facts.) You appear to be upset by the diagnosis. What is distressing you the most?
Client:	That I don't know if it is curable and I may give it to my lover.

Health Care Provider: You have some very normal concerns. Let me help by giving you information that may explain how you got the infection and how to take care of it. (The practitioner then proceeds to synthesize the interview and history data so the patient understands the origin of the change). First let me list the predisposing factors to a candidiasis infection.*

      pregnancy
      diabetes
      oral contraceptive use
      frequent douching
      allergic reactions
      antibiotic therapy
      Metronidazole (Flagyl) therapy
      excessive carbohydrate intake
      psychogenic problems/stress
      obesity
      poor hygiene practices
      debilitation
      hypoparathyroidism

As you can see there are several factors that apply to you. So that you can understand this condition let me explain what candida is.

It is a common ingredient of soil, vegetation, and many dairy products. Vaginal cultures reveal its occurrence in 4 to 6 percent of nonpregnant women and in 10 to 30 percent of pregnant women. It is considered a common vaginal and rectal inhabitant, and infection is attributed to a change in host resistance rather than to a contagious factor. Infection is caused by alteration of the vaginal environment by increasing its glycogen content or by changing its normal acid pH to an alkaline pH.*

Candidiasis is not considered to be a sexually transmitted disease. This suggests that you will not give it to your partner. However, if your partner has symptoms of penis discharge, pain or rash, he should be seen by his health care provider.

Step 5. *Tailor education to the woman's identified concerns.*

    A. At this stage in the client interaction the health care provider can focus on the mode of treatment or on client teaching depending on which the client prefers.

        For the woman presenting with a candidiasis infection, the following table identifies the behavioral objectives associated with the teaching plan and desired outcomes of the client's activities and therapeutic regimen (Table 21–1).

So far three components of the teaching process have been covered. The fourth and possibly most important is the evaluation phase. In the presented case the health care provider either schedules a return appointment for the client to be reexamined for the presence of the microorganism, or has the client telephone with a self-assessment of her response to the treatment regimen. When the evaluation phase is completed, the health care provider can begin to evaluate objectively her care giving abilities for the particular individual.

---

*Source: Neeson & Stockdale, 1981, p. 131.

TABLE 21–1. DIAGNOSIS: ALTERATION IN VAGINAL HEALTH—CANDIDIASIS

Behavioral Objectives	Teaching Guidelines
The client	
1. Identifies the transmitting and predisposing factors	1. Review with client good personal health habits a. Cleanliness, including hand washing, is important prior to sexual activity. b. Cleansing from front to back after a bowel movement decreases potential vaginal contamination. c. Avoid use of feminine hygiene sprays, bath oils, or strong soaps on vulva or in vagina; they may cause an allergic reaction. d. Avoid clothing that promotes moisture retention, for example: pantyhose, nylon underwear, clothes that fit tightly in the crotch. e. Reoccurrence is also noted during periods of increased stress or high carbohydrate consumption for some women.
2. Can describe specific treatment regimen for candidiasis	2. Reinforce the purpose for adhering to a specific treatment regimen a. Stress continuing the ordered medication throughout the menstrual cycle and not stopping treatment when symptoms disappear. b. Advise patients with vulvar irritation to take warm sitz baths. c. Advise patients to have partners use condoms during intercourse at time of treatment. d. Suggest to patients with chronic or recurrent infections to increase personal hygiene and to use medication at bedtime a week before the menses. e. Prescribed treatment may be either Nystatin vaginal tablets: bid for 7 to 14 days or Clotrimazol vaginal tablets or Miconazole nitrate cream: one tablet or applicator full at bedtime for 7 nights, or miconizol nitrate 200mg suppositories at bedtime for three nights.
3. Identifies preventive measures	3. Preventive measures a. Caution against reinfection from contact with bath towels, soiled clothing, used douche tips, or poor hygiene habits. b. "Discuss with the patient the correct method of douching and caution her against its daily use except when infection is present. Once-a-week douching using a vinegar solution when no infection is present is adequate, if at all; overuse can cause drying and changes in the normal vaginal environment" (Neeson & Stockdale, 1981, p. 134). c. Advise that an alternative contraceptive method may be necessary for the oral contraceptive user with recurrent or chronic infection.
4. Can select appropriate self-help remedies	4. Offer self-help remedies: this assists the woman in active participation in her own health maintenance, especially at times when she is unable to obtain immediate medical attention a. Plain yogurt inserted into the vagina with applicator b. Eating 8 ounces of yogurt a day with the onset of symptoms c. Lactobacillus tablets (one or two) placed in the vagina at first sign of symptoms d. Eating increased quantities of garlic e. Daily vitamin consumption can also help prevent the onset; for some women B-complex in large amounts is effective; so are vitamins A, C, and E. (Federation of Feminist Women's Health Centers, 1981, p. 27)

TABLE 21–2. DIAGNOSIS: ALTERATION IN VAGINAL HEALTH—TRICHOMONIASIS

Behavioral Objectives	Teaching Guidelines
The client	
1. Identifies the transmitting and predisposing factors	1. Review personal health habits and means of sexual transmission a. Inform patient that this is a sexually transmitted disease b. "Inform the patient that reinfection may occur after local treatment because the organism remains in 96% of the extra-vaginal sites such as the paraurethral glands, urethra, and endocervix" (Neeson & Stockdale, 1981, p. 138).
2. Can describe the specific treatment regimen for trichomoniasis	2. Reinforce the purpose for adhering to a specific treatment regimen a. Prescribe 2 g stat dose of Flagyl (metronidazole) for both patient and partner. Advise that this drug be taken simultaneously by both partners. When this is not possible, prescribe Flagyl for the woman and instruct her partner to abstain from sexual contact for a week or wear a condom during intercourse for a week. Alcohol consumption is contraindicated due to its antabuse effect during Flagyl therapy. Common side effects from this drug are unpleasant taste in the mouth, nausea, diarrhea, abdominal cramping, headache, vomiting, or dizziness. b. Advise the patient with multiple sexual partners that systemic treatment is inappropriate because reinfection usually occurs. Treatment with a vaginal medication in conjunction with the partner using a condom is recommended. c. Advise the patient to refrain from intercourse during treatment or to have her partner use a condom. d. Advise the patient against using vaginal tampons when treating with a local medication. Tampons interfere with medication absorption and the healing process.
3. Identifies preventive measures	3. Suggest preventive measures a. "Inform the patient that a strongly acidic douche (2 table-spoons of vinegar to 1 quart of warm water) immediately after intercourse with an infected male may be helpful in preventing infection" (Neeson & Stockdale, 1981, p. 138). b. Explain that eating cultured plain yogurt every day during antibiotic therapy may diminish gastric upset c. Advise the patient with a new partner to use condoms
4. Can select appropriate self-help remedies	4. Self-help remedies a. Douching with povidine–iodine (betadine). Greatest success has occurred when this is continued for a week following a menstrual period. Note: pregnant women should not use Betadine b. Garlic clove suppository. To prepare, peel a clove, making sure not to nick the edge, for the juice may cause a burning sensation. In a piece of gauze approximately 1 foot long by 1 inch wide, place the clove. Fold the gauze in half and twist it below the clove, then make a tampon with a gauze tail. The garlic end can then be dipped in a vegetable oil and then inserted. It may be changed every 12 hours for 3 to 5 days (Federation of Feminist Women's Health Centers, p. 26). c. Garlic pearles; take one twice a day for 1 week.

Short- and Long-term Planning

The short-term planning goals are directed toward achieving the health outcome that resolves the presenting problem. As in the previous case, the focus is to identify the client's knowledge base and then supplement it with the pertinent details so the woman can implement the treatment regimen. During this process the long-term planning goals may be identified to include not only prevention measures but also additional educational materials that promote health in general. Publications such as *Our Bodies, Ourselves, Woman's Body in Control, A New View of a Woman's Body*, or *How to Stay Out of the Gynecologist's Office* (see bibliography) could be used during the client's visit and suggested as references or purchasable books to use outside of the health care provider's office.

The succeeding tables (Tables 21–2 to 21–15) outline the behavioral objectives and

TABLE 21–3. DIAGNOSIS: ALTERATION IN VAGINAL HEALTH—HEMOPHILUS, CORYNEBACTERIUM, GARDNERELLA VAGINITIS, OR BACTERIAL VAGINALIS (B. V.)

Behavioral Objectives	Teaching Guidelines
The client	

1. Identifies the transmitting and predisposing factors	1. Review personal health habits and means of sexual transmission
	   a. Tell the patient what her infection is and how it is to be treated.
	   b. Stress good personal hygiene and the need to cleanse from front to back after a bowel movement and to avoid long hours of tampon use.

2. Can describe the specific treatment regimen	2. Reinforce purpose for adhering to specific treatment regimen
	   a. Prescribe Flagyl 500 mg BID for 7 to 10 days. Discuss the use of Flagyl (Table 21–2).
	   b. Advise the patient who has been prescribed tetracycline to take it 1 hour before or 2 hours after meals. Food and dairy products often interfere with its absorption. This treatment is contraindicated in pregnancy.
	   c. Advise the patient to continue treatment even when she has her menstrual period.
	   d. Advise the patient to refrain from sexual intercourse during the treatment or to have her partner use a condom until treatment is complete.
	   e. Suggest the use of a perineal (mini) pad when vaginal creams or suppositories have been ordered to prevent soiling of clothes or prolonged contact with moisture.
	   f. "Explain that eating cultured plain yogurt every day during antibiotic therapy may diminish gastric upset and inhibit a secondary yeast infection of the vagina" (Neeson & Stockdale, 1981, p. 142).

3. Identifies preventive measures	3. Suggest preventive methods a. Advise the patient that her partner will need treatment, or she may be reinfected.

4. Can select appropriate self-help remedies	4. Self-help remedies
	   a. Ingestion of large amounts of all the B vitamins including 100 mg of B_1, B_2, B_6 and 200 mg B_8 and pantothenic acid.
	   b. A tablespoon of vinegar and the oil of one garlic clove in 1 quart of warm water. Use once or twice a day for 3–5 days.
	   c. Also helpful is betadine douche or goldenseal powder in ½ cup warm water twice a day for up to 2 weeks (Federation of Feminist Women's Health Centers, 1981, p. 28).

TABLE 21–4. DIAGNOSIS: ALTERATION IN VAGINAL HEALTH—GONORRHEA

Behavioral Objectives	Teaching Guidelines
The client	
1. Identifies the transmitting and predisposing factors	1. Review personal health habits and means of sexual transmission a. Tell the patient that she has gonorrhea. Explain that this is a highly infectious disease spread by sexual intercourse with an infected person. The contact person needs to be notified so that appropriate examination and treatment occur. Treatment is not successful unless both partners are treated.

2. Can describe the specific treatment regimen for gonorrhea	2. Reinforce purpose for adhering to a specific treatment regimen
	    a. In lower tract disease ambulatory treatment will cure the disease but only when the prescription is taken as directed. Follow-up for test of cure is important and accomplished by having the patient return 1 week after completion of the medication for a repeat cervical, rectal, and throat culture.
	    b. Pelvic rest is important. Patients should not engage in intercourse or any activity that jars the pelvis. Bed rest is encouraged in a semi-Fowler's position which maintains a downward pressure and prevents upward spread.
	    c. Instruct all patients to maintaining an adequate fluid intake and a diet high in protein and vitamins.
	    d. "Explain to the patient who is to be hospitalized why this is necessary. She needs parenteral antibiotic therapy to halt further spread of the infection and peritonitis and close surveillance of her infection to assure proper medication, bed rest, and control of painful symptoms. Swift and conservative action will also enhance her future fertility" (Neeson & Stockdale, 1981, p. 181).

3. Identifies preventive measures	3. Suggest preventive measures
	    a. Help the patient to identify at risk situations. If her sexual partner is not well known to her or has signs of a rash or discharge, she needs to insist that he wear a condom or abstain from intercourse.
	    b. Explain that eating cultured plain yogurt each day during antibiotic therapy may diminish gastric upset.
	    c. Risk of tubal damage is great unless treatment regimen is adhered to.
	    d. Avoid multiple partners.
	    e. Spermicides provide some protection. Use condoms.

4. Can select appropriate self-help remedies	4. Self-help remedies a. Antibiotics are the only sure form of treatment known today.

teaching guidelines for several medical conditions that can be categorized under the heading of Alterations in Vaginal Health and Menstruation. The assessment and planning for women with this diagnosis is short-term because these alterations are not immediately life-threatening. However, there may be long-term physical ramifications if treatment is not successful. The psychological side effects, for example, guilt and embarrassment associated with having a sexually transmitted disease, need to be assessed simultaneously with the physical complaint if successful teaching and treatment outcome are to be achieved.

TABLE 21–5. DIAGNOSIS: ALTERATION IN VAGINAL HEALTH—CONDYLOMATA ACUMINATA: VENEREAL WARTS

Behavioral Objectives	Teaching Guidelines
The client	

1. Identifies the transmitting and predisposing factors	1. Review personal health habits and means of sexual transmission
	  a. Explain what the lesions are and how they were acquired.
	  b. Explain that the warts can be cured, especially if the patient completes treatment and her partner is treated at the same time. Reinfection can occur.

2. Can describe the specific treatment regimen for condylomata acuminata	2. Reinforce the purpose for adhering to a specific treatment regimen
	  a. Advise the patient to maintain a clean and dry vulva. This is an important way to speed recovery; a damp environment enhances the growth of warts.
	  b. When treating vaginitis with a vaginal medication, sometimes spontaneous disappearance of a small condylomata will occur.
	  c. Advise patients treated with podophyllin or Nevitol, to wash it off carefully with soap and water in 4 to 6 hours. Prolonged contact may burn the skin.
	    The lesion may also become painful several hours after this treatment. This pain should not last long. The lesions will start sloughing 2 to 4 days after treatment. Treatment may have to continue every 1 to 2 weeks until all the lesions have cleared (Neeson & Stockdale, 1981, p. 176).
	  d. Warts not able to be treated with podophyllin are treated with cryosurgery or electrocautery.

3. Identifies preventive measures	3. Support preventive measures
	  a. Advise the patient that if she ever sees a lesion on her sexual partner, to refrain from intercourse. Recurrent infections are possible.
	  b. Avoid multiple partners
	  c. Use condoms
	  d. Watch for podophyllin poisoning. Symptoms: lethargy, coma, nausea, and diarrhea

4. Can select appropriate self-help remedies	4. Self-help remedies a. Important to know how to detect these raised lesions so that treatment is begun early

TABLE 21–6. DIAGNOSIS: ALTERATION IN VAGINAL HEALTH—HERPES GENITALIS

Behavioral Objectives	Teaching Guidelines
The client	

1. Identifies the transmitting and predisposing factors	1. Review personal health habits and means of sexual transmission
	   a. Discuss with the woman that this infection is of viral origin and that reoccurrence is possible at any time.
	   b. Advise the client to abstain from sexual intercourse (oral or genital) if either partner has signs of infection. If lesions are confined to the penis, vagina, or cervix, condoms should be used until shedding or all signs of infection have ceased (Neeson & Stockdale, 1981, p. 173).
	   c. Discuss general hygiene measures and life-style changes with the patient to prevent secondary infection and assist in the patients' adaption to their diagnosed condition.

2. Can describe the specific treatment regimen for herpes genitalis	2. Reinforce the purpose for adhering to a specific treatment regimen
	   a. Experimental drugs are now being marketed. Consult PDR for appropriate use. For primary occurrence prescribe Zovorax 200 mg capsules, one every 4 hours.
	   b. Support for pregnant patients includes counseling and information about cesarean section delivery when herpetic lesions are present on vulva, in the vagina, or on the cervix.
	   c. Advise the client with burning during urination to pour warm water over the vulva. If unable to void, contact health care provider for potential need to catheterize.

3. Identifies preventive measures	3. Suggest preventive measures
	   a. Counsel patients with frequent recurrent attacks to seek emotional support for psychological and sociological stressors associated with repeated infections.
	   b. Discuss factors that may be helpful to preventing reactivation of the virus. One common predisposing factor is elevation of body temperature. The following guidelines may be useful to the patient:
	       "Protect self from prolonged exposure to the heat of the sun
	       Avoid overheating and irritation of vulva with hot baths or tight clothing
	       Avoid friction from prolonged intercourse by using a lubricant (K-Y jelly, vegetable oil, saliva)
	       Use aspirin to maintain lowered body temperature before the onset of the menses if reoccurrence is associated with the menstrual period" (Neeson & Stockdale, 1981, p. 173).
	   c. Annual Pap smears

4. Can select appropriate self-help remedies	4. Self-help remedies
	   a. HELP is a national organization formed to assist victims of HVH-2 (HELP, Box 100, Palo Alto, CA 94302). Its newsletter provides information on the latest research (Neeson & Stockdale, 1981, p. 173).
	   b. Increasing vitamins, B-complex, C, E and A at times when one is run down or under stress may help prevent recurrence.
	   c. L-Lysine menohydrochloride and amlive acid have helped speed the healing of herpes. For recurrent herpes: 300–500 mg of lysine daily when active lesions are not visible and 800–1000 mg if sores were present (Federation of Feminist Women's Health Centers, 1981, p. 21).
	   d. Topical applications of zinc oxide, neosporin, Campho-Phenique and Xylocain jelly as well as peppermint tea bags and preparations of golden seal, myrrh, ground comfrey root, sap of aloe vera leaves have been used to relieve discomfort

TABLE 21–7. DIAGNOSIS: ALTERATION IN VAGINAL HEALTH—TOXIC SHOCK SYNDROME (TSS)

Behavioral Objectives	Teaching Guidelines
The client	

1. Identifies the transmitting and predisposing factors	1. Review etiology and good personal health habits
	   a. A rare but serious illness that women may contract during or after their menstrual period primarily associated with the use of tampons
	   b. The bacteria Staphylococus aureus is believed to be the causative agent
	   c. Identifying symptoms are fever, fatigue, weakness, muscle aches, rash (specifically on the hands), severe diarrhea, and rapid shock (extremely low blood pressure)
	   d. Women at greatest risk are:
	     (1) Women who insert tampons with their fingers instead of an applicator
	     (2) Women who have had a chronic discharge in the past year
	     (3) Women with problematic herpes infections

2. Knows the treatment for TSS	2. Reinforce the purpose for adhering to a specific treatment regimen
	   a. Call the health care provider upon first notice of symptoms
	   b. Follow prescribed antibiotic regimen

3. Identifies preventive measures	3. Suggest preventive measures
	   a. Avoid using super plus tampons or those with synthetic abrasive fibers
	   b. Change tampons every 2 to 4 hours. Alternate tampon and pad use so menses washes vaginal lining and prevents abrasions from tampon irritation.
	   c. Wear pads when sleeping to decrease hours of tampon exposure
	   d. Wash hands before inserting a tampon
	   e. Spread the labia lips so tampon is not exposed to external contamination prior to insertion

4. Can select appropriate self-help remedies	4. Self-help remedies a. Antibiotics are the only sure form of treatment known today

TABLE 21–8. DIAGNOSIS: ALTERATION IN MENSTRUAL FUNCTION—AMENORRHEA

Behavioral Objectives	Teaching Guidelines
The client	
1. Identifies the source for this alteration	1. Review normal menstrual cycle and female anatomy a. Differentiate primary from secondary amenorrhea. b. Identify the different levels of dysfunction that can occur—uterus, ovaries, pituitary, and hypothalamus (Fritz & Speroff, 1983; Marut & Dawood, 1983) c. R/O the possibility of pregnancy. d. Establish what level of knowledge the woman has pertaining to her body. e. Explain why diagnostic tests need to be done and which ones will be ordered.
2. Can describe the treatment regimen for amenorrhea	2. Reinforce the purpose for adhering to a specific treatment regimen a. To diagnose the source for the amenorrhea may take time—compliance with the laboratory and clinic visits needs to be explained and understood. b. If drug therapy is to be used, compliance with the schedule is to be reinforced and supported.
3. Identifies preventive measures	3. Suggest preventive measures a. Primary amenorrhea—not applicable b. Clients not desiring a pregnancy need to use contraception (ovulation may occur). Foam, condoms, and diaphragms are preferrable to OCPs that may interfere with diagnostic tests. c. Clients with no physiological basis for lack of periods need further analysis for possible influence of psychologic or stress factors. Counseling appointments may be appropriate.

4. Can select appropriate self-help remedies	4. Self-help remedies
	a. Primary—not applicable
	b. Secondary
	  (1) Clients with asymptomatic post pill amenorrhea need to wait 6 months for their menses to return before seeking evaluation.
	  (2) Obese clients need to be encouraged to lose weight—a factor that is helpful in reestablishing normal menses.
	  (3) Athletes who experience this problem need to be evaluated and if no underlying pathology is present, counseled and given appropriate support in order to cope with this condition.

TABLE 21–9. DIAGNOSIS: ALTERATION IN MENSTRUAL FUNCTION—DYSFUNCTIONAL UTERINE BLEEDING (DUB)

Behavioral Objectives	Teaching Guidelines
The client	

1. Identifies the source for this alteration	1. Review normal menstrual cycle and female anatomy
	  a. Bleeding between periods or heavy bleeding at the time of menses is not normal.
	    (1) Menorrhagia is increased menstrual bleeding.
	    (2) Metrorrhagia is bleeding at time other than during menstruation.
	  b. If no pathological process co-exists, identify the probable cause
	  c. In the differential diagnosis R/O hemorrhage, polyps, or other sources than uterus for origin of bleeding.

2. Can describe the treatment regimen for DUB	2. Reinforce the purpose for adhering to a specific treatment regimen
	  a. Prescribed hormone therapy may take months of treatment to establish regular cycles. Normal function will probably resume at that time with the possible exception of the perimenopausal woman.
	  b. Medication regimens if not adhered to may cause vaginal bleeding to persist.
	  c. When OCPs are used, their effectiveness, use, and side effects as a contraceptive need to be explained.
	  d. Heavy bleeding may occur after the initial treatment for anovulation or after the progesterone withdrawal test.
	  e. Clients who need a D&C need to be given information about the procedure and understand that the reason for this procedure is to scrape the thickened endometrial lining of the uterus. The result is usually a return of normal cycles.

3. Identifies preventive measures	3. Suggest preventive measures
	  a. Underlying stressors (e.g., sexual problems, change in work) are identified so change can be initiated.
	  b. Good dietary habits, a well-balanced diet and one high in iron.
	  c. Good personal hygiene, especially when bleeding to prevent infection or odor.

4. Can select appropriate self-help remedies	4. Self-help remedies
	  a. Understands her normal menstrual cycle so she can detect deviations.
	  b. Modify life-style if DUB is persistent.
	  c. Contact HCP (especially teens experiencing DUB) for reassurance and further information.

TABLE 21–10. DIAGNOSIS: ALTERATION IN MENSTRUAL FUNCTION—DYSMENORRHEA

Behavioral Objectives	Teaching Guidelines
The client	

1. Identifies the source for this alteration	1. Review normal menstrual cycle and female anatomy
	a. Differentiate between primary and secondary dysmenorrhea
	  (1) Primary is painful menstrual cramps without any macroscopically identifiable underlying pelvic pathology.
	  (2) Secondary is painful menstrual cramps due to a macroscopically identifiable underlying pelvic pathology. Causes include endometriosis, IUDs, PID, adenomyosis, cervical strictures or stenosis, ovarian cysts, congenital malformations of the Mullerian system and uterine adhesions, polyps, and/or myomas (Dawood, 1983, p. 719–720)
	b. Identify the onset and quality.
	  (1) Primary—within 2 yr of the onset of menarche. 48–72 hours duration, cramp-like character to the pain, and normal pelvic exam (Webster, 1980).
	  (2) Secondary—not generally associated with onset of menarche except possibly with endometriosis. Diagnosis can be aided by lab findings: complete blood count (CBC), erythrocyte sedimentation rate, pelvic sonograms, and genital cultures.
	c. Have client identify how she has coped with menstrual pain previously and what specific means of relief have been used.
	d. Incidence in the United States was approximately 43% in 1980 (Dawood, 1983, p. 719).

2. Can describe the treatment regimen for dysmenorrhea	2. Reinforce the purpose for adhering to a specific treatment regimen
	a. Primary
	  (1) Clients prescribed oral contraceptives will experience cessation of cramps because of anovulatory cycles.
	  (2) Drug therapy instruction should include dosage, frequency and what side effects may occur. Side effects need to be reported to the HCP. Analgesics (narcotic and nonnarcotic) or prostaglandin synthetase inhibitors Type I are most often used.
	  (3) Explore further the psychosocial problems identified during the visit. Make an appropriate referral for counseling if indicated (Young & Reame, 1983).
	b. Secondary
	  (1) Give instructions regarding the indicated diagnostic procedure: laparoscopy, hysteroscopy, D & C (dilation and curettage).

3. Identifies preventive measures	3. Suggest preventive measures a. Primary Proper diet and routine exercise are important to maintain optimum health. b. Secondary Identify causative agent, treat and prevent reoccurrence.
4. Can select appropriate self-help remedies	4. Self-help remedies a. Contact with HCP for counseling and monitoring of treatment effectiveness is appropriate. b. Clients not taking OCPs are encouraged to assess ovulation by recording events on a calendar. This may also assist clients who need to start medications prior to the onset of menses. c. Specific exercises are helpful: pelvic rock; relaxation method; stretching methods: the Cobra and the bow; mas-

TABLE 21–10. (cont.)

Behavioral Objectives	Teaching Guidelines
	sage direct pressure or polarity. (See either publication by the Federation of Feminist Women's Health Centers for descriptions.) d. Contact warmth: hot baths, heating pads, or hands e. Drink warm liquids: soup or herbal teas—yarrow, peppermint, red raspberry leaf, pennyroyal, mugwort, chamomile, ginger root, parsley, thyme, and spice bush. f. Learning how to use autogenic relaxation training facilitated by vaginal thermofeedback as biofeedback therapy for alleviation of dysmenorrhea (Heczey, 1980, p. 289).

TABLE 21–11. DIAGNOSIS: ALTERATION IN MENSTRUAL FUNCTION—PREMENSTRUAL SYNDROME (PMS)

Behavioral Objectives	Teaching Guidelines
The client 1. Identifies the source of this alteration	1. Review normal menstrual cycle and female anatomy a. A condition characterized by a variety of somatic and psychological symptoms that occur regularly during a particular phase of the menstrual cycle (Neeson & Stockdale, 1981, p. 229). b. Incidence reported to be between 30–50% of menstruating women (Neeson & Stockdale, 1981, p. 229). c. Four patterns of PMS.[a] 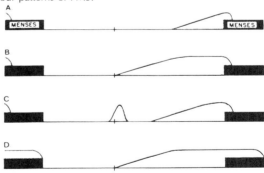 d. Pathophysiology theories: (1) Hypothalamic contribution—progesterone withdrawal or insufficiency resulting in an excess of estrogen may be the precipitating factor. (2) Endocrine contributions—fluid retention previously thought to be dependent on aldosterone and prolactin levels is now felt to be due to increased carbohydrate and salt consumption (Reid & Yen, 1983, p. 712). (3) Hypoglycemia contributions—causal relationships not yet proven but symptoms are evident (Reid & Yen, 1983, p. 712).

(continued)

TABLE 21–11. (cont.)

Behavioral Objectives	Teaching Guidelines
The client	
	(4) Psychosomatic dysfunction—felt to be a dramatization of underlying conflicts with her mother. This theory is not well supported.
	e. Encourage use of a menstrual calendar where client can record symptoms, activities, drug use, and response in the premenstrual phase.
2. Can describe the treatment regimen for premenstrual syndrome	2. Reinforce the purpose for adhering to a specific treatment regimen
	a. Maintain a well-balanced diet and sufficient exercise. Salt restriction needs to be emphasized.
	b. While sufficient exercise is necessary, increased need for rest and relaxation is important during the period of time when symptoms are most severe.
	c. Drug therapy may include OCPs or antiprostaglandins. Analgesics may be helpful to relieve headaches or musculoskeletal pains. Diuretic therapy should be avoided except in the final week of the cycle.
	d. Pyridoxine (vitamin B_6) may be used (25–50 mg), twice per day. Used to help decrease moodiness and irritability, this is under review due to recent investigation (N.E.J.M., Aug. 25, 1983).
3. Identifies preventive measures	3. Suggest preventive measures
	a. Explore what activities and interest beyond work and home the client has.
	b. Encourage discussions and participation of family members during client visits to help facilitate better understanding.
4. Can select appropriate self-help remedies	4. Self-help remedies
	a. Focused on identifying monthly symptoms and preparing for them by appropriate dietary and exercise adjustments.
	b. Contact with HCP for support and reassurance.
	c. See Table 21–10 self-help remedies.

[a]*Source: Reid, R. L., & Yen, S. S. C. The premenstrual syndrome. Clinical Obstetrics and Gynecology, 1983, 26(3), 711, by permission.*

TABLE 21–12. DIAGNOSIS: ALTERATION IN PELVIC HEALTH—CERVICITIS

Behavioral Objectives	Teaching Guidelines
The client	

1. Identifies the source for this alteration	1. Review normal menstrual cycle and female anatomy
	  a. Identify the location of the infection using pictures or diagrams of the female pelvic organs. Direct observation of the cervix, by use of a mirror when the speculum is in the vagina, may add clarity to the explanation.
	  b. Refer to the teaching guidelines for gonorrhea (Table 21–4) when counseling a client with this diagnosis.
	  c. When the infection is not gonoccocal in origin, identify the causative agent if known.

2. Can describe the treatment regimen for cervicitis	2. Reinforce the purpose for adhering to the treatment regimen
	  a. Emphasize to the client who is not to be hospitalized for an acute infection the need for bed rest to prevent spread of infection to her uterus, fallopian tubes, or peritoneum.
	  b. Instruct the client to refrain from sexual intercourse until the infection has cleared, or advise the use of a condom if abstinence is unavoidable.
	  c. To attain optimum recovery, prescribed oral antibiotics or local treatment plans need to be followed as ordered.
	  d. Counseling about the use of cryosurgery or electrocautery includes the procedure, anticipated results, and necessary follow-up postprocedure.

3. Identifies preventive measures	3. Suggests preventive measures
	  a. PAP smears at least once a year help detect the health status of the cervix.
	  b. Condom use with intercourse helps decrease exposure of contaminating agents.
	  c. Recess from the use of OCPs or IUD may be necessary when states of infection, hypoestrogenism, or hypovitaminosis are present.
	  d. Cervical infections are usually cleared with good treatment and follow-up. The mild infection may resolve in 4–8 weeks while severe infections may take 2–3 months.
	  e. Increased production of purulent discharge sometimes coincident with pelvic pain are warning signs that need to be brought to the attention of the HCP.

4. Can select appropriate self-help remedies	4. Self-help remedies
	  a. Antibiotic therapy is the most widely understood and supported means of treatment.
	  b. Home remedies that have shown varying degrees of success.
	    (1) Use of vitamin E oil, honey or aloe vera juice applied to the reddened cervix by use of a cotton swab. (Federation of Feminist Women's Health Centers, 1981, p. 33)
	    (2) Abstinence from coitus or a change in position may alleviate symptoms.

TABLE 21–13. DIAGNOSIS: ALTERATION IN PELVIC HEALTH—PELVIC INFLAMMATORY DISEASE (PID)

Behavioral Objectives	Teaching Guidelines
The client	
1. Identifies the source for this alteration	1. Review normal menstrual cycle and female anatomy a. The most common complication of an untreated or recurrent gonorrheal infection b. Incidence: 10–17% of women with gonorrhea (Fogel & Woods, 1981, p. 235) c. An infectious process that may involve one or more of the following structures—ovaries, fallopian tubes, pelvic peritoneum, pelvic connective tissue, or veins. The most common sites are the fallopian tubes. d. Pain is the most common complaint.
2. Can describe the treatment regimen for PID	2. Reinforce the purpose for adhering to the specific treatment regimen (Table 21–4)
3. Identifies preventive measures	3. Suggest preventive measures (Table 21–4)
4. Can select appropriate self-help remedies	4. Self-help remedies (Table 21–4)

TABLE 21–14. DIAGNOSIS: ALTERATION IN PELVIC HEALTH—ENDOMETRITIS

Behavioral Objectives	Teaching Guidelines
The client	
1. Identifies the source for this alteration	1. Review normal menstrual cycle and female anatomy a. Explain that this is an infectious process affecting the inner lining of the uterus and possibly other adjacent structures. b. With the client who has repeated endometrial infections assess the woman's desire for future pregnancy. Note that with each infection future fertility is compromised. c. Sexual history and consequential counseling is advised.
2. Can describe the treatment regimen for endometritis	2. Reinforce the purpose of adhering to the specific treatment regimen (Table 21–4)
3. Identifies preventive measures	3. Suggest preventive measures (Table 21–4)
4. Can select appropriate self-help remedies	4. Self-help remedies (Table 21–4)

TABLE 21–15. DIAGNOSIS: ALTERATION IN PELVIC HEALTH—ENDOMETRIOSIS

Behavioral Objectives	Teaching Guidelines
The client	
1. Identifies the source for this alteration	1. Review normal menstrual cycle and female anatomy 　a. Assess the client's knowledge of the disease and potential for symptoms, complications, treatment, and fertility. 　b. "Counsel client with mild or moderate disease that with proper hormonal or surgical treatment, 50–80% will have relief from pain and return of fertility" (Neeson & Stockdale, 1981, p. 240). 　c. Explain or reinforce the physician's explanation of surgical procedures to clients who are candidates.
2. Can describe the specific treatment regimen for endometriosis	2. Reinforce purpose for adhering to a specific treatment regimen 　a. Describe drug–therapy; its purpose, the plan and the necessity to follow the prescribed regimen. Drug side effects need to be reported to HCP. All antiprostaglandins need a special prescription. 　b. Support the client in expressing her fears and concerns about surgery. 　c. Reassure the client anticipating radical surgery that for most women the treatment is successful.
3. Identifies preventive measures	3. Suggest preventive measures 　a. Prepare for the client's physical well-being by stressing adequate nutrition prior to surgery. 　b. Offer the client a referral for psychological support or nutrition counseling. 　c. A home assessment for surgical patients will identify the supports necessary when the woman returns home postoperatively.
4. Can select appropriate self-help remedies	4. Self-help remedies 　a. Not appropriate when surgery is indicated. 　b. Encourage the client to contact her HCP whenever she feels anxious or needs clarification, and to keep scheduled appointments.

SUMMARY

This chapter has presented a process framework for approaching women with alterations in gynecological health. Theoretical models, HBM and Bermosk and Porter, which organize care and support a holistic approach to client's needs assessment, were illustrated so health care providers could enhance the organization of short-term and long-term health care goals for their clients. The teaching process was identified as a means to address an individual client's needs and to complement her health promoting behaviors. Furthermore, three specific areas where an alteration in gynecological health status occur were delineated and the health promoting activities were outlined in the teaching guidelines. It is anticipated that when the health care provider utilizes this theoretical and practice framework approach to women's health care, then the goals of increasing self-help activities and health promoting behaviors will culminate in a happier, healthier woman while also strengthening the effectiveness of the health care provider/client relationship.

BIBLIOGRAPHY

Argüelles, J., & Argüelles, M. *Mandala*. Berkley, Calif.: Shambala, 1972.

Beachman, D. W., & Beachman, W. D. *Synopsis of gynecology* (10th ed.). New York: C. V. Mosby, 1982. *(Medical text with readily understandable medical information.)*

Becker, M. H. (Ed.). *Health belief model and personal health belief*. Thorofare, N.J.: Charles B. Slack, 1974. *(This book describes the theory base for the health belief model and devotes several chapters to the application of the model in practice. The cost to benefit ratio for monitoring changes in health behaviors is emphasized. Charts and diagrams are used to help explain the theory.)*

Becker, M. H., Haefner, D. P., Kasl, S. V., Kirscht, J. P., Maiman, L. A., & Rosenstock, I. M. Selected psychosocial models and correlates of individual health-related behavior. *Medical Care Supplement*, 1977, *15*(5), 27–46.

Bermosk, L. S., & Porter, S. E. *Women's health and human wholeness*. New York: Appleton-Century-Crofts, 1979. *(This book offers health care providers of women a language and philosophical foundation for their practice. The chapter "The Women's Healing Model" contains the mandala, the organizing symbol that depicts the process and parts of the human wholeness philosophy. The book reviews both eastern and western philosophies and practices of medicine.)*

Ceccio, J. F., & Ceccio, C. M. *Effective communication in nursing: Theory and practice*. New York: John Wiley & Sons, 1982. *(This book is a useful guide for all nurses who teach and practice. Written communication is emphasized. Creative suggestions are illustrated by exercises and diagrams. Utilizes principles of the Roy Adaptation Model.)*

Chalker, R. (Ed.). *A new view of a woman's body*. New York: Simon & Schuster, 1981. *(A basic reference book that every woman should own. Put together by the Federation of Feminist Women's Health Centers, it can boast excellent pictures and diagrams, and presents good self-care suggestions for when one is experiencing an alteration in pelvic health (refer to chapter, Universal Health Problems of Women).)*

Chin, R. The utility and system models and developmental models of practitioners. In J. P. Riehl & C. Roy (Eds.), *Conceptual models for nurse practice*. New York: Appleton-Century-Crofts, 1974. *(The author discusses three models of change a practitioner can utilize: the system model, the developmental model, and the model for "changing." The models are outlined and compared. This chapter defines terminology and gives the base from which later sections of the book explore specific conceptual models.)*

Dawood, M. Y. Dysmenorrhea. *Clinical Obstetrics and Gynecology*, 1983, *26*(3), 719–727. *(Current article giving the diagnostic, physiological, and medical management ramifications of this health condition. Good illustrations.)*

Dukes, Sr. M. E. M. The need for autonomous choice. In H. Yura & M. B. Walsh (Eds.), *Human needs 2 and the nursing process*. Norwalk, Conn.: Appleton-Century-Crofts, 1982. *(The author defines the nature of humans philosophically and the inherent need to attain autonomy throughout his/her life. Nursing implications regarding this theory and examples of the nursing process are described.)*

Federation of Feminist Women's Health Centers. *How to stay out of the gynecologist's office*. Culver City, Conn.: Peace Press, 1981. *(Another sophisticated publication from the Federation of Feminist Women's Health Care Centers. Excellent illustrations by Suzann Gage. Includes a medical terminology dictionary.)*

Fogel, C. I. The gynecologic triad: Discharge, pain, and bleeding. In C. I. Fogel & N. F. Woods (Eds.), *Health care of women—A nursing perspective*. St. Louis, Mo.: C. V. Mosby, 1981. *(The author discusses medical diagnosis of altered gynecological health from the symptoms of discharge, pain, and bleeding. Very thorough and with good descriptive pictures and charts. Addresses some teaching needs in the sections titled "Preventive Measures.")*

Fritz, M. A., & Speroff, L. Current concepts of the endocrine characteristics of normal menstrual function: The key to diagnosis and management of menstrual disorders. *Clinical Obstetrics and Gynecology*, 1983, *26*(3), 647–689. *Excellent synopsis of endocrine physiology of menstrual regulation. A must for practitioners to know prior to teaching menstrual cycle information to women.)*

Heczey, M. D. Effects of biofeedback and autogenic training on dysmenorrhea. In A. J. Dan, E. A. Graham, & C. P. Beecher (Eds.), *The menstrual cycle* (Vol. 1). New York: Springer, 1980. *(Analysis of a research study that found that by giving women positive communications regarding the menstrual period during their menses an increase in the positive affects would occur.)*

Hongladarom, G. C., McCorkle, R., & Wood, N. F. *The complete book of women's health.* Englewood Cliffs, N.J.: Prentice Hall, 1982. *(This book covers the gamut of women's health issues, physical needs, behaviors, and resources. Chapters 1, 3, 6, and 23 are especially well organized and relevant to the education process.)*

Kandzari, J. H., & Havard, J. R. *The well family: A developmental approach to assessment.* Boston: Little, Brown, 1981. *(This book is based on the concept that family wellness is the key to healthy individuals and a healthy society. Wellness goals and behaviors can be learned. The role of the nurse is supportive and complementary during the process of enhancing family wellness. The first two chapters outline this process and the remainder of the book examines specific applications.)*

Klaus, B. Sexually transmitted diseases and vaginitis. In L. Sonstegard, K. Kowalski, & B. Jennings (Eds.), *Women's health: Ambulatory care* (Vol. I). Englewood Cliffs, N.J.: Prentice-Hall, 1982. *(The author describes a variety of STDs and vaginitis in a format that correlates with the nursing process excluding the formal evaluation. Each gynecological problem is defined and followed by the relevant subject data, objective data, diagnosis and treatment.)*

Knowles, M. *The adult learner: A neglected species* (2nd ed.). Houston: Gulf Publishing, 1978. *(This book is an overview of many learning theorists and their theories. An examination of different learning styles and developmental factors is presented in text and table format. A helpful reference for the person with lack of familiarity with adult learning.)*

Latta, W., & Wiesmeier, E. Effects of an educational gynecological exam on women's attitudes. *Journal of Obstetric and Gynecologic Nursing,* 1982, *11*(4), 242–245. *(This article discusses a research study that analyzed women's attitudes concerning the speculum examination for female students ages 18 to 25. The attitudes were compared between the group that had a traditional examination and a group that encouraged women's participation and learning through specific teaching methods. Statistical significance was noted in this study.)*

Marieskind, H. I. *Women in the health system: Patients, providers, and programs.* St. Louis, Mo.: C. V. Mosby, 1980. *(This book presents historical and persistent data about women's health and why women obtain health care. Chapter 2 contains information on the characteristics of women's health care utilization and types of care they seek. Chapter 4 assesses "women in the health care work force." The impacts of today's technologies and women's health issues are also covered.)*

Marut, E. L., & Dawood, M. Y. Amenorrhea (excluding hyperprolactinemia). *Clinical Obstetrics and Gynecology,* 1983, *26*(3), 749–761. *(Current medical diagnosis and management succinctly summarized.)*

Maslow, A. H. *Motivation and personality.* New York: Harper & Row, 1954. *(A classic. This book needs to be read by all health professionals, especially the two chapters that address human motivation theory.)*

Neeson, J. D., & Stockdale, C. R. *The practitioner's handbook of ambulatory OB/GYN.* New York: John Wiley & Sons, 1981. *(The book covers problems in obstetrical and gynecological ambulatory care. Content in the chapters on gynecological infections and menstrual disorders were utilized in this chapter. Each chapter is clearly organized, giving definition of the problem, etiology, clinical features, differential diagnosis, necessary diagnostic studies, management and treatment, and complications and patient teaching.)*

Nicassio, P. M. Behavioral management of dysmenorrhea: An overview. In A. J. Dan, E. A. Graham, & C. P. Beecher (Eds.), *The menstrual cycle* (Vol. 1). New York: Springer, 1980. *(Differentiates treatment interventions into physiological affective and cognitive domains. Suggests ways to incorporate into a therapeutic approach to patient control management.)*

Notman, M. T., & Nadelson, C. G. *The woman patient* (Vol. 1). New York: Plenum, 1978. *(This book focuses on the diagnostic problems for obstetrical and gynecological patients. The first chapter, "The Woman Patient," brings to light the character changes in the doctor–patient relationship within the recent past. The changes in women as health care consumers are again implicated in Ch. 14, "Medical Gynecology: Problem and Patients.")*

Reid, R. L., & Yen, S. S. C. The premenstrual syndrome. *Clinical Obstetrics and Gynecology,* 1983, *26*(3), 710–718. *(Gives a good pathophysiology review, good illustrations, and stresses education and reassurance in the management regimen.)*

Sandelowski, M. *Women, health, and choice.* Englewood Cliffs, N.J.: Prentice-Hall, 1981. *(This book discusses in great depth the practice and philosophical needs and choices women have regarding their health. Part 1 gives a strong conceptual interpretation of women's health behaviors, status, and beliefs. Physiology, health issues, and health altering agents are also covered.)*

Schaumburg, H., Kaplan, J., Windebank, A., Vick, N., Rasmus, S., Pleasure, D., & Brown, M. J. Sensory neuropathy from pyridoxine abuse. *New England Journal of Medicine,* 1983, *309*(8), 445–448. *(A discussion of pyridoxine abuse and guidelines established for safe use.)*

Smith, J. P. *Nursing science in nursing practice.* London: Butterworths, 1981. *(This book has great versatility in covering the philosophical, practical, and conceptual issues nursing is researching and exploring today. Nursing concepts are defined, philosophical perspectives are challenged, educational processes are critiqued, the nursing process is expanded, and the science of nursing is cross-compared with other disciplines. A British publication with significant relevance to nursing in the United States.)*

Smitherman, C. *Nursing actions for health promotion.* Philadelphia: F. A. Davis, 1981. *(This book is divided into three parts. The first part, The Nursing Process, delineates the following aspects of the nurse–patient relationship: communication, helping, problem-solving, teaching, and leadership. Content is well-organized and case studies described, but the format-style is cumbersome.)*

Spellacy, W. N. Abnormal bleeding. *Clinical Obstetrics and Gynecology,* 1983, *26*(3), 702–709. *(Emphasizes need for good data base via history. Differentiates physiological from pathological DUB.)*

Thibodeau, J. A. *Nursing models: Analysis and evaluation.* Monterey, Calif.: Wadsworth Health Sciences Division, 1983. *(A comprehensive book on the analysis and evaluation of nursing practice models. Diagrams and explanations of theory building relationships make this book very versatile.)*

Webster, S. K. Problems for diagnosis of spasmodic and congestive dysmenorrhea. In A. J. Dan, E. A. Graham, & C. P. Beecher (Eds.), *The menstrual cycle* (Vol. 1). New York: Springer, 1980. *(Developed a table for recording specific menstrual feelings that would then diagnose the kind of dysmenorrhea a patient presented with.)*

Yaengo, D. D., & Reame, N. Psychosomatic aspects of menstrual dysfunction. *Clinical Obstetrics and Gynecology,* 1983, *26*(3), 777–784. *(A fascinating article that legitimizes the mind–body interrelationship and the impact of stress on normal menstrual functioning.)*

Extensive Gynecological Surgery

22

Ann Marie Dozier

Extensive gynecological surgery refers to procedures that not only involve much tissue removal and recuperation, but that cause dramatic alterations in the physical appearance and functioning of the woman's body. In concert with this, the psychological and sociological sequelae can be substantial. Special attention is needed for this group of women because of the complex actual and potential problems each must face and adapt to. This chapter focuses on the radical vulvectomy and pelvic exenteration as the two main extensive gynecological procedures. Although this discussion is addressed to health care professionals, much of the content is employed primarily by nurses. Therefore, the word nurse is used throughout the chapter.

The need for women to undergo these interventions has evolved over time. The principal agent responsible for this evolution is cancer. As researchers and clinicians learned more about cancer, radical procedures were introduced to arrest its spread. Subsequently, experiences in clinical practice along with research results led to revisions regarding the conditions for which utilization of these procedures is warranted.

The circumstances surrounding any recommendation to proceed with such radical surgery are complex but must be well understood by the nurse. It is only through this understanding that thorough care and teaching can be rendered to the patient. After reviewing the rationale and outcomes of the surgery, this chapter explores the patient's preoperative and postoperative needs, presents teaching methodologies, and discusses special considerations.

Patient education or teaching has been integrated into health care for a number of years. For patients facing surgery, it is important to determine what they know and expect about the upcoming procedure as well as the recuperative period. Awareness of their physiological, sociological, and psychological states is also needed. Appropriate interventions, based on the knowledge deficits encountered, are then implemented. Evaluation of the patients' responses follows. This process is well known and has been applied to diverse populations. A myriad of patient benefits has been identified. Thus preoperative preparation as a health care intervention is the right of every patient.

Women who agree to undergo procedures such as a radical vulvectomy or pelvic exenteration require extensive preoperative preparation. For these women, facing a surgery that will dramatically alter their bodies, the preparation expands in scope, depth, and time. They require an integrated plan that allows them to face and begin to adapt to the anticipated outcomes of surgery (Crosson, 1981; Hamilton & Schlapper, 1974; Springer, 1982; Yarbrough, 1981). See Chapter 2 for additional information about the planning process.

Adaptation to the events and outcomes of extensive surgery for cancer is an ongoing process. According to one scheme, which outlines the stages of this process, each cancer patient faces a series of issues and associated adaptive tasks (Table 22–1). Successful completion of the tasks enables the patient to function effectively (Mages & Mendelsohn, 1979). The remainder of this chapter utilizes this scheme to examine how the nurse can best help the woman face and complete these tasks.

RADICAL VULVECTOMY

Discovery of Cancer
To help the woman with her adaptive tasks, the nurse must first understand the indications for doing a radical vulvectomy, as well as the characteristics of the disease. This knowledge can then be used in preparing the woman for the surgery and recuperation.

Cancer of the vulva most commonly originates from the squamous epithelium. Although other types such as basal cell or melanoma do occur, treatment considerations are similar to those of squamous cell cancer (Cavanaugh, Praphat, & Ruffolo, 1982; Krupp, 1981).

Typically vulvar cancer presents as a palpable nodule or rash, exophytic in nature.

TABLE 22–1. ISSUES AND ADAPTIVE TASKS OF CANCER PATIENTS: A PERSONOLOGICAL APPROACH

Issue	Adaptive Task
Discovery of cancer	Appraise significance of discovery Initiate appropriate treatment
Primary treatment	Recognize and deal with realities of situation Regulate the emotional reactions Integrate the experience of illness with the rest of one's life
Damage to one's body from cancer and/or treatment	Mourn the loss Replace or compensate for lost parts or functions where possible Maximize other potentials to maintain sense of self-esteem and intactness
Maintaining continuity	Understand and communicate one's changed attitudes, needs, and limitations that permit formation of a new balance with environment
Possibility of recurrence and progression of disease	Live with fear; one must be able to put it out of mind most of time and yet remain aware of realities to continue appropriate medical follow-up and take it into consideration in making long-range plans
Persistent or recurrent disease	Exercise choice where possible Accept one's helplessness and dependence where necessary without excessive regression or turning to a magical solution

(Source: *Adapted from Mages, N. L., & Mendelsohn, G. A. Effects of cancer on patients' lives: A personological approach. In* G. Stone & F. Cohen (Eds.), Health and psychology: A handbook. *San Francisco: Jossey-Bass, 1979, pp. 255–284.*)

The patient is usually postmenopausal and has had a long standing history of pruritus. Occasionally the area may be infected or have ulcerated; exudate or blood may have been noticed (Friedrich & Wilkinson, 1982; Krupp, 1981). The growth of vulvar tumors has been described as slow, eventually extending to proximal structures, such as the urethra, vagina, and rectum. Involvement of the lymph nodes can also occur, usually at the inguinal and femoral groups first (Krupp et al., 1973).

This spread pattern is the basis for staging vulvar cancers. Since 1971 the FIGO (International Federation of Obstetricians and Gynecologists) has accepted the tumor–nodes–metasteses (TNM) system. Thus, as seen in Table 22–2, the larger the tumor, the higher the stage. Unfortunately, the 2-centimeter cut off point is arbitrary, the intraepithelial cancers are not included, and only the clinical palpation of lymph nodes is used. Staging is therefore imprecise and its prognostic usefulness dubious (Krupp, 1981). Several authors have developed their own systems, but none has yet received enough acceptance to replace the FIGO system.

As far as has been determined there are not definitive risk factors for the development of vulvar cancer. There is an increased incidence with age, but the exact relationship is unclear. In addition several authors have described a potential relationship between vulvar cancer occurrence and granulomatous infections of the vulva (Lash & Zibel, 1951; Saltzstein, Woodruff, & Novak, 1956) and neoplasia of the anogenital tract or both (Buchler, 1975; Jimerson & Merrill, 1970).

A discussion of the adaptive tasks associated with discovery of cancer follows. Although these may appear to have little bearing on preoperative preparation, they in fact do. It is essential that the nurse (1) understand the discovery process and (2) recognize its impact on the establishment of rapport and on the patient's ability to learn. A patient who is not permitted this opportunity to put her experiences into perspective may not be ready to become involved in her recuperation.

At this point the patient is facing the possibility of discovering a cancer. Most commonly the woman finds the lesion herself. Then she begins the task of appraising the discovery. Even though it presents as a lump, delay in seeking consultation from a health care provider is common. One study reported that 37 percent of the women waited over 12 months before seeking help (Cavanaugh, Praphat, & Ruffolo, 1982). Other studies had similar findings (Boutselis, 1972; Garcia & Boronow, 1972; Rutledge, 1970).

A variety of reasons have been forwarded to explain this behavior. Certainly, the woman's fears about the outcome or diagnosis may be the main factor. In addition the intimate or private nature of the genital area may deter some women from seeking attention. This can be further complicated by the woman's belief that the itching or lump are normal phenomena of age; the serious nature of the lesion is not fully appreciated. An alternative perspective is proposed by Weisman (1979). Delay may be an indication of the woman's independent self-reliance. She may not want to become dependent. Having cancer may be equated with such dependence. As will be seen, these possibilites must be taken into account as the woman finally seeks attention for her symptoms.

As the woman moves to her next task, initiation of appropriate treatment, another difficulty may be encountered. Her delay is oftentimes extended by what is termed physician or provider delay. Treatment in the form of salves or lotions is tried before the lesion is biopsied. Only if the symptoms continue or the lesion has not responded is a biopsy done. Unfortunately, these efforts can delay the initiation of appropriate treatment from several months to a year (Parker, 1975).

By the time the woman is facing the treatment alternatives, she has already completed the tasks associated with discovery. Allowing her to describe the events and what

TABLE 22–2. CARCINOMA OF VULVA: INTERNATIONAL FEDERATION OF OBSTETRICIANS AND GYNECOLOGISTS (FIGO) METHOD OF STAGING

TNM Classification

T Primary tumor

T1	Tumor confined to the vulva—2 cm or less in larger diameter.
T2	Tumor confined to the vulva—more than 2 cm in diameter.
T3	Tumor of any size with adjacent spread to the urethra and/or vagina and/or perineum and/or to the anus.
T4	Tumor of any size infiltrating the bladder mucosa and/or the rectal mucosa or both, including the upper part of the urethral mucosa and/or fixed to the bone.

N Regional lymph nodes

N0	No nodes palpable.
N1	Nodes palpable in either groin, not enlarged, mobile (not clinically suspicious of neoplasm).
N2	Nodes palpable in either one or both groins, enlarged, firm and mobile (clinically suspicious of neoplasm).
N3	Fixed or ulcerated nodes.

M Distant metastases

M0	No clinical metastases.
M1a	Palpable deep pelvic lymph nodes.
M1b	Other distant metastases.

Definitions of the Different Clinical Stages in Carcinoma of the Vulva (FIGO)

Stage I

T1 N0 M0	Tumor confined to the vulva—2 cm or less in the larger diameter. Nodes are not palpable or are palpable in either groin, not enlarged, mobile (not clinically suspicious of neoplasm).

Stage II

T2 N0 M0	Tumor confined to the vulva—more than 2 cm in diameter. Nodes are not palpable, or are palpable in either groin, not enlarged, mobile (not clinically suspicious of neoplasm).

Stage III

T2 N0 M0 T3 N1 M0 T3 N2 M0 T1 N2 M0 T2 N2 M0	Tumor of any size with (1) adjacent spread to the lower urethra and/or the vagina, the perineum, and the anus, and/or (2) nodes palpable in either one or both groins, enlarged, firm and mobile, not fixed (but clinically suspicious of neoplasm).

Stage IV

T4 N0 M0 T4 N1 M0 T4 N2 M0 T1 N3 M0 T2 N3 M0 T3 N3 M0 T4 N3 M0	Tumor of any size (1) infiltrating the bladder mucosa, or the rectal mucosa, or both, including the upper part of the urethral mucosa, and/or (2) fixed to the bone or other distant metastases. Fixed or ulcerated nodes in either one or both groins.

(Source: *Krupp, P. J. Invasive tumors of vulva: Clinical features and management. In M. Coppleson (Ed.),* Gynecological oncology. *Edinburgh: Churchill Livingstone, 1981, pp. 329–338, by permission.*)

decision-making processes she undertook allows the nurse to gain insight into her understanding and thought processes, while at the same time beginning the establishment of rapport and support, both required during the remainder of the woman's treatment and recuperation. This review also affords the woman an opportunity to seek validation for appropriate actions, gain understanding for inaction, and begin to focus on who or what to blame for her present situation. This opportunity for dialogue frequently can be missed.

Sometimes, the woman may not want to discuss past events, feeling embarrassed about describing the area or not having come sooner. By being an active nonjudgmental listener, however, the professional can provide support (Koile, 1977). Reassurances can and should be offered in that there was nothing the woman did or did not do to cause the cancer. In addition it is important to move the woman's focus from past events to the present decisions about treatment. This can be facilitated by the nurse's acknowledgment of the client's past actions and positive reinforcement for having come, no matter how long the delay.

Primary Treatment

Once the diagnosis of vulvar cancer has been biopsy-confirmed, the treatment of choice is surgery. The cancer's location and usual spread pattern make radiation therapy difficult both for the therapist to treat and the patient to tolerate. Chemotherapy has not been shown to be effective. Because the goal of treatment is disease removal, the extensiveness of the procedure is determined by the degree of cancer invasion and metastasis.

Current thinking separates in situ and invasive vulvar cancer. The former occurs in women during the second and third decades of life, whereas the latter is more commonly found in women in their sixth, seventh, or eighth decade. Because in situ means on the surface, the question is whether a lesser procedure is as effective as a more extensive one (Kolstad, 1981). This is the subject of some debate. The gynecology–oncology literature recommends surgical interventions ranging from wide-local incision to total vulvectomy (Cavanaugh et al., 1982; Choo, 1982; Kneal, Elliott, & McDonald, 1981). An increasing number of oncologists advocate that no more than a hemivulvectomy be done for women with localized disease. This should not only be an effective treatment, but in many cases preserves the function of the clitoris while maintaining a more cosmetically appealing result (Kolstad, 1981). Additional discussion and research is required to thoroughly evaluate the criteria for and results of such procedures.

For women with superficially invasive (microinvasive) disease and for those with frankly invasive disease, but not metastases, the nearly universal treatment is a radical vulvectomy with bilateral groin node dissection. This procedure may seem extreme, but by removing the lesion and the surrounding tissues the chance of recurrence is virtually eliminated. For women who wish to preserve clitoral function, alternatives are considered (Choo, 1982; Krupp, 1981; Lash & Zibel, 1951).

Dissection of the groin lymph nodes is undertaken to evaluate disease spread. In the past, a pelvic lymphadenectomy was also done. This is now advocated only for selected patients, such as those with positive groin nodes or those with cancer of Bartholin's gland or clitoris or melanoma of the vulva (Cavanaugh et al, 1982; Cavanaugh & Shephard, 1982; Morley, 1981; Nelson, 1977; Way, 1948). Some clinicians, however, continue to utilize pelvic lymphadenectomy for all invasive squamous lesions stages I through II (Krupp, 1981).

A related issue questions whether groin node dissections need to examine the deep and superficial (inguinal) nodes. Some clinicians advocate dissection of the superficial nodes first then, if positive, consider deep node treatment. They believe that the likelihood of positive deep nodes being found in the absence of positive inguinal nodes is rare (Cavanaugh et al, 1982; DiSaia, Creasman, & Rich, 1979). This issue remains unresolved.

Patient outcomes in terms of survival indicate that 90 percent of women with invasive vulvar cancer, who at the time of surgery have negative lymph nodes, are disease-free 5 years later. If positive inguinal (superficial) nodes were found, however, only 65 percent of the women will be without disease at the 5-year point (Friedrich & Wilkinson, 1982). These figures are a further indication of the lethality of vulvar cancer and the effectiveness of radical surgery for treating women with invasive squamous cell cancer of the vulva.

Preoperative Assessment. According to the scheme being used here, the next adaptive task for the woman is to recognize and deal with the choices. The nurse must understand what choices are available and utilize a methodology for teaching and discussion that the woman will be able to comprehend.

To accomplish this the nurse must first learn more about the woman from a subjective and objective standpoint (see Chapter 2). In addition to a description of recent events and decisions, this assessment should include the items noted in Table 22–3.

This information allows the nurse to attain a holistic view of this patient, her roles, relationships, and needs. In addition, insight into her self-perception, esteem, and body-image is gained. This information helps the nurse individualize teaching to the needs of this patient.

To help the woman the nurse must know the type of cancer, its spread, and the treatment options offered. A good approach is to hear in the patient's words what she already understands about her disease. It is best to use the word the patient uses. Be aware whether or not she says the word cancer. Use of the words "disease," "growth," or "tumor" is recommended unless you know the patient well. Ask her if anyone has given a name to the disease. This helps establish a trusting relationship with her. Because some patients cannot bear the thought of having cancer or, even worse, talking about it, employing a less frightening word can be an adaptive response to a stressful situation. This does not mean that you avoid discussing the serious nature of the patient's condition or avoid talking about her fears. During this discussion take time to clarify any misconceptions she has stated.

Often, after hearing the description of the treatment, the patient focuses on "if" questions such as "What if I did not have the surgery?" or "How will I look if I am operated on?" Being honest is important; however, sharing all the details about cure

TABLE 22–3. ASSESSMENT CONTENT AREAS

Demographic information, particularly marital status and living situation
Previous personal or familial experiences with hospitalization and illness, especially cancer
Educational or intellectual level
Present level of activity, especially mobility, self-care, and interests
Knowledge about normal anatomy and physiology of the pelvis and perineum
Health beliefs and practices
Ongoing and past health problems, current medications, and personal hygiene habits, particularly bowel and bladder
Available support persons are used
Sexual beliefs and practices (see also Table 22–6)
Personal insights
   Relationships with others
   Response to prior stressful events (physical and emotional)
   Identification of thoughts/feelings about the present event(s)
   Identification of personal assets

rates can be overwhelming and is usually *not* what she really wants to know. Statements such as, "We have had good results using this procedure with patients who have problems similar to yours" or "If the cancer is not treated thoroughly, it will come back or grow" are likely to be what she is really asking for. The woman may also be seeking information regarding any functional changes that could happen such as ability to have intercourse or to void normally. Reassure her that these functions should not change. Many vulvectomy procedures do, however, remove the clitoris.

Frank discussion about its removal and the availability of alternative measures to achieve erotic or orgasmic satisfaction must be undertaken (see Table 22–8). Because discussion at this time merely sets the stage for additional discussion during the recuperative period, excessive detail is not necessary.

As a patient advocate, the nurse must insure that the woman is aware of the surgery's potential outcomes and the recuperative course ahead. Extended hospital stay, complications such as wound breakdown, and long-term concerns such as loss of clitoral function or leg lymphedema must be mentioned. This discussion should treat these items as serious, but not insurmountable obstacles. The patient must be reassured that her providers will be there to help her throughout recuperation and not abandon her if complications or problems ensue.

These actions contribute toward maintaining the patient's psychological equilibrium. It is appropriate to mention that the physical changes may affect the way she feels about herself as a woman and how she feels about herself in her other roles and relationships. Even though she may deny such feelings now, early mention legitimizes the topic for discussion during or after recovery.

The family's needs cannot be overlooked during the assessment. Although the focus of this chapter is on the woman with cancer, the family must also be involved. The degree and extent of involvement for each family will vary. For details about assessment of the family's needs see Lewis, 1983.

The second reality this woman must face is consenting to the surgery. Here it is important *not* to make unrealistic assurances. There are no guarantees and no patient should be assured otherwise. This honesty helps bridge the gap between nurse and patient.

Preoperative Preparation. The next step in dealing with the realities of the situation is preparing the woman for the actual surgery and recuperation. This contributes to the completion of her other two tasks: regulating emotional reactions and integrating the experience into the rest of her life. The preparatory statements previously made to the patient now become more specific. Caution must be exercised to prevent her from becoming overloaded with stimuli. It is preferable for hospitalization to commence several days before the scheduled surgery. This allows time to adjust to the environment, its personnel, and processes. It also affords the nurse an excellent opportunity to determine what teacher role is effective, identify the critical behavior changes that are needed, and initiate preoperative teaching and subsequent review and reinforcement.

The content of this preparation is extensive, including standard procedures such as administration of pain medication and pulmonary exercises. The interventions and expected outcomes are summarized in Table 22–4. In addition, the patient should be aware of other postoperative limitations and additional drainage tubes that will be attached. These last two items will vary depending on the wound closure techniques used by the surgeon. Should the area be closed primarily, then the first 2 to 5 days of recuperation will probably require the patient to be on complete bedrest, able to log roll from side to

TABLE 22–4. PATIENT UNDERGOING RADICAL VULVECTOMY BEHAVIORAL OBJECTIVES FOR TEACHING

Objectives	Intervention
The patient will be able to:	
1. State disease, type and goal of surgery pointing to diagram or self	Using drawings (preferably not photos) show patient area to be operated on: Labia (folds of skin) will be removed Groins (frontal folds at hips) will be opened, examined and tissue removed Goal is cure (in most cases)
2. State routine preparation procedures and their purposes	Review procedures, indicating that they are routine: shave and prep NPO—MN Preoperative injection
3. State the routine recovery procedures	Review: Transport to recovery room Return to room VS monitoring Where family can wait Presence of Foley Groin drainage tubes IV
4. Describe expected discomfort and availability of relief medications	Using the word discomfort with adjectives (mild—moderate—severe), explain that: Discomfort and/or pressure will be felt—this is to be expected Location of discomfort—groin, hips, lower torso Ambulation and dressing changes will cause discomfort Medication is available—it will be offered but that she should also ask (preferably before it becomes severe) Until she can eat/drink, it will be a shot It is normal to regularly require medication for at least the first week Bending at the waist/hips can cause discomfort as can sitting.
5. State wound closure technique that will be used and cleaning/care necessary (depending on surgeon's preference)	Discuss: Wound closure/dressing will be closed/dressed Need for dressing changes, and observations That it will look red and swollen at first That patient can look at it via a mirror After several months of healing it will look like normal skin, minus the folds Hair regrowth often covers perineal scars and groin scars will blend into "cracks" at hips Wound care (after catheter removed) needed after each void; staff will do care, eventually patient will do with little staff assistance Wound breakdown most common complication—dressing changes may be required Use drawings Fig. 22–1 and 22–2
6. State the purpose and importance of getting up to sit and walk; demonstrate how to get up	Discuss ambulating in terms of: Preventing blood clots, lung congestion, and mobility and recuperation problems Improves general sense of well-being and promotes healing Show patient and have patient practice how to get out of bed (rolling on side, pushing self up from bed)

510

TABLE 22–4. (cont.)

Objectives	Intervention
The patient will be able to:	
	Assure patient that medication will be available before or after ambulating Discuss expected distances to be walked
7. State rationale and sequence of diet progression	Review chronologically intake limitations: NPO to clear liquids then solid food anesthesia effects on peristalsis; need for moderation as limits are removed

8. State purpose of urinary catheter	Discuss catheter, placed during surgery, to drain urine:
	  may feel urge to void
	  tube necessary to keep wound clean
	  usually removed once patient able to sit comfortably

9. State purpose of and demonstrate lung exercises	Discuss risk of lung problems after surgery and goal of prevention Instruct patient how to use incentive spirometer and effectively turn, cough, deep breathe Have patient demonstrate
10. State that she will assume self-care activities beginning on the second postoperative day	Clarify that an important part of recovery is resumption of normal activities She will be encouraged to do for herself (beginning with bathing) once she becomes alert and able to do the activity Assure her that she will be assisted as long as is necessary
11. Identify her concerns/fears about adjusting to the physical changes resulting from surgery	Clarify what changes are expected Identify that concerns are normal Create environment in which patient feels free to discuss these concersn—privacy and an attentive listener are key Assure her that staff will always be available to her for assistance/support Determine her risk for nonadjustment based on her age, length of present relationship, and gender role definition (Derogatis, 1980)
12. Identify her concerns about how these changes could/might effect her return to everyday activities	Allow patient to mourn loss, express concerns/fears Identify strengths and supports available to patient
13. State the actual and potential changes in her sexual functioning; state how these changes may alter her concept of herself as a sexual person; identify methods to ameliorate alterations	Identify baseline behavior Clarify if/how this surgery will alter functioning; explore alternatives as necessary Discuss with partner and patient jointly: use of lubrication easing penetration of vagina, exploring alternative erotic areas

14. State the possible long-term problems of the surgery	Mention that:
	  Leg swelling can continue for years—(this is particulary problematic for patients who stand for long periods of time)
	  Urinary stream may be diverted
	  Discomfort when sitting for long periods of time or when restrictive clothing is worn
	  Reduced rotation of hips
	  Possible return of cancer (itching, bump)

side. Once ambulation is initiated, she may need to walk in a semi-flexed position. Some surgeons prefer to let the wound heal by secondary intention. Thus the open area is covered by a dressing soaked with saline, betadine, or even honey (Cavanaugh & Ostapowicz, 1970). It is changed several times a day. Ambulation for these women begins the day after surgery.

Although the informational aspect of preoperative teaching is important, the nurse should not just focus on the facts. The goal of this preparation is to bring the patient's expectations into line with reality. Thus, prior to any teaching, the nurse must assess the patient's level of knowledge. It is imperative to determine what the patient understands about the surgery and recuperative period. Also, asking what or how much she would like to know will help the nurse determine what to include in the preparation. Another concern related to teaching is what kind of information is necessary to share. The facts alone regarding what will happen should be supplemented by descriptions of the sensory stimuli the patient is likely to experience.

A successful approach developed by Johnson (1972, 1973) and Johnson and Rice (1974) incorporates sensations into the preparation. She found that by sharing this kind of information with patients they were able to develop appropriate expectations, reduce stress, and achieve improved outcomes. Her findings also indicated that sharing just factual information can increase patients' distress. To integrate sensations into the preparation, the nurse must present each topic from the standpoint of how it will feel to the patient. For example, the nurse might say:

> The day after surgery you will be helped out of bed to walk a short distance. You may feel light-headed, but if you take it slowly, keeping your head up and eyes open, that feeling will pass. The area around your surgery may also be uncomfortable—your hips may feel stiff and your skin taut. The medication should help reduce this. After several days this stiffness or discomfort will improve.

In this integration you have combined both fact and sensation. The patient can then have an idea of what to expect.

The actual content you should include is extensive (Table 22–4). The following descriptions include details regarding this content along with hints to share with patients. It is helpful to divide the information into several sections, discussing each at a different sitting. This allows the patient time to think and review what was said. Including a significant other in the preparation should also be considered. Later, this person will be able to help reinforce what was said or even assist the patient as she carries out a particular recuperative activity. Traditionally, preoperative teaching has been organized chronologically, beginning with a review of routine presurgery procedures. Although this may seem appropriate, it is not necessarily the best way to approach teaching. Asking what the woman would like to know about first allows her some control in a situation in which she feels powerless. It also may relieve her mind about a particular circumstance (see Chapter 2). For example:

> Mrs. T. remembers that when she had a cholecystectomy, her nasogastric tube was inserted while she was still awake. She describes the experience as "horrible. I kept gagging and fighting it."

Reassurances that these tubes are not usually needed, and would be placed only when she is under anesthesia, help dissipate her fears. This allows her to focus on what else is said.

As the teaching is planned, another aspect to consider is to begin with the content that will need to be reinforced at a later opportunity. Furthermore, if the patient is told in the beginning about a shot or enema, she may focus on that unpleasant, though relatively minor event, instead of the larger picture of recovery.

Teaching about the postoperative period should be done from the patient's frame of reference. Instead of describing things that nurses will do to or with her, describe events in a way that identifies how she is expected to participate or feel. This can have a dramatic effect on facilitating learning and on improving or easing recovery.

Postoperative pulmonary exercises are an excellent example of this. Teaching should include why the respiratory system needs special attention (effects of anethesia, secretion build up, and lessened use of lung capacities) and the complications that could result (e.g., pneumonia, atelectasis). Emphasize that the exercises are preventative (Table 22–4). By having her learn and practice preoperatively she can become an effective participant in her recovery. The other subjects included in preoperative preparation should be taught from a similar focus, including sensations and what the patient can do to help herself (Table 22–4).

One procedure, which also warrants mention, is postoperative wound care. The surgeon may have explained what is going to be removed, but, as is the case with many procedures, the patient cannot easily visualize or imagine what the wound will look like. Therefore, what is said must take into account the procedure planned as well as the patient's desire to know. The easiest way to describe the end result is to say that the labia or folds of skin around the vagina and urethra will be removed. Using diagrams (Fig. 22–1) is helpful (Table 22–4 also).

The preparation should also include mention of the meticulous wound care required after surgery. Wound breakdown and infection is the most common (45 percent of patients) complication of vulvar surgery (Nelson, 1977). If primary closure is used, then the wound cleaning and dressing changes may be done only once or twice a day. Drains into the groin area may be used to promote closure and healing (Fig. 22–2). For the patient whose wound is left to close by secondary intention or whose suture line has broken down, the need for dressing changes at least three times a day becomes paramount (Table 22–4).

Before the patient's participation in wound care is discussed, it is necessary to determine how much she will actually be able to do. Her mobility, body weight, and ability to understand and follow directions are factors to consider. For example, J. D. was a 69-year-old married housewife who, prior to admission, led a physically active life including gardening and cleaning. She was able to learn how to do her wound care and

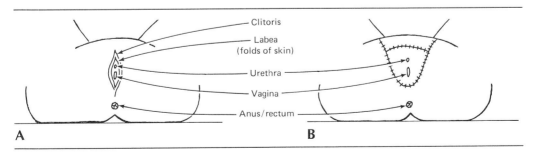

Figure 22–1. Simplified representations of anatomy before (**A**) and after (**B**) radical vulvectomy with groin dissection.

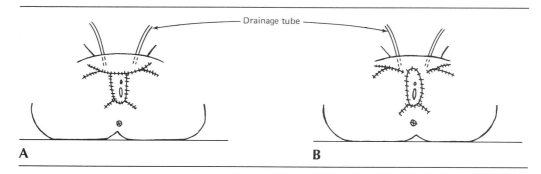

Figure 22–2. Vulvectomy after primary closure. **A.** Groin dissection incision contiguous with perineal incisions. **B.** Groin incisions separate from perineal incisions.

had recovered enough to assume responsibility for it, but because of her large frame and body weight (270 pounds) she could not reach the perineal area or even aim the irrigating bottle correctly. Because her preoperative preparation had led her to expect to do this, she became frustrated and irritated with herself when she was unable to do the cleansing independently. This situation might have been avoided had the preparation taken her physical limitations into account.

Preoperative preparation can be the critical element in physical recovery. Teaching methodologies and teacher resources are discussed in Chapters 2 and 3. Incorporation of the ideas presented here into a framework suitable to your teaching style cannot help but improve the patient's ability to recognize and deal with the realities of recovering vulvar surgery.

Obviously if the patient is admitted several days prior to surgery, the nurse can implement a thorough teaching plan. If time constraints exist, however, the nurse must select the critical content to include in the teaching. This selection must be based on assessment of the patient as well as knowledge of the potential problems oftentimes experienced during recovery. For example, previous respiratory difficulties would necessitate emphasis on pulmonary exercises. In contrast someone with poor preoperative hygiene would require instruction emphasizing the skin and wound care aspects.

The remaining two tasks associated with primary treatment are integrating the experience into one's life and regulating emotional reactions. Patients facing surgery begin to focus on these tasks preoperatively, but usually do not complete them until after surgery. The woman facing a radical vulvectomy is still usually asking the unanswerable question "Why me?" The search for an answer leads her to examine her past: roles and relationships with friends and family; beliefs in the supernatural; past decisions; and life events. Even though an answer is not usually found, this review allows the woman to put her present situation into perspective. The nurse may participate in this process as a listener or someone with whom the woman can validate or share her perceptions. Frequently remarks such as "I've lived through (some experience), this cannot be as bad as that" or "Nothing can be worse than living with this itching" or "God is punishing me for . . ." all reflect this integration. This is an ongoing process that is likely to continue throughout her hospitalization. The review may also be utilized to the patient's benefit. If she is having difficulty facing the surgery, it is helpful to ask her what helped during difficult situations in the past. This information can be used to assist the patient in meeting the challenge of the present situation.

The review can also help you prepare the woman for surgery. Her verbal and nonverbal cues may indicate, for example: (1) what kinds of experiences upset her, (2) how she dealt with previous distressing events, or (3) if she has an internal or external locus of control (see also discussion of Readiness in Chapter 2). This information can be used to determine the approach employed. Validate observations with the patient: "You seem more upset about this subject than when we talked before" or "You haven't asked anything about. . . . Do you have any concerns about that?" In responding the nurse should recognize the patient's anxiety and offer realistic reassurances. Capitalizing on how this woman faced a past loss or accident will help gear the teaching to her coping style. The woman who views life events as occurrences over which she has no control may be less likely to want to assume responsibility for self-care activities. Thus your efforts to discuss these activities may need to focus on them not as her responsibility but as expectations the nurse has for her.

As with the other adaptive tasks, this regulating goes on throughout the treatment and recuperation phase. The patient's emotional state will determine to what degree the nursing staff needs to be involved with the regulation. Regardless of this, every patient needs nursing support. This should include frequent visits to the patient's room as well as physical contact such as touch. This reassures the patient of her humanness and conveys an empathy necessary for the ongoing development of rapport.

Impact on body image is another aspect of dealing with the realities of the situation. For the woman with vulvar cancer, incomplete knowledge of anatomy complicates her preoperative understanding and, therefore, her readiness to hear and understand the observable differences she will undergo. To many women, their first look, with the assistance of a mirror, is 3 to 5 days after surgery. The healing vulva is still swollen, reddened, and, if left open, bloody looking. The patient is usually shocked and disgusted. Easing the shock of this first look can be started preoperatively (Table 22–4).

The patient's emotional state (Table 22–3) or psychological readiness for the surgery must also be taken into account as she is prepared for surgery (see discussion of anxiety in Chapter 2). For example, preoperative preparation becomes complicated if she is not ready or able to understand the information. Some patients are exceedingly anxious. Sharing information about what to expect should only begin once the source of the anxiety has been identified and resolutions implemented. This may be impossible. Determining whether the observed behavior is this person's coping style when faced with stressful situations gives insight about whether or not the behavior is adaptive or maladaptive. One patient who fretted about every detail to extremes (but did not deal with the fact that she had cancer) was questioned about how she had behaved after her husband had died. She proceeded to describe exactly the same behavior being observed. This distinguished her present behavior as part of her coping style not as abnormal and potentially maladaptive behavior.

For those patients whose anxiety will not allow them to "hear" explanations, the nurse must become more directive (pedagogical) and determine the critical content *for* the patient. The decision about this can be made jointly with the patient, being sure to take into account what postoperative problems this patient is likely to experience. Thus if during a past hospitalization this woman had problems with lower extremity phlebitis, emphasis on measures to prevent phlebitis would be critical. If the woman is obese and a heavy smoker, then pulmonary exercises information would be critical. Again, the patient herself may indicate how much she should be told. Comments such as "I always worry about things ahead of time" or "Telling me about what will happen just makes me more nervous" are clear messages to keep in mind as the preparation is done.

The Recuperation Period. Preparation and teaching must continue throughout hospitalization. The recuperation process in the hospital must be facilitated by review of the information shared before surgery. Additional information, individualized to each patient, should also be incorporated. This individualization must be based on the recuperative course. For example, the patient may not be moving or coughing well enough after surgery, thus increasing her risk for pulmonary difficulties. Intensifying the teaching about the pulmonary regimen is essential. Contracting with the patient regarding appropriate frequency of coughing and turning should also be undertaken.

Other areas discussed in general terms preoperatively will assume greater importance after surgery. Individualization is a key here also. Resumption of normal activities is based on the woman's functional level before surgery in addition to the surgical procedure, amount of retraction, level of discomfort, ability to move, and orientation to reality. These factors lead to a wide variation among patients as they move to self-care. Patient teaching at this point should focus on clarification of expectations along with agreement with the patient about her day to day progress toward self-care.

More attention is also given to the patient's coping with the actual and perceived changes resultant from surgery. Knowledge about the patient's beliefs and practices regarding her female role and sexual functioning determines the nurse's interventions. Derogatis and Kourlesis (1981) state that older women in longer and, presumably, more stable relationships are less threatened by this surgery. They do not fear the loss of their partner as much as younger women whose relationships have been of shorter duration. The women who see themselves as very "feminine" similarly have more difficulty adjusting to the actual or perceived changes brought about by the vulvectomy procedure. As the woman begins to resume self-care, the realities of what these changes are may begin to have an impact. The nurse should initiate discussion of these concerns by mentioning that "many women are upset when they first see the wound. Some wonder if they will ever feel normal or if their husband (partner) will see them as an attractive person anymore." This legitimizes the subject, indicating to the patient that this is an acceptable subject to discuss. Often the woman is afraid of rejection or of spreading the cancer to her partner or husband. Reassurance about what is and is not changed is necessary here. Similar fears may be shared by her partner. Discussions between patient and partner should be facilitated.

Interestingly, as Derogatis and Kourlesis (1981) observed, some older patients do not feel the impact of these changes. Their satisfaction comes more from affection and physical contact than from intercourse. Other older women do not feel free to discuss with their partner or spouse the surgery or the changes it brings. Intercourse may continue as always, whether the patient's needs are satisfied or not. Still other women are able to have frank discussions with their partners. It is this group that benefits the most from the discussion and support the nurse can offer. (See Tables 22–6 and 22–8 for guidelines about sexual assessment and alternatives for sexual expression.)

Summary

Preparing a woman to undergo radical vulvectomy surgery is a process that must be started at her initial outpatient visit. The establishment of rapport, understanding, and support begins as the woman faces the adaptive tasks of appraising the discovery and initiating appropriate treatment. As she recognizes and deals with the realities of her situation, her preoperative preparation is focused to help her accomplish this task. Adapting and implementing the strategies described here prepare the patient for radical vulvectomy surgery and recovery.

PELVIC EXENTERATION

The pelvic exenteration has been described as ultraradical, "an innovation made possible by advances in the ancillary sciences [improved instrumentation and capacity for physiologic support]" (Coppleson, 1981, p. 523). It is most commonly undertaken to treat the woman with locally advanced or recurrent squamous cell cervical cancer. The indications for this procedure are very specific. Because many women, considered as candidates, are eliminated during the evaluation process, the following discussion focuses first on the indications for and purpose of the procedure.

The goal of the exenterative procedure is *cure*. It involves removal of the pelvic viscera including the bladder and the rectosigmoid. The patient's excretions are diverted to urinary and fecal stomas. Some women undergo a radical vulvectomy simultaneously (Barber, 1982). For women with disease outside the pelvis, it has been demonstrated that quantitative survival is not improved by this procedure (Hass, Buchsbaum, & Lifshitz, 1980). One suspects that it would not improve their remaining life qualitatively either. Consequently, any woman being considered for a pelvic exenteration must undergo careful scrutiny to determine that the cancer is not outside of the pelvis. This involves a physical examination, tests, and, at the time of surgery, paraaortic and pelvic lymph node evaluation. Should any of these steps yield positive results, the exenterative procedure would not be carried out. The remaining option for these women, who had previously undergone radiation therapy, is limited to palliative chemotherapy.

Usually women who are evaluated for an exenterative procedure were initially diagnosed with stage I cervical cancer (limited to the cervix). Oftentimes the disease was termed bulky, meaning it completely encompassed the cervix, but did not extend into other tissues. The original treatment these women underwent consisted of either surgery or radiation therapy, or both. Cervical cancer recurrence can be classified as distant (34 percent), lymph node metastasis (36 percent), or central (30 percent). The local or "central" lesion is often found on follow-up examination at the vaginal apex. Commonly, the patient is asymptomatic. This local spread pattern, typical of cervical cancer, lends itself to radical resection (Coppleson, 1981). In contrast, recurrence in the form of metastases is not treated with exenterative surgery.

A second group who also should be evaluated for exenterative surgery are those women who present initially with advanced disease. The spread of cancer to contiguous tissues, as Figure 22–3 demonstrates, means that even though advanced, the disease may still be localized or limited to the pelvis. A pelvic exenteration is then a treatment option.

Before detailing the preoperative preparation process, it is important to be aware of the main controversies associated with this radical procedure. The need for a partial exenteration in selected cases has been advocated (Barber, 1982; Symmonds, Pratt, & Webb, 1975). When the patient's disease has penetrated the bladder or the rectum, not both, would not an anterior or posterior exenteration alone be adequate if the dissection left free margins? This position, although logical, has been resisted by some gynecological oncologists because of the risk of incomplete resection, particularly in the radiated patient. They also cite the multiple complications apparent in the preserved organ, due mainly to radiation effects combined with compromised blood flow or trauma during the operative procedure (DiSaia & Rich, 1981).

A second controversy surrounds the decision about whether positive *pelvic* lymph nodes contraindicate proceeding with the exenteration (Barber, 1982). This evaluation takes place on the operating table. First the extrapelvic areas are examined. If malignant cells are found, the exenteration is not undertaken. The pelvic area is explored and the

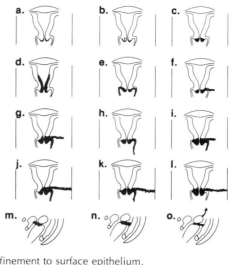

a.	Stage 0	Confinement to surface epithelium.
b.	Stage Ia	As in "a" plus microinvasive histologic pattern.
c.	Stage Ib	Invasive cancer confined to the cervix.
d.	Stage Ib	Invasion confined to the cervix but also involving the fundus of the uterus.
e.	Stage IIa	Cervical and upper vaginal involvement without parametrial extension.
f.	Stage IIb	Cervical plus parametrial extension but not to the pelvic side wall.
g.	Stage IIb	Cervical, parametrial, and upper vaginal involvement.
h.	Stage IIIa	Cervical plus involvement of the lower third of the vagina.
i.	Stage IIIa	"h" plus parametrial involvement but not to the side wall.
j.	Stage IIIb	Involvement of cervix, pelvic wall, and lower third of the vagina.
k.	Stage IIIb	Cervical, pelvic side wall, and upper vaginal involvement.
l.	Stage IIIb	Cervical, pelvic side wall, and upper vaginal
m.	Stage IVa	Bladder involvement.
n.	Stage IVa	Rectal involvement.
o.	Stage IVb	Extension beyond the pelvis.

Figure 22–3. Staging of carcinoma of the uterine cervix: patterns of extension. (Source: *Copple-son, M. (Ed.). Gynecologic oncology. Edinburgh: Churchill-Livingstone, 1981, p. 477, by permission.)*

peritoneum opened. Present thinking considers pelvic lymph nodes not to be, by themselves, an indication for deferring the surgery. However, the pelvis must be thoroughly evaluated to assure that the lymph node metastasis and the central recurrence can be resected. Only then should the surgery be pursued (Symmonds & Webb, 1981).

The third and most common controversy asks whether the patient is truly benefiting from a procedure that permanently and drastically alters her normal functioning. To answer this question it is important to examine both the statistics and the human issues. Nonsurgical treatment for the previously radiated person is limited to chemotherapy. Less than 10 percent of these patients are alive 2 years later. For all recurrent cancer patients, none are alive 5 years after recurrence. Survival statistics for exenteration patients vary, but, since 1948 when Brunschwig introduced it, 5-year survival has been improving (due mainly to changes in selection criteria and improvement in operative and postoperative techniques and support). These statistics can be improved by "excluding the elderly, the obese, the heavily irradiated and other high risk patients" (DiSaia & Rich, 1981, p. 525). Similarly work at M.D. Anderson has shown that patients who at the time of recurrence are symptom-free, have a normal intravenous pyelogram (IVP), and whose recurrence is *more* than 5 years after their primary treatment will be more likely to be alive 5 years after exenteration (Rutledge et al, 1977). Table 22–5 indicates that the 5-year survival overall varies between 20 and 62 percent. The high point of this range drops to 38 percent if series with less than 100 patients are excluded. These rates must be contrasted with the grim numbers depicting survival of patients with recurrences.

The human issues cannot be as easily quantified. The clinical viewpoint emphasizes that "the true test for the justification of the pelvic exenteration are the results that have been achieved" (Barber, 1982, p. 166). The survival statistics compare favorably with other cancer sites and patients' survival 5 years after recurrence (Barber, 1982). This part of the controversy is, therefore, based on anecdotal experiences and treatment philosophies. Some would argue that preservation of life is the goal regardless of the means employed. Others look to using quality of life as a parameter. The question remains unanswered. What is clear, however, is that the choices acceptable to the health care provider may not be acceptable to the patient and her family. Frank discussions about postrecovery limitations, stoma care, and so on must be undertaken.

Confirmation of Recurrence

The following describes the process, based on Mages and Mendelsohn's (1979) tasks, that the woman with a cervical cancer recurrence deals with (Table 22–1). Typically, the woman is accompanied by a family member to hear whether the suspected recurrence is confirmed. This is followed by a discussion of options focusing primarily on the exenterative procedure and its goal (cure). Details such as the creation of urinary and fecal stomas, removal of pelvic tissues (including vagina), and extended recuperation are included. Sexual rehabilitation is initiated as well. The decisions regarding whether to proceed with surgery are reviewed. Other options, such as chemotherapy, and should the surgery not be done, are discussed. Regardless of what information is shared, you can expect the woman to hear only a few of the details. Rarely should decisions be made

TABLE 22–5. PELVIC EXENTERATION: TREATMENT RESULTS

Author	Institution	No. of Patients Treated	No. of Operative Deaths	No. Surviving 5 Years[a]
Douglas R. 1957	New York Hospital	23	1 (4.3%)	5 (22%)
Parsons, L. 1964	Boston	112	24 (21.4%)	24 (21.4%)
Brunschwig, A. 1965	Memorial Hospital	535	86 (16%)	108 (20.1%)
Bricker, E. 1967	Washington University	153	15 (10%)	53 (34.6%)
Kreiger, J. 1969	Cleveland Clinics	35	4 (11%)	13 (37%)
Ketcham, A. S. 1970	National Cancer Institute	162	12 (7.4%)	62 (38.2%)
Symmonds, R. 1975	Mayo Clinic	198	16 (8%)	64 (32.3%)
Rutledge, F. 1977	M.D. Anderson	296	40 (13.5%)	99 (33.4%)
Morley, G.	University of Michigan	34	1 (2.9%)	21 (62%)
Total		1548	199 (12.8%)	449 (29%)

[a]*Note:* In almost every series both the operative death rate and the 5-year survival rate were dramatically improved in the later years.
(Source: *Coppleson, M. (Ed.). Gynecologic oncology. Edinburgh: Churchill-Livingstone, 1981, p. 525, by permission.)*

immediately. The woman needs time and space to consider what has been said. Family members are commonly consulted. Fortunately when the details are being shared, the physician(s), nurses, and staff are usually familiar to the patient. This allows her to feel more at ease in expressing her feelings about the information, her fears, and the future. Once at home, many questions arise. The woman should feel free to contact the staff to seek any needed clarification.

During this process the woman is facing the issue of persistent or recurrent disease. The tasks here are for the woman to (1) exercise choice where possible and (2) accept helplessness and dependence where necessary (Mages & Mendelsohn, 1979).

Exercising Choice. The first choice is whether or not to proceed with the work-up. This puts the woman in a difficult position. Should she agree to undergo the procedure, she then must begin facing how to accept and live with the procedure's results. Concomitantly, she is undergoing an evaluation that *at any time* may eliminate surgery as an option. Because the remaining option, chemotherapy, is done for palliation not cure, a situation of ambivalence is created within the patient. This can reduce the effectiveness of the teaching strategies employed and the ability of the woman to exercise choice.

Supporting the woman during this adaptive task is a challenging but critical role for the nurse. The challenge comes from the continuity that must be maintained. The critical aspect comes from the physical and psychological evaluation that must be undertaken. The following describes these processes.

Because this patient's physical work-up can take place both within and outside the confines of the hospital, special efforts to maintain continuity must be in place. The plan of care must be known to all involved and explanations about upcoming procedures and rationale be exactly done. It is helpful to identify two or three individuals to be responsible for the coordination, planning, and teaching. This reduces fragmentation and inaccuracies (Yarbrough, 1981).

Scrutiny of the patient's physical state is undertaken, focusing first on the pelvis to determine if the central recurrence has spread to either pelvic sidewall, lymph nodes, or ureters. A physical examination initially evaluates this. A symptom triad of ureteral obstruction, leg edema, and sciatic pain is synonymous with unresectable disease (DiSaia & Rich, 1981). Other symptoms, such as leg or lower abdominal pain, would indicate disease spread but not resectability. An IVP is also done. Any suspicious areas, such as enlarged lymph nodes, are aspirated. Should these tests reveal ureteral obstruction or malignant cells outside the pelvis, the option of surgery is eliminated.

Once pelvic spread is delineated, evaluation of systemic spread begins. A scalene node biopsy is done. This usually entails hospitalization. If metastases are not found, chest tomograms are completed to insure that the disease has not spread there. A computerized tomography (CT) scan of the thorax or abdomen or both may be done to evaluate disease spread. Depending on the technician's skill and radiologist's interpretive abilities these examinations may or may not yield accurate or useful results.

During the medical work-up, evaluation of the patient's psychological readiness must also be undertaken. The responsibility for this assessment varies among institutions. A provider trained in psychiatry is not essential (Krant, 1981). In fact, a multidisciplinary approach is preferable. This allows input from different professionals and does not limit the scope of assessment. Regardless of who completes the assessment, it must be thorough. For any gynecological cancer patient, Edlund (1982) recommends utilizing the psychological assessment tool developed by Snyder and Wilson (1977). In addition she recommends inclusion of a sexual health assessment (Woods, 1981) (Tables 22–3 and 22–6).

TABLE 22–6. QUESTIONS AND GUIDELINES FOR SEXUAL ASSESSMENT

Questions

Are you physically close or intimate with someone?
    If yes, how satisfactory is this relationship?
    Do you think your partner is satisfied with it?
    How does your relationship differ from what you expected (better, not as good, has changed over the years)?
    Are you and your partner able to talk about your relationship?
    If no:
    Are you able to find a release for your sexual desire, drive, or energy (jogging, physical activity, masturbation)?
    Are you satisfied with this? If no, is this a problem to you?
    Has intercourse been part of your sexual experience?
    If yes:
    Has intercourse ever been painful for you? If yes, can you relate this to anything? (lubrication, penetration, position)
Are pelvic examinations painful for you?
Have you ever experienced orgasm by any means?
Has there been a change in your sex drive?
Do you have difficulty:
    Becoming aroused?
    With lubrication?

If patient has a male partner:
    Does your partner have any difficulties such as maintaining an erection or ejaculating too soon?
    If yes, what have you done to try to overcome this? Is there anything else you think we should know?
    How do you see your disease/treatments effecting your ability to be intimate or achieve satisfaction?

Guidelines for Sexual Assessment

Provide privacy and time[a]
Use language patient understands[a]
Progress from less sensitive to more sensitive issues[a]
Refer to ubiquity of sexual practices (use "how" and "when" not "did you ever")
Avoid assumptions about patient's sexuality or sexual practices[a]
Correct misconceptions and clarify terminology during interview[a]
Be an active listener
Assume responsibility for initiating discussion (thereby legitimatizing it as a topic for discussion)
Allow the patient to refuse to talk about it
Combine open and closed-ended questions
Emphasize the acceptability of behavior

[a]From *Woods, N. F. Human sexuality in disease and illness. St. Louis, Mo.: C. V. Mosby, 1981.*

For the woman facing a pelvic exenteration these same elements apply. Fortunately, the relationship established with the patient during previous admissions or visits allows the nurse to make comparisons between the patient's past and present behavior, beliefs, and thought processes. Using Snyder and Wilson's (1977) tool provides a holistic psychological profile of the patient. Several elements deserve special mention.

Any premorbid comments or fears regarding dying during surgery or not going home or living any more must be explored. Certainly all patients face, to some degree, their own mortality as they prepare for surgery. Exploring these fears will help determine if they are based in reality. This, in turn, may indicate if the patient is employing adaptive or maladaptive coping mechanisms to a situation where there is a perceived loss of control (Edlund, 1982; Weisman, 1979).

Evaluation of the support systems available to the patient is another critical aspect of this assessment. A primary family member, the woman's partner, or other significant person, should be involved from the outset. This person(s) should be aware of the expected recuperative process in the hospital and after discharge. Discussion about the patient's limitations is also necessary to plan for help after discharge. This discussion should be initiated in the presence of both patient and partner. Additional discussion can take place together or separately at the discretion of the couple and the provider.

The exact requirements necessary to pass the pre-exenterative psychological assessment have not been researched. Retrospective information is available in anecdotal form, but has little predictive value. Based on information available in the literature, the following questions are proposed. Each should be answered positively before an exenterative procedure is undertaken:

1. Has the patient accepted being a cancer patient?

   • Does she use the word cancer?
   • Can she explain the rationale for her decision(s)?

2. Is she able to carry out her prediagnosis activities?

   • Has she resumed work or household activities?
   • Is she functioning in all of her pretreatment roles (e.g., mother, worker, wife, friend, lover)?

3. Does she view the results of this surgery as something(s) she can overcome or adjust to?

   • Is she asking questions or seeking information? Is she expressing concerns regarding possible future problems?
   • Is she employing an adaptive* coping mechanism?
   • Is she talking and behaving optimistically, but not naively about the future?
   • Is she talking and acting in a manner that expresses hope and faith (as opposed to helplessness or hopelessness)?

4. Is she expressing her fears, concerns, feelings?

   • Are they realistic?
   • Is she using resources or other support persons to talk about what is facing her?

If the physical and psychological evaluations indicate that the exenterative procedure can be undertaken, the preoperative preparation must begin. In most cases this discussion will have begun during the evaluation process. It is presented here to reduce fragmentation of the information.

This preparation accompanies the woman's move to the next adaptive task, i.e., accepting helplessness and dependence.

Accepting Helplessness and Dependence. Mages and Mendelsohn (1979) originally depicted this task for the person who is terminally ill. Although the woman facing exenterative surgery is terminally ill from the standpoint of recurrence, she is facing a potentially curative surgery. This may seem contrary to the essence of the task. However, she is in a

---

*Defined by Weisman as finding "good solutions for old problems, adequate solutions for new problems, and resourceful solutions for unexpected problems" (1979, p. 15).

position where some degree of dependency will be a necessary part of recovery. This includes being dependent on professionals, family members, and friends. (For additional discussion about dependence–independence, see Derdiarian, 1983.)

Prior to initiating any teaching, it is imperative to assess the patient's level of understanding. Based on this, priorities for teaching can be set to insure that content is not overlooked (see section under Radical Vulvectomy for additional discussion).

Fortunately, there is much written information about preparing patients for exenterative surgery. Yarbrough (1981) published a teaching plan for the professionals working with these patients. It is presented in Table 22–7 as a reference for the remainder of this discussion. Note that six different professionals are involved in the teaching process. This will differ depending on the individual institution's resources and division of responsibilities. Nevertheless, the objectives and content delineated by Yarbrough are universal and can be applied to patients at other institutions. Other information is also available for professionals regarding care for these patients (Dericks, 1974; Hamilton & Schlapper, 1974; Miller, 1962).

Individualization of teaching methodology is critical. The patient is still facing the possibility that the exenteration would not be undertaken. Anxiety about the unknown can dramatically reduce how well she is able to understand and integrate the teaching content into her expectations. In terms of the adaptive tasks, the patient should be aware of the need to be dependent during the initial recuperative period. Later she will move into tasks discussed under the radical vulvectomy section of this chapter.

Before exploring the body image and sexuality concerns associated with exenterative surgery, mention of some guidelines about preoperative preparation and support are necessary. Including a significant other in the teaching should be done. In addition, plan time for reinforcement and review, taking into consideration the patient's readiness to learn. Also, have an operating room and recovery room nurse visit the patient preoperatively. A visit to the intensive care unit is also in order. The patient and family must also know the visiting hours, location of waiting room, and expected length of operative time. (See also discussion in Lewis (1983) about family support.)

Using written information as a supplement to teaching and reinforcement must be considered. A number of pamphlets about ostomies are available (see written material resource list at end of chapter). These should be used with discretion depending on the patient's literacy and intellectual level. Show the patient drawings of the internal changes the surgery will create along with how her abdomen will look (Fig. 22–4). This is usually the most difficult part of the procedure for the patient to visualize or imagine. One example of written information was published by M.D. Anderson Hospital (Resource A). Regardless of what is used, remember that written information is only a supplement to other teaching.

The physical changes this woman will face after surgery can be overwhelming. The health care professional must present them to the patient as *surmountable* obstacles. Demonstrating that the health care professional believes she can learn to care for the stomas as a part of her life is important. Simultaneously, empathy must be conveyed toward the patient and her family. Recognize that the information can be overwhelming and that it will take her time to adjust. Assure her that she will not be discharged until she can care for herself. Again her acceptance of dependency will be necessary initially, as she relearns self-care.

Adjustment to the stoma care and the concomitant physical changes may be complicated by the patient's reaction to her changed body. This is further multiplied by her perceptions about changes in her sexuality. These issues are a part of body image and

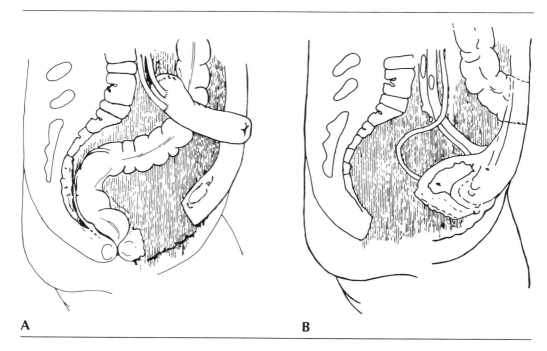

A   **B**

Figure 22–4. Anterior (**A**) and posterior (**B**) exenteration. (Source: *Hamilton, M. S., & Schlapper, N. J. Nursing care of patients with extensive surgery: Pelvic exenteration. In* Nursing care of patients with ostomies and pelvic exenterations. *American Cancer Society, 1974. Reprinted from proceedings of the National Conference on Cancer Nursing, by permission.)*

self-image concepts. Norris (1978) views body image as the "somatic ego." It is the "information, perceptions about one's body as different and apart from all others" (Norris, 1978). It is the frame of reference through which each person perceives and compares herself with others. Self-image or self-concept incorporates body image; it is the sum of other's reactions to the individual in concert with the individual's beliefs, background, and physical status. It is in essence who an individual is. Exenterative surgery forces each patient to ask and answer the question "Who am I?" This questioning forces a reexamination of past decisions, current beliefs, and priorities. Usually this leads to a distinction between the physical self and the intangible self (e.g., personality, beliefs, values).

The nurse can help the woman face these questions. Being available to talk, initiating discussion about sensitive subjects, identifying subjects she is avoiding, and recognizing/confronting nonverbal cues are ways in which the nurse can help. However, the patient's timeline to work through these issues may be different from that of the nurse. The patient cannot be forced to adapt psychologically at the same speed that she is adapting or adjusting physically, nor should she be expected to. The full ramifications of the changes may not become apparent for months following surgery. The health care professional should be available during this time. Watch for signals regarding her readiness or need for discussion. This ongoing support helps the patient believe that her body, though changed, is still acceptable (Woods, 1979). Preoperatively the patient should be

TABLE 22–7. GYNECOLOGY DEPARTMENT TOTAL PELVIC EXENTERATION PATIENT TEACHING PLAN

Team Member	Objective	Content	Teaching Action	Outcome Criteria
Physician	1. Patient will be able to define a total pelvic exenteration and explain briefly why it is performed.	A total pelvic exenteration includes removal of the bladder, the lower part of the bowel, and the female reproductive organs including uterus, ovaries, fallopian tubes, and vagina.		Patient defines a pelvic exenteration and explains why it is performed.
Clinic nurse	2. Patient will be able to identify selected parts of the anatomy and indicate the pelvic changes that will occur as a result of the surgery.	Indicate the following organs on the anatomical illustration: uterus, fallopian tubes, ovaries, and vagina. Explain that lymph nodes and blood vessels in the pelvic cavity will also be removed.	Introduce patient handbook, Pelvic Exenteration, and use handbook illustrations of the female anatomy for clarification.	Patient identifies parts of the female anatomy affected by the surgery when presented with an anatomical drawing.
	3. Patient will be able to verbalize ways in which the total pelvic exenteration will alter body image, excretory and sexual functions.	Discuss scope of the operation, removal of the rectum, bladder, reproductive organs, stomas on abdomen for bowel and bladder function and vaginal reconstruction.		Patient explains how the surgery will alter her body image and excretory and sexual function.
	4. Patient will be able to identify members of the health care team involved in her care and their roles	Introduce all members of the health team to the patient and ask that they provide a brief explanation of their responsibilities to the patient.		Patient identified team members and their roles.
	5. Patient will be able to generally explain the sequence of tests and treatments she will be receiving.	Review the length of hospital stay, sequence of tests and treatments.	Make arrangements for the patient to tour the inpatient area.	Patient explains the sequence of tests she will be receiving.
Social worker	6. Patient will be able to identify support systems among her family and friends.	Discuss with patient home environment, family relationships, and financial situation.		Patient's family members and friends provide emotional support during the patient's illness.

(continued)

525

TABLE 22–7. (cont.)

Team Member	Objective	Content	Teaching Action	Outcome Criteria
	7. Patient will be able to identify local resources she can rely on for home care and financial assistance.	Review patient's home, family, and employment situation. Refer to appropriate agencies.	Provide patient with a list of local resources.	Patient seeks financial assistance and home care assistance at the local level as needed.
	8. Patient will be able to discuss sexual rehabilitation.	Review how the total pelvic exenteration will effect and alter sexual function. Discuss the vaginal reconstruction and explore the patient's and partner's feelings.		Patient indicates post surgery needs when they arise.
Enterostomal therapist	9. Patient will be able to identify anatomical changes effecting gastrourinary and gastrointestinal tract.	Discuss and reinforce what has been discussed by other multidisciplinary team members.	Distribute: "Colostomies, A Guide," "Caring for Your Ileal Conduit." Show equipment and appliances used by the ostomate.	Patient identifies anatomy changes on model of gastrourinary or gastrointestinal tract.
Dietitian	10. Patient will be able to discuss the importance of proper nutrition prior to surgery.	Discuss weight maintenance or weight gain, high intake of protein, basic four food groups and discourage weight loss.	Distribute: "Guide to Good Eating," and "Nutritional Build-Up."	Patient identifies high protein foods; states the names of the basic four food groups and which groups contribute protein to the diet and verbalizes the importance of weight maintenance and weight gain.
	11. Patient will be able to explain the importance of NPO status postoperatively.	Discuss necessity of adequate bowel function prior to initiation of feeding	Discuss content.	Patient states rationale for NPO status.
	12. Patient will be able to explain rationale for intravenous solutions even though patient is not eating.	Explain that CHO, PRO, and FAT, vitamins, minerals, electrolytes will be fed into her subclavian vein in a form that requires no digestion by the intestinal tract, so the bowels are kept at rest.	Show model of IVH solution.	Patient verbalizes that nutritional needs will be met after surgery via IV route.

13. Patient will be able to explain need for nutritional assessment (where applicable).	Explain skin test, anthropometrics, and diet history, obtain weight history, and note recent weight loss of 10lbs in 1 month or 10% of body weight.	Show calipers, measurement tubes and explain rationale for each component of assessment and its relationship to readiness for surgery.	Patient states at least 2 components of nutritional assessment.
14. Patient will be able to define a total pelvic exenteration and how it will alter body image, excretory and sexual functions.	Discuss scope of operation removal of rectum, bladder, reproductive organs, stomas on abdomen for bowel and bladder function; vaginal reconstruction.		Patient defines the pelvic exenteration and discusses altered body functions excretory and sexual functions.
15. Patient will be able to describe her treatment plan and the diagnostic tests she will be receiving.	Discuss purpose of procedure or test, bowel prep, blood work, pulmonary toilet activity, diet restrictions, betadine douche, skin care, stoma marking, x-rays, lymph-angiogram, subclavian line, IVH, TED hose.		Patient describes the tests she will undergo and the sequence of the treatment plan.
16. Patient will be able to carry out postoperative activities as taught.	Stay in PCU, Monitor NG Tube, IV, pain control, activity deep breathing, coughing, ankle and leg exercise, proper medication.		Post-operatively, the patient deep breathes, coughs, and does ankle and leg exercises as taught.
17. Patient will be able to recognize possible complications and how to prevent them.	Review importance of pulmonary toilet activity, wound and perineal care so as to prevent pulmonary and circulatory complications and to prevent wound infection and skin breakdown. Review signs of wound infection; redness, increased soreness, swelling, foul odor, drainage, increased temperature, and general malaise. Discuss ileal or sigmoid conduit complications, perineal skin irritation, excessive leakage around pouch, abnormal color of urine and change in color of stoma or retraction.		Patient describes possible complications and what can be done to prevent them.

In-patient nurse

(continued)

TABLE 22–7. (cont.)

Team Member	Objective	Content	Teaching Action	Outcome Criteria
Dietitian	18. Patient will be able to verbalize the importance of obtaining or maintaining ideal body weight.	Discuss the fact that there will be fewer complications postoperatively if patient maintains IBW and is adequately nourished. For underweight patient, caloric intake and weight gain will assure proper healing. For the obese patient, stress that weight loss, after adequate healing, will enable patient to care for stomas more easily. For patient with appetite problems, suggest commercial supplements, PRO supplemental drink recipes and small frequent feedings.	For underweight patients and those with appetite problems distribute: "Nutritional Build-up— Supplementary Beverages."	Patient states at least 2 components of nutritional assessment. Underweight patients are able to plan 6 feedings, High Protein meal plan. Obese patient accurately designs a low caloric meal plan for 1 day.
	19. Patient will be able to explain the importance of normal bowel movements.	Stress that bowel movement patterns will be individual. Dietary modification in most cases can provide control of constipation, diarrhea, gas, irritation, and blockage. Remind that emotional upsets can lead to disturbance of normal bowel patterns. Suggest residue dietary principles and increased fluid, Nat and KT rich food if patient experiences chronic diarrhea.	Explain dietary means of controlling bowel movements. Give: "Dietary Guidelines for Ostomy Patients." Explain low residue diet, if pertinent.	Patient lists 2 foods that help achieve normal bowel function and states their mode of action.
	20. Patient will be able to explain the importance of consuming an adequate diet.	Review basic 4 food groups to insure adequate nutrient intake. Skipping meals may increase gas production. Keep food record of those foods that cause discomfort and try them again at a later date.	Review illustrations on "Guide to Good Eating."	Patient designs a daily meal pattern including the recommended servings from the "Guide to Good Eating."

	Objective	Content/Intervention	Outcome
	21. Patient will be able to explain the importance of nutrition even after recovery from surgery.	Assess achievement of dietary and nutritional goals; provide alternative ways to obtain ideal body weight, (i.e., other weight reduction regimens for weight loss). Encourage experimentation with foods once avoided to assure wide variety.	Patient is instructed on maintaining ideal body weight. Dietary recall assessed for nutritional quality.	Patient states need to maintain weight. Patient accurately plans corrections in daily intake to satilfy nutritional needs.
Enterostomal therapist	22. Patient will be able to properly irrigate colostomy.	Discuss how to set-up equipment and check stoma condition.	Demonstrate steps in setting-up equipment. Distribute instructional sheet, "Colostomy Irrigation."	Patient irrigates colostomy properly.
	23. Patient will be able to demonstrate how to apply and care for equipment.	Explain how to measure and change pouch sizes. Discuss how to place pouch. Explain how to keep all equipment clean.	Distribute: "How to Apply Pouch" and "How to Apply Urinary Equipment." Initiate a demonstration with the patient participating.	Patient applies and cares for equipment.
	24. Patient will be able to identify community health resources specific to her needs.	Discuss where to purchase equipment and supplies. Discuss the role of the community nurses in the continuing care of the patient. Describe the services of national ostomy societies and the American Cancer Society.	Distribute a list of Houston area and home area equipment supplies. Provide patient with the name of an ET in his/her community. Give patient your name and the phone number of the MDAH ET Department.	Patient makes contact with appropriate community health resources, as needed.
In-patient nurse	25. Patient will be able to follow instructions for home care.	Not to drive car for _____ weeks. No sexual activity until _____, douching with _____, no heavy housework or lifting, dietary information given, prescriptions, return appointment given, VNA referral, may shower.	Review Discharge Instructions in patient education handbook.	Patient follows do's and don'ts of home care.

Main goal: The patient will be able to return to her home and occupation with the ability to deal with an altered body structure.

This teaching plan was prepared by the Gynecology Patient Education Committee, M.D. Anderson Hospital and Tumor Institute, The University of Texas System Cancer Center. Committee members include: Dr. Jan Seski, Michael Loeffler, Eutemia Chua, Laura Griffinberg, Nancy Stewart, Lisa Smith, Beverly Hampton, Kathy Crosson, and Betty Yarbrough. This plan may be reproduced and distributed.
(Source: Oncology Nursing Forum, 1981, 8(2), 37–40.)

introduced to the support persons that will be available to her postoperatively and postdischarge, e.g., the community health nurse or team.

Psychosexual adjustment is a vital part of her postsurgical recovery, and adaptation to changed body image. This begins with an assessment of the meaning and expression of sexuality by patient or the couple prior to recurrence. Involvement of the partner is essential here. Be aware, however, that the spouse may not be the woman's sexual partner. The assessment yields information about the meaning and importance of vaginal intercourse and patterns of foreplay and communication. Loss of a functional vagina and clitoris must not be glossed over in preoperative preparation. Although the full impact of the loss may not be felt for 6 months or more, early discussion provides the couple with information about options. This must include normal reactions to loss. Often they parallel Kubler-Ross's stages of grief. The partner may withdraw from the woman because of fear of injury to her or guilt about his own feelings. This is perceived by the patient as rejection. She then withdraws. A maladaptive cycle is created. Anticipatory guidance in the form of information often prevents this from happening. For those couples who cannot have vaginal intercourse or who need to develop other erotic areas, a number of techniques are available. (See Table 22–8 and Chapter 5 for additional details about

TABLE 22–8. TECHNIQUE AND OPTIONS FOR SEXUAL EXPRESSION/INTIMACY FOR THE COUPLE TO CONSIDER

Maximize potential of touching	Insure privacy and time. Avoid perineal contact; tissue thinning there may cause pain. Caress and fondle each other. Touch upper back, thighs, breasts/nipples, and buttocks. Method of touch (to stimulate light pressure nerve endings): feather light touch increasing gradually in pressure and rapidity. Have each partner learn how to stimulate the other. Experiment. Explore pleasurable sensations. Use mechanical devices for stimulation.
Stimulate other senses	Be imaginitive. Use erotic clothing. Describe or provide olfactory cues; describe in detail sexual fantasy. Use erotic pictures.
Decrease visual impact of stomas or scars	Provide reduced or soft lighting. Use of lingerie or covers over stomas and appliances. Prior to sexual expression, avoid foods that stimulate colostomy function.
Maximize energy	Avoid timing sexual expression after heavy eating or drinking or after tranquilizing or narcotic medications. Employ relaxation response technique. Early morning after a full night's sleep is best.
Maximize understanding	Prior to and after sexual expression discuss what happened or did not happen. Share feelings and sensations. Make "I . . ." statements as opposed to generalizations.
Minimize discomfort during intercourse	Avoid male superior position. Minimize vaginal penetration by using lateral decubitus position or by keeping thighs closely adducted or by the male approaching from behind. Avoid penile thrusting. Use intrathigh or intramammary intercourse. Have woman hold penis as it begins to penetrate to simulate vaginal wall tightness.

approaches and techniques available.) In discussing this with the couple do not focus on intercourse or orgasm as the goal. This can set up a performance anxiety that undermines sexual expression. Keep in mind that orgasmic capacity is not necessarily obliterated by pelvic exenteration (Lamont, DePetrillo, & Sargeant, 1978); other erogenous zones can be developed. The need for open communication between partners is the critical element necessary to satisfactorily resolve this problem. Remember patients welcome information about what they *can* do (Woods, 1979). Depending on the provider's skills and the preexisting problems in the patient's sexual relationship, it may be useful to involve a sex counselor or therapist.

Summary

The pelvic exenterative procedure is traumatic to the patient's physical and psychological well-being. Ongoing evaluation of physical and psychosocial adaptation prior to and after hospitalization is, therefore, essential. Valuable assets in this process are knowledgeable personnel available by phone and at clinic visits to discuss potential problems and changes. Health care providers can ease the trauma of this surgery by anticipating problems and giving the patient and partner the tools with which to work—accurate information, time, and sustained support.

Less Extensive Procedures. Although the discussion in this chapter has focused on radical, extensive surgery, many of the principles presented apply to less radical procedures such as a hysterectomy. Teaching plans and sample patient education materials are available in the literature. One example is in Resource B. An abbreviated listing of the resources available is in the Resources section. Appendix C contains generic care plans developed at the University of Rochester Strong Memorial Hospital for patients undergoing nonradical procedures. The interventions pre- and postoperatively can be used as a guide for developing the teaching plan content. By combining them with the teaching principles in this book, an effective preparation plan can be developed and implemented.

CONCLUSION

Within the framework of Mages and Mendelsohn, this chapter has reviewed the techniques and content necessary to prepare the woman undergoing a radical vulvectomy or a pelvic exenteration. The actual content and approach must be individualized to the patient's needs, the teacher's skills, and the institution's practices. Use of a schemata to understand how the patient is reacting to the diagnosis and treatment is recommended.

RESOURCE A

PELVIC EXENTERATION

Your doctor has found that you need to have several of the organs in your lower abdomen removed because they have been invaded by cancer. The name given this surgery is pelvic exenteration.

The average hospital stay for a pelvic exenteration patient is 3–4 weeks.

There are three types of pelvic exenterations—total, anterior, and posterior. In each of these all the female reproductive organs are removed during surgery. Therefore, you will no longer be able to have children nor will you have menstrual periods.

Depending on which of the three types you have and whether you decide to have your vagina surgically rebuilt, your sexual ability and sensitivity may be altered greatly or not at all. Your doctor will talk with you and your partner about this before surgery.

A total pelvic exenteration includes removal of the bladder, the lower part of the bowel (descending colon and rectum) and the female reproductive organs, including the uterus, ovaries, fallopian tubes and vagina.

If you have this procedure, you will have two stomas. A stoma is a small opening in the abdomen that lets your body eliminate waste, either stool or urine, when the bladder or the lower part of the bowel has been removed. The stoma that will drain your bowels is called a colostomy and probably will be on the lower left side of your abdomen. The stoma that will drain your bladder will be on the right side and is called a urinary conduit.

In an anterior pelvic exenteration, the bowel is left alone, leaving it to work normally. Patients needing this procedure have only one stoma, a urinary conduit.

In the posterior pelvic exenteration, the bladder is left alone and the patient can urinate normally. Patients needing this procedure have only one stoma, a colostomy.

Although several organs will be removed during your surgery, the way you look will not change greatly, except for having one or two stomas on your lower abdomen. Special, odor-free bags have been designed to be worn over the stomas to collect the stool or urine. The collection bags are comfortable to wear and when you are dressed no one will notice any change in the way you look.

The prospect of living with a stoma often is the most dreaded fact faced by patients having pelvic exenterations. Thousands of persons are living completely normal, active lives with stomas, differing only in that they eliminate wastes from their bodies through small openings in their abdomens. Specially trained nurses, enterostomal therapists, will teach you to care for yourself and your stoma before you leave the hospital so that you will go home confident and able to care for yourself.

Preparation

When you are first scheduled for a pelvic exenteration, start doing whatever you can to help improve your general health. Such things as eating a well-balanced diet, staying active and stopping or reducing your smoking (if you smoke) will help you recover from surgery as quickly as possible.

You probably will be asked to check into the hospital a few days before the time of your surgery. This allows time for routine blood and urine tests, as well as any other tests you might need. You will be given a special soap called Phisohex or an iodine solution called Betadine to bathe with. This will prevent local infection. During these days before your surgery, please feel free to ask any questions you have about your surgery.

Two to three days before your surgery, you will be given an enema to cleanse your bowels. You may not want to eat or drink anything after noon the day before your scheduled surgery. Before bedtime the evening before your surgery, your abdomen and genitals (external sex organs) will be shaved. You may be given a sleeping pill to make sure you get a good night's sleep.

A day or so before your surgery a needle will be placed in a vein near your collarbone. After your surgery you will not be able to eat. You will be fed through this needle with a solution of water, protein, sugar, fat, minerals and vitamins.

A small tube will be placed in your stomach to drain it and keep your stomach empty. The tube will be inserted through your nose, down your throat and into your stomach (nasogastric tube) and/or a small incision will be made on the side of your abdomen and the tube placed directly into your stomach.

You will be taught deep breathing and coughing exercises to help clear your lungs and prevent pneumonia. You also will be taught "splinting" methods to help ease any pain you might feel when doing the exercises.

The anesthetist who will put you to sleep for your surgery will review with you what is going to take place during the surgery and answer any questions you may have. You will be given medicine to help you

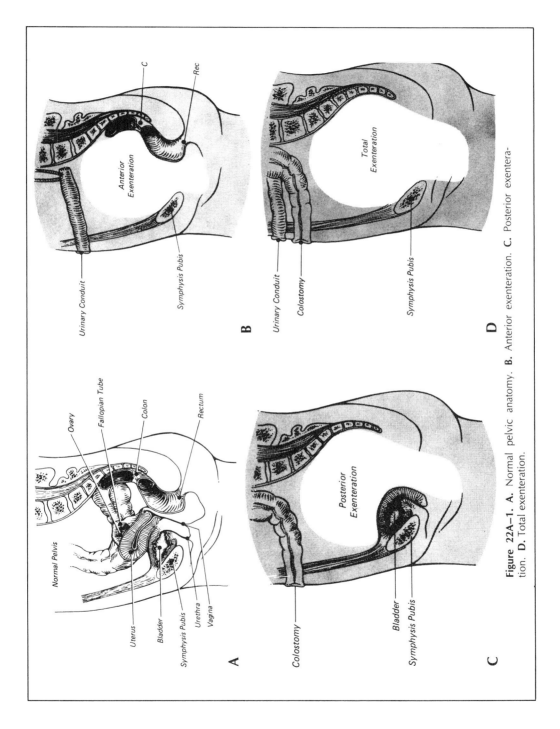

Figure 22A–1. A. Normal pelvic anatomy. **B.** Anterior exenteration. **C.** Posterior exenteration. **D.** Total exenteration.

533

relax and a needle will be placed in a vein in your arm through which you will be given a mixture of sugar and water, as well as some antibiotics to help prevent infection.

The Procedure

During your surgery, the anesthetist who gives you the drug that puts you to sleep will keep constant watch on your condition. The surgery usually lasts 5–6 hours.

The organs are removed through an incision made in the lower abdomen. If you have a total pelvic exenteration and have decided to have your vagina rebuilt so that normal sexual activity can continue, it will be done as part of the surgery.

Postoperative Care

You can expect some discomfort for about 48 hours after your surgery. This is normal. You can be given medicine to ease any pain or extreme discomfort, so ask for it. You will be given medicine to help prevent infection while your body is recovering from the immediate shock of the surgery. You will also be given a medicine called heparin to prevent blood clots from forming.

You will stay in the postoperative recovery room for 1–2 days before going back to your hospital room. After surgery, your bowels will be very sluggish and will not accept food. You may need to be fed through the needle near your collarbone for 2–3 weeks. The tube draining your stomach will stay in place for 7–21 days after surgery. It will be removed as soon as your bowels become active again.

During surgery, a tube will be placed in your pelvic cavity to drain any fluid that may collect. One end of this tube will come out through the closed incision. This tube will be removed 6–7 days after surgery.

Your stoma or stomas will already have temporary collection bags in place. These will be checked and changed regularly by your enterostomal therapist until you can begin learning to care for your stoma or stomas yourself.

If you have had a posterior pelvic exenteration, your bladder may be weak even though it was not touched by the surgery. For a while it may not empty well. To prevent infection, a small, soft tube (a catheter) may be placed in the opening that leads to your bladder to make certain your bladder drains completely. The outside end of the catheter drains into a plastic bag that holds the urine. The catheter may have to stay in your bladder for a few days.

You will be expected to be up and moving about shortly after surgery. It probably will be uncomfortable to get up and walk the first few times, but the exercise will help you get well faster. Your nurse will help you as needed.

Do the deep breathing exercises you were taught every 2–4 hours after your surgery.

Discharge

Do not expect to be able to do everything you did before your surgery as soon as you leave the hospital. Your body will need several months to fully recover. You probably will find that you get tired easily. Do not let yourself get too tired. Take breaks and rest periods often. Avoid strenuous physical activities such as driving a car, heavy housework (vacuuming), heavy lifting (grocery bags) or active sports until your doctor says it is OK.

However, do get some exercise, such as walking.

Your genitals may still be swollen. The swelling will go down in time, but you may wish to keep taking hot sitz baths three times daily. (You will learn about sitz baths while in the hospital.)

Your doctor will tell you when you can start having sexual relations again. If you have your vagina rebuilt, you may need to avoid sexual intercourse for 4–6 weeks after leaving the hospital. However, you can douche, using a solution of hydrogen peroxide or a vinegar/water/Betadine solution twice a day.

Since your ovaries have been removed, your body will no longer make female hormones and the symptoms of the "change of life" (menopause) may appear. These symptoms can be corrected by taking a hormone pill prescribed by your doctor. Do not take any hormones unless told to by your doctor.

You may begin bathing again as soon as the stitches are removed, about 3 weeks after your surgery. Showers are preferable, but you may take baths. Be very careful not to slip and fall. Clean the incision area with soap and water.

You will have no dietary restrictions other than those you might have had for other medical reasons before your surgery. Begin eating your usual diet unless your dietitian has told you otherwise. Eat a well-balanced diet to help healing.

Avoid wearing any tight clothing such as a girdle or knee-high hose.

There are some symptoms that should be reported to your doctor if they occur:

1. Redness, swelling, drainage or increased soreness along the incision or at the graft site (if you had your vagina rebuilt).
2. A temperature of more than 100°F.

It is important that you take all your medicine the way you were told by your doctor or pharmacist and that you return to the clinic for your follow-up appointments. You will have frequent check-ups for the first few years and then will be placed on a schedule of yearly visits.

If you have any problems or questions about the care of your colostomy and/or urinary conduit, or any other problems or questions, call your doctor at these numbers:

This patient education booklet was prepared at the University of Texas M. D. Anderson Hospital and Tumor Institute at Houston, Texas. This material may be reproduced and distributed.

(*Source:* Pelvic exenteration. *Oncology Nursing Forum*, 1981, 8(4), 53–56, by permission.)

RESOURCE B

A PATIENT'S GUIDE TO RADICAL HYSTERECTOMY

Women who are about to undergo a radical hysterectomy have many questions about the procedure and its effects. This booklet attempts to answer some of the initial questions by describing the surgery itself, the patient's experience in the hospital, and the recommended follow-up care. A further discussion with your physician will serve to expand this information and to clarify the differences that may apply to your individual case.

Description of Radical Hysterectomy
A radical hysterectomy is designed to treat not only the malignant tumor in the uterine cervix, but also the adjacent areas into which the tumor may have spread. The structures that are removed in this procedure are the uterus and the uterine cervix, the nearby supporting tissues, the uppermost part of the vagina and the pelvic lymph nodes. All the removed tissues are examined carefully under a microscope to determine precisely the extent of the disease.

The following illustrations will help you visualize the area of surgery.

With any surgery there are risks of bleeding, infection and unusual anesthetic reactions. In more extensive surgery such as a radical hysterectomy additional risks must be anticipated. Such risks relate to the more extensive areas of operation and include damage to the adjacent organs such as the bowel, bladder, ureters (tubes that drain urine from the kidneys to the bladder) or the large vessels and nerves in the field of surgery. Blood clot formation, nerve damage and prolonged leg swelling may all occur but are fortunately quite rare. Damage to the urinary tract with resultant urine drainage through the vagina also can rarely occur but is usually correctable by additional surgery. These risks are a necessary price for the aggressive treatment of cancer but should be discussed carefully with your physician.

Initial Evaluation
The initial evaluation includes a review of your medical history and a physical examination. The pathology slides are reviewed as well as any pertinent past medical records. X-ray studies of the kidneys and bladder (intravenous pyelogram) and of the bowel (barium enema) are often obtained to determine if there is any abnormality in these organs possibly related to pressure by the tumor. A chest x-ray, electrocardiogram and blood and urine studies are routinely performed. With this information at hand, the surgeon will discuss all the findings with you. Alternative methods of treatment that might be available will be discussed with you as well as the anticipated events that occur with a radical hysterectomy. Your questions will be answered and then with your consent, the hospitalization is planned.

Hospital Admission
The Patient Care Coordinator will schedule the day of surgery, the time of hospital admission and any further tests requested by your physician. She can answer many initial questions about hospital routines, financial coverage or other services you might want. Your Gynecologic Nurse Oncologist is a specialist in caring for women with gynecological cancer and will be available to you throughout your hospitalization and recovery from surgery. A registered Primary Care Nurse will help coordinate your care on the hospital unit. The orientation booklet given to you in the Admitting Department details other resource personnel available to you and your family.

You will become acquainted with several physicians during your hospital stay. In addition to your staff physician who will perform the surgery, other resident gynecologists, anesthesiologists and possibly medical students will compose a team specifically involved in your care. In this way there will always be physicians in the hospital who are familiar with your care.

At the time of hospital admission, personnel in the Admitting Department may direct you to several areas for routine testing. Urinalysis, chest X-ray, electrocardiogram, and blood studies may be performed at this time. Your family may accompany you to these various departments and stay with you in the waiting areas.

When you are settled on the hospital unit, a resident gynecologist will review your records, perform a physical examination and write initial orders for your hospital care. Hospitalization generally lasts from 7 to 10 days.

The Day Before Surgery
The day before surgery your resident physician will review the plans initiated by your staff physician, answer any questions you may have, and ask you to sign the standard operative consent form for the surgery.

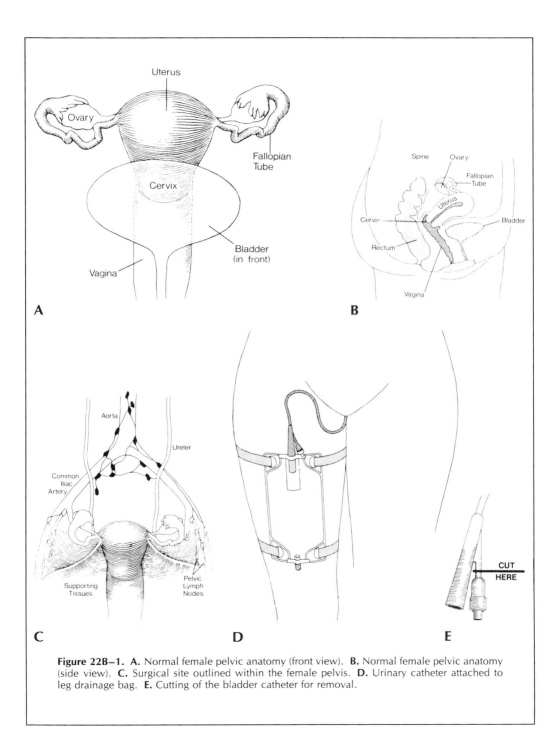

Figure 22B–1. **A.** Normal female pelvic anatomy (front view). **B.** Normal female pelvic anatomy (side view). **C.** Surgical site outlined within the female pelvis. **D.** Urinary catheter attached to leg drainage bag. **E.** Cutting of the bladder catheter for removal.

The anesthesiologist will meet with you for an examination and discussion of the surgical anesthetic. He will order medications for sedation before surgery including sleeping medicines for the night if you wish. These medicines are part of your total anesthetic plan; they will make you drowsy and relaxed.

Your nurse will instruct you in postoperative routines. She will teach you breathing exercises that prevent lung congestion and limb exercises that improve blood circulation while you are less active. Walking will be encouraged soon after surgery for early mild activity stimulates the body's return to normal function. Your family is welcome during this orientation.

On the evening before surgery, the surgical area will be cleaned and shaved and you will have a vaginal douche and enema. You may have a regular dinner but nothing to eat or drink from midnight until after surgery. Family members may visit with you in the morning before surgery but have them come early since you will be taken to the operating room about an hour before the scheduled time.

Hospital Care After Surgery

The operative procedure will usually take 5 to 6 hours followed by 2 to 3 hours for recovery from the anesthetic. There is a room near the operating room where your family may wait. Your doctor will talk with them after the surgery to let them know how you are doing.

As you awaken, you will become aware of the nurse checking your condition frequently. Your blood pressure, pulse and temperature will be monitored and you will have an intravenous line (I.V.) until you are able to drink and eat normally. Two catheters (hemovacs) are placed below the incision to drain excess fluid from the surgical site and these will be attached to a suction machine. You will also have a urinary bladder catheter. Do not be alarmed if you are receiving oxygen or a blood transfusion upon awakening as these are not uncommon immediately after surgery.

You will be encouraged to take deep breaths and to cough deeply every 2 to 3 hours and periodically to turn in bed and exercise your feet and legs. You will be urged to sit on the edge of the bed in the evening or the following morning and to begin walking as soon as possible. Ambulation will be continually encouraged throughout your hospital stay. After any surgery these activities may be painful, and there will be medicine ordered for you to allay your discomfort. Your nurse will work with you on scheduling medications for adequate pain control and rest balanced with progressive increase in your activity.

Periodic injections of a blood-thinning medicine are usually given to prevent the formation of blood clots. These injections are discontinued when you are fully ambulatory.

Bowel function is normally sluggish after any abdominal surgery as an effect of the anesthetic and because of manipulation during surgery. Adjustment to drinking and eating, therefore, will be gradual. As this improves you will switch from a clear liquid to a regular diet and intravenous fluids will be discontinued.

Persistent slowed bowel function following radical hysterectomy can be secondary to the unavoidable cutting of tiny nerve fibers in the surgical sites. Techniques of dietary management (daily prune juice, high fiber or high bulk diets) or other bowel programs (stool softener medications or mild laxatives) help prevent difficulties. An increased daily fluid intake augments bowel function. Once your normal diet and activity are reestablished, bowel function usually becomes more normal.

The hemovac drainage catheters will be left in place until there is only a minimal amount of fluid coming from them. Removal of these catheters does not generally cause any significant discomfort.

The urinary bladder catheter will be left in place for an extended time—usually 3 to 6 weeks after the surgery. This not only relieves pressure on the surgical site but allows for greater healing of the tiny nerves to the bladder that are inevitably cut at the time of surgery. These nerves help control the bladder fullness sensations and without the catheter you might not exactly appreciate when to empty your bladder and over distention might result. As you improve, you will be taught to care for the catheter and learn how to remove it prior to your first postoperative clinic visit. (See Recovery at Home Section)

Drinking fluids (6 to 8 glasses a day) is important to prevent any bladder infection while the catheter is in place. It is permissible to take tub baths while the catheter is in once the incision is healed.

Stitches will usually be removed 7 to 10 days after surgery. There may be a reddish to brown discharge from the vagina for several days and a scab-like crust may be passed from the vagina about 1 week after surgery. This is part of the normal healing process.

Any major surgical procedure of this magnitude consumes a great deal of physical and emotional energy. The increased fatigue, hospital confinement and temporary physical limitations may lead to feelings of nervousness or frustration and even anger. These personal reactions may distress you and it often helps to share your concerns with a close family member or friend or staff member. These reactions are normal and temporary.

Recovery at Home

Before your hospital discharge you will be examined and told what to expect in the coming days. Although it is unusual to encounter complications after the hospital discharge, do inform your doctor if you have any of the following:

Excessive bleeding, fever or chills, unusual pain or swelling, unusual vaginal or wound discharge, disturbing emotional reactions, or indeed any other related problems that concern you.

Clinic or office telephone:

After hours, call:

Light activity is encouraged in the first 2 weeks after surgery or until you are seen in the clinic for the first time. Driving or prolonged sitting should be delayed for 3 or 4 weeks since this increases congestion in the pelvic blood vessels. Isometric (tightening) exercises of the abdomen may begin after 3 or 4 weeks. Heavy lifting and strenuous activity should be avoided for 2 to 3 months.

A balanced diet with an emphasis on high protein foods will help to build up your strength and will aid wound healing. Foods from the four basic food groups (milk products, meat or fish foods, fruits and vegetables, and bread, cereal or grain foods) provide essential nutrients and important vitamins and minerals. Foods rich in protein are meats, fish, cheese, milk, soybean products, legumes and eggs. Your physician may prescribe iron supplements if you are anemic. A dietitian is available to offer suggestions about your diet if you prefer.

In general, adequate rest and nutrition balanced with mild physical and diversional activities form the recommendations for your recovery period.

At your first clinic visit (generally 3 or 4 weeks after surgery) your urinary bladder function will be tested. If bladder sensation and function has returned enough for you to be able to empty your bladder completely, the catheter can be permanently removed.

Two to three hours before your scheduled appointment, remove the catheter as you were instructed in the hospital:

1. Cut the catheter near where it attaches to the bag (Figure 22B–1E).
2. Wait for fluid to drain out (about a teaspoonful).
3. Pull the catheter out gently. You should feel no resistance and no discomfort.
4. Drink several glasses of liquids (juices, carbonated beverages, water, etc.), and
5. Bring the urinary drainage leg bag with you to the clinic.

When you arrive at the clinic, you will be asked to urinate. Then, another catheter will be placed to see if the bladder is empty. (If you are uncomfortable with the pressure of a full bladder after you take the catheter out and before your appointment, empty your bladder and continue to drink fluids.) If after the second catheter is placed, the bladder is found to contain only minimal amounts of urine, the catheter will be permanently removed. There may be a continued loss of full sensation which may require you to empty your bladder "by the clock" every 2 to 3 hours. This will be discussed further with you if there should be any delay in return of sensation. This is unusual but manageable.

If large amounts of urine remain in the bladder at the time of second catheterization, the second catheter will be allowed to remain for 1 or 2 weeks longer. The procedure for removing the catheter is the same. Do *not* be discouraged if the catheter must remain a while longer. It is a function of return of nerve sensation and sometimes just takes longer. Please report any unusual bleeding from the catheter or unusual pain or irritation associated with it.

Personal Impact and Sexuality

Each woman reacts to the procedure of radical hysterectomy in her own way. There may be a temporary period when you will feel anxious or insecure in reflecting about its effect on you, your husband, or the way you live. This is normal and to be expected. Cancer is a stressful disease and radical hysterectomy is a complicated treatment. Talking with someone close can help release tension but do allow yourself time to adjust physically and emotionally. Most women do feel confident and comfortable in resuming their normal activities within a few weeks or months.

Many women believe that a hysterectomy will cause menopausal (change of life) symptoms such as hot flashes, night sweating or mood changes. However, it is removal of the ovaries, not the uterus, which will produce these symptoms in younger women and removal of the ovaries can often be avoided at the time of a radical hysterectomy. Removal of the uterus causes only a cessation of menstrual periods and, of course, loss of childbearing function.

Sexual feeling should not be altered as a result of this surgery. Sexual intercourse as well as vaginal douching or use of tampons should be delayed, however, for 3 to 6 weeks after surgery depending on wound healing. Personal concerns related to sexual activity of you or your husband may be discussed with your physician or nurse at any time.

Follow-up Care

Despite treatment, there is always a risk that cancer can recur. Further treatment then might be required and therefore follow-up examinations are recommended every 3 months for the first year and at 6-month intervals during subsequent years. A negative examination is always very reassuring to you. It is frequently possible to arrange some of these follow-up examinations with your local or referring physician but the staff and the facilities at the University Hospital will continue to be a resource to you.

Conclusion

This booklet has provided the basic information regarding the surgical procedure of radical hysterectomy, the patient's experience in the hospital and the follow-up care after surgery. Knowing what is normal and expected from this procedure can be reassuring to women facing it. Further discussion by you and your family with the physician or nurses is welcome at any time.

This patient education booklet was prepared by Katy Jusenius formerly Gynecologic Nurse Oncologist at the Division of Gynecologic Oncology, Department of Obstetrics and Gynecology, University of Washington School of Medicine, Seattle, Washington. It was reviewed in preparation by David C. Figge, MD, and Hisham K. Tamini, MD, at the same facility. Illustrations are by Jan Norbisrath. It is reprinted with permission of the author and may be reproduced and distributed.

(*Source:* A Patient's Guide to Radical Hysterectomy. *Oncology Nursing Forum,* 1983, *10*(1), 72–75, by permission.)

WRITTEN MATERIAL RESOURCES

Written Material Available for Patient Teaching

Managing a Urostomy. Hollister, 1974. *(Aimed at professionals. Can be used for patients. Thorough discussion of possible problems/situations that an ostomate could encounter.)*

The following are from the Office of Cancer Communications, Patient and Professional Education Materials for Ostomates: Selected Annotations. *NIH Publications No. 81-1512, U.S. Dept. HHS, May, 1981.*

A Guide for the Urinary Ostomate. C. R. Bard, Inc., 1977, 14 pp; brochure. *(This guide to the day-to-day management of a urinary ostomy supplies information on appliances, skin care, diet, and sources of professional help. Cost: $1.50. Source: Coloplast Brand Ostomy Products, Bard Home Health Products Division, 50 Industrial Road, Berkeley Heights, NJ 07922. Telephone: (201) 277-8320.)*

Booklet of Instructions for Persons with a Colostomy. V. C. Dericks, 13 pp; brochure. *(This booklet explains self-care to colostomy patients, using a question and answer format. Source: Director of Nursing Services, The New York Hospital, 525 E. 68th Street, New York, NY 10021.)*

Care of Your Sigmoid Colostomy—A Patient's Handbook. 1979, 16 pp; brochure. *(The booklet briefly explains colostomy surgery, management, and equipment. It also offers hints for living with a colostomy and lists sources for information and assistance. Source: The American Cancer Society, local units.)*

Caring For Your Ileal Conduit. 1977, 12 pp; brochure; 2 inserts. *(Basic self-care is described for the cystectomy patient. Included are simple, illustrated explanations of the ileal conduit, the stoma, skin care, and various types of appliances. The brochure also contains an appliance and skin care checklist, and two inserts describing the attachment of appliances, using either cement or self-sticking discs. Cost: free, single copies; bulk rates. Source: The University of Texas System Cancer Center, M.D. Anderson Hospital and Tumor Institute, Dept. of Nursing, 6723 Bertner Avenue, Houston, TX 77030. Telephone: (713) 792-7134.)*

Changing Your Colostomy Bag. N. Woods, 1975, 14 pp; booklet. *(Changing the colostomy appliance is explained in simple terms, through text and informal illustration. Ancillary procedures that can be used to avoid discomfort and other complications are also described. Self-evaluation questions are included. Cost: $2. Source: Patient Education Center, The North Carolina Memorial Hospital, Box 515, Manning Drive, Chapel Hill, NC 27514. Telephone: (919) 966-1091/2.)*

Colostomies: A Guide. E. Lenneberg & A. N. Mendelssohn, Rev. 1974, 32 pp; brochure. *(The booklet explains the different types of colostomies and the techniques for managing them. The ostomate is encouraged to return to work and to resume normal social and physical activities. Recommendations are included on diet, travel, and clothing, and the procedure for irrigation is outlined step-by-step. Also available in Chinese or Spanish. Cost: $3; inquire about bulk rates. Source: United Ostomy Association, Inc., 2001 W. Beverly Blvd., Los Angeles, CA 90057. Telephone: (213) 413-5510.)*

Ileal Loop: A Self-Care Manual. C. L. Blackmon, J. R. Bengel, & M. M. Schuster, Revised 1980, 16 pp; brochure. *(New ostomates with an ileal loop (urinary diversion) receive specific, practical suggestions for stoma and skin care and management of the appliance. Instructions are given for assembling, attaching, and cleaning the permanent appliance. Equipment manufacturers are listed. Cost: $0.25. Source: Milner-Fenwick, Inc., 2125 Greenspring Drive, Tumonium, MD 21093. Telephone: (301) 252-1700.)*

Living Comfortably With Your Colostomy. D. Larson, 1970, 22 pp; brochure. *(Line drawings explain the results of colostomy surgery, the application and drainage of stoma bags, maintenance of the stoma, and coping with minor problems. Also included are a diet for colostomy patients advice on clothing and physical activity, sources of colostomy supplies, and addresses of ostomy societies. Cost: $1.50 plus handling. Order No. 717. Source: Sister Kenny Institute,*

Publications-Audiovisuals Office, 2727 Chicago Avenue, Minneapolis, MN 55407. Telephone: (612) 874-4175.)

Managing Your Colostomy. 1978; brochure. *(The brochure describes changes in normal anatomy and physiology created by a colostomy. All aspects of self-care, such as irrigation, diet, skin care, activity, and emotional and sexual adjustment, are also described. Included are lists of ostomy supplies and sources of assistance. To help the patient live with a colostomy and return to a meaningful, active life, the pamphlet includes charts for patients to record irrigation, activities, problems, diet, medical information, and phone numbers. Cost: $19.95/25. Source: Robert J. Brady Co., Bowie, MD 20715. Telephone: (301) 262-6300.)*

Odor. S. Williams. *Metro Maryland* (United Ostomy Association) 4(4), 4–5, Dec. 77. *(In a society very conscious of body odors, ostomates develop anxieties about their special odor problems. The article gives advice on how to minimize the leakage of odors from stoma devices by emphasizing hygiene, scrupulous care of the device, avoidance of odor-producing foods, adequate fluid intake, and use of specially-designed deodorants. Source: local medical libraries.)*

Ostomy Review II. 1974, 77 pp; selected articles. *(Included are reprints or condensations of selected articles from the Ostomy Quarterly (1968–1973). (Following a general section are sections on colostomy, ileostomy, and urostomy. The full range of ostomy topics is covered: stoma and appliance management, the care of children with ostomies, sex after surgery, odor barriers, diet, and employment. A glossary of ostomy terms, a section of "helpful hints," and a list of equipment manufacturers are also included. Cost: $3.50. Source: United Ostomy Association, Inc., 2001 W. Beverly Blvd., Los Angeles, CA 90057. Telephone: (213) 413-5510.)*

Recognizing, Treating, and Preventing Ostomy-Related Skin Problems. P. Lazar, J. D. Sarbacker, & M. Kowlaski, 1978, 20 pp; brochure. *(Many of the dermatological aspects of ostomy management are described. The most important issues are recognizing, treating, and preventing ostomy-related skin problems. Cost: free. Source: Hollister, Inc., 211 E. Chicago Avenue, Chicago, IL 60611. Telephone: (312) 751-7800.)*

So You Have—Or Will Have an Ostomy. 1972, 6 pp; brochure. *(The brochure answers the major questions that ostomates or potential ostomates may have about the physical and psychological adjustments they must make. It stresses that ostomates can live a full, normal life with a few changes in their habits or life-styles. Cost free/single copy. Source: United Ostomy Association, Inc., 2001 W. Beverly Blvd., Los Angeles, CA 90057. Telephone: (213) 413-5510.)*

The Ostomy Book: Living Comfortable with Colostomies, Ileostomies and Urostomies. B. D. Muller, & K. A. McGinn, 1980, 236 pp; book. *(Ostomy surgery is not uncommon, yet it remains shrouded in secrecy and taboos. This book, written by an ostomate, aims to dispel the myths and fears surrounding the subject. Directed at the average person, it gives thorough, factual information on the physical and emotional aspects of ostomy, in a sensitive and often humorous way. It includes the personal experiences of many ostomy patients and their families and will give hope and confidence to those in the same predicament. Cost: $7.95. Source: Bull Publishing Company, P.O. Box 208, Palo Alto, CA 94302. Telephone: (415) 322-2855.)*

Urinary Diversion Care. D. C. Broadwell, & S. L. Sorrells. 1980. 41 pp; brochure. *(The brochure describes self-care techniques after urinary colostomy surgery. Stoma and skin care, colostomy irrigation, diet, medication, daily activities, and sex are discussed. Also listed are descriptions of organizations and enterostomal therapy follow-up programs are given. Cost: $1. Source: Emory University Clinic, Enterostomal Therapy Dept., 1365 Clifton Road, N.E., Atlanta, GA 30322. Telephone: (404) 321-0111, ext. 321.)*

Urinary Ostomies: A Guidebook for Patients. K. F. Jeter, Revised 1978, 31 pp; brochure. *(This is a comprehensive guide for patient self-care following a urinary ostomy. Among the subjects discussed are the definition of a urinary ostomy. Preparation for surgery, the postoperative period, the stoma, skin care, appliances, and physical and social rehabilitation. Numerous photographs of urinary ostomates of all ages engaged in sports and other physical activities provide encouragement for the new ostomate. Drawings illustrate steps in the procedure of attaching the appliance. A glossary, a list of equipment manufacturers, and titles of other ostomy publications are also included. Cost: $3. Source: United Ostomy Association, Inc., 2001 W. Beverly Blvd., Los Angeles, CA 90057. Telephone: (213) 413-5510.)*

REFERENCES

American Cancer Society. *The psychological impact of cancer*. New York: American Cancer Society, 1974, 1–16, 55–94.

Anderson, P. L., & Hacker, N. F. Psychosexual adjustment of gynecologic oncology patients: A proposed model for future investigation. *Gynecologic Oncology*, 1983, *15*, 214–223.

Barber, H. Relative prognostic significance of preoperative and operative findings in pelvic exenteration. *Surgical Clinics of North America*, 1969, *49*, 431–447.

Barber, H. Surgical procedures in gynecologic malignancies. In J. vanNagell & H. Barber (Eds.), *Modern concepts of gynecologic oncology*. Boston: John Wright PSG, 1982, pp. 469–486.

Boutselis, J. G. Radical vulvectomy for invasive squamous cell carcinoma of the vulva. *Obstetrics and Gynecology*, 1972, *39*, 827–836.

Brown, R. S., Haddox, V., Posada, A., & Rubins, A. Social and psychological adjustment following pelvic exenteration. *American Journal of Obstetrics and Gynecology*, 1972, *111*, 162–171.

Brunschwig, A., & Brockvnier, A. Jr. Surgical treatment of squamous cell carcinoma of the vulva. *Obstetrics and Gynecology*, 1972, *29*, 362–368.

Buchler, D. Multiple primaries and gynecologic malignancies. *American Journal of Obstetrics and Gynecology*, 1975, *123*, 376–381.

Cavanaugh, D., & Ostapowicz, F. Radical operation for carcinoma of the vulva: A new approach to wound healing. *Journal of OB/GYN of the British Commonwealth*, 1970, *77*, 1037–1040.

Cavanaugh, D., & Shepard, J. The place of pelvic exenteration in primary management of advanced carcinoma of the vulva. *Gynecologic Oncology*, 1982, *13*, 318–322.

Cavanaugh, D., Praphat, H., & Ruffolo, E. H. Cancer of the vulva. In R. M. Wynn (Ed.), *Obstetrics and gynecology annual* (Vol. 11). Norwalk, Ct.: Appleton-Century-Crofts, 1982.

Choo, Y. C. Invasive squamous carcinoma of the vulva in young patients. *Gynecologic Oncology*, 1982, *13*, 158–164.

Christiano, M. Y. Hysterectomy. In E. D. Smith (Ed.), *Women's health care*. Norwalk, Ct.: Appleton-Century-Crofts, 1981, pp. 122–135.

Coppleson, M. *Gynecologic oncology* (Vols. 1&2). Edinburgh: Churchill Livingstone, 1981.

Creasman, W. T., & Rutledge, F. Preoperative evaluation of patients with recurrent carcinoma of the cervix. *Gynecologic Oncology*, 1972, *1*, 111–118.

Crosson, K. Patient education: A patient teaching aid for the pelvic exenteration patient. *Oncology Nursing Forum*, 1981, *8*, 53–56.

Dericks, V. C. Nursing care of patient with an ostomy. *American Cancer Society*, 1974.

Derdiarian, A. K. Dependence—independence behavioral changes in cancer surgical patients. *Cancer Nursing*, 1983, *6*(6), 453–462.

Derogatis, L. R., & Kourlesis, S. M. An approach to evaluation of sexual problems in the cancer patient. *CA-A Cancer Journal for Clinicians*, 1981, *31*, 46–49.

DiSaia, P. J., & Rich, W. M. Advanced and recurrent carcinoma of cervix. In M. Coppleson (Ed.), *Gynecologic Oncology* (Vol.1). Edinburgh: Churchill Livingstone, 1981, pp. 517–527.

DiSaia, P. J., Creasman, W. T., & Rich, W. An alternate approach to early cancer of the vulva. *American Journal of Obstetrics and Gynecology*, 1979, *133*, 825–832.

Donahue, V. C. Sexual rehabilitation of gynecologic cancer patients. In M. Coppleson (Ed.), *Gynecologic oncology*. Edinburgh: Churchill-Livingston, 1981, pp. 1050–1053.

Donahue, V. C. Office guide to sexual counseling of gynecologic oncology patients. *Medical Aspects of Human Sexuality*, 1978, *8*, 51–52.

Donahue, V. C., & Knapp, R. C. Sexual rehabilitation of gynecologic cancer patients. *Obstetrics and Gynecology*, 1977, *49*, 118–121.

Edlund, B. J. The needs of women with gynecologic malignancies. *Nursing Clinics of North America*, 1982, *17*, 165–178.

Fisher, S. G. Psychosexual adjustment following total pelvic exenteration. *Cancer Nursing*, 1979, *2*, 219–225.

Friedrich, E. G., & Wilkinson, E. J. The vulva. In A. Blaustein (Ed.), *Pathology of the female genital tract*. New York: Springer-Verlag, 1982, pp. 13–53.

Gallagher, A. M. Body image changes in the patient with a colostomy. *Nursing Clinics of North America,* 1972, *7*(4), 669–667.

Garcia, C., & Boronow, R. Carcinoma of the vulva: Anatomic and histologic prognostic factors. *Southern Medical Journal,* 1972, *65*(2), 237–240.

Gelfant, B. B. Preoperative teaching of gynecological patients. *Point of View,* 1984, *21,* 4–7.

Green, T. H. Carcinoma of the vulva—A reassessment. *Obstetrics and Gynecology,* 1978, *52,* 462–469.

Hamilton, M. S., & Schlapper, N. J. Nursing care of patients with extensive surgery: Pelvic exenteration. In *Nursing care of patients with ostomies and pelvic exenterations,* American Cancer Society, 1974, pp. 7–17.

Hass, T., Buchsbaum, H., & Lifshitz, S. Nonresectable recurrent pelvic neoplasm: Outcome in patients explored for pelvic exenteration. *Gynecologic Oncology,* 1980, *9*(2), 177–181.

Holden, L. S. Helping your patient through her hysterectomy. *RN Magazine,* 1983, *46,* 42–46.

Humphries, P. T. Sexual adjustment following a hysterectomy. *Health Care of Women,* 2(2), 1980, 1–14.

Iverson, T., Abeler, V., & Aalders, J. Individual treatment of stage I cancer of the vulva. *Obstetrics and Gynecology,* 1981, *57,* 85–89.

Jimerson, G., & Merrill, J. Multicentric squamous malignancy involving both cervix and vagina. *Cancer,* 1970, *26,* 150–153.

Johnson, J. The effects of accurate expectations about sensations on the sensory and distress components of pain. *Journal of Personality and Social Psychology,* 1973, *27,* 261–275.

Johnson, J. The effects of structuring patients' expectations on their reactions to threatening events. *Nursing Research,* 1972, *21,* 499–504.

Johnson, J., & Rice, V. H. Sensory distress and the components of pain: Implications for the study of clinical pain. *Nursing Research,* 1974, *23,* 203–209.

Jusenious, K. A teaching aid for the radical hysterectomy patient. *Oncology Nursing Forum,* 1983, *10*(1), 71–75.

Jusenious, K. Sexuality and gynecologic cancer. *Cancer Nursing,* 1981, *4,* 479–483.

Kneale, B. L., Elliott, P. M., & McDonald, I. A. Micro-invasive carcinoma of the vulva: Clinical features and management. In M. Coppleson (Ed.), *Gynecologic oncology* (Vol. 1). Edinburgh: Churchill Livingstone, 1981, pp. 320–338.

Koile, E. *Listening as a way of becoming.* Waco, Tx.: Regency Books, 1977.

Kolstad, P. Conservative surgery for invasive carcinoma of vulva. In M. Coppleson (Ed.), *Gynecologic oncology* (Vol. 2). Edinburgh: Churchill Livingstone, 1981, pp. 838–839.

Krant, M. J. Psychosocial impact of gynecologic cancer. *Cancer,* 1981, *48,* 608–612.

Krueger, J. C., Hassell, J., Goggins, D. B., Ishimaatsv, T., Pablico, M. R., & Tuttle, E. J. Relationship between nurse counseling and sexual adjustment after hysterectomy. *Nursing Research,* 1979, *28,* 145–150.

Krupp, P. J. Invasive tumors of vulva: Clinical features and management. In M. Coppleson (Ed.), *Gynecologic oncology.* Edinburgh: Churchill Livingstone, 1981, pp. 320–338.

Krupp, P. J., Lee, F. Y., Batson, H. W., & Collins, J. H. Carcinoma of the vulva. *Gynecology Oncology,* 1973, *1,* 345–362.

Lagasse, L. D., Berman, M. L., Watring, W. G., & Ballon, S. C. The gynecologic oncology patient: Restoration of function and prevention of disability. In L. McGowan (Ed.), *Gynecologic oncology.* New York: Appleton-Century-Crofts, 1978, pp. 398–415.

Lamb, M. A., & Woods, N. F. Sexuality and the cancer patient. *Cancer Nursing,* 1981, *4,* 137–144.

Lamont, J. A., DePetrillo, A. D., & Sargeant, E. J. Psychosexual rehabilitation and exenterative surgery. *Gynecologic Oncology,* 1978, *6,* 236–242.

Lash, A. F., & Zibel, M. Carcinoma of the vulva in a young woman. *American Journal of Obstetrics and Gynecology,* 1951, *62,* 216.

Leiber, L., Plumb, M. M., Gerstenzang, M. L., & Holland, J. The communication of affection between cancer patients and their spouses. *Psychosomatic Medicine,* 1976, *38*(6), 379–389.

Lewis, F. M. Family level services for the cancer patient: Critical distinctions, fallacies and assessment. *Cancer Nursing*, 1983, *6*(3), 193–200.

Mages, N. L., & Mendelsohn, G. Effects of cancer on patients' lives: A personological approach. In G. Stone, F. Cohen, & M. Adler (Eds.), *Health and psychology—A handbook*. San Francisco: Jossey-Bass, 1979, pp. 255–284.

Magrina, J. F., Webb, M. J., Gaffey, T. A., & Symonds, R. E. Stage I squamous cell cancer of the vulva. *American Journal of Obstetrics and Gynecology*, 1979, *134*, 453–459.

Martin, N. Self-care model for patients experiencing radical change in body image. *Journal of Gynecological Nursing*, 1978, *7*, 9–13.

McIntosh, D. Sexual attitudes in a group of older women. *Issues in Mental Health Nursing*. 1981, *3*, 109–122.

Merkatz, R., Smith, E., & Seitz, P. Preoperative teaching for gynecological patients. *American Journal of Nursing*, 1974, *74*, 1072–1074.

Miller, O. Nursing care after pelvic exenteration. *American Journal of Nursing*, 1962, *62*, 106–107.

Moran, A. J., & Perry-Jones, E. The surgical treatment of invasive squamous carcinoma of the vulva using a modified incision. *Irish Medical Journal*, 1980, *73*, 426–431.

Morley, G. Cancer of the vulva: A review. *Cancer*, 1981, *48*, 597–601.

Morley, G. W., Lindenauer, S. M., & Youngs, D. Vaginal reconstruction following pelvic exenteration: Surgical and psychological considerations. *American Journal of Obstetrics and Gynecology*, 1973, *116*, 996–1002.

Nelson, J. H. *Atlas of radical pelvic surgery*, (2nd ed.). New York: Appleton Century Crofts, 1977.

Norris, C. M. Body image. In C. E. Carlson, & B. Blackwell (Eds.), *Behavioral concepts and nursing intervention* (2nd ed.). New York: J. B. Lippincott, 1978, pp. 5–36.

Orr, J. W., Shingleton, H. M., Hatch, K. D., Taylor, P. T., Austin, J. M., & Partridge, E. M. Urinary diversion in patients undergoing pelvic exenteration. *American Journal of Obstetrics and Gynecology*, 1982, *142*, 883–889.

Paritzky, J. F., & Overby, B. A. Preoperative teaching on a gynecology unit. *Journal of Gynecological Nursing*, 1982, *11*, 384–386.

Parker, R. T., Duncan, I., Rampone, J., & Creasman, W. Operative management of early invasive epidermoid carcinoma of the vulva. *American Journal of Obstetrics and Gynecology*, 1975, *123*, 237–240.

Reimer, B. L. A guide to understanding hysterectomy. *Patient Information Library*, Daly City, Ca.: PAS, 1979.

Rutledge, F., Smith, J. P., & Franklin, E. W. Carcinoma of the vulva. *American Journal of Obstetrics and Gynecology*, 1970, *8*, 106–108.

Rutledge, F., Smith, J., Wharton, J., & O'Quinn, A. Pelvic exenteration: Analysis of 296 patients. *American Journal of Obstetrics and Gynecology*, 1977, *129*, 881–892.

Saltzstein, S., Woodruff, J., & Novak, E. Postgranulomatous carcinoma of the vulva. *Obstetrics and Gynecology*, 1956, *7*, 80.

Simmons, K. N. Sexuality and the female ostomate. *AJN*, 1983, *83*(3), 409–411.

Smith, E. D. (Ed.). *Women's health care: A guide for patient education*. New York: Appleton-Century-Crofts, 1981.

Snyder, J. C., & Wilson, M. F. Elements of a psychological assessment. *American Journal of Nursing*, 1977, *77*, 235–239.

Springer, M. Radical vulvectomy: Physical, psychological, social and sexual implications. *Oncology Nursing Forum*, 1982, *9*(2), 19–21.

Stanfill, P. H. The psychosocial implications of hysterectomy. *Journal of Gynecological Nursing*, 1982, *11*, 318–320.

Stillman, R. E., Goodwin, J. M., Robinson, J., Dansak, D., & Hilgers, R. D. Psychological effects of vulvectomy. *Psychomatics*, 1984, *25*(10), 779–783.

Stoklosa, J., Bullard, D., Rosenbaum, E., & Rosenbaum, I. *Sexuality and cancer: Comprehensive guide for cancer patients and their families*. Palo Alto: Bull, 1980.

Symmonds, R. E., & Webb, M. F. Pelvic exenteration. In M. Coppleson (Ed.), *Gynecologic oncology*. Edinburgh: Churchill-Livingstone, 1981.

Symmonds, R. E., Pratt, J. H., & Webb, M. J. Exenterative operations: Experience with 198 patients. *American Journal of Obstetrics and Gynecology*, 1975, *121*, 907–918.

van Nagell, J. R., & Barber, H. (Eds.). *Modern concepts of gynecologic oncology*. Boston: John Wright PSG, 1982.

Way, S. The anatomy of the lymphatic drainage of the vulva and its influence on the radical operation for carcinoma. *Annual Report of The College of Surgery of England*, 1948, *3*, 187.

Weinberg, J. S. Psychosexual impact of treatment in female genital cancer. *Journal of Sex and Marital Therapy*, 1974, *1*, 155–157.

Weisman, A. D. *Coping with cancer*. New York: McGraw-Hill, 1979.

Wise, T. N. Effects of cancer on sexual activity. *Psychosomatics*. 1978, *19*, 796–875.

Woodruff, J. D., Julian, C., Puray, T., Mermut, S., & Katayama, P. The contemporary challenge of carcinoma in situ of the vulva. *American Journal of Obstetrics and Gynecology*, 1973, *115*, 677–686.

Woods, N. F. *Human sexuality in disease and illness*. St. Louis: C. V. Mosby, 1981.

Yarbrough, B. Teaching plan for patient undergoing total pelvic exenteration. *Oncology Nursing Forum*, 1981, *8*(2), 36–40.

Breast Cancer and Surgery: Education for Recovery

23

Geri LoBiondo-Wood and Patricia Clancy

Currently, much controversy surrounds the extent of surgery for operable breast cancer. Up until the end of the sixties the radical mastectomy was considered by most the treatment of choice. Now surgeons and women are exploring a variety of surgical and nonsurgical options. Yet, even with newer options and choices for treatment, breast cancer still claims the highest percentage of cancer deaths in women. It is predicted that carcinoma of the breast will develop in 1 out of every 11 women at some period in their life (American Cancer Society, 1982), thereby making it a major concern for women and their health care providers.

The breast takes on various meanings for a woman depending on her culture, self-esteem, and body image. Health providers, when assisting a woman through the encounter with breast cancer, are not only concerned with the physiological measures but also the psychological, supportive, and educational measures. About 90 percent of breast lumps are discovered by women themselves (Breast Cancer Digest, 1980). The finding of a breast lump triggers diverse emotional responses even though the majority of breast lumps are benign. Various diagnostic procedures are necessary to either confirm or disprove the presence of carcinoma. If the lump proves to be carcinoma, the treatment of primary breast cancer can be the standard surgical approach or minimal surgery plus radiation. This is generally not complicated and not life threatening. Nonetheless, the disease at the optimal minimal stage and size (1½ to 2 cm) may be silently attacking part of a woman's feminine self. What makes the diagnosis of primary breast cancer difficult is that there may have been no insistent alarms, no feelings of "illness," or threats such as that posed by a gallbladder attack. If she is one of the many who has not been able to recognize or accept the silent message from her body, whose insistent denial has caused a delay of professional evaluation, she has the added burden of fear that her treatment may be too late (Schain, 1978).

Therefore, the interventions that health professionals offer the woman and her family facing breast cancer treatment are based on her learning readiness and a recognition of the psychological issues grounded by the sequential events in the clinical course of breast cancer. These issues have been elucidated by various clinicians (Giaquinta, 1977; Holland, 1976; Schain, 1978; Scott, 1983; Thomas, 1976). The stages, as described by these care providers from three major health care disciplines, have their own inherent series of events, tasks, and behavioral responses. These stages generally fall into a sequential pattern but may be altered by the unpredictable course of the disease. Thomas (1976) formulated a table of factors and critical events in the psychosocial adjustment to breast cancer. These are presented in Figure 23–1.

Responses to Cancer: Developmental Stages

The prodromal or first stage is believed to be a developmental phase occurring when a woman develops her conceptions of health, self, and illness (Holland, 1976; Scott, 1983; Thomas, 1976). The concepts formed during this period are believed predictive of a woman's response to cancer. In the next stage, the prediagnostic stage, the woman becomes attuned to the warning signs of cancer in her body. Her response for action or delay is influenced by internal and external forces as well as ego defenses. The type of action and length of time before response are critical to the outcome of the disease (Scott, 1983).

During the third or diagnostic stage the woman seeks medical consultation and explores options. This stage is characterized by highly charged emotions. Holland (1976) states that this is a time of fear, one in which women use various coping mechanisms, which may include repression, denial, fatalism, and prayer. During this sensitive period, the skills of an astute, supportive health care provider are needed to establish an open communication system and rapport with the woman so that her own particular needs can be recognized.

The next three stages, the operative, the immediate postoperative, and the extended postoperative, evolve from the surgical procedures and hospitalization. During these stages, the individual and her family's fears are most intensely felt. Scott (1983) found the preoperative period to be one of high anxiety with diminished levels of critical thinking ability. These results suggest that a woman and her family need an assessment of their coping abilities; additional clinical interventions may be indicated. Optimal rehabilitative practice would begin the information process during the preoperative period. The woman should be evaluated for the amount and type of information most helpful to her and most congruent with her personality. It is important for the patient and her family to receive comprehensive care as early in the operative phase as possible to promote the highest level of both physiological and psychological recovery. A well-managed hospitalization can ease the stress of discharge and postoperative rehabilitation.

The adjuvant stage is postdischarge. This may encompass further treatment: chemotherapy, hormonal therapy, radiation, and possible immunotherapy if indicated. This period as in all others has its inherent stresses. During this time the woman begins to recover from surgery, yet faces the trauma of added therapies and their possible side effects (Scott, 1983).

After this extended postoperative stage, the disease will take one of two courses. The woman will either experience recurrence or recovery. If there is a recurrence the woman faces further emotional morbidity (Schain, 1978). The progression of disease brings increased discomfort, further hospitalization, treatment, metastases, and death. During this phase, as the woman becomes ever more self-absorbed, the family assumes the weight of maximizing the utilization of life (Giaquinta, 1977; Thomas, 1976). Both the woman and her family need the support and caring of the health care team to assist them with the poignant difficulties of separation and loss.

Whether the woman advances to recurrence or recovery is affected by variables such as extent of pathology, overall health status, genetic predisposition, and functioning level of the immune system. The recovery phase is a positive stage. Thomas (1976) states that this is a time of reordering of values and priorities and an incorporation of the loss of the breast. As with this and all other stages, continued psychological support and an open communication system are needed for resolution of crisis and extended rehabilitation periods.

These stages elucidate the developmental psychodynamics that a woman may experience with a diagnosis of breast cancer. One needs to recognize that movement from one stage to another is affected by multiple factors brought to bear by the disease itself as well as each individual's psychological, social, and physiological background. A schematic developed by Scott (1983, p. 23) of the stages in the course of breast cancer provides a concise outline of these events (Table 23–1).

Etiology of Breast Disease. Breast cancer may be seen as multifactorial in its etiology. Factors such as age, sex, genetics, hormonal environment, diet, and national origin have all been implicated. Although breast cancer is seen in men, it is much less frequently a problem. There is one carcinoma of the breast in men for every 100 carcinomas of the breast in women. Cancer of the breast is almost unknown in prepubertal females and is very rare in women under 20 years of age (Rush, 1984). After age 20, there is a gradual increased incidence that reaches a plateau between 45 and 55 years of age. A sharp rise in the incidence of breast cancer occurs after 55 years of age, the annual risk of developing breast cancer for women 80 to 85 years being twice as high as for women 60 to 65 years of age. Genetically, if the mother has breast cancer, her daughter has a two to three times greater chance of developing breast cancer than women in the general population, but no specific pattern of inheritance is evident.

It has also been found that Jewish women who are descendants of European Jews are at a somewhat greater risk. In the United States and Northern European countries the incidence of breast cancer is five to six times higher than in Asian and African countries. This has been in part attributed to the consumption of animal fat and protein (Breast Cancer Digest, 1980).

Breast cancer often is a multicentric disease; there may be multiple foci of carcinoma in a single breast, or in the opposite breast. Certain types of breast cancers tend to be especially multicentric, e.g., lobular carcinoma. Thus, a woman who has had one breast cancer is at a higher risk for developing another. This risk has been estimated to be 1

TABLE 23–1. STAGES IN THE CLINICAL COURSE OF BREAST CANCER

Stage	Description
Prodromal	Predetection, developmental concepts of health, cancer, breast, self, intellect, coping strategies/abilities, family interactions
Prediagnostic	Problem detection, delay or action period
Diagnostic	Medical evaluation, presurgical clinical diagnosis, consideration of options
Operative	Presurgery preparation, education, period of high anxiety, and disruption of life-style, surgery
Immediate	Postoperative, in-hospital, beginning rehabilitation, contact with others Postoperative emotional scale
Extended	Postdischarge, continuing rehabilitation, maintenance, restructuring living Postoperative and home priorities
Adjuvant	Adjuvant therapy, treatment, suspension of recovery priorities
Recurrence	Metastatic breast cancer, advancing disease, terminal
Recovery	Reintegration of self-body image, reconstruction options

(Source: *Adapted from Scott, D. W. Quality of life following the diagnosis of breast cancer.* Topics in Clinical Nursing, *1983, 4(4), 23.*)

I PRODROMAL PERIOD

PATIENT EXPERIENCE

1. History of prior serious illness, especially cancer
2. Experience with health care system
3. Information about breast cancer
4. Relationship with breast or other cancer patient

PATIENT VARIABLES	FAMILY VARIABLES
1. Personality	1. Stability
2. Coping patterns	2. Number and age of members
3. Health beliefs and practices	3. Proximity and intimacy
4. Affective state	4. Interdependence
5. Intellectual and cognitive abilities	5. Resources
6. Biographical data	6. Roles and responsibilities
7. Attitudes toward breast cancer	7. Cultural/ethnic background
8. Self-concept	

PURPOSE: Help toward formulation of planned interventions as patient and family go through critical events

II PREDIAGNOSTIC PERIOD
(confusion, conflict)

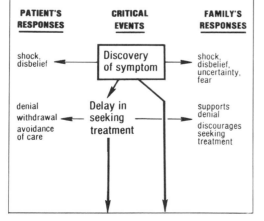

PATIENT'S RESPONSES	CRITICAL EVENTS	FAMILY'S RESPONSES
shock, disbelief	Discovery of symptom	shock, disbelief, uncertainty, fear
denial withdrawal avoidance of care	Delay in seeking treatment	supports denial discourages seeking treatment

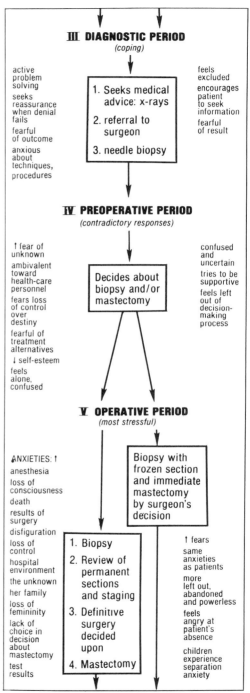

III DIAGNOSTIC PERIOD
(coping)

active problem solving

seeks reassurance when denial fails

fearful of outcome

anxious about techniques, procedures

1. Seeks medical advice: x-rays
2. referral to surgeon
3. needle biopsy

feels excluded

encourages patient to seek information

fearful of result

IV PREOPERATIVE PERIOD
(contradictory responses)

↑ fear of unknown

ambivalent toward health-care personnel

fears loss of control over destiny

fearful of treatment alternatives

↓ self-esteem

feels alone, confused

Decides about biopsy and/or mastectomy

confused and uncertain

tries to be supportive

feels left out of decision-making process

V OPERATIVE PERIOD
(most stressful)

ANXIETIES: ↑

anesthesia

loss of consciousness

death

results of surgery

disfiguration

loss of control

hospital environment

the unknown

her family

loss of femininity

lack of choice in decision about mastectomy

test results

Biopsy with frozen section and immediate mastectomy by surgeon's decision

1. Biopsy
2. Review of permanent sections and staging
3. Definitive surgery decided upon
4. Mastectomy

↑ fears

same anxieties as patients

more left out, abandoned and powerless

feels angry at patient's absence

children experience separation anxiety

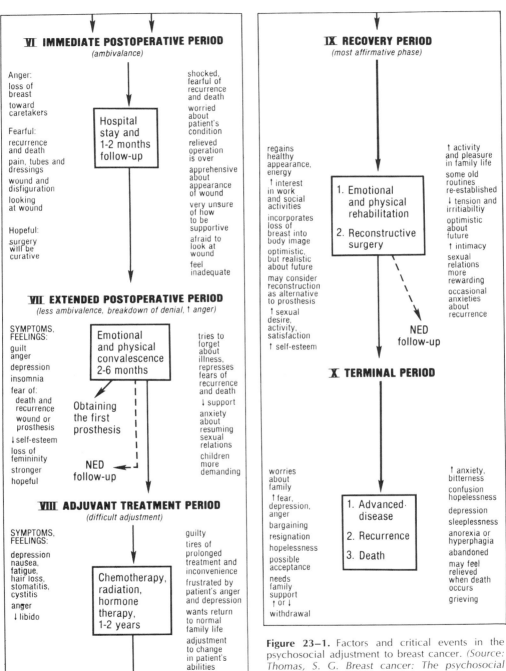

Figure 23–1. Factors and critical events in the psychosocial adjustment to breast cancer. *(Source: Thomas, S. G. Breast cancer: The psychosocial issues.* Cancer Nursing, *1978, 1(1), 53–60, by permission.)*

percent per year for the life of the woman (Rush, 1984). No one factor has been isolated as the cause of breast cancer and its development is still seen as a result of interlinked factors. Therefore, researchers recommend treating all women as being at risk for breast cancer (Cancer Communications, October 1982).

Malignant Diseases of the Breast. With few exceptions, malignant neoplasms of the breast are adenocarcinomas. Histologically, the lesions vary greatly and a number of classification systems are used. Consistent classification and staging is highly recommended so that clear conclusions regarding prognosis and treatment can be made. The system being promoted is devised by the American Joint Committee in Cancer Staging and End Results Reporting, which is based on a system developed by the International Union against Cancer in 1958 (Rush, 1984).

TABLE 23–2. CLASSIFICATION OF BREAST CANCERS

Type	Occurrence (%)	Description
A. Paget's disease of the nipple	1	Primary carcinoma of the mammary ducts of the nipple that has invaded the skin. It appears on the nipple as a scaling and eczematoid lesion.
B. Carcinomas of mammary ducts		
1. Noninfiltrating carcinoma of the mammary ducts	1	Carcinoma in situ, confined within the ducts.
2. Infiltrating a. Papillary carcinoma	5	These lesions produce a soft to palpation mass. Bulky, slow growing, soft cystic mass.
b. Carcinoma with productive fibrosis (Infiltrating adeno-carcinoma with fibrosis)	78—most common	Lesion also called scirrhous carcinoma, fibro-carcinoma, and sclerosing carcinoma. Hard fibrous lesion with uneven serrated edges. Lesions may be scattered, well differentiated, clusters to dense cellular aggregates.
c. Medullary carcinoma with lymphoid infiltrate	5	Lesions are soft, bulky, and often large. Lesions are freely movable on palpation.
d. Comedocarcinomas	5	Usually found in association with other forms of adenocarcinomas that result in productive fibrosis.
e. Colloid	1	Soft and ill-defined and may be quite bulky before detection.
f. Tubular	1.2	Also known as well-differentiated or "orderly" carcinoma
C. Carcinomas of mammary lobules 1. Noninfiltrating 2. Infiltrating	Less than 5	These lesions arises from the cells of the acini and the terminal ducts in the mammary lobes. The in situ stage is the noninfiltrating lesion. If not recognized early the lesion becomes infil-trative. Multicentricity and bilaterality are important features of lobular carcinoma.
D. Sarcomas	Very rare	Lesions have a firm and rubbery consistency and average 5 to 10 cm in size
E. Inflammatory carcinomas	1–2	Presents acutely with redness, pain and swelling of the breast. Breast appears hot and cellulitic. Diagnosis made by demonstrating carcinoma invading dermal lymphatics; prognosis is grave.

In addition to staging, breast cancers as previously mentioned are also classified histologically. Table 23–2 summarizes the classification system proposed by Foote and Stewart (1946) and as discussed by Rush (1984). As mentioned, the classification and staging sytems are highly important for selection of treatment and prognosis.

TREATMENT OF BREAST CANCER

Much has been written in recent years in both the popular press and in the medical literature regarding the changing options in the treatment of breast cancer. The original Halstead mastectomy, long the standard treatment for breast cancer, provided the first surgical procedure that resulted in increased survival rates. However, the operation was conceived at a time when most breast carcinoma was diagnosed at a very advanced stage. The ability to diagnose breast cancer at earlier and earlier stages resulted in the development of a variety of new treatment options and more hopeful statistics.

Presently, there exists controversy in both the medical and lay communities regarding the precise role of these new treatment options. Beyond this controversy, certain factors exist that limit the application of treatment options. These factors include the woman's age, her past and present medical history, the extent of the disease, and her personal decision about the surgery. The surgeon's training, knowledge, and personal biases also have a profound influence on a woman's treatment. In this uncertain climate it is extremely important that the woman and her physician discuss the various treatment options and decide on the one that best fulfills the woman's needs. Also, health professionals in attempting to help their clients sort through current treatment options for primary operable breast cancer need to be aware of the benefits that a thorough staging of disease may provide. Such staging yields information with both short- and long-term implications. Hayward (1981) enumerates these as follows:

1. The removal of sufficient tumor tissue during diagnostic surgery to allow for determination of the tumor's protein (estrogen and progesterone) status. These hormone assays indicate important prognostic predictions as well as guidelines for treating recurrent disease.
2. Similarly, full axillary lymph node dissection provides information regarding the necessity for adjuvant chemotherapy, removes foci for local recurrence, and provides prognostic data. The prognosis deteriorates arithmetically when more than four lymph nodes are involved.
3. Certain trials indicate that women at higher risk benefit from adjuvant chemotherapy and hormonal therapy by decreased recurrence and possibly improved survival.
4. A higher risk category may be determined by knowledge of lymph nodes status.

Mastectomy. Any operation that removes breast tissue is termed a mastectomy (Rush, 1984). The various types of breast surgery may be classified in the following manner:

Less Than Total Removal of the Breast. These procedures are variously titled local excision, lumpectomy, tumorectomy, or quadrantectomy (Stehlin et al., 1979). The amount of breast tissue removed varies with the extent and type of disease and the judgment of the surgeon. These procedures are primarily used for very early carcinomas, those usually found by mammography with or without a palpable lump in the breast. Usually, radiation

with or without chemotherapy is instituted following the excisional process. These procedures produce varying degrees of breast deformity but rarely require reconstruction. This
surgery should also obtain tissue for the previously mentioned staging information. Several
studies using limited resection coupled with radiation therapy have shown results that
compare favorably with those obtained with more extensive resection. Many surgeons feel,
however, that further study is needed before adopting these techniques.

Removal of the Breast Only. There are a variety of techniques that involve removal of all
breast tissue without removal of the axillary nodes or chest muscles. The subcutaneous,
total or simple mastectomy involves removal of the entire breast and nipple except the
subcutaneous mastectomy that leaves the nipple intact (Rush, 1984; Teicher et al., 1978).
These procedures are most often used for early carcinomas. They are also used in certain
high-risk individuals where prophylactic mastectomy is felt to be indicated, even when
the breast in clinically free of cancer. Prophylactic mastectomy is currently a highly
controversial issue. Most surgeons agree that with certain types of cancer the total
mastectomy provides the best means of treatment. Because these procedures leave the
chest musculature intact, reconstruction is a possible option. The use of postoperative
chemotherapy or radiation depends on the extent of disease and type of tumor.

Removal of More Than the Breast Proper. At the present time the most common operation for breast cancer is the modified radical mastectomy (Maddox et al., 1983; Rush,
1984). It is perhaps more properly termed a total mastectomy with complete axillary
dissection. In this procedure the entire breast is removed including the fascia of the
pectoralis major. The pectoralis minor may or may not be taken to allow a more complete
removal of the axillary lymph nodes. Removal of this muscle, however, produces no
deformity or disability. The contours of the chest remain. This allows for either immediate or delayed reconstruction as desired by the woman. The major advantage in this
procedure is the information gained about the spread of the tumor to the axillary lymph
nodes. This has been shown to be necessary for informed decision regarding adjuvant
therapy. Surgeons who use this procedure feel that the added time required for the
lymph node dissection is justified by the information gained. Provided the major nerves
are not injured during the operation there is little permanent disability. The woman must
exercise the involved side to prevent shoulder stiffness, however.

The standard Halstead or radical mastectomy involves the en bloc removal of the
breast and axillary content as described but also includes removal of pectoral muscles
(Maddox et al., 1983; Rush, 1984). This procedure, although still advocated by a number
of surgeons, is probably best reserved for women with tumors that have grown into the
chest musculature. There is a considerable degree of deformity following this procedure
and skin grafts may be required to close the wound. Reconstruction surgery, while still
possible, is more involved; good results are more difficult to achieve. The so-called
extended radical mastectomy, which included sternal resection, was utilized for central
or medial breast lesions that drained to the sternal lymph nodes. Local recurrence to this
area is now controlled by radiation therapy.

Radiotherapy. The purposes of preoperative or postoperative radiotherapy in conjunction with one of the types of mastectomies are to reduce the incidence of local recurrences, to preoperatively shrink large tumors, and to destroy metastatic cancer in lymph
nodes. There are also advocates of primary radiation therapy for breast cancer (Prosnitz
et al., 1977; Wallner et al., 1976). Those who use this approach advocate it for small

lesions after excision. Long-term follow-ups to evaluate the risk of developing subsequent carcinoma are lacking but preliminary data appear somewhat promising (Levene et al., 1977, 1978).

If radiotherapy is used as the primary treatment of cancer the goal is a cure. External and/or internal radiotherapy may also be used as adjuvant therapy or as palliative therapy. It is a localized treatment and affects only the area included in the radiation field. The therapeutic dose of radiotherapy is fractionated, that is, given in small doses over a fixed period of time. According to Leahy and colleagues (1979), the rationale of dividing dosage is based on the theory that normal cells have a greater ability to recuperate from the radiation effects than do cancer cells, the goal being the creation of a hostile environment for the cancerous cell. Currently, radiotherapy has four specific applications in the treatment of breast cancer:

1. As primary treatment for inflammatory breast cancer, for local control of inoperable breast cancer, for clients who cannot undergo surgery for medical reasons, for clients who refuse surgery, or as an alternative to mastectomy in women with early disease
2. As an adjunct to mastectomy or local excision
3. To shrink a large tumor to an operable size
4. A palliation to alleviate pain caused by distant metastasis, especially bone metastasis (Breast Cancer Digest, 1980)

With increasing sophistication of the radiation equipment, the side effects, especially radiation pneumonitis and severe skin necrosis, are much less frequent. Other side effects include sunburnlike reaction of the skin, general malaise, nausea, and vomiting. Therefore, the woman and her family will require preprocedure teaching and support similar to the process of preoperative teaching.

Chemotherapy. Chemotherapy, alone or in combination with either hormonal manipulation or radiation, is a standard method of dealing with metastatic breast cancer. Early reports documenting the effectiveness of adjunctive chemotherapy were done by Bonadonna and colleagues (1978) and Henderson and Canellos (1980). These researchers showed a significant increase in 5-year survival rates, and a lower recurrence rate in premenopausal women treated with multidrug chemotherapy regimens. Similar studies have also shown some benefit among postmenopausal women treated with chemotherapy, although the results have not equaled those in premenopausal women. Most oncologists would not use chemotherapy in clients without evidence of metastatic disease, as the agents themselves are not without significant side effects, including a possible carcinogenic potential. Other side effects may include tissue damage at injection site, stomatitis, nausea and vomiting, diarrhea, loss of appetite, inflammation of the oral mucosa, and loss of hair. Potentially troublesome for the younger woman is chemo-induced amenorrhea with loss of vaginal lubrication. These side effects can be especially traumatic to a woman's self-esteem and body image after mastectomy. Chemotherapy is administered either orally, intramuscularly, or intravenously. Most chemotherapy regimens consist of a combination of drugs. There are four major types of drugs used. These are alkylating agents, antimetabolites, antibiotics, and inhibitors of mitosis. The precise role of chemotherapy as an adjunctive treatment depends on further prospective randomly controlled studies. Pretreatment teaching and supportive care to assist the woman and her family in coping with these side effects is imperative. It is important for woman to know that most patients are able to maintain their life-styles during their treatment period.

Hormonal Therapy. Hormonal manipulation, usually of the ablative variety, has been used for a number of years in treating women with recurrent or widely disseminated breast cancer. The ablative hormonal therapies include oophorectomy, adrenalectomy, and hypophysectomy. There are also additive (drug) hormonal therapies. These are agents such as androgens, progestins, glucocorticoids, estrogens, and antiestrogens.

In the past there was no method to determine if a woman's tumor was hormonally dependent. Presently the use of hormonal therapy has been revolutionalized through the determination of the presence or absence of hormonal receptors in the tumor. These include estrogen and progesterone receptors. Over 60 percent of clients with estrogen receptor positive tumors respond to hormonal manipulation (Rush, 1984). Concurrent with the discovery of these receptors has been the development of the antiestrogen drug therapies, especially tamoxifen. Tamoxifen is presently the drug of choice for clients with estrogen receptor positive metastic cancer (Carbone & Davis, 1978; Plotkin et al., 1978). The use of antiestrogen therapy is the first line treatment with chemotherapy held in reserve for those clients who fail to respond or for those with estrogen receptor negative tumors. The side effects of tamoxifen and other additive hormonal therapies may include nausea, vomiting, hot flashes, fluid retention, tender breasts, urinary incontinence, hypercalcemia, and masculinizing effects such as deepening of voice, increased facial hair, and changes in psyche and libido (Breast Cancer Digest, 1980). The future role of hormonal manipulation for both metastatic and recurrent breast cancer is yet to be defined but offers a potentially much less toxic and more specific therapy for women with breast cancer.

Biopsies—One-Step Versus Two-Step Procedures. Any clinically suspicious finding in the breast merits a biopsy with histological examination. Only a pathologist can diagnose if the tumor is benign or malignant. Often, this is possible from the frozen section done immediately after the biopsy; but frequently the final diagnosis cannot be made until the permanent slides are reviewed by the pathologist. This confirmation may take from 2 to 4 days. The following conditions mandate a biopsy:

1. All three-dimensional lumps that do not shrink or swell dependent on the phase of the menstrual cycle. Cysts may be aspirated but must be biopsied if they recur, if the fluid is bloody, and if the entire lesion does not disappear after aspiration.
2. Suspicious lesions discovered by diagnostic aids, such as mammography.
3. Serosanguinous or bloody nipple discharge.
4. Other suspicious signs, such as eczema of the nipple, enlarged axillary nodes, inflamed breast skin, unexplained dimpling of the skin, and nipple deviation or retraction (Gallagher, 1978, p. 75).

If the frozen section on the biopsy is obviously positive for malignancy there is a choice. The surgery may be postponed, or the surgeon may proceed immediately with definitive surgery. Proceeding with the surgery immediately subjects the woman to one procedure, one anesthesia, lower costs, decreased chances of infection, and no anxious days of waiting between events. It is important to note that any surgery is accompanied by a degree of risk, therefore the two-step procedure exposes a woman to the risks of surgery twice. Kinne (1982) recommends the one-step procedure. He cites evidence that there may be a poorer prognosis with the two-step procedure, particularly with a prolonged delay between biopsy and mastectomy when (1) the regional nodes are positive and (2) when there is evidence of trauma at the biopsy site.

On the other hand, Margolese (1982) saw no evidence to support the contention that the two-step procedure is unsafe as long as there is a limit to the interval between biopsy and treatment. Schain (1976) notes that some women find the two-step procedure a more preferable choice, so that they may have time to prepare for the changes in their own life and those of their family. The most important benefit is that the woman feels she has some control over her destiny, has specific information, and can make a fully informed decision. Scott (1983) indicates that the period between the procedures would be a fruitful time for teaching and counseling.

EDUCATIONAL PROCESS

The impact that the health professional may have along the continuum of the clinical course of breast cancer may be influenced by many factors, including availability of personnel, level of knowledge and clinical expertise, health care setting, and territorial imperatives or who has the right to impart what information to whom. During the earliest and most uncertain period, the woman is generally seen only in outpatient settings such as the physician's office and testing areas. As she struggles with her worst fears and fantasies, she may feel fragmented within the health care system (see Chapter 2, Crett's Health–Illness Stages). Spletter (1981) makes the suggestion that a family member, husband, or good friend, be present during early discussion sessions with the physician. This concerned person can listen, ask questions, remember, and help clarify issues raised during medical evaluation. She quotes one woman as saying, "It is critical that a woman be able to go through the experience with a good friend . . . someone who is willing to become informed and participate in discussions with your doctor. At times, I just stopped listening, and got choked up. Having my husband there really helped reexplain things. . . . Don't go through it alone, no matter what" (Spletter, 1981, p. 110).

During the diagnostic period a woman may seek information from several sources such as others with personal experience or from publications of the medical or lay community. It is therefore important to remember that the process of dealing with the disease has begun before she first becomes hospitalized (Moetzinger & Dauber, 1982). Each stage has its own particular educational needs and is affected by the woman's response to each period, as well as her assessed individual needs (see Chapter 2 for detail).

Immediate Preoperative Period. Many clients require a great deal of information to understand and integrate the whole treatment process. During the immediate preoperative period it is vital to evaluate the prodromal personality of the woman in terms of understanding how receptive she may be to the teaching and learning process. It is important to assess what kind of coping patterns she has used on previously stressful events. Morris, Greer, and White (1977) suggest early supportive interventions for women who are especially at risk for long-term problems. These include women clinically depressed immediately prior to mastectomy, emotionally labile women, and premenopausal women who may be experiencing sexual maladjustment.

Schain (1978) points out that it is most important at this time for physicians to discriminate between women who perceive facts as anxiety reducing and those who find information overwhelming (see Chapter 25, Anxiety section). This discrimination is important for all health professionals. Therefore, one must be able to identify the woman who seeks out information and wants to know all about the preoperative procedures and various diagnostic routines. This person can deal with ample pretreatment education and reinforcement. On the other hand, the woman who avoids, denies, or does not listen to important information because of psychological distress should only receive minimal information and be gently guided through the required procedures. Information for this type of woman can be provided when she is receptive from the professional with whom she seems to have the best rapport. The variations in readiness to learn during the hospitalization period are due in part to the woman's psychosocial adaptation to illness as well as educational, cultural, and personality factors (see Chapter 3, Decision Making). The typical hospital experience of a woman admitted for treatment of breast cancer is usually of short duration but fraught with tension. The affect is one of extreme anxiety and apprehension, particularly just prior to surgery.

The general admission protocols of most hospitals recognize the comfort measures provided for the patient and those with her by a thorough orientation to the hospital unit, including introduction to hospital personnel, explanation of how the day is divided, and when meals are served. The emphasis should be on an overall attempt to demystify what may be a totally foreign social system. In addition, a thorough review and reinforcement of the preoperative protocols concerning preparation for surgery is a teaching imperative, bearing in mind previously mentioned factors affecting learning readiness. Experience with women who have breasts cancer confirms the high levels of anxiety, this has implications for learning. The information to be imparted should be short and basic although amplification of information may be possible and desirable for family or a concerned companion.

Postoperative Period. The first postoperative day often provides a marked and startling contrast to the fears of the previous day. Many women are almost euphoric in their relief that the surgery is over. Many are pleased to be able to get up and walk around, talk with their families, and resume basic biological functions without too much difficulty. This is a good period during which to explain to the woman the list of important information embodied in the postmastectomy guidelines (Table 23–3). The information is designed to help ease and hasten surgical recovery. This knowledge may answer questions or encourage more questions.

It is important not to lose time in clarifying the patient's understanding of her surgery. One should not cover all of the details in the first teaching session unless the patient is very receptive. The woman should be gently assisted with proper positioning and elevation of the affected arm. Additionally, the woman needs an explanation of the reasons for the elevation, shown how to flex the forearm muscle while the arm is in the elevated position. This assists with control of possible arm edema. The wound drainage system (e.g., Reliavac, Hemovac) is tolerated with less annoyance if the benefits are explained. Although the patient may be feeling better the first postoperative day, she should understand it will be normal for her to experience mood swings and fluctuations of physical stamina. The nurse should also bear in mind that the patient's atttention span will likewise vary because of pain, fatigue or weakness, depression, denial, or anger. Accordingly, the nurse should introduce the remainder of the topics when the patient is reasonably alert.

A particularly useful time to discuss the incision is during morning care when there is privacy. To accustom the woman to the loss of her breast, the incision should be described when the dressing is changed and she should be gently encouraged to view the incisional areas as soon as she is ready. This may well promote tears. Reassure her that it is a normal reaction to grieve the loss of this potent symbolic body part. This may be a

TABLE 23–3. TEACHING GUIDELINES FOR POSTMASTECTOMY AND/OR POST-AXILLARY LYMPH NODE DISSECTION

Desired Outcome	Learning Goals	Evaluation
1. Knowledge of surgical procedure	1. a. General rationale for particular surgical procedure. b. Refers specific questions to surgeon. 2. Understands verbal or pictorial descriptions of anatomy involved. 3. Understands function of breast lymphatic drainage and nodes. 4. Understands significance of histo-pathological screening of axillary lymph nodes including the fact that medial or inner quadrant lesions may involve sternal nodes. 5. Is aware of necessity for tumor tissue sampling to determine estrogen and progestrone receptor proteins. (ERP and PRP status)	1. Can verbalize reason for her own type surgery. 2. Identifies anatomical structure involved and what has been removed. 3. Perceived relationship of lymphatic system to breast cancer surgery. 4. Verbalizes that recommendation for adjuvant therapy is based on outcome of lymph node pathology report. 5. Understands that future treatment and prognosis based on knowledge of this hormonal response.
2. Knowledge about incisional area and change in body in age	1. Understands incisions differ depending on treatment option. a. Breast conservation. Will see incision breast (maybe defect in chest contour) plus axillary incision. b. Knows mastectomy incision is usually transverse running from tip of sternum toward or into the axilla. Chest wall is flat as in prepuberty. Radical mastectomy, loss of anterior chest wall contour. 2. Learns what type of closing materials are used on the incision: sutures, steri-strips, clips. Approximately how long in place. That the skin flaps are well approximated with no raw open areas.	1. Identifies extent of incisional areas and anatomical alterations. 2. Can verbalize what incisional area may look like.

(continued)

TABLE 23–3. (cont.)

Desired Outcome	Learning Goals	Evaluation

	3. Knows simple post-op care of incision.
	  a. Keeps new incisional area dry, does not disturb dressings.
	  b. Does not use any type of deodorant or powder on affected axilla.
	4. Understands importance of beginning to deal with incision and change in body image.
	5. Knows what the incision looks like. There may be skin discoloration, unevenness along the incisional line.
		3. a. Will check with physician before resuming a full shower.
		  b. Understands she may resume using customary toilet articles after full wound healing.
		4. a. May or may not be able to view incision with support.
		  b. Expression of feelings is encouraged.
		5. a. Understands it is all right to start with a small quick look.
		  b. She realizes superficial skin abnormalities will disappear. Chest will be flat, covered with normal skin.

	6. Care of incision at discharge from hospital usually minimal.
	  a. Dry sterile dressing pad placed over area.
	  b. Comfortable bra with temporary prosthesis in cup to keep dressing in place. Use little safety pins on the outside of bra to secure the temporary prothesis.
	7. Review signs and symptoms of infection, inflamation around incisional area: heat, swelling, pain, redness, drainage.
	8. Inform woman that healed incisional area or scar may be gently massaged with cream of choice to help keep area soft and supple.
		6. Demonstrates dressing change.
		
		7. Can state signs and symptoms of infection and why this must be reported to physician immediately.
		8. Understands that scar contracture is a normal phenomenon; softing of tissue will occur in time.

3. Acknowledges boundaries of incisional pain and related sensory alterations in terms	1. Understands that incisional pain or pulling should limit fresh post-op activity. 2. Review phenomena of referred pain or sensory discomfort due to incised nerve endings. These are experienced as sensations	1. Verbalizes location of incisional area and need to ask for pain relief p.r.n. to maintain comfort and promote activity. 2. Understands that range of motion (ROM) exercises and activities of daily living (ADL) with affected area help work through

of pain relief and activity levels	to shoulders or arm on side of surgery: heaviness, tingling, aching, trickling water, phantom nipple, and breast. 3. These sensations subside over time (over a year) after incision heals.	and relieve referred sensations. Also sensations more pronounced during damp weather and stress. 3. Understands that she is experiencing the worst of these sensations while in hospital.
4. Knowledge of purpose of wound draining systems	1. Describe placement of drainage catheters under skin flaps on chest wall. Serosanguineous drainage collects in small plastic container usually pinned to gown. 2. Drainage is monitored for daily amount. 3. It may take 5 to 14 days for drainage to subside. Minimal amount prompts removal of system. 4. Understands that fluid may continue to collect under skin after the drainage system is removed; look for soft swelling.	1. Understands that body produces sub-cutaneous fluid postsurgery. 2. She is aware that a dry incisional area promotes faster, less painful healing. 3. Will prepare for discharge from hospital when drain is removed. 4. Woman understands that this is not unusual. The fluid may be easily aspirated with needle and syringe, not usually painful due to area's surgical numbness.
5. Knowledge of rationale for postoperative arm elevation	1. Review that loss of function and interruption of axillary lymphatics due to breast surgery predisposes to temporary postoperative arm lymphedema. 2. Initiate 5–10 tight fist clenchings while arm in elevated position; note flexing of forearm muscle.	1. Will elevate arm while supine with arm on pillow, wrist higher than elbow, elbow higher than shoulder. Will maintain position several times a day and at night. 2. Observe muscle flexing action of forearm increasing venous return and thus decreasing fluid in upper extremity. 3. Will practice this strategy for ½ hour any time arm swelling is noted.
6. Knowledge of hand and arm precautions to be maintained following axillary lymph node dissection and for life because lymph nodes do not re-	1. Will not allow venipuncture nor bloods to be drawn from affected arm or hand. 2. Will not allow constricting bands around any part of affected arm: clothing, bracelet, watch, blood pressure cuff. 3. Bilateral mastectomies may have necessary medical diagnostic work done on a previously operated mastectomy arm with	1. Verbalizes cause and effect between break in skin, infection, and lymphedema. 2. Verbalizes relationship between constriction and lymphedema. 3. Understands occasional necessity of using affected arm for essential medical reasons.

(continued)

561

TABLE 23–3. (cont.)

Desired Outcome	Learning Goals	Evaluation
generate (see table on Hand and Arm Precautions)	no circulatory problems, or either arm or legs depending on discretion of physician.	

7. Has realistic expectations of post-discharge activities	1. Understands that postsurgical anemia and shock to system predisposes to lack of physical and emotional stamina.
	2. Understands that it is safe and good to resume intimate relations including sexual intercourse with her partner.
	3. Understands that it is wise to check with surgeon before:
	  a. Driving a car
	  b. Undertaking strenuous activities such as sports.
	  c. Going back to work
		1. a. Plan ADL to each days tolerance.
		  b. Plan for rest between activities during convalescence.
		2. a. Covers and protects incisional area with a padded dressing when first home.
		  b. Gentle lovemaking is reassuring to both partners.
		  c. Delay may foster unwholesome barriers.
		3. Understands that healing rate and stamina vary; do not compare self to others.
		  a. Depends on incisional healing and type of care.
		  b. Depends on presurgical level of competance and stage of recovery.
		  c. Depends on the activity level of the job; kindergarten teaching vs. desk work.

8. Knows that it will be possible to achieve a symmetrical, normal looking appearance when clothed.	1. Understands that the postoperative incisional chest area needs 4–6 weeks for thorough healing before wearing permanent breast prosthesis.
	  a. Understands that the Reach to Recovery Volunteer, a recovered post-mastectomee, is a helpful and knowledgeable resource regarding breast forms and readjustments following a mastectomy. If possible, she will be contacted to visit.
	2. Understands many retailers are prepared to fit postmastectomy breast prostheses: lingerie department, corset shops, mastectomy boutique, surgical supply store.
		1. Knows that a light weight temporary form to fill bra cup is necessary for first few weeks. The best is:
		  a. The temporary dacron fluff filled form supplied in a kit by the RRV from the American Cancer Society (A.C.S.).
		  b. Light, temporary form purchased from a lingerie department or shop.
		  c. If the above not available, use fluffed kerlex or cotton in gauze to fill bra cup until a suitable one is obtained.
		2. May browse in shops as soon as strength permits to investigate selection but awaits full healing before purchase. See text.

9. Knowledge of rationale for Range of Motion Exercises (with concurrence of physician) See table of exercises.

10. Expects incisional healing, and return of shoulder ROM and own strength within weeks but understands a return to emotional equanimity may take several months to a year.

11. Strong belief in importance and practice of Breast Self-Examination (especially because remaining breast is at increased risk for developing cancer)

---

3. Prepared to inquire of her surgeon her option regarding breast reconstruction (if she has not done so already).

1. Understands that goal of exercises is maintenance of normal ROM for shoulder and strengthening of arm on affected side.
2. Understands that exercises should be limited by endurance and incisional discomfort.
3. Understands that exercises should be continued until there is a return to pre-surgical mobility. *Exception:* discontinue limp swing exercise after 2 weeks to avoid lymphedema of the affected arm.

1. Understands that diagnosis of cancer and loss of body part are tremendously stressful events that may result in varied, intermittent emotional symptoms: depression, insomnia, mood changes, recurring nightmares, difficulty concentrating, exhaustion, anger, crying spells, denial, fear of recurrence.

1. Understands need to examine breast and contralateral chest wall including the incisional area systematically on a regular basis. (See Ch. 4 for procedure).
2. Woman understands that familiarity with her own body landmarks will aid in recognizing possible changes that may be medically significant.

---

3. Realizes breast reconstruction is a choice she can make for herself in her own time, at her own convenience, providing she is not involved in chemotherapy or radiation therapy at the time.

1. Demonstrates set of exercises.
2. With practice will see gradual improvement in levels of endurance and ROM.
3. Perceives these exercises as something she can do for herself. By restoring body function and strength she enhances self-esteem.

1. Realizes that intermittent mood changes are not indicative of long-term mental breakdown but rather normal reactions to having had breast cancer surgery.
2. Will seek postmastectomy group in community and share experience. Call A.C.S.
3. Perceives that return to structure of normal activities enhances well-being and self-satisfaction and recovery.

1. Demonstrates and explains technique. Understands importance of promoting this vital self-hygiene measure to other females she cares about.
2. Realizes that a conscientious program of BSE along with regular medical follow-up provides the best defense against future breast disease.

good time to describe the potential mood swings that are normal for postmastectomy women. Depression, grief, and anger come and go, usually subsiding by the end of the first postoperative year (see Chapter 24 on Depression).

Most women patients enjoy and benefit from group teaching and "rap" or support sessions if they can be arranged. Group sessions can help women share a multitude of concerns: fear about cancer recurrence, grief and anger at losing the breast, doubts about their femininity. A group can mutually explore how and what to discuss with friends, family and children and they also can provide much needed emotional support (also see Chapter 3 on Group Process). If not possible, encourage the patient to seek a qualified support group such as the YMCA program ENCORE when she leaves the hospital. Table 23–5 offers suggestions for community-based programs.

Exercises and Precautions. It is imperative that the woman has a clear understanding of her role in maintaining the integrity of the circulation and skin of the hand and arm on the side where there has been surgical removal of the axillary lymph nodes. She should thoroughly understand hand and arm precautions (Table 23–4) and her response to any infection on the affected arm. This teaching can be easily validated by patient response to selected cue words or phrases. "What would you do if . . . you are scrubbing pots and pans . . . you see a red sore or a hang nail on the affected hand."

TABLE 23–4. PRECAUTIONARY MEASURES TO AVOID LYMPHEDEMA IN AFFECTED SHOULDER, ARM, AND HAND

1. Minimize possibility of infection by maintaining skin barrier; prevent breaks in skin. If break in skin occurs, wash with mild soap and water, cover with protective dressing. Check under bandage for signs and symptoms of infection.
   A. Wear rubber gloves when using strong cleaning agents, steel wool or drying detergents.
   B. Use gardening gloves when gardening or doing maintenance work.
   C. Use cream on hands to maintain softness and avoid cracks especially in cold weather.
   D. Manicuring nails. Avoid cutting cuticles, keep soft with cream, push back with orange stick, use cuticle remover.
   E. Avoid diagnostic bloodwork, injections, or finger prick in affected arm.[a]
   F. Use insect repellent to avoid insect bites.
   G. Groom underarm on affected side with an electric razor. Do not use straight razor to remove hair, armpit may be numb. Use cream depilatory only if nonirritating to skin.
   H. When sewing use a thimble.
   I. Any unusual soreness, redness, or swelling of affected arm or hand should be reported to your physician.
2. Avoid burns
   A. When cooking use long padded oven mitts.
   B. If a smoker, try to hold cigarette in unaffected hand.
   C. Avoid sunburn, use sun blocker and acquire a gradual tan.
3. Maintain unimpeded circulation
   A. Avoid constriction in affected arm by wearing loose bracelets, avoid tight watchbands, tight sleeves and clothing.
   B. Use unaffected arm for blood pressures.[a]
4. Carry heavy objects, packages, and purse with unaffected arm. Especially right after surgery, before muscle strength in affected arm has returned.

[a]Restrictions may need to be modified for bilateral mastectomies. Physician should indicate extremity for diagnostic work. (Source: *Adapted from Dietz, J. H. Rehabilitation and readaptation for patient with breast cancer. In E. Gallagher, H. Leis, R. Snyderman, & J. Urban (Eds.), The breast. St. Louis, Mo.: C. V. Mosby, 1978; American Cancer Society. Reaching to recovery: A concerned approach for women who have had breast surgery (3rd ed.). New York: American Cancer Society, New York City Division, & Memorial Sloan-Kettering Cancer Center, 1980.)*

The range of motion exercises (Table 23–5) may or may not be approved by the patient's surgeon as there is controversy that they may promote wound drainage if started in the early postoperative period. These exercises should be demonstrated to the woman. It should also be explained that these exercises, both in the early postoperative period and in the long-term, may prove beneficial in returning the woman more rapidly to her previous level of activity. As with any exercise program, it is best to start slowly and build up tolerance and endurance. The woman should be warned not to push or pull past incisional pain. These exercises promote easing and limbering of stiff arms and shoulders. Women should be reminded not to continue the limp swing exercise beyond one week at home. Physical activity and exercise help to promote circulation, physical well-being, and a better feeling about one's body.

Appearance and Sexuality. Set aside several periods near the time of discharge from the hospital, as there are a host of concerns that should be addressed before the woman is discharged. There are two topics that may be uppermost in her mind and are interrelated: concern with her appearance and sexuality. The topic of sexuality may be broached by mentioning that sexual partners often wonder when it is safe to resume sexual intercourse. This lets the patient know that others have been concerned also. It is important to stress that a mastectomy does not physically impair sexual functioning. Sexual activity can resume upon discharge (Dulcey, 1980). It may be reassuring for both partners if at first the mastectomy incision is protected and covered by a padded dressing. This may ease both partners' worries of inadvertently harming a tender area and worries over having to cope with the alteration of her body image. Experimentation should be encouraged to reveal the most comfortable and least taxing position, possibly side by side with the mastectomy incision uppermost. Couples should be warned of possible barriers to intimacy. The mate may fear appearing too demanding of the weaker partner even though there is a strong desire to physically express caring and tenderness. The woman may fear she is undesirable and reject her partner's advances even though she longs to be reassured. Couples, therefore, should be encouraged to be open and caring with one another, striving for a wholesome sexual relationship, and strengthening intimacy. Depending on the couple's relationship and needs this can be accomplished through the privacy of their own relationship, or through discussion with a health care professional as a couple or within a group setting with couples in similar circumstances.

Prostheses. If possible a Reach to Recovery Volunteer (RRV) from the American Cancer Society may be the most reassuring and valuable resource for the mastectomy patient about to be discharged. She may be able to relate to the patient in a special, meaningful way, because she has undergone a mastectomy herself. The Reach to Recovery volunteer can provide information about breast prostheses. She may also provide the patient with a lightweight temporary breast prosthesis. If it is not possible to contact a Reach for Recovery volunteer the woman should be sent home with some kind of padding in her empty bra cup, such as fluffed kerlex. It is vital that she look balanced and symmetrical in her clothes. She should be reassured that a temporary, light breast form may be purchased in a corset or lingerie shop.

The woman will not be ready to purchase a permanent breast prosthesis until full incisional healing has taken place. This may be 4 to 6 weeks after discharge from the hospital. The reason for the delay is that the permanent breast form is designed to provide a balancing weight for the remaining breast. Therefore, the weight and the nonporous nature of silicone make it inappropriate next to healing tissue. There are many

TABLE 23–5. POSTMASTECTOMY EXERCISES

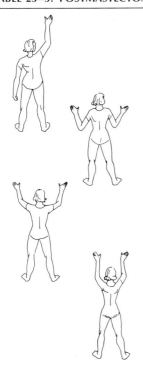

1. Wall Climbing Exercise
   a. To mark the goal, face the wall, reach as high as possible with unaffected arm, make a mark at that level. Goal may be modified by preexisting shoulder problem or bilateral mastectomy. Reach for the highest extension possible.
   b. Start the exercise facing the wall. Standing about 6 inches away, place palms against the wall at shoulder level.
   c. Using the wall for support and keeping hands parallel to each other, inch up the wall until incisional pulling or pain is experienced. Stop. Deep breathe. Work hands back down to starting position. Do not drop hands.
   d. Eventually by doing this exercise three to five times a day, five repetitions each session, the maximum extension will be attained. It is important to keep hands and shoulders even while doing the exercises. Maintain good posture. Bilateral mastectomies perform the exercise process with each arm, keeping within pain limitations.

2. Limp Swing Pendulum
   Use a chair with a medium high back. Bending the torso forward, place the unaffected arm across the chair back. Rest the forehead on that arm. Relax the affected arm. Allow to hang loosely.
   a. Start exercise by gently swinging the whole arm from the shoulder. Swing crossways from left to right. Keep the elbow straight.
   b. Next describe small circles. Keep arm loose and straight. Reverse the circling motions.
   c. End the exercise with a forward to backward swinging of the arm. Motion coming from the shoulder, not the elbows. When finished, stand up slowly to avoid feeling dizzy. The goal of this exercise is shoulder relaxation. No exact number of repeat arm movements is required. The range of motion will increase as the shoulder relaxes. Do this set once during the exercise session. *Note:* Do NOT continue this arm dependent exercise beyond 1 week home from the hospital.

3. Deep Breathing Exercises
   Sit in a comfortable chair, both feet flat on the floor, shoulders back. Place either hand over the center of the chest area. Watch for hand movement to gauge chest expansion. Take slow breath through the nose until chest fully expands. Then exhale letting shoulders drop and relax. Repeat five times. This is beneficial and relaxing throughout the whole day.

TABLE 23–5. (cont.)

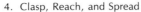

4. Clasp, Reach, and Spread
   a. Sit up straight in a chair. Clasp hands together in front.
   b. Slowly raise clasped hands to the forehead, keeping elbows adducted. If there is incisional pulling or pain stop at that point. Take several deep breaths, if incisional pulling subsides, continue. If not, postpone the exercise until incisional pulling is not troublesome. Continue by raising clasped hands to top of head. Deep breath.
   c. Let clasped hands slide toward nape of neck.
   d. Goal is to gradually open and spread arms apart. Keep shoulders and arms even and symmetrical. Maintain good posture. Keep relaxed by periodic deep breathing. It is helpful to hold the most advanced position for as long as possible. This exercise can be done lying in bed while watching television. When returning to normal position return in same fashion as going up. Keeping hands clasped, bring hands over head slowly down to the lap. One repetition each session.

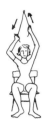

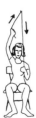

5. Pulley Exercise
   For this exercise obtain approximately 6 feet of a stout rope such as a clothes line. Place the rope over a secure clothes or plant hook. Position a straight back chair in front of the rope.
   a. Sitting up straight in the chair, reach the unaffected arm up as high as possible. Grasp the rope, loop it around the fingers. Keep that arm up. At the lower free end of the rope start inching the affected arm up as far as possible until incisional pulling or pain is felt. Stop. Loop the rope around the fingers. Now let both arms hang limply, supported by the rope. Do deep breathing.
   b. If discomfort is relieved by deep breathing, continue and stretch the affected arm even higher by gently pulling down on the rope with the other hand. Eventually full arm extension or whatever presurgery ROM was possible will be obtained.
   The highest position of arm extension should be held until the hands tire. At that point unloop both hands and gently slide down the rope to the lap. Do not abruptly release the rope and let the hands drop, this would cause pain. Bilateral mastectomy patients should do this exercise with both arms. Start with the first position by reaching up the rope as high as possible with the stronger or less sore arm. Stop at the point of incisional pain or pulling. Loop the rope around the fingers and follow the described exercise. Repeat the process with the other arm. Do this exercise once each session.

(Source: Exercises and figures adapted from: *Reach to recovery: A concerned approach for women who have had breast surgery (3rd ed.). New York: American Cancer Society and Memorial Sloan-Kettering Cancer Center, 1980, by permission.)*

retailers who stock breast prostheses and have trained fitters. Lingerie departments, corset shops, mastectomy boutiques, and surgical supply houses also carry prostheses. The local American Cancer Society may have a list of shops or the Reach for Recovery volunteer may provide information on the nearest shops. It is helpful for the woman to investigate several stores before making a purchase. When ready to try on breast forms and make a purchase she should wear a snug-fitting top or sweater. Some women feel reassured if a good friend or family member accompanies them on the shopping trip. It can be a truly helpful experience for your patient if the hospital purchasing agent can procure a demonstration prosthesis. The woman then has an opportunity to feel the consistency and weight (very firm jello in saran wrap), see the shape, and prepare herself before having to face these foreign objects alone in a public place. Silicone breast forms are costly; the woman should be alerted to inquire how much her insurance coverage will provide. Also, these purchases are classed as a medical deduction on income taxes.

The silicone forms have a slightly adherent nonslippery quality so they may be worn directly on the skin in a regular bra provided it is supportive and fits well. The secret to feeling comfortable and secure with the prosthesis is to use a bra that fits well under the arm and neckline and holds the form snuggly against the body even when bending over. Women have recommended the sport or jogging bra as giving excellent support. Some women object to the feel of silicone next to the skin. Many forms come with soft knitted covers. Another alternative is to construct an inner pocket into the bra or buy a feminine-looking mastectomy bra with ready-made pockets. Many women feel more secure with their prostheses tucked into a pocket. Although the average size range is medium to large, the small-breasted woman will be relieved to note the availability of small breast forms that fit in soft light bras. Another alternative for her is simply to purchase a padded bra. A small light form may be useful in covering the defect from a lumpectomy or quadrentectomy. Actually, there are different types of prostheses with varying prices. The woman should be able to choose from a selected variety.

Women are curious about the different types of bras that may be worn. Long-lines and all-in-ones are excellent, especially when wearing the light temporary prosthesis: they will not "ride up." An underwire bra can be worn only if the wire is not in contact with the incision; it may be comfortable only after the incision is healed and with extra padding. It may be necessary to secure the bra edge and the temporary form with a piece of elastic attached to the panties to keep it from riding up.

There are many different sizes, styles, and prices of breast forms. There should be a breast prosthesis that provides comfort, peace of mind, and the security of a natural look for each woman.

Extended Postoperative and Adjuvant Period. Based on the pathology report, a woman's physician may recommend further adjuvant therapy. This therapy may include chemotherapy, radiation, or hormonal therapy. This prospect can incite uncertainty and fear, often fed by ignorance, imagination, and hearsay. It is recognized that fear of the unknown usually presents greater stress than reality. It may therefore be reassuring for the woman to talk with a chemotherapy clinician who can give her an idea of the range of side effects of the various therapies. Most women receiving adjuvant therapy are able to function at about 70 to 80 percent of normal capacity.

Recovery Period. Recovery implies not only restoration of physical well-being but also an optimistic reconsideration of life's goals. Among those goals for a postmastectomy woman may well be the desire to explore the options for breast reconstruction. She may have reached a stage where her temporary breast prosthesis represents a continued annoyance, a daily reminder of her cancerous breast, and a hinderance to an active life-style. Woods (1980, p. 874) states that "treatment of cancer of the breast as with any other disease may be considered optimal only when maximum rehabilitation has been achieved. Satisfactory restoration of contour is now possible with most postmastectomy patients."

The health care professional then needs to have useful and practical knowledge about reconstruction to provide information and counseling to the woman reaching this stage in the recovery process. Actually, the information may be even more important for the female community at large. The fact that breast reconstruction is a valid and many times an aesthetic option may encourage the woman with a potential undiagnosed breast problem to seek medical evaluation more quickly.

Data from 1978 indicate that only 15,000 of one million postmastectomy women chose reconstruction. Today, problems with reconstruction have been largely overcome (Spletter, 1981). In the past, reconstruction attempts were often heroic procedures employing fat grafts from the woman's own body or multistaged procedures such as the time consuming tube pedicles from the abdomen. These were unsatisfactory procedures causing extensive scarring.

One impetus to an increased interest in performing reconstruction was the development of medical grade silicone gel implants in the 1960s. These products have continued to improve and now provide an extremely lifelike simulation of breast tissue. Also the less radical procedures for breast cancer have allowed for earlier less involved reconstruction procedures. In addition, advances in surgical technique have seen the development of procedures that involve the transposition of soft tissue to cover chest wall defects and to be used in place of foreign material, thus correcting an area previously inhospitable to reconstruction.

The present range of reconstructive possibilities is quite broad and the majority of women can benefit, including women with advanced disease, if their interest is strong enough. There may be certain medical conditions that prohibit reconstruction in any form. There are many variables that influence a woman's prognosis and each woman's case needs to be considered individually. Therefore, the woman interested in reconstruction should be free to explore the full range of reconstruction possibilities. Besides medical groups, there are volunteer groups who provide information (see the resource list at the end of the chapter).

Financing. A very important factor influencing the consideration of reconstruction is one of cost and family finances. Here again, pressure from women's groups has motivated the matter of insurance remuneration. Many companies are now following an enlightened policy of according breast reconstruction a rehabilitative status eligible for coverage as opposed to cosmetic surgery. New York, Connecticut, and California presently have state laws mandating coverage (Rutledge, 1982).

Expectations. What may a woman expect from reconstruction? Realistic goals would include replacement of the breast contour on the chest wall. Many times this contour may be quite aesthetically pleasing even in the nude. At the least there would be a restoration of cleavage, normal appearance in a bra, bathing suit, and a low cut evening dress. Finally, the freedom to pursue an active sports life without the worry and annoyance of a foreign body pounding on her chest wall while jogging or playing tennis.

Timing. Even though it is possible for a breast prosthesis to be implanted at the time of mastectomy, most reconstructive surgeons prefer a 3- to 6-month delay (Dinner & Peters, 1978; Lynch, Madden, & Franklin, 1977; Thomas & Yates, 1977). During this time the scar softens, vascularity of skin flaps improves, and the skin becomes more supple on the chest wall. Actually, a woman can decide on reconstruction at any propitious time for her, even years later. Radiation or chemotherapy pose restrictions while therapy is in progress. After radiation the chest skin may need to be evaluated for the possibility of soft tissue transfer prior to implant. Chemotherapy cytotoxicity may cause delay in wound healing, which would postpone reconstruction 6 to 12 months (Ruetschi et al., 1980).

Fear of Recurrence. The woman can be reassured that the implant elevates muscle and skin improving palpation for superficial recurrence. However she needs to understand the importance of continued vigilance and follow-up by her surgeon. This is particularly true when there has been soft tissue transfer covering the chest wall.

Reconstruction. Reconstruction of the breast is either performed simultaneously with a mastectomy or delayed until pathology results are available, until healing is complete, or until adjuvant therapy is completed. Immediate reconstruction offers a woman a sense of "wholeness" immediately. The best candidate for immediate reconstruction is a woman whose tumor is small and who has a minimal risk of local recurrence (Jurkiewicz & Stevenson, 1984). Immediate reconstruction has not achieved widespread acceptance, but in the future the plastic surgeon will likely work with the general surgeon in planning the mastectomy to achieve the best reconstructive results. For optimal results most breast reconstruction requires two or even three procedures several months apart. This is accomplished by the creation of a breast mound with a prosthesis, the reconstruction of the nipple areola complex if desired, and establishment of symmetry with the other breast. If the skin flaps on the chest wall are tight, a temporary expandible implant may be utilized.

The simplest procedure possible, when there is sufficient tissue on the chest wall, is insertion of a silicone implant into a pocket created under the pectoralis major muscle. This particular method helps reduce the incidence of contracture and capsule formation around the prosthesis. This side effect can be reduced by a program of massage to the area after surgery. This requires a hospital stay of 3 days and a return to work in 10 days.

Reconstruction after a radical mastectomy is more complicated but nonetheless can provide very satisfactory results (Dinner & Peters, 1978). Many women are satisfied with their appearance and feel the effort is justified. New techniques involving development of soft tissue over the thin-skinned chest wall have made gratifying results possible. Preferred methods of soft tissue reconstruction presently used are skin or muscle flaps or both, obtained from the woman's chest, abdomen, back, or buttock (Jurkiewicz & Stevenson, 1984). Of these methods, the latissimus dorsi musculocutaneous flap is presently the preferred method. This more complicated surgery requires 5 to 7 days of hospitalization. The woman can return to work in 3 weeks but should refrain from heavy physical exercise of the involved arm for 6 to 8 weeks.

The second part of the reconstruction involves creation and placement of the nipple areola complex by skin grafting procedures with skin donated from the other nipple, upper thigh, or labia. At the same time the other breast is adjusted in size and placement. The remaining breast may be modified in one of three ways: breast augmentation, breast reduction, or mastopexy. This procedure requires 3 days of hospitalization and return to work in a week.

Between the two stages of reconstruction any disparities between the two breasts are masked by wearing a bra. Reconstruction is a viable and acceptable option for many women, especially those with an active life-style. In the future women facing reconstruction surgery will have the choice of improved methods of breast reconstruction.

Follow-up Care. A woman who has undergone any of the discussed treatments for breast cancer should have at least a bi-yearly physical examination and a mammography at least once per year. The examinations are necessary to check for recurrence or development of cancer in the opposite breast.

Educational Approach

As with any life experience, all women react individually. As previously discussed, many women react with a great deal of anxiety but many also seem resolved and react with lesser degrees of anxiety. Before any educational process is begun the woman should be fully assessed. Most breast cancer surgery is carried out in a general surgical setting, therefore most education will be on a one-to-one basis. Inclusion of partner or close friend, if amenable to the woman, is highly recommended. When possible, small groups of women postmastectomy can be supportive, informative, and provide an atmosphere for sharing similar experiences.

Children of women with breast cancer often do not understand the procedure. If possible, some explanation of the procedure, dependent on the child's age and development level should be provided to allay fears and fantasies. If there are daughters or sisters past puberty, breast self-examination should be taught due to the higher incidence of breast cancer in this group of women (see Chapter 4). Health care providers in addition to breast cancer rehabilitation teaching also have a primary responsibility for teaching breast self-examination. The role of early detection is a known factor. Therefore, the health care providers' role in preventive care is clear despite the controversy over which type of intervention or surgical procedures are optimum.

COMMUNITY BASED INFORMATION SOURCES*

AFTER—Ask a Friend to Explain Reconstruction, 1378 Third Avenue, New York, NY 10021, (212) 472-0400.

American Cancer Society, National Office, 777 Third Avenue, New York, NY 10017. *(Offers basic service programs to cancer patients. Contact them for Reach to Recovery Volunteers. Look in white pages of phone book for local unit.)*

American Society of Plastic and Reconstructive Surgeons, 233 E. Michigan Avenue, Suite 1900, Chicago, IL 60601. *(Call (312) 856-1818 for information regarding availability of reconstructive surgeons by geographic location.)*

AWEAR—A Woman Educating About Reconstruction, 1-800-552-7996 (toll-free).

Breast Cancer Advisory Center, 11426 Rockville Pike, Suite 406, Rockville, MD 20850. *(Volunteer group. Mails information sheets. Answers questions about all aspects of cancer diagnosis.)*

ENCORE, YWCA, National Board, 600 Lexington Avenue, New York, NY 10022. *(Postoperative breast cancer patients. Exercise, may include swimming and discussion group. Call local YMCA branch or write to the National Board for regional programs.)*

---

*Source: Spletter, M. *A woman's choice: New options in the treatment of breast cancer.* Boston, Mass.: Beacon Press, 1981.

IMAGES and OPTIONS, San Francisco Bay Area, (415) 522-2924.

Make Today Count, Inc., P.O. Box 303, Burlington, IA 52601, (319) 753-6521. *(Psychological assistance to patients with advanced career and their families. Over 300 chapters located throughout the country. Check local directory or write to above address.)*

RENU—Reconstruction Education for National Understanding, Cleveland, OH (216) 444-2900 (24-hour answering service), Washington, DC (202) 483-2600.

BIBLIOGRAPHY

American Cancer Society. *Cancer facts and figures: 1982.* New York: American Cancer Society, 1982.

Bonadonna, G., Valagussa, P., Rossi, A., Zucali, R., Tancini, G., Bajetta, E., Bramilla, C., DaLena, M., DiFronzo, G., Banfi, A., Rilke, F., & Veronesi, V. Are surgical adjuvant trials altering the course of breast cancer? *Seminars In Oncology,* 1978, *5*(4), 450–463.

Carbone, P. P., & Davis, T. E. Medical treatment for advanced breast cancer. *Seminars in Oncology,* 1978, *5*(4), 417–427.

Clancy, P. *The postmastectomy rehabilitation class: Nursing section.* Prepared by P. H. Clancy for the Memorial Sloan-Kettering Cancer Center Breast Rehabilitation Program, unpublished, January 1982.

Dinner, M. I., & Peters, C. R. Breast reconstruction following mastectomy. *Surgical Clinics of North America,* 1978, *158*(4), 851–868.

Dulcey, M. P. Addressing breast cancer's assault on female sexuality. *Topics In Clinical Nursing,* 1980, *1*(4), 61–68.

Foote, F. W., & Stewart, F. W. A histologic classification of carcinoma of the breast. *Surgery,* 1946, *19*(1), 74–99.

Gallager, E. (Ed.) *The breast.* St. Louis, Mo.: C. V. Mosby, 1978.

Giaquinta, B. Helping females face the crisis of cancer. *American Journal of Nursing,* 1977, *77*(10), 1585–1588.

Hayward, J. L. Conservative surgery in the treatment of early breast cancer. In E. F. Lewison & A. C. W. Montague (Eds.), *Diagnosis and treatment of breast cancer.* Baltimore: Williams and Wilkins, 1981, pp. 127–128.

Henderson, I. C., & Canellos, G. P. Cancer of the breast—The past decade. *New England Journal of Medicine,* 1980, *302*(1), 17–30.

Holland, J. The clinical course of breast cancer: A psychological perspective. *Frontiers of Radiation Therapeutic Oncology,* 1976, *11*, 133–145.

Jurkiewicz, M. J., & Stevenson, T. R. Plastic and reconstructive surgery. In S. Schwartz (Ed.), *Principles of surgery* (4th ed.). New York: McGraw-Hill, 1984, pp. 2101–2150.

Kinne, D. W. Opinion: The case of the one-step biopsy procedure for breast cancer. *Cancer: A Cancer Journal for Clinicians,* 1982, *32*(1), 46–50.

Leahy, I., St. Germaine, J. M., & Carriciogg, G. *The nurse and radiotherapy,* St. Louis, Mo.: C. V. Mosby, 1979.

Levene, M. B., Harris, J. R., & Hellman, S. Primary radiation therapy for operable carcinoma of the breast. *Surgical Clinics of North America,* 1978, *58*(4), 767–776.

Levene, M. B., Harris, J. R., & Hellman, S. Treatment of carcinoma of the breast by radiation therapy. *Cancer,* 1977, *39*(6), 2840–2845.

Lynch, J. B., Madden, J. J., & Franklin, J. D. Breast reconstruction following mastectomy for cancer. *Annals of Surgery,* 1977, *5*, 490–501.

Maddox, W. A., Carpenter, J. T., Laws, H. L., Song, S. J., Cloud, G., Urist, M. M., & Balch, C. M. A randomized prospective trial of radical (Halsted) mastectomy versus modified radical mastectomy in 311 breast cancer patients. *Annals of Surgery,* 1983, *198*(2), 207–212.

Margolese, R. G. Response: The case for the two-step breast procedure for breast cancer. *Cancer: A Cancer Journal for Clinicians,* 1982, *32*(1), 51–57.

Moetzinger, C. A., & Dauber, L. G. The management of the patient with breast cancer. *Cancer Nursing*, 1982, *5*, 287–292.

Morris, T., Greer, H. S., & White, P. Psychological and social adjustment to mastectomy: A two-year follow-up study. *Cancer*, 1977, *40*, 2381–2387.

Pelnik, S., & Leis, H. P. Clinical diagnosis of breast lesions. In E. Gallagher (Ed.) *The breast*. St. Louis, Mo.: C. V. Mosby, 1978.

Plotkin, D., Lechner, J. J., Jung, W. E., & Rosin, P. J. Tamoxifen flare in advanced breast cancer. *JAMA*, 240(24), 1978, 2644–2645.

Prosnitz, L. R., Goldenberg, I. S., Packard, R. A., Levene, B., Harris, J., Hellman, S., Wallner, P. E., Brady, Z. D., Mansfield, C. M., & Kramer, S. Radiation therapy as initial treatment for early stage cancer of the breast without mastectomy. *Cancer*, 1977, *39*, 917–923.

Reutschi, M. S., Kovachev, D., Kinne, D. W., & Chaglassian, T. A. Breast reconstruction after mastectomy: Part I. *Memorial Sloan-Kettering Cancer Center Bulletin*, 1980, *10*(2), 53–61.

Ruetschi, M. S., Kovachev, D., Kinne, D. W., & Chaglassian, T. A. Breast reconstruction after mastectomy Part II. *Memorial Sloan-Kettering Cancer Center Bulletin*, 1980, *10*(3), 102–108.

Rush, B. F. Breast. In S. Schwartz (Ed.), *Principles of surgery* (4th ed.). New York: McGraw-Hill, 1984, pp. 522–555.

Rutledge, D. N. Nurses' knowledge of breast reconstruction: A catalyst for earlier treatment of breast cancer? *Career Nursing*, 1982, *5*(6), 469–474.

Schain, W. Psychological impact of the diagnosis of breast cancer on the patient. *Frontiers of Radiation Therapeutic Oncology*, 1976, *11*, 77.

Schain, W. Guidelines for psychological management of breast cancer: A stage related approach. In E. Gallager, H. Leis, R. Snyderman, & J. Urban (Eds.), *The breast*. St. Louis, Mo.: C. V. Mosby, 1978.

Schwartz, S. (Ed.). *Principles of surgery* (4th ed.). New York: McGraw-Hill, 1984.

Scott, D. W. Quality of life following the diagnosis of breast cancer. *Topics in Clinical Nursing*, 1983, *4*(4), 20–27.

Scott, D. W. Anxiety, critical thinking and information processing during and after breast biopsy. *Nursing Research*, 1983, *32*(1), 24–28.

Spletter, M. *A woman's choice: New options in the treatment of breast cancer*. Boston: Beacon Press, 1981.

Stehlin, J. S., Evans, R. A., Gutierrez, A. E., Cowles, J., de Ipolyi, P. D., & Greeff, P. J. Treatment of carcinoma of the breast. *Surgery, Gynecology & Obstetrics*, 1979, *149*, 911–922.

Teicher, I., Ariel, I. M., Stone, A., Tinker, M. A., & Wise, L. The treatment of potentially curable breast cancer. *Resident & Staff Physician*, 1978, *24*(9), 55–72.

Thomas, S. G. Breast cancer: The psychosocial issues. *Cancer Nursing*, 1976, *1*(1), 57.

Thomas, S. G., & Yates, M. M. Breast reconstruction after mastectomy. *American Journal of Nursing*, 1977, *77*(9), 1438–1442.

U.S. Department of Health and Human Services. *The Breast Cancer Digest*. National Cancer Institute, Bethseda, Md.: NIH Publication No. 81-1691, 1980.

Wallner, P. E., Brady, L. W., Jr., Loughend, J., Matsumoto, T., Antoniades, J., Prasavinichai, S., Glassburn, J. R., Asbell, S. D., & Damsker, J. I. Subtotal mastectomy and radiation therapy in the definitive management of localized breast malignancy. *American Journal of Roentgenography*, 1976, *127*, 505–507.

Woods, J. E. Breast reconstruction after mastectomy. *Surgery Gynecology and Obstetrics*. 1980, *150*, 869–874.

Psychosocial Problems: Education for Prevention

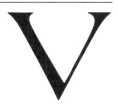

Women have an increased incidence of depression and anxiety. They are also victims of abuse in the area of family violence. In addition, women have a higher rate of medical and surgical intervention. Chapters 24, 25, and 26 address these problems and propose that education aimed at prevention and coping with the stresses of life may assist women to more positive mental health and/or appropriate use of health care services and providers. Chapter 25 proposes that education aimed at women's understanding of their socialization and society's view of women can assist women in avoiding the role of victim. The authors for the chapters in Part V are psychiatric nurses and a psychiatrist. The nurse authors also have backgrounds in women's health or obstetrics and gynecology.

What Women Should Know About Depression

24

Geri LoBiondo-Wood

Depression as a mood or a feeling is felt by all at some time during one's life, but depression as a health care problem for women is of considerable importance. Descriptions of depressed individuals can be found in the Bible as well as in ancient mythology. Depression as a clinical entity was first described by Hippocrates who coined the term melancholia. Despite similar descriptions of the symptoms of depression across all eras, each generation has had its own theories as to the etiology of depression and the best methods of treatment.

Most authors agree that women suffer from a higher incidence of depression than men (Klerman & Weissman, 1980; Radloff, 1980). This chapter describes some of the theories of depression in women and attempts to highlight those contributing factors that may be responsible for the higher incidence of depression in women. Health care practices and preventive strategies for dealing with depressed women are suggested based on the unique needs and rights of women. These strategies are geared toward the primary and secondary level of prevention. Tertiary level strategies or severe clinical depression are beyond the scope of this chapter.

It is difficult to accurately assess the incidence of depression in women within the general population. Nevertheless, data are available on the utilization of mental health facilities by both women and men and how they differ in primary diagnosis. The three most frequent mental health diagnoses between the ages of 18 and 64 years are depressive, schizophrenic, and alcohol disorders. According to the latest figures (Table 24–1), with only a few exceptions in various age categories, men were more often treated for alcohol-related disorders than women. Review of schizophrenia reveals only minor differences between the sexes for rates of occurrence. The age-adjusted rates for depressive disorders show women to have a higher incidence of depression. This holds true even when comparing public and private hospitals. The only age group in which men surpass women in the diagnosis of depression is 65- to 74-year-olds. Depression also occurs more frequently among whites than nonwhites for all age groups (Table 24–2).

Depression, as a nonclinical entity, has been described as a mood, a feeling, an affect, or a reaction to a loss. As an emotional state, depression is not a discriminating concept. Depression as a feeling or a mood is a component of human existence. In short, transient periods of depression can be felt at various times in one's life cycle. These normal reactions are usually short-lived and rarely disrupt one's ability to work and carry

577

TABLE 24–1. AGE-ADJUSTED RATES BY DIAGNOSIS, SEX, AND TYPE OF MENTAL HEALTH FACILITY IN THE UNITED STATES

	Sex	
Diagnosis	Male	Female
Public facility		
Alcohol disorders	10.9	2.4
Depressive disorders	11.8	19.1
Schizophrenia	26.4	21.6
Nonpublic hospitals		
Alcohol disorders	14.8	6.6
Depressive disorders	48.8	102.0
Schizophrenia	30.0	39.5

(Source: U. S. Department of Health, Education and Welfare/Public Health Service/Alcohol, Drug Abuse and Mental Health Administration, Division of Biometry (Statistical Note No. 137) Washington, D.C.: U.S. Government Printing Office, August, 1977.)

out everyday life. The true incidence of episodes of depression in the average woman's life is unknown. Depression as a nonclinical entity may manifest itself with what DeRosis and Pellegrino (1976) termed "garden variety symptoms." These symptoms are similar to those described in Table 24–3 but may be manifested in lesser or more suppressed ways. It can only be inferred from the data on depression as a clinical illness that women may experience more episodes of nonclinical depression than men.

Depression can also be associated with sadness and also suggests a departure from the normal response to sadness (Areti & Bemporad, 1978). Sadness, which results from an unplanned circumstance, is most often considered a negative experience; however, it may result in positive outcomes. It can be a motivating force that influences one to correct the situation. Once a remedy is found the "sorrow work" (Areti & Bemporad, 1980) is done and the sadness decreases or disappears. This type of sorrow work is most often seen in situations of grief and loss. Some depression can thus be seen as adaptive or growth-promoting.

TABLE 24–2. DIAGNOSED DEPRESSIVE DISORDERS AS A PERCENTAGE OF TOTAL DISCHARGE BY AGE, SEX, RACE AND NONGOVERNMENT PSYCHIATRIC INPATIENT UNITS IN THE UNITED STATES

Age	Both Sexes	Male	Female	White	All Other Races
Under 18	17.7	10.9	23.6	19.3	10.8
18–24	27.0	16.7	36.6	29.1	17.3
25–34	34.6	25.3	41.1	37.7	19.1
35–44	44.6	33.7	50.5	46.4	28.4
45–54	47.6	43.4	50.2	49.0	24.2
55–64	50.6	44.6	54.7	54.4	5.0
65–74	53.2	53.9	52.8	55.2	5.0
75+	33.4	25.8	37.7	34.2	5.0
All ages	37.7	28.8	43.9	40.5	18.4

(Source: U.S. Department of Health, Education and Welfare/Public Health Service/Alcohol, Drug Abuse and Mental Health Administration, Division of Biometry (Statistical Note No. 137) Washington, D.C.: U.S. Government Printing Office, August, 1977.)

TABLE 24–3. COMMON CHARACTERISTICS AND SYMPTOMS OF DEPRESSION

1. Affect of sadness, grief, hopelessness, blue, emptiness, and loneliness.
2. A lack of ability to experience pleasure in activities previously enjoyed.
3. Appetite changes, usually loss of weight (or can be an increase also).
4. Lethargy, slowness of speech, movement, and thoughts.
5. Low self-esteem and personal devaluation.
6. Loss of interest in self, feelings of worthlessness and guilt.
7. Outlook of gloom and pessimism, loss of interest in family, work, and friends.
8. Anxiety, feelings of dread.
9. Decreased sexual interest.
10. Change in appearance and self-care habits: grooming, dress, posture, and facial expression.
11. Hostility or anger may be present but suppressed.
12. Psychomotor agitation or retardation.
13. Difficulty in concentration, which may lend itself to doubt, indecision, rumination, or confusion.
14. Somatic complaints.
15. Sleep disturbances, usually insomnia and complaints of feeling worse in the morning.
16. Sense of helplessness and futility, tearfulness.
17. Thoughts of death or suicide.

Distinguishing depression as a normal mood from depression as a mental health disorder is difficult. Each individual's tolerance and ability to deal with depression varies greatly. Futhermore, the etiology of depression in women is multifactorial and interrelated to sociological, psychological, and physiological factors. The presence or absence of a precipitating event may further complicate the picture of depression. Depression can be seen on a continuum from mild, to moderate, to severe or clinical psychosis. A clear discrimination among the points on this continuum is not possible as there is considerable overlap between the various points. Clinically, four criteria are used to diagnose depression: intensity of symptoms, duration of symptoms, a precipitating event, and psychopathology factors such as weight loss and suicidal ideation. The common characteristic symptoms of depression are listed in Table 24–3. The diagnostic categories in which depression is a primary component and those in which depression may be a factor are listed in Table 24–4. Many views exist on the etiology of depression. To understand the roots and the current treatment of depression some of the major theoretical viewpoints are reviewed.

Theories of Depression

Biological View/Physiological View. The biological or physiological view of the development of depression has been of great interest in the recent past. In the early 1950s, serendipitously, there was found to be a depletion of norepinephrine (NE) and serotonin (5-HT catecholamines) in clients with symptoms of depression. Concurrently, it was discovered that clients with tuberculosis treated with isoniazid displayed elevated moods. It was found that isoniazid blocked the destruction of NE and 5-HT by inhibiting the production of monoamine oxidase (MAO), an enzyme that metabolizes these amines. From these and other developments antidepressant drugs or MAO inhibitors were developed to treat depression. These antidepressants have been very helpful in treating some but not all clients with clinical depression. Several biological tests have also been devel-

TABLE 24–4. CLINICAL DISORDERS IN WHICH DEPRESSION IS A COMPONENT

Major depression, recurrent
Major depression, single episode
Bipolar depression, depressed
Bipolar depression, mixed
Atypical depression
Adjustment disorder with depressed mood
Primary degenerative dementia, senile onset with depression
Dysthymic disorder

Depression may also be a component in the following:

Drug and alcohol dependence
Schizophrenia
Personality disorders
Medical illness
Obsessive–compulsive neurosis
Sexual dysfunction

oped to assess depressive illness that suggest that depression has more than simply a psychological etiology. Moreover, it is important to highlight that the physiological makeup cannot be separated from the psychological picture of an individual in attempts to explain depression. Genetic studies have also suggested a genetic link to the development of depression (Kety et al., 1975; Klerman & Barrett, 1973) but this is difficult to assess due to other influences such as learning and environment.

Psychodynamic View. Numerous theorists and clinicians have attempted to explore the etiology of depression within a psychodynamic viewpoint. Abraham (1911/1960) was probably the first psychoanalyst to explore depression. Abraham felt that a deep repression of libidinal satisfaction, an ambivalence, and an inability to love were significant aspects of depression. What Abraham did not touch on was object loss, which is now considered to be the cardinal concept in this framework. In Freud's classic work *Mourning and Melancholia* (1917/1957), he proposed that during early childhood the child formed an intense object relationship (with the parent), which was thwarted because of a disappointment with the love object. When these negative feelings are unresolved, the feelings toward the lost love object become internalized. These internalized feelings give rise to anger and pervasive ambivalence in all relationships and predispose one to depression.

Many have expanded on the psychoanalytical theory (Adler, 1961; Bonime, 1976; Chadoff, 1970) by adding such concepts as stress. These authors believe that depressive personalities have their roots in early childhood and are a result of a lack of nurturance or interactive difficulties with the love object. This results in internalized aggression, ambivalence, and a strong sense of narcissism. The early theorists (Abraham, 1911/1960; Freud, 1917/1957) stress the instinctual roots of depression, whereas the later theorists stress the interpersonal components and the resultant dependency needs and low tolerance for frustration.

Current psychoanalytical thinking is also influenced by the concepts of self-esteem and ego. Areti and Bemporad (1978), Bibring (1953), and Sandler and Jaffe (1965), albeit using dissimilar systems, focused on the individual's inability to regulate self-esteem adequately as the core concept of depression. More specifically, depression relates to the regulation of self-esteem and reflects a discrepancy between the actual state of self and a desired ego ideal (Rush, 1982). According to Bibring (1953), one experiencing depression has suffered from a severe loss of self-esteem. This loss results in a conflict between an actual or an imaginary helplessness and high goals that one feels unable to achieve. This situation is further aggravated by the original feelings of dependency and deprivation felt in childhood, which were repressed. Therefore, one who experiences depressive episodes is seen as having difficulties with autonomy and intimacy.

Cognitive View. Beck (1970, 1974, 1976) described cognitive changes as the core of depression and labeled three specific distortions as the triad of depression. These are a negative view of oneself (low self-esteem), a negative view of the world, and a negative perspective of the future. One who is depressed manifests the triad by seeing oneself as deprived, frustrated, rejected, and punished. Individuals who fit the triad make systematic errors of cognition and negatively distort in such a way that external events are constructed to depict loss or deprivation. These errors include: arbitrary inference, in which a conclusion is drawn despite inadequate or contrary evidence, selective abstraction, or focusing on a single detail rather than the whole context of a situation (Beck, 1974). These distortions in a person's judgment take on a causal relationship between perceived defects and judgments of unworthiness. Operationally, these distortions take the form of personal criticism and a negative view of oneself. Experiences with the world and the future seem overly demanding and obstructive. Experiences and outlook are constructed as evidence for defeat and loss. This evidence gives the depressed person support for feelings of rejection, deprivation, and increased dependence (Rush, 1982). Depressed individuals arrive at the conclusion that they are inadequate and a failure.

Another theorist, Seligman (1974), proposed a cognitive model of depression based upon the phenomenon of learned helplessness in animals. In his early studies, Seligman noted helplessness in dogs, characterized by passivity in the face of stress and difficulty in learning a response that produces relief. A naive dog given escape–avoidance training in a shuttle-box soon learned to jump a barrier or cue to avoid the forthcoming mild electric shock. However, a naive dog, pretreated with inescapable shock (Seligman & Maier, 1967), responded to escape–avoidance training by sitting down and taking the shock passively. The dog failed to learn that jumping the barrier produced termination of the painful shock. More recent studies by Seligman and others on human subjects support the learned helplessness model (Miller & Seligman, 1973; Thornton & Jacobs, 1981).

The symptoms of learned helplessness and depression closely parallel each other. Passivity, a symptom of depression, is the central symptom of learned helplessness (Seligman, 1981). Mendel (1970) described a loss of interest, a decrease in energy, an erosion of motivation, and an increasing inability to cope with work and responsibility as symptoms associated with depression.

Depressed patients not only make fewer responses, but they are "set" to interpret their own responses as failures or as doomed to failure (Seligman, 1981). This helplessness and pessimism coincides with the negative cognitive set described by Beck.

Interpersonal View. The interpersonal view is based on the belief that depression, regardless of the symptoms, severity of symptoms, or personality traits occurs within an interpersonal and a psychosocial context (Klerman et al., 1974; Paykel et al., 1969; Weissman et al., 1974; Weissman & Paykel, 1974). In this view interpersonal experiences in the individual's family of origin will be reflected in current interpersonal interactions and attitudes. The development of depression is seen as having three component process: (1) symptom formation: which includes the development of a depressive effect and negative symptoms and may arise from psychobiological and/or psychodynamic mechanisms,

(2) social and interpersonal relations: based on childhood experiences will affect interactions in social roles, social reinforcement, competency, and personal mastery, and (3) personality: personality traits and patterns developed such as anger, guilt, poor communication patterns, and poor self-esteem will effect interpersonal experiences (Rush, 1982).

The interpersonal view implicity recognizes interpsychic factors but does not explicitly deal with them. The goal of this view when used in therapy is on current problems, frustration, and conflict.

Weissman and Paykel (1974) testing the interpersonal view found in a comparison study of depressed women and their normal neighbors that depressed women were considerably more impaired in all aspects of social functioning, as wives, workers, mothers, family, and friends. This impairment was greatest with family, with whom poor communication and anger were evident. This interpersonal view contributes to our understanding of depression in women.

Moreover, as with most aspects of mental illness and disequilibrium patterns, no one theory or concept completely explains the problem or gives conclusive solutions to the puzzle of depression. It seems that even though the symptomatology may be fairly stable along a continuum from mild to severe, the causes are multifactorial and varied from individual to individual.

For women the roots of depression seem to be even more complex. There may also be a link between depression and women's disadvantaged social and economic status, and a lack of positions of power and authority. Women in the past have been rewarded for developing traits of submissiveness, helplessness, and passivity.

Virginia Woolf stated, "It is obvious that the values of women differ very often from the values which have been made for them by the other sex" (1929, p. 76). Therefore, women have defined themselves in terms of men. Gilligan (1982) purports that psychology has persistently misunderstood women in their psychological growth by using a male standard to explain female psychology. Her work, even though it focused on morality, rights, and responsibility, can be extrapolated and applied to depression. Women's roles have been that of nurturer, caretaker, and helpmate, the weaver of networks of relationships on which she relies (Gilligan, 1982). Whereas women have been assuming these roles, men in theories of psychology have tended to devalue these roles.

Miller (1976) feels that the groundwork for depression in women is laid in their development. Women develop within a context of affiliations and attachments. Their sense of self-esteem becomes focused on their capacity to develop and preserve relationships. Miller believes that women when faced with the loss of affiliation cannot rely on their own individual achievement and therefore may become depressed. She further suggests that women need the power of self-determination and the restructuring of the nature of relationships to avoid such problems.

Other critics of various psychodynamic views (Chesler, 1972; Franks & Burtle, 1974; Masling & Harris, 1969) have pointed out that psychiatry is dominated by male theorists and the stereotypical roles of women continue to hold women in a stance of submissiveness and passivity. A major work on sex role stereotypes by Broverman, Broverman, Clarkson, Rosenkrantz, and Vogel (1970) documented the presence of sex role stereotypes among mental health professionals. The studies indicated a negative assessment of women. A healthy woman was considered to be submissive and dependent, whereas in men these traits were considered to be unhealthy.

The juggling of traditional and new roles in the business, professional, and personal environment may also contribute to higher rates of depression in women. Equally important is the stress of inequality and discriminatory practices of both the social and the employment environments. Klerman and Weissman (1980) suggest that a model for the development of depression in women should incorporate the views of learned helplessness and life-event stresses with the consideration of concurrent physiological changes. This model should also integrate loss, social order, and alterations in the biogenic amines. Because no one theory completely explains the origins of depression, the health care provider must be aware of the variety of causes of depression and the various treatment options.

Prevention of Depression

Reducing the risks of certain predictable events that occur in all individuals and that may affect one's mental health and coping skills is the goal of prevention. Events of separation, loss, grief, developmental crises, and transitional situations as well as interpersonal styles and social factors may be preludes to depression. Prevention, as defined by Caplan (1970), aims at reducing the incidence, duration, and residual effects of mental disorders. Caplan emphasizes primary prevention or reduction of the incidence of new cases of mental disorders and the promotion of mental health. To accomplish these goals in reference to women, high-risk populations for depression need to be identified and anticipatory guidance needs to be given in the form of health education and supportive community services.

The fact that women more commonly experience depression and, therefore, are identified as a high-risk population is the first step of primary prevention. A further consideration then is to understand and assess the similarities of situations and individuals in whom depression is a problem. A number of studies reflect the types of individuals and types of situations that can be classified as high risk. Radloff (1980) found that women were more depressed among the divorced–separated group, the never-married who were not head of a household (mainly young adults living with parents) group, and the widowed group. When women were compared to men, women who were often married, divorced–separated, and never-married (not head of a household) were more depressed. Investigation of social factors linked with depression for both groups revealed that youth (18 to 24 years), low education, low income, low status employment, and physical illness were high-risk factors. Radloff also analyzed the social factors by sex and found similar results. Radloff suggests that susceptibility and precipitating factors result from certain biological and social factors. Futhermore, this susceptibility is a learned habit or helpless coping style triggered by problems or stresses. Using a learning theory model, she suggests that the cognitive (susceptibility) dimension needs to be altered. In this formulation depression occurs when the woman feels as if she has no ability to influence goals or expectations. Depression then develops sequentially. For example, in a situation in which one feels powerless to cope, this feeling reinforces cognitions of helplessness and low self-esteem. Subsequently, appetite and sleep disturbances cause a sense of "low" feelings and sadness. The sadness and lack of motivation interferes with daily living, causing a cycle of depression. To prevent such occurrences, learning or cognition needs to be altered.

This formulation of learned control is further enhanced by Maccoby and Jacklin (1974). They found that the actions of boys more frequently had consequences than did the actions of girls. Similarly, others have found that the traditional female role has been described as dependent, nonassertive, passive, and emotional (Bardwick & Douvan, 1972; Bem 1974; Horner, 1970). The traditional female role may be part of the explanation of the high rates of depression. The women's movement in the past two decades has given rise to what has been termed the liberated woman; this can mean anything from a working professional mother who still keeps modified traditional roles in the home to a frank feminist who rejects all notion of the traditional woman. Expectations and the roles of women today are fluid. Probably, there will never be a set idea of what is meant by the liberated or traditional woman. Yet, each woman within her own setting needs to be able to achieve a degree of assertiveness to have her own needs and rights met.

In the recent past women have recognized their lack of assertiveness and the need to express themselves openly and directly. This has led to the development of many assertive training courses for women (Tolor, Kelly, & Stebbins, 1976). The learning of assertive techniques and the assuming of assertive roles is a means for women to clarify their rights as individuals as well as a means to express needs. Learning of assertiveness or social effectiveness can assist women when they experience helplessness or an inability to affect their environment, both of which may lead to feelings of depression.

Direct stress, such as a predictable life event, for instance marriage or loss, changes in life conditions such as poverty, or unpredictable life events such as divorce, sexual abuse, physical abuse, and sexual discrimination may place individuals whether male or female at a higher risk for depression. But, for a woman, who has learned feelings of helplessness, dependence, and self-doubt, the anxiety triggered by these situations may be more hazardous. Therefore, the probability that one will experience some form of depression depends on one's susceptibility to it and the presence of precipitating factors. The precipitating factors can be social, biological, or developmental. Studies have shown which of these risk factors favor the development of depression in women. It has also been suggested that women have learned over time to be more susceptible to depression through stereotyped sex role socialization (Radloff, 1980). The implications for prevention and treatment of depression are evident.

The increased awareness of the differences in rates of depression between the sexes should lead health care providers to include in their health assessment a careful appraisal of personality styles and roles that a woman assumes as a individual and vis-a-vis friends, family, and environment. This assessment also needs to consider if the woman is experiencing a milder depression that she herself can stem through education on improved self-care habits, or a more severe or clinical depression that may need direct clinical interventions. Assessment of the extent or severity of depression can be accomplished by a review of the characteristics and symptoms as discussed in Table 24–3. These symptoms can be posed in the form of questions during the total health assessment. The degree of severity of the symptoms would include length of time experienced, continuous versus intermittent course, as well as if there is any relationship to life events. Some women are unaware of their depression. Lack of awareness can occur with denial of feelings, fatigue, restlessness, or inability to make decisions. This may be related to a low level of depression. As an example, relocation to a new area, even though planned and desired, results in a transient low level of depression.

DeRosis and Pellegrino (1976) identified three types of depression-prone women. The first is the over-compliant, self-efficacious, love-addicted woman who is not guided by her own needs and wants but experiences life through the acknowledgment she obtains from others, especially men. These women cannot express anger or criticism without feeling guilty or remorseful. Feelings of this nature can lead to dependence, helplessness, and a lack of joy with self and activities. The second type identified is the detached uninvolved woman. The uninvolved woman is conceptualized as dependable but aloof. Her sense of self is found in her sameness and noncompetitive behavior. These women are depicted as having a low tolerance for anxiety and have a sense of hopelessness or resignation about the future. The third type, called the domineering woman, is one who wants to achieve mastery over all. This woman is aggressive and competitive; one who always wants to be the best. The domineering woman needs to be in control and fears feeling helpless. The problem with this style is that this woman must constantly compete to maintain her superiority. Many of the qualities displayed by all three types of women are not poor qualities. The problem arises when these styles become either consciously or unconsciously obligatory and rigid modes of behavior. Therefore, assessment should be aimed at evaluating if a woman has the qualities outlined and if she experiences them in a negative way. If she does, then based on her learning needs, the practitioner can help her to assess when, what, and how these tendencies become problematic. This is one way for the practitioner to better know the client and for the woman to better know herself.

Roles like personality styles can also contribute to depression. The roles that one assumes do not cause depression in and of themselves. A woman in her life time can assume up to a dozen roles each with its own stressors at any one given time. These roles may all be well managed and the number of "hats" that one wears may go unnoticed. But a new stressor or an unexpected change in one role may cause an inability to carry out the other roles. When this occurs one may not be able to live up to either her own or the expectations of others, and she may develop some type of depression. A combination of events, roles, physiological parameters, personality characteristics, societal expectations, and biases can influence the development of depression. From the above discussion it is obvious that no one component can be overlooked when considering assessment or prevention. There are many circumstances that may not be easily amenable to change, such as a loss or some of society's biases against women. What is amenable to change are feelings. The feelings of depression can be mastered or prevented with the development of problem solving, assertiveness, and by knowing oneself well enough to be able to recognize and stem the development of depression. To accomplish this, mechanisms for prevention should be offered to women at an early age.

It is during the adolescent years that the seeds of how to prevent depression could be taught. During the adolescent years young women begin to confront key developmental tasks. During these years adolescents are also a more captive audience because they are in school. Helping young women accept the idea of universality of feelings and sharing of insights within school settings and networking can serve them well in later years.

Intervention Strategies

When prevention is not attempted or has not succeeded, the health care provider needs to directly address the problem of depression. Assessment and definition of the problem precede care strategies. The assessment not only takes into consideration the level of depression, but should also assess the woman's perception of the problem. One also needs to evaluate the woman's coping skills and the presence or absence of environmental, social, and interpersonal support systems. The identification of individuals who are already in the health care system for other problems or in the community at large who would benefit from assistance in dealing with depression, is also important if health care providers focus on primary prevention. Women as individuals and as a group gather in many diverse places such as churches, their own or their children's schools, charitable and political organizations, and work areas. As individuals, they are seen in all facets of the health care system. It is in these places that health care providers can provide education for prevention and intervention for women with early signs of depression so as to promote mental health.

If the presence of depressed feelings is to be recognized early, the care provider must become sensitive to both verbal and nonverbal cues from the client. The attention to such cues should be undertaken, even when other symptoms and problems bring the woman to the health care facility. The communication and understanding of these feelings bring to light other issues that may affect care. Care providers should be aware of their own attitudes and values toward the depressed as well as their own mood level. For example, if the care provider feels that people should have more or better control over themselves, these feelings may interfere with or hinder any therapeutic interventions. It has been suggested that those who care for depressed individuals should have working structures through which they may receive validation of their experiences and communicate concerns about their approach with clients (Swanson, 1982). This can be accomplished through clinical supervision and team meetings. This networking is very important in dealing with the depressed client because much of the initial assessment and intervention includes the processing of the affect and cognition of the client.

Based upon the need of the individual woman, a decision should be made as to whether individual or group intervention is necessary. Individual and group interventions are discussed here only in the broadest sense. If it is assessed that a woman has a severe level of depression, referrals should be made for a more formal psychotherapeutic group or individual interventions. Clients with less severe depression may benefit from an array of group strategies such as supportive groups, networking, women's groups, assertiveness training, or activity-related groups such as health collectives or short-term crisis groups. Individual interventions can also include supportive strategies based upon approaches derived from cognitive or systems theory. It is in these settings and with appropriate strategies that health care providers can give information and interventions that promote mental health.

Once the assessment is done, the development of strategies for dealing with depressed individuals can be accomplished using the taxonomy of objectives as outlined in Chapter 2. The symptomatology of depression affects the cognitive, affective, and psychomotor domains. The following are interventions for each of these domains. The use and alteration of the strategies depend on the individual assessment of each woman and where her needs lie based on the teaching continuum (see Chapter 2).

Psychomotor Domain. The psychomotor domain is a key and probably the first domain to which assistance should be geared. This domain is where feelings and cognition manifest themselves with feelings of lethargy, inability to function at one's best level, in sleeping disturbances, and in general retardation of activity. This may also result in varying degrees of social withdrawal and isolation. The depressed woman, either consciously or unconsciously, adapts her psychomotor activity to deal with feelings of depression.

The psychomotor domain may be the easiest domain within which to develop strategies for a woman who has some degree of motivation. This is the one area where women who experience a mild or moderate form of depression can be encouraged to begin alternative or self-help strategies.

To begin with, clients should be encouraged to establish a daily routine. This routine should include adequate rest, nutrition, and exercise. Goals should be set for type and complexity of routine dependent upon the needs of the woman, her life-style, and level of depression. A regular sleep pattern should be established. A well-balanced nutritional status should also be a goal. Meals and food patterns can have many meanings for individuals. Additionally, women have changing nutritional needs throughout their life cycle. Poor nutritional status does not cause depression but can bear on a woman's general health status, body image, and feelings of well-being.

Exercise and setting time aside for oneself has been recognized as critically important. This time should result in relaxation. A regular exercise program has shown to produce chemical and psychological changes that aid mental well-being. Additional benefits of a regular exercise program are a sense of accomplishment, control over one's life, and probably some physical body trimming that can improve one's body image. Increasing these positive feelings can aid in decreasing feelings of worthlessness, helplessness, and hopelessness. Suggested activities include walking, jogging, yoga, aerobic dancing, or swimming. The important point is to choose one and do it daily. Competitive activities should probably be limited during periods of depression.

Cognitive Domain. It is important for women to know and be able to describe the signs and the symptoms of depression and realize that these signs and symptoms can be subtle as well as overt. Time should also be taken to help the woman identify what the "shoulds" are in her life. The "shoulds" are those expectations that one has of herself in relationship to herself (personality and roles), to the environment, and to others. By developing this combination of knowledge and comprehension, a woman has the basic tools to be able to cognitively structure her thinking in such a way that she could apply her knowledge in situations that may be highly stressful and, therefore, conducive to the development of depressive feelings.

When one is depressed, the thought processes can be labeled as having cognitive distortions. These distortions are breakdowns of communication that need to be recognized, analyzed, and evaluated. Burns (1980) has identified ten cognitive distortions:

1. All or Nothing Thinking. One sees circumstances in "all or none" categories. "If I am not perfect, I am a total failure."
2. Over Generalization. This is the view that one single negative event is the beginning of a never-ending pattern.
3. Mental Filter. This is the choosing of one negative point and dwelling on it to the exclusion of other details of reality.
4. Disqualifying the Positive. This is the rejection of a positive experience so that a negative belief about self or an event can be harbored.
5. Jumping to Conclusions. One negatively interprets events, without supporting data by either assuming others are reacting negatively to them or by convincing oneself that events will have negative outcomes before they happen.
6. Catastrophizing or Minimization. This is either the maximizing or minimizing of one's own qualities or deficits with the focus of making oneself look negative.
7. Emotional Reasoning. One supposes that one's feelings reflect reality. An example is "I made an error, so I must be stupid."
8. Should Statements. This is setting oneself up with should statements based on other's expectations or unreal expectations of self.
9. Labeling. This is an extreme example of over generalization involving emotional content. An example of this is when one makes a mistake and instead of describing the mistake one labels oneself as being "stupid."
10. Personalization. This is seeing oneself as the cause of a negative external event for which one is in fact not responsible.

Burns (1980) recommends that the care provider explain these distortions to the client and have the client make a chart of these distortions, fill it out, and bring it back to the provider. A review of these can assist both the client and the care provider to become aware of the cognitive patterns of the individual which may have led to the development of depression.

Affective Domain. The affective domain of the depressed woman can be fairly problematic and complex. The feelings of one who is depressed can not be easily separated from her cognitive distortions. This domain is affected by anxiety, one's ability to receive, perceive, respond, and express oneself well enough to have one's needs met. To assist one, effective value clarification is also necessary. The values one holds also affect all domains. By assisting her to understand her own values the care provider can work with the client to organize those values that are helpful and those that may be affecting how she feels about herself.

When developing affective strategies, it is helpful to review with the woman any feelings of ineffectiveness, helplessness, or powerlessness. Does the woman see life as totally gloomy or is it one specific aspect or role about which she is depressed? It has been previously noted that depressed individuals demonstrate a lack of pleasure from previously enjoyed activities. When this occurred and what specific activities are affected need to be identified. Depressed individuals also may experience anxiety, hostility, or anger. Those affects may be directed toward self, toward others, or suppressed.

Special Strategies

Work. Whether work is a full-time job outside the home or full-time mothering, or a combination of both, women develop certain ideas of how best to achieve success. These roles have seen a great deal of change over the past two decades and will continue to evolve over time. Generally, full-time mothers have fewer major roles than their working mother counterparts. The power of separate roles can be a source of identity and self-esteem (Gergen & Marecek, 1976). Women who perceive their existence to be lived within a single role may experience paralyzing blows to their self-esteem whenever they fail to meet their expectations for this role (Marecek, 1978). Yet, the combination of the major roles of worker and mother can be a double-edged sword when a woman attempts to be both super-mom and super-worker. DeRosis and Pellegrino (1976) give suggestions for full-time mothers and working women that can be adapted to the individual woman's needs. These suggestions are presented in Table 24–5. The important overall goal should be the development of the woman's own self-help learning.

Assertiveness Training. Assertiveness training is a behavior therapy that has as its goal the reduction of anxiety in social situations and the development of social skills in order to express oneself directly and honestly in interpersonal situations (Alberti & Emmons, 1974; Wolpe, 1958). There are various models of assertiveness training. The most popular one, the skill-deficit model, assumes that an unassertive individual has an assertion skill-deficit (Lindhan & Egan, 1979). The elements of this training include response practice, coaching, and modeling.

Jakubowski (1977), using Seligman's (1974) theories of depression, developed a four-stage assertion training program:

1. Assisting clients to focus on and differentiate assertive, aggressive, and nonassertive behavior with the goal of motivating assertive behavior.
2. Assisting clients in identifying their own interpersonal rights and to develop a belief system supportive of their assertiveness.

TABLE 24–5. SUGGESTIONS FOR DEPRESSED WOMEN IN THEIR WORK ROLES

Mothers	Working Women
1. Arrange time for yourself free of any usual responsibilities.	1. If your problems are job related, it may be helpful to keep in mind that many other women may experience the same problems. Try meeting with other women to discuss problems and solutions. Check YWCA or local women's organizations for such groups.
2. Set up a babysitter pool with parents in your area.	
3. Get together with other mothers to discuss common problems and frustrations.	
4. Do not give up your interests; take courses, go to the library, keep up with an area of interest or your significant male person.	2. Locate a successful man or woman with whom you can talk. Her or his experience can be invaluable in problem solving.
5. Plan at least one day a month to be alone with your significant male person.	3. Try to examine your "shoulds" that can be causing your job dissatisfaction. Find a role model on whom you can pattern new behavior.
6. Get information on your local free or inexpensive entertainment or other related activities.	
7. If you have the time, do volunteer work.	4. If you are married and in conflict because of conflict between roles, explore new solutions with your family. Make a chart and divide up the tasks.
8. Deepen friendships with other women and do things together regularly.	
9. Try to locate one or two couples who you are compatible with and plan activities.	5. Make time for yourself; exercise, shopping, meditating are some suggestions.
10. When planning a family vacation build in some leisure time for yourself.	6. The loneliness of a single working woman has a quality all its own. This loneliness may be one of the most difficult features in depression to surmount. Quick solutions do little good here. The best solution is companionship. Companionship needs to be cultivated over time.
11. Try exchanging weekend baby-sitting with friends periodically.	
12. Examine your shoulds of motherhood. Mothers are not totally responsible for their children's intelligence and success in life. It is all right to be angry with children at times.	

(Source: Adapted from DeRosis, H., & Pellegrino, V. Y. The book of hope: How women can overcome depression. New York: Macmillan, 1976, pp. 125–126, 171–173.)

3. Assisting clients in removing or reducing hindrances that prevent the use of assertive behavior.
4. Assisting clients in practicing assertive techniques through modeling, coaching, and rehearsing.

The core of assertiveness is one's ability to know one's own human rights. Nonassertive behaviors promote a cycle of helplessness. Knowing one's rights in interpersonal situations can assist in promoting self-esteem and integrity. Bloom, Coburn, and Pearlman (1975) compiled a list of women's rights in conjunctions with their assertiveness training program. These are:

1. The right to be treated with respect.
2. The right to have and express one's feelings and opinions.
3. The right to be listened to and taken seriously.
4. The right to set one's own priorities.
5. The right to say no without feeling guilty.
6. The right to ask for what one wants.
7. The right to get what one pays for.
8. The right to ask information from professionals.

9. The right to make mistakes.
10. The right to choose not to assert oneself.
11. The right to change one's mind.

Dependent on a woman's background, the development of assertive behavior requires a reorganization of perceptions of self and interpersonal interaction. Assertive training techniques are used widely. Groups are often held in adult continuing education programs. Health care providers who wish to learn and apply these techniques can do so through course work and the review of professional sources on the subject (see Bibliography section at the end of the chapter).

Groups. The process of treating individuals in groups is known as group therapy. A number of theories and methods of group therapy have evolved throughout the years. Groups range from informal groups, such as supportive and self-help groups, to formal groups that are highly structured like psychotherapy groups. Yalom (1975) suggests that group interventions offer therapeutic change through an intricate interplay of guided experiences. These guided experiences used in group therapy are referred to as curative factors. These are:

1. Instillation of hope
2. Universality
3. Imparting of information
4. Altruism
5. Corrective recapitulation of the primary family group
6. Development of socializing techniques
7. Imitative behavior
8. Interpersonal learning
9. Group cohesiveness
10. Catharsis
11. Existential factors

Groups, as more formal care strategies, using the above schema, offer several advantages over individual strategies. Groups provide an interpersonal environment where individuals can learn through feedback and self-observation how their strengths and limitations of their behavior impacts on oneself and others. This type of intervention can also provide members with a cohesive and supportive setting for developing more adaptive and satisfying behaviors and thereby an increase in self-esteem. In less formal groups or self-help groups learning also occurs, but the learning is usually topic-related and leaders act as resource persons rather than as guiders of group process. Group interventions for depressed women can serve both as a mechanism for gaining information and development of interpersonal skills.

For women who throughout their lives have lacked information, felt a sense of learned helplessness, and felt as if they were alone in their experiences, a variety of groups are available. Various types of groups which can be suggested are listed in Table 24–6; see also Chapter 3 and Yalom (1975), Loomis (1979), and Marram (1978). Groups may either be the sole care strategy or part of an overall treatment plan. It is important for the care provider to be aware of community service agencies and also to contact such groups as community health nurses to learn the type and availability of groups in the community.

TABLE 24–6. TYPES OF GROUPS FOR DEPRESSED WOMEN

Therapy groups: Usually aimed toward improvement of insight so as to begin behavior change. Can use various theories for approaches.

Crisis groups: Usually short-term issue oriented, e.g., divorce, loss, death, rape.

Assertive training groups: Usually short term; skill development.

Work/task groups: Can be a group of mothers who organize to share responsibilities.

Didactic: This type of group presents fixed content such as prevention of depression by a group leader.

Self-help groups: Usually issue related, e.g., stress management, widows groups, parenting groups, parents of SIDS.

Networking groups: Can be business, professional, social, or political such as women's action groups for equal rights.

Self-awareness groups: These usually assist in development of interpersonal strengths.

Summary

Overall, for various reasons women seek more assistance for depression than men. The various stages of the life cycle from adolescence to old age require the use of different approaches. Scarf (1980), in her research on women and depression, noted the relatively systematic themes and issues of depressed women consistent with the various life cycle stages. Depression at any stage may make adaptation and coping difficult, and also effects the individual's total picture of herself both physically and psychologically. Growth and a sense of well-being cannot flourish in the face of depression. Health care providers need to be cognizant of the very early signs of depression as well as ways to prevent depression through individual and group strategies. The strategies suggested in this chapter focus specifically on depression but there are many other ways in which prevention of depression can be accomplished through general health information, client participation in definition of attainable health and personal goals, care providers' support to develop necessary health maintenance skills, and direct specific strategies. Currently, health care providers have the necessary tools to work toward assisting women in the development of a satisfying mental health status based on women's unique needs.

BIBLIOGRAPHY

Abraham, K. *Notes on the psychoanalytic treatment of manic–depressive insanity and allied conditions*. Selected papers on psychoanalysis. New York: Basic Books, 1960 (original 1911).

Adler, K. A. Depression in the light of individual psychology. *Journal of Individual Psychology*, 1961, *17*, 56–67.

Alberti, R. E., & Emmons, M. L. *Your perfect right: A guide to assertive behavior* (2nd ed.). San Luis Obispo, Calif.: Impact, 1974.

Areti, S., & Bemporad, J. R. The psychologial organization of depression. *American Journal of Psychiatry*. 1980, *11*(137), 1360–1365.

Areti, S., & Bemporad, J. R. *Severe and mild depression*. New York: Basic Books, 1978.

Bardwick, J. M., & Douvan, E. Ambivalence: The socialization of women. In V. Giernick & B. K. Moran (Eds.), *Women in sexist society*. New York: Basic Books, 1972.

Beck, A. T. *Cognitive therapy and the emotional disorders*. New York: International Universities Press, 1976.

Beck, A. T. The development of depression: A cognitive model. In R. Friedman & M. Katz (Eds.), *Psychology of depression: Contemporary theory and research*. Washington, D. C.: Winston-Wiley, 1974.

Beck, A. T. Etiologies of depression: The analytic spectrum. In D. Hill & L. E. Hollisters (Eds.), *Depression*. New York: Medom, 1970, pp. 17–20.

Beck, A. T., & Breenberg, R. Cognitive therapy with depressed women. In V. Franks & V. Burtle (Eds.), *Women in therapy*. New York: Brunner/Mazel, 1974.

Beck, A. T., & Breenberg, R. Cognitive therapy with depressed women. In V. Franks & V. Burtle (Eds.), *Depression*. New York: Medom, 1970.

Bem, S. L. The measurement of psychological androgyny. *Journal of Consulting and Clinical Psychology*, 1974, *2*(42), 155–162.

Bibring, E. The mechanism of depression. In P. Grunacre (Ed.), *Affective disorders*. New York: International Universities Press, 1953.

Bloom, L., Coburn, K., & Pearlman, J. *The new assertive woman*. New York: Dell, 1975.

Bonime, W. The psychodynamics of neurotic depression. *Journal of American Acadamy of Psychoanalysis*, 1976, *4*, 301–326.

Broverman, I. K., Broverman, D. M., Clarkson, F. E., Rosenkrantz, P. S., & Vogel, S. R. Sex-role stereotypes and clinical judgments of mental health. *Journal of Consulting and Clinical Psychology*, 1970, *34*(1), 1–7.

Burns, D. D. *Feeling good: The new mood therapy*. New York: Signet Books, 1980.

Caplan, G. *The theory and practice of mental health consultation*. New York, Basic Books, 1970.

Chesler, P. *Women and madness*. New York: Doubleday, 1972.

Chadoff, P. The care problem in depression. In J. Masserman (Ed.), *Science and psychoanalysis*. New York: Grune & Stratton, 1970, p. 17.

DeRosis, H. A., & Pellegrino, V. Y. *The book of hope: How women can overcome depression*. New York: Macmillan, 1976.

Franks, V., & Burtle, V. (Eds.). *Women in therapy: New psychotherapies*. New York: Brunner/Mazel, 1974.

Freud, S. *Mourning and melancholia* (Standard ed.). London: Hagarth Press, 1957, (original 1917).

Gergen, K. J., & Marecek, J. *The psychology of self-esteem*. Morristown, N.J.: General Learning Press, 1976.

Gilligan, C. *In a different voice*. Cambridge, Mass.: Harvard University Press, 1982.

Horner, M. S. Feminity and successful achievement: A basic in consistency. In J. M. Bardwick, E. Douvan, M.S. Horner, & D. Guttman, (Eds.), *Feminine personality and conflict*. Belmont, Calif.: Brooks/Cole, 1970.

Jacobson, E. The self and the object world. *Psychoanalytic Study of the Child*, 1954, 9, 75–84.

Jakubowski, P. Self-assertive training procedures for women. In E. Rawlings & A. D. Carter (Eds.), *Psychotherapy for women: Treatment toward equality*. Springfield, Ill.: C. C. Thomas, 1977.

Kety, S. S., Rosenthal, D., Wender, P. H., Schulsinger, F., & Jacobsea, B. Mental illness in the biological and adaptive families of adopted individuals who have become schizophrenic: A preliminary report based on psychiatric interviews. In R. R. Fieve, D. Rosenthal, & H. Brill (Eds.), *Genetic research in psychiatry*. Baltimore, Md.: Johns Hopkins University Press, 1975.

Kiev, A. *Somatic manifestations of depressive disorders*. New York: Elsevier, 1974.

Klerman, G. L., & Barrett, J. E. The affective disorders: Clinical and epidemiological aspects. In S. Gershorn & B. Shopsin (Eds.), *Lithium: Its role in psychiatric research and treatment*. New York: Plenum, 1973.

Klerman, G. L., & Weissman, M. M. Depressions among women: Their nature and causes. In M. Guttentag, S. Salasin, & D. Belle (Eds.), *The mental health of women*. New York: Academic Press, 1980.

Klerman, G. L., DiMascio, A., Weissman, M. M., Prusoff, B. A., & Paykel, E. S. Treatment of depression by drugs and psychotherapy. *American Journal of Psychiatry*, 1974, *131*, 186–191.

Lindhan, M. M., & Egan, K. J. Assertion training for women. In A. S. Bellack & M. Hersen (Eds.), *Research and practice in social skills training*. New York: Plenum Press, 1979.

Loomis, M. E. *Group process for nurses*. St. Louis, Mo.: C. V. Mosby, 1979.

Maccoby, E. E., & Jacklin, C. N. *The psychology of sex differences*. Stanford, Calif.: Stanford University Press, 1974.

Marecek, J. Psychological disorders in women: Indices of role strain. In I. H. Frieze, J. E. Parsons, P. B. Johnson, D. N. Ruble, & G. L. Zellman (Eds.), *Women and sex roles*. New York: W. W. Norton, 1978.

Marram, G. D. *The group approach in nursing practice* (2nd ed.). St. Louis, Mo.: C. V. Mosby, 1978.

Masling, J., & Harris, S. Sexual aspects of TAT administration. *Journal of Consulting Clinical Psychology*, 1969, *33*, 166–169.

Mendel, J. *Concepts of depression*. New York: Wiley, 1970.

Miller, J. B. *Toward a new psychology of women*. Boston: Beacon Press, 1976.

Miller, W. R., & Seligman, M. E. Depression and the perception of reinforcement. *Journal Abnormal Psychology*, 1973, *82*, 62–73.

National Institute of Mental Health, Department of Health, Education and Welfare, Division of Biometry and Epidemiology (Mental Health Statistical Notes, No. 137 & 138). Washington, D. C.: U.S. Government Printing Office, August, 1977.

Paykel, E. S., Myers, J. K., Dienelt, M. N., Lerman, G. L., Lindenthal, J. J., & Pepper, M P. Life events and depression: A controlled study. *Archives of General Psychiatry*, 1969, *21*, 753–760.

Radloff, L. S. Risk factors for depression: What do we learn from them? In M. Guttentag, S. Salasin, & D. Belle (Eds.), *The mental health of women*. New York: Academic Press, 1980.

Rush, A. J. *Short term psychotherapy for depression*. New York: Guilford Press, 1982.

Sandler, J., & Jaffe, W. G. Notes on childhood depression. *International Journal of Psychoanalysis*, 1965, *46*, 88–96.

Scarf, M. *Unfinished business*. New York: Ballantine Books, 1980.

Seligman, M. E. P. A learned helplessness point of view. In L. P. Rehm (Ed.), *Behavior therapy for depression: Present status and future directions*. New York: Academic Press, 1981.

Seligman, M. E. P. Depression and learned helplessness. In R. J. Griedman & M. M. Katz (Eds.), *The psychology of depression: Contemporary theory and research*. Washington, D.C.: Winston & Sons, 1974.

Seligman, M. E. P., & Maier, S. Failure to escape traumatic shock. *Journal of Experimental Psychology*, 1967, *74*, 1–12.

Swanson, A. R. Depression. In J. Haber, A. M. Leach, S. M. Schudy, & B. F. Sidelean (Eds.), *Comprehensive psychiatric nursing* (2nd ed.). New York: McGraw-Hill, 1982.

Thornton, J. W., & Jacobs, P. D. Learned helplessness in human subjects. *Journal Experimental Psychology*, 1981, *87*, 367–377.

Tolor, A. Kelly, B. R., & Stebbins, C. A. Assertiveness, sex-role stereotyping and self-concept. *Journal of Psychology*, 1976, *93*, 571–664.

Weissman, M. M., Klerman, G. L., Paykel, E. W., Prusoff, B. A., & Hanson, B. Treatment effects on the social adjustment of depressed patients. *Archives of General Psychiatry*, 1974, *30*, 771–778.

Weissman, M. M., & Paykel, E. S. *The depressed women: A study of social relationships*. Chicago: University of Chicago Press, 1974.

Wolpe, J. *Psychotherapy by reciprocal inhibition*. Stanford, Calif.: Stanford University Press, 1958.

Woolf, V. *A room of one's own*. New York: Harcourt, Brace & World, 1929.

Yalom, I. *The theory and practice of group psychotherapy*. New York: Basic Books, 1975.

Anxiety Disorders: Identification, Treatment, and Prevention

25

Theresa A. Caffery and Laurence B. Guttmacher

Anxiety is an ubiquitous problem of living. The psychological and physical signs of anxiety are experienced when an individual perceives a threat to her physical or psychological well-being. Mild to moderate amounts of anxiety are normal and may be beneficial when confronting a new or stressful event. These feelings alert the individual to danger and mobilize coping and adaptive responses to the stressful event, thereby decreasing distress. Some individuals experience overwhelming feelings of anxiety, however, that can incapacitate, immobilize, and lead to maladaptive responses and anxiety disorders.

Anxiety disorders are common. Zung (1980) estimated a 9 percent prevalence of anxiety states in the normal population and a 32 percent prevalence for individuals who seek medical treatment in family practice settings. One only has to observe that in 1979, 50 million prescriptions were written for anxiolytic agents in the United States to realize the scope of the problem (Cooperstock & Parnell, 1982; Hollister, 1978; Institute of Medicine, 1979).

The purpose of this chapter is to assist health care professionals to educate women about anxiety disorders, to recognize when women are experiencing anxiety, and to identify various options for the treatment of anxiety. We will be discussing generalized anxiety disorders and to a lesser extent panic disorder. The diagnostic criteria as noted in the *Diagnostic and Statistical Manual,* 3rd edition (DSM III) of the American Psychiatric Association are listed in Tables 25–1 and 25–2.

When an individual perceives a threat, anxiety occurs, triggering somatic and visceral responses through the autonomic nervous system and the hypothalmic–pituitary–endocrine system (Rickels, 1980). Anxiety represents a symptom cluster with diverse central and peripheral manifestations, including motor tension, autonomic hyperactivity, apprehension, and hypervigilance. It is based upon the anticipation of danger and is, therefore, future-oriented. The perceived danger may be either internal or external (Guttmacher, Murphy, & Insel, 1983). Anxiety may also represent a response to unconscious forces from the individual's past. It may be triggered by seemingly innocent events that reawaken old unresolved conflicts. The pathophysiology of anxiety is not clear and it is not understood how individuals differ in their subjective experience and regulation of anxiety (Schweitzer & Adams, 1979).

An individual's particular symptomatology is characteristic and consistent over time and reflects, in its manifest content, the operation of many interacting factors. "These

TABLE 25–1. DSM-III: DIAGNOSTIC CRITERIA FOR GENERALIZED ANXIETY DISORDER

A. Generalized, persistent anxiety is manifested by symptoms from the following four categories:
  1. Motor tension; shakiness, jitterness, jumpiness, trembling, tension, muscle aches, fatigability, inability to relax, eyelid twitch, furrowed brow, strained face, fidgeting, restlessness, easily startled.
  2. Autonomic hyperactivity, sweating, heart pounding or running, cold clammy hands, dry mouth, dizziness, light-headedness, paresthesia (tingling in hands or feet), upset stomach, hot or cold spells, frequent urination, diarrhea, discomfort in the pit of the stomach, lumps in the throat, flushing pallor, high resting pulse and respiration rate.
  3. Apprehensive expectation, anxiety, worry, fear, rumination, and anticipation of misfortune to self or others.
  4. Vigilance and scanning, hyperattentiveness resulting in distractability, difficulty in concentrating, insomnia, feeling "on edge," irritability, impatience.

(Source: American Psychiatric Association. Diagnostic and statistical manual of mental disorders (3rd ed.). Washington, D.C.: APA, 1980, p. 233, by permission.)

include physiological diathesis, early emotional experiences, and social or cultural norms characteristic for that individual. Thus the expression of anxiety is the result of several forces and will differ from individual to individual according to age, sex, socioeconomic status, and culture" (Schweitzer & Adams, 1979, pp. 32–34).

Any discussion of anxiety is reminiscent of Alice's discussion with Humpty Dumpty. " 'That's a great deal to make one word mean,' Alice said in a thoughtful tone. 'When I make a word do a lot of work like that,' said Humpty Dumpty, 'I always pay it extra.' " Zung (1979, 1980) has suggested that the assessment of anxiety is made difficult by the vagueness of the term. Anxiety as a term has been used to describe a dysphoric affect, an etiology, a drive, a situational response, a personality trait, and an emotional disorder.

Treatment of anxiety would be made far easier if we had some understanding of the pathophysiology of the disorder. All too often, commentators on anxiety write from their own positions of bias. We shall present some of the theories of how anxiety evolves and discuss various treatment approaches.

TABLE 25–2. DSM-III: DIAGNOSTIC CRITERIA FOR PANIC DISORDER

A. At least three panic attacks within a 3-week period in circumstances other than during marked physical exertion or in a life-threatening situation. The attacks are not precipitated only by exposure to a circumscribed phobic stimulus.

B. Panic attacks are manifested by discrete periods of apprehension or fear, and at least four of the following symptoms appear during each attack:

  1. Dyspnea
  2. Palpitations
  3. Chest pain or discomfort
  4. Choking or smothering sensations
  5. Dizziness, vertigo, or unsteady feelings
  6. Feelings of unreality
  7. Paresthesias (tingling in hands or feet)
  8. Hot and cold flashes
  9. Sweating
  10. Faintness
  11. Trembling or shaking

(Source: American Psychiatric Association. Diagnostic and statistical manual of mental disorders (3rd ed.). Washington, D.C.: APA, 1980, p. 231, by permission.)

Psychological Theories of Anxiety

Psychoanalytical Theory. Freud's original theory of dammed libidinal energy emerging as anxiety went through several significant revisions before his death. Since that time elaborate psychoanalytical theories have been developed to explain the meaning of anxiety. These theories are unproven, but health care providers need an understanding of these theories because they are widely accepted by professionals and lay people. Modern psychodynamicists argue that the ego (that rational part of the mental apparatus that mediates with the outside world) reacts to unacceptable impulses, feelings, or thoughts nearing consciousness with anxiety. This represents the concept of signal anxiety, a dysphoric affect that is sufficiently unpleasant as to cause avoidance of the stressor. The individual responds by rallying her most effective defense mechanisms (Nemiah, 1981).

According to psychodynamic theory any unconscious impulse that has been associated with the threat of disapproval, punishment, or retaliation would be perceived as dangerous or unacceptable on a conscious level. The appraisal of the relative danger of expressing an unconscious impulse may be supported by realistic considerations or may be entirely based on childlike or irrational thoughts regarding the anticipated response of others. This assessment of the risk of expressing an impulse is not a conscious or deliberate activity but rather an automatic, unconscious judgment (White & Gilland, 1975). When unacceptable near conscious awareness anxiety is experienced, defense mechanisms are utilized to prevent expression. White and Gilland (1975, p. 3) define "defense mechanisms as the various automatic, involuntary and unconsciously instituted psychological activities by which human beings attempt to exclude unacceptable impulses from conscious awareness." When unacceptable impulses are successfully excluded from conscious awareness, they are no longer threatening and anxiety diminishes. Preventing an unacceptable impulse from reaching conscious awareness, however, does not lessen or destroy the impulse. Instead considerable psychic energy must be employed to prevent the impulse from resurfacing and generating future anxiety.

Raskin and colleagues (1982) observed a high incidence of early separation and separation disorders of childhood in anxious adult patients. Patients diagnosed with panic disorders had a significantly higher incidence of grossly disturbed childhood environments.

Behavioral and Cognitive Models. Unlike personality or psychodynamic theories that describe psychological disturbance as a reflection of a maladaptive mental apparatus, behaviorists pay no attention to intrapsychic conflict or early childhood experiences in the formation of symptoms. Behaviorists view anxiety as an inappropriate response to stimuli that are threatening and are experienced as symptoms of physiological arousal.

Cognitive Therapy. Cognitive therapists have emphasized the importance of thought patterns in influencing emotions and behaviors. Epstein (1983, p. 55) describes this interaction stating that "human emotions and impulses are almost invariably mediated by cognitions, often in the form of a chain of verbal responses or images that can alleviate or retard the development of an emotion or impulse." Epstein (1983, p. 55) further observed "that individuals are usually unaware that their perceptions of an event is what generates the emotional response. Instead, individuals tend to attribute the events as the stressor and experience uncomfortable feelings of helplessness, loss of control and anxiety."

Beck, Laude, and Bohnert (1974) have observed that anxious patients have a constant pattern of thoughts and fantasies typically anticipating physical harm and public humiliation or ostracism. Beck (1976) described anxiety disorders as an overactive alarm system; the patient is so sensitive to the possibility of harm that she constantly worries about harm and is unable to realistically appraise the potential for danger in new situations.

Anxious individuals fixate on the signal (fear) and develop irrational fearful thoughts that they are unable to reason with, causing maladaptive coping responses. These thoughts may in turn be followed by stimulus generalization such that there are an ever increasing number of anxiety provoking stimuli. Beck, Laude, and Bohnert (1974) and Ellis and Harper (1977) believe that helping anxious patients examine the reality of these thoughts and teaching them to more realistically appraise the dangerousness of situations mobilizes more effective coping and alleviates anxiety.

Biological Theories of Anxiety. Family studies of anxious individuals provide inferential evidence of a genetic predisposition to anxiety. Cohen (1951) observed that when one parent was affected, 37.7 percent of the children also experienced anxiety and when both parents were anxious the percentage of children affected was 61.9 percent. Other family studies indicate a strong genetic component. Interviews with families of individuals with panic disorders reveal a 41 percent concordance rate for this disorder. This is as high a concordance rate as any in the psychiatric literature. Interestingly, there was not an unusually high incidence of generalized anxiety disorders among problem families, suggesting that they have different genetic backgrounds (Crowe et al., 1980).

The implications of the genetic data are important for the health care provider because they suggest that whenever one member of a family is anxious, other family members may be at risk to develop anxiety disorders. Schweitzer and Adams (1979) have suggested that early intervention to the anxious individual may prevent morbidity in other family members, especially children. Early recognition, stress management, and environmental change are suggested strategies to reduce tension in these families.

The recent discovery of the benzodiazepine receptors has greatly assisted our understanding of the biology of anxiety (Tallman et al., 1980). Benzodiazepines are highly effective treatment for many of the signs and symptoms associated with anxiety (Rickles, 1980). They seem to exert their effect through binding on to a specific macromolecular receptor, which also interacts with a neurotransmitter, gamma-aminobutyric acid (GABA). Differences between individuals in the number and sensitivity of benzodiazepine receptors have been posited to explain differing vulnerabilities to stress.

Further support for differing biological vulnerability to anxiety is provided by the lactate infusion model (Guttmacher, Murphy, & Insel, 1983). Intravenous sodium lactate when given rapidly to patients with panic disorder will precipitate a panic attack, but similar effects are not noted with normal controls.

It is clear, then, from these various sources of data that some people are at higher risk than others for the development of anxiety. The best marker for this high-risk group is a past history of anxiety or anxiety avoiding behavior (e.g., substance abuse). The astute health care provider will also obtain a careful family history to identify high-risk patients who would warrant extra intervention.

WOMEN AND ANXIETY

A review of the psychiatric and sociological literature suggests that women are at increased risk of being diagnosed and treated for psychiatric illness. Studies of anxiety disorders reveal an increased incidence among women (Dohrenwend, Neugebauer, &

Dohrenwend, 1980). Women are more likely to be diagnosed with anxiety disorders whereas men are more often treated for personality disorders and alcoholism (Howell, 1981).

Several theories have been advanced to explain women's supposed vulnerability to psychopathology. Behaviorists have postulated that women experience greater anxiety and depression because of their sex role characteristics. According to Wolfe (1979, pp. 196–197) "women are taught to inhibit aggression, to be passive, and to maintain emotional responsiveness to others, thus denying their own needs. Commonly, women encounter a double bind of either accepting the prescribed passive stereotypical roles and getting little satisfaction for themselves or asserting themselves and experiencing further rejections by not living up to others' expectations." When women's behavior deviates, they often experience feelings of anxiety, guilt, and depression.

Role theory has been a popular explanation for psychopathology in women. Role theorists postulate that women experience increased rates of psychiatric illness secondary to assuming lower status and ascribed roles that provide fewer options for behavioral expression (Marecek, 1978; Moulton, 1977).

There is little disagreement that the women's movement has brought about an increased awareness of the discrimination inherent in women's status. What is less clear is whether this awareness has created new opportunities or appreciably changed the average woman's status.

Although there is the illusion of more career and educational opportunities that have been traditionally assigned to men, many women lack the necessary resources and opportunities to acquire new skills. When women attain higher status jobs, they continue to earn less money than their male colleagues (Oakley, 1974; Rapoport & Rapoport, 1976). This apparent opportunity when combined with limited success can give rise to cognitive dissonance and may contribute toward anxiety and depression.

Role change is stressful and may produce anxiety, conflict, and dissonance with other concurrent roles. Most women have been programmed throughout life to avoid competition and conflict. As one female attorney related, "I don't know how to compete against a middle-aged male attorney. Nothing has prepared me for what it would be like."

As women change their priorities and attempt new behaviors, other concurrent roles will be altered. Support from their partners may be threatened. Research has indicated that although more women are working, they are still expected to provide the majority of household and child care services. Failure to adequately perform these expected roles has been identified as a major cause of marital stress in dual career relationships (Rapoport & Rapoport, 1976).

Other sources of potential stress for women are the unique biological events of menarche, pregnancy, childbirth, and menopause. Our society values women capable of producing children, and failure to exercise one's reproductive potential is still frequently considered a rejection of femininity and deviant. All of these normal biological events have been identified as transitional stages that may produce anxiety and place women at risk of psychiatric illness. These events may not just be experienced as anxiety at the time they first occur, but may also be reexperienced with further reproductive milestones.

Finally, anxiety and depression may serve a homeostatic function in our society because these traits or experiences lend credence to the idea that women should be maintained at the status quo and not given equal rights because they are incapable of demonstrating competence secondary to their hormones or emotionality.

Although many studies (Gove & Tudor 1973; Greenly & Mechanic, 1976; Lewis & Lewis, 1977) have reported increased rates of psychiatric illness in women and theories have been advanced to explain these observations, major methodological flaws exist in regard to the research design and the criteria for determining psychiatric illness.

The true incidence and prevalance of psychiatric disorders is unknown and most of the available information concerns only women who present for treatment. These data underrepresent the true prevalence of psychopathology. The alternative approach is to do a community-based study interviewing random samples of the general population.

Epidemiological studies based on identified patients also have the problem that the decision to seek treatment is made on subjective and personal grounds. Individuals vary on what they consider a psychological problem and whether they believe that discussing their problems is useful. Although more women request psychiatric treatment, it is unclear whether this is a reflection of higher rates of psychiatric problems or a reflection of socialization in that women are encouraged to talk about their problems.

Lack of diagnostic specificity has been a problem. This problem has been somewhat ameliorated by the specificity afforded by DSM III. Diagnostic standards may also be applied in a different fashion as a function of race, sex, and social class (Adebimpe, 1981). Future research needs to be done to clarify whether women are, in fact, at increased risk for mental illness, what factors interact to produce this disturbance, and what measures are effective for the prevention of illness.

Assessment of Anxiety

Women with anxiety often present to non-psychiatric health care providers for treatment. Brown (1979) estimated that 70 percent of the patients that experience psychiatric symptoms seek treatment from a nonpsychiatric practitioner and that approximately 32 percent of these patients experience anxiety disorders.

Clients typically complain of "nervousness" or "tension." These complaints may be the final common pathway for a wide variety of disorders. They most typically reflect underlying fear, anger, or anxiety. Catastrophic illnesses, medical disorders, and various chronic illnesses may mimic a primary anxiety disorder. Thus, the assessment of anxiety may be difficult and time consuming. Anxiety reactions vary from individual to individual and may be expressed differently by the same individual at different times. Frequently, women present with physical complaints. This occurs because the somatic stigmata of anxiety are more easily identified than the underlying effect, and physical illnesses are more socially acceptable than emotional illnesses.

Techniques useful in assessing anxiety include:

1. Providing a supportive environment for the individual to freely discuss her concerns.
2. Utilizing an open-ended interview format that allows the patient to describe symptoms, the circumstances present at the onset, when symptoms reoccur, the methods the patient has utilized to alleviate distress, as well as the patient's thoughts about the meaning of the symptoms.
3. Exploring the stressful events in the patient's life. Common stressors for women are problems balancing the multiplicity of roles of worker, lover, and mother. Contraceptive use with worries about side effects and delaying childbirth for a career may be stressful as well. Utilizing a developmental framework or knowledge of stressors throughout the life cycle can alert the practitioner to potential areas of stress. Again, the area is often best explored utilizing open-ended questions such as "How is work? How are your children?"
4. Collecting a past medical history and review of systems to identify other health

problems. A drug history is especially important as some medications precipitate an anxiety response and patients may self-medicate themselves with a variety of pharmacological agents, including alcohol.

5. Completing a physical examination and performance of laboratory work based on physical findings.

Differential Diagnosis. A wide variety of physical disorders can present with anxiety. Symptoms of anxiety may represent a variety of physical disorders or may reflect a response to a chronic illness. Schuckit (1983) has reported that physical causes of anxiety, separate from the patient's psychological reaction, are seen in 10 to 40 percent of patients presenting to nonpsychiatric practitioners with anxiety or depression (Table 25–3).

The most common physical disorders that present with anxiety would probably include hyperthyroidism, arrhythmia, withdrawal syndromes, and the use or misuse of certain medications (Table 25–4).

Anxiety is also a common feature of some primary psychiatric disturbances. Differential diagnosis includes:

1. Transient situational disturbances that result from maladaptation to stressful life events.
2. Character disturbances in individuals often resulting in chronic anxiety secondary to their inability to successfully adapt to stress.
3. Psychotic disturbances may be associated with anxiety and panic, particularly as patients experience decompensation, increased disorganization, or a relapse of their illness.
4. Withdrawal from alcohol or other CNS depressants may have anxiety as a prominent symptom early in the process.

As is obvious, some of the difficulty in determining the best treatment for the symptoms of anxiety can be minimized by remembering that what we call anxiety is a "set of symptoms, not a diagnosis; effective therapy is aimed at treating the underlying

TABLE 25–3. ORGANIC CAUSES OF ANXIETY SYMPTOMS

Organic Basis	Anxiety Symptoms
Cardiovascular	Angina pectoris, arrhythmia, congestive heart failure, myocardial infarction, syncope (multiple causes), valvular disease, i.e., mitral valve prolapse, vascular collapse
Dietary	Caffeinism, monosodium glutamate, tyramine containing food and monoamine oxidase inhibitors, vitamin deficiency disease
Drug-related	Akathesia, anticholinergic toxicity, digitalis toxicity, withdrawal syndrome
Hematologic	Anemias
Immunologic	Anaphylaxis, systemic lupus erythematosis
Metabolic	Cushing's disease, hypercalcemia, hyperkalemia, hyperthermia, hyperthyroidism, hypocalcemic menopausal symptoms, porphyria, thyrotoxicosis
Neurologic	Encephalopathies (infectious, metabolic and toxic), essential tremor, intracranial mass lesions, postconcussion syndrome, seizure disorders (especially temporal lobe), vertigo
Respiratory	Asthma, chronic obstructive pulmonary disease, pneumonia, pneumothorax, pulmonary edema, pulmonary embolus
Secreting tumors	Carcinoid, insulinoma, pheochromocytoma

(Source: Rosenbaum, J. Anxiety. In A. Lazarre (Ed.), Outpatient psychiatry: Diagnosis and treatment. *Baltimore, Md.: Williams & Wilkins, 1979, pp. 252–256, by permission.)*

TABLE 25–4. DRUGS THAT MAY CAUSE SYMPTOMS OF ANXIETY

Class	Example
Anticholinergic	Cogentin, Artane
Antihistamine	Ornade, Actifed, Benadryl
Antipsychotic	Thorazine, Haldol, Mellaril
Benzodiazepine	Valium
Caffeine	Over the counter decongestants and analgesics
Cardiovascular agents	Epinephrine
Central nervous system stimulants	Amphetamines
Corticosteroids	Cortisone
Drug withdrawal	Alcohol, narcotics, beta-blockers, barbiturate withdrawal
Monoamine oxidase inhibitors (MAOIs)	Parnate, Nardil
Beta-blockers	Inderal
Sympathomimetics Bronchodilators, decongestants, tocolytic	Theophylline, Brethine, Vasodilan, Sudafed, Yutopar

(Source: Adapted from Erman, M., & Guggenheim, F. Psychiatric side effects of commonly used drugs. Drug Therapy, 1981, 6(11), pp. 55–64.)

cause and problems rather than merely responding to the symptoms. The correct diagnosis is paramount in treatment planning, because there are various treatment options and what works well for one anxiety disorder may not work well for another" (Shader & Greenblatt, 1983, p. 22).

Learning to Cope with Anxiety

Many women learn about anxiety only after experiencing the troublesome signs and symptoms of this normal emotional response. Learning in this fashion is negative and problematic as the cognitive and behavioral concomitants of anxiety disorders are known to inhibit an individual's learning abilities.

Anxiety disorders and panic attacks represent a major health problem for women. Studies concerning anxiety disorders and panic attacks indicate that women develop these disorders two to three times more frequently than men and are the major users of anxiolytic drugs (Cooperstock, 1978).

Although anxious feelings are a normal response to novel or stressful events, there has been little formal effort expended in teaching women how to cope with anxiety. As a society we have exerted limited effort to prepare individuals with the skills to cope with psychological feelings. This lack of preparation to cope with feelings may be due to the fact that our society (1) values self-reliance and (2) interprets the expression of negative or uncomfortable feelings as a sign of weakness.

A review of the literature on the theory and treatment of anxiety suggests that learning plays a crucial role in individual responses to stressors, formation of anxiety symptoms, and the treatment of anxiety disorders. Further evidence is offered in the studies of prepared childbirth education in which many investigators observed that women who receive education about labor and delivery were observed to be less anxious and had lower rates of analgesic use than women who did not attend childbirth education class. Caplan (1976) and others have suggested that educational intervention, such as anticipatory guidance and self-help groups, enhances coping responses to stressful events. Future research is necessary to determine whether education prevents anxiety disorders.

Learning how to adapt to stressors prior to experiencing the negative effects of anxiety may be beneficial. Education about anxiety should include a definition of anxiety, a description of the symptoms, how to recognize and cope with anxious feelings, and guidelines to help individuals determine whether professional help is needed.

The process of education may use an individual or a group format. Refer to Chapters 2 and 3 for an excellent discussion of the principles of adult learning and various educational modalities.

Content should include a discussion that (1) anxiety is a normal emotional response to a stressful event, and (2) that anxiety may be understood as a positive feeling state as it alerts the individual of an internal or external threat. Individuals also need to appreciate that it is not the feeling per se but the degree and patients' response to the threat that cause difficulties. Use of parables help the patient appreciate the universality of this response and may help her identify events that precipitate anxiety in her ecology.

As many women do not understand the role of emotions in the formation of symptoms, a review of the signs and symptoms of anxiety and a simple explanation of the pathophysiology of the symptom often alleviates stress. The ability to recognize and understand that their symptoms occur as a result of anxiety often alleviates fear and facilitates understanding.

Once patients gain understanding and are able to place their signs and symptoms in perspective, new coping mechanisms need to be learned. Coping mechanisms involve a variety of operations that patients use to alleviate stress. Health maintenance is extremely important for the individual to cope with anxiety. Education about proper nutrition, exercise, and the need to plan for leisure activity are essential to emotional health. Often under stress patients employ self-destructive behavior such as smoking, poor eating, and substance abuse to alleviate their distress. The behaviors are known to be detrimental to health and in themselves may produce anxiety.

Individuals need to learn an alternative behavior to cope with anxiety as it is an ever present reality of life. Relaxation by exercise, yoga, or meditation often alleviates tension that is associated with anxiety. Exploring the patients' life-styles helps them to recognize potential stressful events. Anticipatory guidance about what to expect in potentially stressful events fosters mastery and decreases the potential for anxiety responses. Social skill training helps patients develop more appropriate behaviors to cope with interpersonal stress and career stress. There are also many groups that women can join to learn how to cope with anxious feelings. Groups are helpful as they decrease isolation, provide support networks, and reinforce changing behaviors.

Finally, women need guidelines to determine when they should seek professional help. In general, when patients are so affected by their symptoms that they are unable to perform tasks of living or anxiety is not relieved by the above measures, professional help may be needed and psychiatric consultation should be considered appropriate. Providing information about resources in the community helps women to become active participants in their care.

Treatment of Anxiety

To recapitulate, anxiety may be a natural response to stressful life events. When present in a mild to moderate degree, it signals the individual of imminent danger and motivates her to mobilize defense mechanisms appropriate for adaptation and provides an opportunity for personal growth. Excessive anxiety, however, immobilizes individuals who often respond with ineffectual or inappropriate coping mechanisms that increase distress. Dennis and Hendrie (1980) have estimated that pathological anxiety is the most common of all psychiatric disorders, with the prevalence rate for lifelong anxiety neurosis approaching 5 percent.

Regardless of the etiology of the anxious feelings, individuals attempt to avoid or reduce their distress. Several factors influence how an individual responds to stressful events. These include the individual's genetic background, personality structure, previous experience with stressful events, other concurrent stressors, social support systems, and community and economic resources. When an individual is able to gain mastery over stress, anxiety is reduced and equilibrium is reestablished. If the individual is unable to adapt successfully, her anxiety increases. She may often employ maladaptive responses such as substance abuse, further increasing the anxiety. Often after an unsuccessful response to stress an individual may seek medical treatment for the physical symptoms of anxiety. She may have little or no insight as to the precipitants of the symptoms or to the relationship of anxiety to the formation of the experienced distress.

In the primary care setting, discriminating between normal and pathological anxiety may be difficult and require several patient visits before the distinction is clear. It is helpful to consider anxiety on a continuum and to identify whether these feelings interfere with the patient's daily living.

Although some patients will complain of the emotional symptoms, i.e., "bad nerves," "tension," or a "nervous breakdown," the majority of patients will complain of a variety of somatic symptoms. The preponderance of somatic complaints will often lead the health care provider to order a number of laboratory tests to discriminate among diseases that mimic anxiety reaction and to rule out an organic etiology. This testing is not only time-consuming and expensive, but may iatrogenically enhance the patient's stress. To further complicate the assessment, the cognitive changes that accompany anxiety disorders may inhibit the patient's ability to provide an accurate description of the symptoms, inhibit the patient–practitioner relationship, and interfere with the patient's ability to comply with and comprehend treatment.

Once the practitioner has determined that the patient's symptoms represent an anxiety disorder, this formulation must be shared with the patient and a treatment plan developed. Communication is the first step in the treatment of anxiety. The provision of realistic information about the nature of the symptoms, especially the physical concomitants, fosters intellectual mastery and effective coping.

According to Steinmuller (1978), the provision of concrete information that is as unambiguous as possible, often accompanied by drawing or written instructions, is very important. Communication of information and reassurance may need to be repetitive as anxiety alters cognitive function and limits an individual's ability to process and use information. The practitioner is in an excellent position to teach more effective communication skills and provide the patient with feedback about her communication style. Effective communication is necessary to enable the patient to become an active participant in her care.

Availability of the health care provider is extremely important as a means of support, reassurance, and problem solving. As cognitive changes interfere with the patient's ability to understand and learn new skills, the availability of the practitioner is extremely reassuring.

Education is important to modify individual perception and dysfunctional responses to stressors. Many individuals lack basic understanding of their physiological functioning, of means to maintain health, and an awareness of the adverse effects of stress on health.

Education about anxiety needs to include information about the pathophysiology, the recognition, the relief, and the prevention of anxiety disorders. The goals of education are to facilitate an individual's ability to recognize stress and adapt in a healthier manner when confronting future stressors.

As anxiety is involved in many patients' symptoms, the health care provider should determine the role of stress in the individual's symptom formation. A teaching plan must be developed based on the patient's insight, level of understanding, ability, and motivation to learn.

Often a detailed explanation of the role of anxiety in the formation of symptoms will alleviate distress. Selected written information is often helpful. Written information affords the patient an opportunity to review information that she may have been unable to understand during the office visit. More frequent follow-up, and the health care provider's availability to answer questions, is often helpful.

Clients can be taught to recognize stress and their response by keeping a diary or activity log in which they record daily events, their response, and what action was taken to alleviate distress. These logs can be reviewed to help women become more aware of what events are stressful and what activities alleviate their discomforts. Utilization of a public health nurse home visit is often valuable in assessment of the home to determine social supports, provide education, and reinforce adaptive behavior.

There are a variety of self-help educational and supportive groups available that alleviate anxiety (see Resources). Although these groups differ in their objectives, they share common curative features. Membership in a group decreases individual isolation, provides support, and an opportunity to learn alternate coping skills (see Chapter 3). Clients most likely to benefit from groups are those that recognize a problem, are motivated to change their behavior, and are not so compromised by their symptoms as to be unable to function in a group.

Groups vary in their focus. Educational groups such as parent effectiveness training, childbirth education, assertiveness training, and social skill groups operate on the notion that by education, anticipatory guidance, and support, anxiety responses are prevented. Other groups are designed to modify anxiety through changing the behavior or the attitude of their members. Examples of this form of group include Alcoholics Anonymous, Recovery for patients who have had mental illness or nervousness, and Parents Without Partners. Membership in these groups is dependent upon the patient admitting that she has a specific problem and having the motivation to work on that problem. Another evolving form of group focuses on a particular life crisis such as death, for example, or bereaved parents groups.

Some patients will be so compromised by their symptoms that they will not respond to educational interventions, reality testing, and supportive measures. In such cases consultation with a mental health specialist is appropriate. Mental health consultation provides evaluation, treatment, and referral for patients who require more intensive psychotherapy and psychopharmacological treatment. Mental health consultants can also be used for supervision by the health care practitioner once a decision is reached that the patient should receive treatment in the primary care setting. The need for mental health consultation services is dependent on the primary care provider's repertoire of skills, the availability of psychiatric consultation, and the patient's willingness to participate in the consultative process.

When consultation is indicated, it is critical that the primary health care practitioner explore the patient's feelings about the need for psychiatric consultation, provide education and guidance about the consultation process, and how it may be of use. Without education, patient resistance may be encountered as many anxious individuals do not recognize or acknowledge that psychological factors may be important in the formation of their symptoms. When appropriate, it is wise to counsel patients that psychiatric referral does not mean that they are "crazy." When patients are allowed to actively participate in their treatment a sense of responsibility is fostered and feelings of dependence and loss of control can be lessened.

The treatment goals for anxious patients regardless of the treatment model utilized are (1) to restore equilibrium and (2) to facilitate patient's learning of more adaptive coping mechanisms for future stress. Common treatment approaches for anxious patients are: (1) psychotherapy, (2) behavioral management, (3) psychopharmacological therapy, and (4) social engineering. None of these approaches are mutually exclusive and often it is beneficial to utilize an eclectic approach.

The selection of treatment for anxiety disorders is dependent on patient and health care provider factors. Patient factors that are important in selecting treatment modalities are the type of anxiety disorder, the level of distress, the client's personality, the client's personal and economic resources, the client's ability to tolerate insight, and the motivation. Health care provider factors are the individual's level of psychotherapeutic skill, their philosophy, the level of interest, and the availability to treat the client with anxiety disorders.

Psychotherapeutic Intervention. Psychodynamic psychotherapy, crisis intervention, and supportive therapy are three major psychotherapeutic interventions available. Although these therapies differ with regard to focus and technique, these models share common themes. According to Frank (1978), all therapies should offer a relationship with a practitioner who provides competence, caring, concern, empathy, compassion, and the opportunity for ventilation, clarification, and reassurance. The goals of psychodynamic psychotherapy are to relieve anxiety through the exploration and resolution of the patient's unconscious conflicts and to modify those aspects of the individual's personality structure that prevent her from realizing her full potential.

Psychodynamic theorists believe that anxiety is alleviated in two stages. First, the individual gains insight into the conflict, and second, the individual is able to consider and mobilize more appropriate defense mechanisms. Techniques used in psychodynamic psychotherapy are ventilation, interpretation, and free association to work through unresolved conflictual feelings, which then allow the patient to adapt more creatively.

Patients most likely to benefit from psychodynamic psychotherapy are intelligent, psychologically minded, highly motivated individuals, able to verbalize their feelings, tolerate interpretation, and not so impaired or psychotic as to be unable to form an effective relationship. This form of therapy is time consuming, expensive, and requires a high level of training so that general practitioners would need to refer the patient to a psychotherapist.

Crisis intervention therapy has been very effective in alleviating acute anxiety states. Each individual has a specific tolerance for stress, which is dependent on the general level of adjustment, the internal and external resources available to that person, and the degree and type of stress being experienced.

The primary focus of crisis intervention therapy is to resolve the presenting problem utilizing a combination of psychotherapy and problem-solving techniques. Crisis intervention usually involves a brief course of therapy. Past problems are not addressed and personality reconstruction is not attempted in this model; however, the patient may gain considerable insight and personal growth by successful resolution of the current crisis (Burgess & Baldwin, 1981).

Crisis intervention therapy is a useful treatment approach for anxiety disorders because it is short term, less costly than psychodynamic approaches, and patients do not need to meet the rigid selection criteria necessary for psychodynamic therapy. As this model incorporates problem-solving skills, support, education, and basic psychotherapeutic principles, it can often be utilized by the generalist. For an excellent review of crisis intervention theory and application of techniques, the reader is directed to the Burgess and Baldwin (1981) text.

Supportive therapy is an effective approach to anxiety. Although every model of psychotherapy utilizes an element of support, the amount of support conveyed differs. Supportive psychotherapy is aimed at helping clients consider life-style changes to decrease stress and identify more realistic life goals. Fiore (1979) suggests that supportive therapy also aids patients to recognize and better cope with any resistance to giving up the secondary gains acquired from their illness. In the supportive therapy model, the major activity of the therapist is to foster a strong positive relationship in which the patient feels strong support. The therapist utilizes this relationship to guide the patient to more adaptive problem-solving skills. Education, sympathetic listening, empathic understanding, and anticipatory guidance are utilized in this form of therapy to alleviate anxiety symptoms.

The therapist takes a much more active stance than in psychodynamic psychotherapy. No attempt is made to change the personality structure of the patient; instead the supportive therapist accepts the personality structure as is. The patient is actively supported in attempting new coping skills with positive reinforcement and guidance. Supportive therapy is the most common type of therapy utilized in medical settings and is easily mastered by health care practitioners. It is also a useful model because it can be helpful for all patients regardless of their level of functioning.

Behavioral and Cognitive Therapy. Relief of acute tension states and elimination of avoidance behavior is accomplished by the application of learning principles to modify specific identified maladaptive responses.

When utilizing a behavioral approach several assumptions are made. These are: (1) that all behaviors are a learned response to stimuli; (2) that behaviors are reinforced or extinguished by cultural and social factors; (3) that resolving past experiences or intrapsychic conflict is not necessary for behavioral change; and (4) that all behaviors are fluid and can be modified through education, skill training, modeling, and other behavioral techniques (Suinn & Deffendacher, 1980).

Behavioral therapies have distinct stages. Assessment of the current problem in behavioral terms occurs first, treatment goals are then formulated, and intervention strategies are delineated. Assessment is concrete and explicit. Treatment goals are defined as target behaviors. In designing a program to retrain the patient, the program specifies which techniques will be utilized to modify behavior and identifies the specific tasks of the therapist and the patient. The therapist and the patient contract to implement the plan. New adaptive responses are learned, practiced, and reinforced, and the patient is supported to transfer these new skills to current life situations. Evaluation of the treatment plan is accomplished by measuring outcomes of target behaviors.

Behavioral interventions attempt to educate an individual as to how to recognize stress and cope with stressful stimuli more effectively so as to prevent future anxiety disturbance. Common behavioral techniques used to treat anxiety disorders are desensitization, stress management, and cognitive therapy.

Systematic desensitization has been found effective for reducing anxiety associated with a specific stimulus, e.g., phobias. Phobics learn to associate anxiety with previously neutral situations. Patients attempt adaptation to these phobic stimuli by avoidance. Although avoidance behavior removes the individual from the fearful stimuli, it makes future exposure to the same stimuli more distressing.

According to Wilson and Lazarus (1978), the basic assumption behind desensitization procedures is that the fear evoked by subjectively threatening situations can be reduced by a guided and progressive exposure to a hierarchy of anxiety generating situations. Systematic desensitization is based on the assumption that a patient cannot experience the affect of anxiety if physically relaxed. Systematic desensitization is a three-step process:

1. The patient is instructed in relaxation training. Muscular relaxation can be effected by a deep muscle relaxation model (Bensen, 1975; Jacobson, 1938), hypnosis, biofeedback, meditation, or by medication.
2. Once the patient has been able to master relaxation techniques, the therapist and the patient develop a list of phobic stimuli ordering them from minimally to maximally feared.
3. Relaxation and phobic stimuli are paired through imagery and the patient is guided to visually experience fearful situations in a relaxed state (in vitro desensitization). Then the patient is able to transfer gradually relaxation techniques to stressful events outside the therapy session.

Other desensitization techniques include in vivo desensitization and implosion therapy. The former is quite similar to the technique described above, differing only in that the patient is assisted in going out into the world, gradually experiencing the feared stimuli on her hierarchy. Implosion differs in that the patient is told to experience the most feared item on the hierarchy first. This sink-or-swim approach is currently in some disfavor, both for ethical reasons and because of questionable outcomes.

Biofeedback techniques have been used to induce relaxation and reduce tension. Biofeedback techniques enable patients to attend to and to control autonomic signs of arousal. Biofeedback for anxiety disorders often uses skin temperature, information, and control. In general, anxiety disorders produce vasoconstriction, which patients are taught to recognize as skin temperature changes. Electromyographic biofeedback has also been used for anxiety disorders. This method provides the patient with a mechanism for recognizing muscle tension. Patients learn that anxiety is incompatible with muscular relaxation. In the area of inducing relaxation, biofeedback techniques are useful but have not been proven to be superior to the standard relaxation exercises. Furthermore, Holroyd (1979) has suggested that biofeedback and relaxation may be effective because these techniques indirectly induce patients to modify their environment rather than enabling patients to control problematic physiological responses. Relaxation training, through a standardized exercise program or by biofeedback, is an important intervention for anxiety disorders; however, it provides only one coping mechanism for tension relief.

A broader behavioral treatment approach to anxiety disorders is cognitive therapy. Cognitive therapy encompasses a set of operations employed to modify individual maladaptive feelings, thoughts, and behaviors by thought restructuring and behavioral manipulations. Cognitive therapy for anxiety disorders is based on the observation that patients who are anxious have common irrational, nonproductive thought patterns that prevent effective coping (Beck, 1976; Janis, 1983; Meichenbaum, 1983).

Cognitive interventions are based on changing an individual's perceptual processes. Janis (1971, 1983) and Meichenbaum (1983) have suggested that the provision of education and anticipatory guidance may modify an individual's response to an anticipated stressful event. Based on his work with prospective surgical patients, Janis (1971, 1983) has suggested three counseling procedures to prepare patients for stressful events. These include giving realistic information, which challenges the person's ignorance and denial, to reassure so as to make her able to confront her vulnerability, and to motivate her "to plan preparatory actions for dealing with subsequent crises." "Feelings of helplessness, hopelessness, and demoralization" are minimized by calling attention to the individual's personal and social coping mechanisms, thus enabling the patient to feel confident about surviving and recovering from the stressful event. Dress rehearsals are utilized, thus enabling the patient to work out strategies for coping (Janis, 1983, pp. 78–84). Janis postulates that newly learned coping skills can also be utilized to cope with future stressors.

Meichenbaum (1983, p. 151) has defined treatment goals to promote enhanced coping. These are:

1. To teach patients the role that cognitions and emotions play in the formation of a stress response.
2. To train patients to self-monitor and block nonproductive thoughts, feelings, and behaviors.
3. To train patients in the fundamentals of problem solving (how to identify a problem and consequences).
4. To model and practice coping mechanisms such as relaxation techniques, communication skills, and use of social supports to alleviate stress.
5. To give patients behavioral homework assignments to practice stress management.

In summary, behavioralists view anxiety as a natural consequence of selecting inappropriate responses to stressful situations. Faulty perceptions of an event, lack of behavioral skills, and avoidance of stressors have been identified as the precipitants of anxiety reactions. All behavioral interventions utilize learning theory to modify behavior.

Pharmacological Management of Anxiety Disorders. In 1979 50 million prescriptions were written in the United States for diazepam (Valium) (Cooperstock, 1982). This antianxiety agent was used by 7.5 percent of American men and 14.1 percent of the women. Fifteen percent of these anxiolytic users had taken anxiolytic drugs on a daily basis for the preceding year (Cooperstock, 1982; Mellinger & Butler, 1983). Fortunately, in the last decade there has been an encouraging trend of fewer prescriptions being written.

How do we account for the overwhelming popularity of these agents? Some part of their use may be explained by nonanxiolytic uses, because all are effective hypnotics, muscle relaxants, and anticonvulsants as well. Nonetheless, almost half of these prescriptions are written for anxiety. Clearly, the drugs must be perceived positively by a significant number of patients and physicians.

Acute anxiety is generally a self-limiting phenomenon. Because of this, a placebo or no treatment will be effective in 80 percent or more of patients (Rickels, 1980, 1983). The value of these drugs becomes apparent when discussing more chronic anxiety.

There are several problems with benzodiazepines. Patients may be less motivated to seek other, more long-term solutions. There is risk of withdrawal upon discontinuation. Withdrawal symptoms including increased anxiety, gastrointestinal complaints, and in more serious cases seizures can occur with prolonged use of normal doses (Lader, 1983). Because of these withdrawal phenomena, any patient on benzodiazepines for more than several months should have the medication tapered upon discontinuation.

It should be emphasized that use of anxiolytic medication should only be for a short time and viewed as an adjunct to other, more lasting forms of therapy. Continuous demands for benzodiazepines may be an indication for referral to a psychiatrist or specialist in substance abuse.

Risks with these drugs also include interaction and synergy with other CNS depressants, especially alcohol. Patients on benzodiazepines must be cautioned to severely limit alcohol intake. Use of these drugs during the first trimester of pregnancy is associated with the development of cleft lip and cleft palate in the fetus, so they should not be prescribed to reproductive-age women in the absence of effective contraception. Patients must also be warned about the risk of sedation when using these drugs.

Other drugs have been used in generalized anxiety disorders. Barbiturates pose the same risks as benzodiazepines, except that the withdrawal syndrome is far more serious and, unlike benzodiazepines, they are quite lethal when taken as an overdose. Beta-blockers, such as propranolol, have been widely used in Great Britain. The English distinguish between central and peripheral anxiety; the former representing the sense of dread and fear, the latter being the peripheral autonomic symptoms associated with anxiety. Beta-blockers are quite effective in muting the peripheral manifestations (Noyes, 1982).

The choice of medication is dependent on the patient's age, diagnosis, medical status, drug history, personality, and social context (Shader & Greenblatt, 1983). In general anxiolytics are taken for general anxiety disorders and mixed anxiety disorders, whereas antidepressants are more effective for panic disorders.

Psychosocial Prophylaxis. Individuals are continuously stressed by the complexities of modern life and are vulnerable to change, uncertainty, ambiguity, and interpersonal conflict. The stress generated from such events can be acute in nature but is usually episodic and recurrent in nature (Shader & Greenblatt, 1983).

Research has identified a number of factors that produce a vulnerability to stress. Poverty, crowded environments, hunger, lack of employment and education, and a lack of access to medical care produce stress and increased morbidity and mortality. Personal habits of smoking, overeating, alcohol, and recreational drug use are all known to cause increased risk for illness.

Epidemiological studies suggest that life events can be stressful and precipitate anxiety disorders. Common life events such as pregnancy, childbirth, divorce, single parenting, loss of a significant other, and geographic relocation have been associated with stress disorders. Increased morbidity has been associated with workers on jobs involving high levels of responsibility and interpersonal or role conflicts (Elliott & Eisdorfer, 1982; Hamburg, Elliott, & Parron, 1982).

Although it is now possible to predict risk populations vulnerable to increased morbidity, there has been a lack of preventive services to promote healthy adaptation to the common stressful life events.

Regardless of the practitioner's theoretical framework, the prevention of anxiety disorders is crucial to the promotion of health. At a basic level, whether anxiety is caused by psychodynamic factors, maladaptive behaviors, errors in cognition, or a neurochemical mechanism, anxiety is a learned response and intervention must focus on teaching patients more adaptive responses.

The goals of psychoprophylaxis are to decrease the psychological stress in a community and to increase individuals' personal and social resources. Because our environment may play a role in developing stress and anxiety related illness by presenting stressors and reinforcing maladaptive behaviors, intervention strategies must be developed to decrease environmental risk.

As our culture positively values individualism, competition, and self-reliance, there is a need for acceptance of stress as a normal part of life and to prepare individuals to adapt and cope creatively to prevent anxiety disorders. Although some individuals are overwhelmed and disabled by anxiety, not all individuals who experience stress become ill. Future research is necessary to determine why some individuals in similar circumstances develop anxiety disorders and others are able to cope effectively.

Educational strategies must be developed to change our concepts, attitudes, and behavioral responses to stress. As responses to stress are learned early, stress management should be incorporated early in educational experiences. Individuals need to learn not only basic skills to cope with life, but, also, to learn how to cope with their emotional feelings. Further development and refinement of preventive programs for stress management must be designed and implemented to decrease the risk of developing inappropriate stress responses and anxiety disorders.

The following case history explores the multiple factors that may interact to form anxiety disorders. The following case ultimately required psychiatric intervention. This very complex history was chosen because it underscores the importance of the biopsychosocial paradigm. The patient was unresponsive to intervention focusing on any single component of this model, but did very well when all aspects were approached in a coordinated fashion. Although such comprehensive treatment might be beyond the scope of many primary practitioners, this case does demonstrate how anxiety can evolve and how treatment can be developed once the pathogenesis is elucidated.

Case History

Ms. F, a 28-year-old woman, presented to a psychiatrist's (LBG) office accompanied by her mother after 9½ years of panic attacks. During these episodes she would sense that her stomach was tied in knots. She would hyperventilate with tingling paresthesia in her extremities as a result. She sensed her heart pounding and would break into a sweat with gross tremor of her hands. She would become intensely fearful of fainting and would feel totally out of control during these episodes.

Her life had become more and more circumscribed since the development of these episodes. She was only able to leave home if accompanied by her mother. She would not allow her mother to leave home without her as she was quite certain that this would invoke an episode. Whenever she thought about being alone, she would become quite anxious, but did not experience the autonomic symptoms characteristic of her panic attacks. She had quit her last job 8 years previously.

She reported feeling depressed and frustrated about her social isolation from friends and her inability to work. Her sleep was within normal limits. With the help of a dieting group, she had managed to go from 220 to 130 pounds during the preceding 2 years. She reported normal appetite. She had occasional thoughts that she would be better off dead, but had no active plans of suicide. She was occasionally tearful. Her affective symptoms and irritability would significantly increase in the 5 days prior to the onset of her menses, then would abate as her flow began.

She reported a relatively idyllic childhood, punctuated on several occasions by her father's depression. He would, during these times, become withdrawn but not abusive. He was hospitalized twice and responded to ECT. She was an acceptable student, popular with her peers, although with some transitory school phobia in first grade. She became a key punch operator upon graduation from high school and continued to live at home as did most of her friends.

When she was 19, her only sister married. Two weeks later she had her first episode of panic while shopping alone. It was quite similar symptomatically to her current episodes. Her second episode was several months later. She was convinced she would die and was taken to a hospital emergency room. This pattern was repeated on numerous occasions as the episodes became more frequent.

She became involved in almost continuous psychiatric treatment over the next 9 years, involving many different therapists and modalities of treatment including supportive and insight therapy, behavior therapy, family therapy, group therapy, and treatment with antipsychotics, low doses of antidepressants, and Valium. The only treatment that seemed to make any difference, and that only transitorily, was a clinic for agoraphobics that included contact with other similarly afflicted patients and behavior therapy.

Her past medical history and review of systems were unremarkable. Her physical examination was within normal limits. There was no click or murmur on auscultation suggestive of mitral valve prolapse. Her family history revealed an extraordinary diathesis for both affective disorder and untreated agoraphobia.

She was initially seen individually with her mother staying in the waiting room. Considerable time in the first several sessions was spent with patient education. A multifactorial model of panic disorders was presented and the importance of insight, of biological treatments, of behavioral techniques, and most importantly, of approaching her feared stimuli in an orderly fashion were all underscored.

Because of the significant anticipatory anxiety superimposed upon her panic attacks, she was begun on alprazolam, ultimately reaching a dose of 6 mg per day. Her panic attacks ceased, but she remained severely compromised by her anticipatory anxiety. A hierarchy of feared situations was developed. The first four sessions were spent individually, principally exploring her relationship with her family. The patient felt that her illness gave her mother a purpose in life and that her mother gave her clear messages discouraging any independence. As the extent of the symbiosis became apparent it seemed clear that joint sessions would prove necessary.

Ms. F and her mother worked on developing a behavioral hierarchy and began a program of in vivo desensitization. The first step involved Ms. F's mother driving around the block alone. While there was some resistance to this program, they were able to advance nonetheless. Over the next month Ms. F began to appreciate that she had not had a panic attack, although her anxiety was quite high whenever she was faced with a new task. Slow progress continued with Ms. F going out with a friend for an hour and letting her mother go down the block for 15 minutes alone.

During the tenth session, Ms. F revealed that she had had an abortion at age 19. She had wanted to continue the pregnancy, but gave in to her mother's pressure to terminate it. She was filled with guilt and rage toward her mother around this event. Although she had had one panic attack prior to the abortion, they significantly accelerated afterward. She thought frequently of the loss. The next several sessions were spent mourning the loss and working through their feelings toward one another around this issue. We can only speculate, but it seems entirely plausible that abortion counseling might have averted many years of guilt and self-punishment.

The picture that began to emerge was one of a young woman at extremely high biological risk who had an abortion shortly after her only sister married and left home. She was filled with guilt about an act she found to be morally wrong and with rage toward her mother. Her agoraphobia functioned to punish her mother, helped her to avoid men and sex, and gave her a way to "atone."

As this became clearer to the F's, there was a sudden and dramatic increase in their activities. Ms. F was able to travel independently, leave home for prolonged periods, to date, and to enter a job training program. She remains on medication, but sees her life as in no way currently impaired.

This case clearly illustrates the necessity of adopting multiple approaches to treatment. Simple behavioral or insight-oriented approaches had failed in the past. Successful treatment was predicated upon the assessment that Ms. F's agoraphobia was multiply determined.

From a biological standpoint, it was clear that Ms. F was at extraordinarily high risk. Her family history is rife with alcoholism, major depression, and agoraphobia. This vulnerability contributed to the generalization from panic attacks which many people occasionally endure, to panic disorder, to frank agoraphobia.

Ms. F appears to have gone through the sequence common to most phobics. Her panic attacks were extremely noxious and she wished to avoid them at all costs. Phobics learn to associate the panic attacks with certain environmental stimuli and work very hard to avoid these at all costs. Classic agoraphobics learn that the panic attacks occur outside the home and refuse to leave these safe boundaries. Ms. F varied slightly in that she associated her mother, not her home, with safety. Frequent panic attacks, whenever away from her mother, led to the development of anticipatory anxiety whenever she even thought of being away from her mother.

How do we understand the choice of her mother instead of her house as the safe object? This requires the use of a family systems perspective. Unconsciously, she was enraged with her mother and her role in encouraging Ms. F to have an abortion. She soon became an albatross around her mother's neck, following her everywhere and wreaking almost a decade's vengeance. She was, on the other hand, filling many of her mother's needs, giving her mother a function in life.

Intrapsychically, her prolonged removal from the world and its pleasures can be seen as a self-punitive act, an unconscious attempt to redeem herself from what, at least in part, she regarded as a sinful act.

Socially, it is easy to see how agoraphobia can become a self-perpetuating disorder. Ten years of absenting herself from the world left her with dated job skills and peers who had moved onto very different developmental stages.

Her treatment incorporated many approaches to understanding her disorder. In the beginning a careful history was obtained and considerable time was spent in teaching about the disorder. Ms. F was a fairly sophisticated consumer, undoubtedly reflecting the many different types of therapy she had attempted over the years.

The next, and simplest, step was the biological treatment of the panic disorder. Alprazolam was chosen instead of a more traditional antidepressant because of her significant anticipatory anxiety. Her panic attacks promptly abated and her anticipatory component diminished slightly.

Graduated in vivo desensitization was begun almost as soon as the panic attacks stopped, based upon the belief that all of the theorizing and understanding in the world would be of little benefit unless accompanied by actual testing in the patient's own environment.

As soon as the symbiosis with her mother became apparent, it was decided to enter into family therapy. Ms. F's illness was fulfilling too many of both their needs to allow this to be ignored. Insight-oriented work was also necessary to understand the dynamics surrounding the abortion and its ramifications. Environmental supports were shored up through the use of a job training program, sponsored by the local Office of Vocational Rehabilitation.

This case was chosen because it so clearly underscores the need for using many different approaches and early intervention to adequately understand and help these very challenging patients.

CONCLUSION

Our time period has been termed "The Age of Anxiety." It seems clear that anxiety is an all too common feature of modern American life. Although it is frequently a normal response and can at times be helpful, it can also lead to significant morbidity. Health care providers need to develop awareness that anxiety may be a feature in each client's symptoms and be prepared to assess women's anxiety potential and refer them for consulation when necessary.

Our understanding of anxiety is still in its infancy. We are only now beginning to be able to differentiate different subtypes and to develop some understanding of causation. Although there is currently no research to document that education and early intervention can serve to avert or minimize anxiety, logic dictates that these measures should help and they are clearly ethically desirable. Future research is necessary to determine the impact of preventive efforts on anxiety disorders or in helping women cope effectively with anxiety in daily living.

CLIENT RESOURCES

Audiovisual—Relaxation

Bernstein, D. A., & Borkove, T. D. *Progressive relaxation training*. Champaign, Ill.: Research Press, 1973. *(Audio recording set that includes written instructions for learning relaxation response. Is best used as an adjunct to individual or group learning as deep muscle relaxation technique can be complex and patients often benefit from initial evaluation and teaching by a practitioner.)*

Mulrey, R. *Tension management and relaxation*. St. Louis, Mo.: C. V. Mosby, 1981. *(Relaxation through exercises and guided imagery.)*

Audiovisual—Stress

Selye, H. *Stress anxiety and the cardiovascular system*. New York: Pfizer Inc., 1976. *(1 to 10 cassettes outlining stress effects on the body.)*

Mental Health Association. *Learning to cope: How to deal with your tensions*. Screenscope, Inc., 1022 Wilson Blvd, Arlington, VA 22209. *(25 min (16 mm color) film focuses on management of tension associated with daily living.)*

Pandora's bottle & drinking women. Motivational Media, 6855 Santa Monica Blvd., Los Angles, CA 90038. *(This film explores the impact of social attitudes and misconceptions on the identification and treatment of alcoholic women and concludes with a discussion of fetal alcohol syndrome.)*

Center for Multicultural Awareness, 2925 Columbia Pike, Arlington, VA 22204. (703) 979-6100. *(Offers a selection of multicultural prevention films developed by National Institute of Drug Abuse.)*

Pamphlets

There are a large variety of printed materials developed for the patient and public that offer education and awareness about stress and stress related disorders. Information and copies of available material may be obtained from:

National Association of Mental Health, 1800 N. Kent St., Arlington, TX 76011.

National Clearing House for Mental Health Information, 22400 Rockville Pike, Rockville, MD 20857.

Books

Bensen, H. *The relaxation response*. New York: Morrow, 1975. *(Well-written descriptions of attaining relaxation through exercises and guided imagery.)*

Carlson, D. (Ed.). *Staying well*. Chicago, Ill.: Contemporary Books, 1982. *(Blue Cross and Blue*

Shield guide to promoting wellness through good nutrition, physical fitness and stress reduction. Easily read, provides concrete examples on how to identify and prevent stress and anxiety.)

Schaffer, M. *Life after stress.* Chicago, Ill.: Contemporary Books, 1983. *(A practical guide to stress management with good examples of the effect of stress and how to cope.)*

Sindons, D. E. *Controlling stress and tension: A holistic approach.* Englewood Cliffs, N.J.: Prentice-Hall, 1979. *(Practical guide to the multifactors that cause stress and intervention to alleviate tension. Practiced techniques for self-assessment and monitoring of stress are provided. Excellent discussion of utilizing transcendental meditation, biofeedback, and stress reduction and prevention through physical activity and nutrition.)*

Groups Appropriate for Alleviating Stress

Alcoholics Anonymous. *(Provides support and education for alcoholics who cannot control their alcohol use. Also offers programs for spouses and siblings. Provides hotline, pamphlets, and speakers. Membership is free and often members are assigned a sponsor to help them cope better with daily stessors. For information regarding group meetings contact:*
1. *National Headquarters at 468 Park Ave. S., New York, NY 10016.*
2. *a local community mental health service.*
3. *a phone book or newspaper.)*

Compassionate Friends, National Office, P.O. Box 1347, Oak Brook, IL 60521. *(Peer support for bereaved parents.)*

Emotions Anonymous, P.O. Box 4245, St. Paul, MN 55014 *(Approach to individuals with emotional conditions.)*

La Leche League. *(For nursing and other new moms. Offers hotline for breast feeding problems and support.)*

National Association for Retarded Citizens, National Office, 2709 Ave. E. East, Arlington, TX 76011 *(Offers a variety of support systems for retarded individuals and their families.)*

Neurotic Anonymous, National Office, 1341 G. Street North West, Washington, DC 20005. *(Support for individuals with emotional problems.)*

Parents Anonymous, National Office, 22330 Hawthorne, Torrance, CA 90505. *(For parents of abused children. Offers peer support, crisis intervention and information.)*

Recovery Inc., National Office, 7910 Woodmont Ave., Washington, DC 20014. *(Support and education for patients recovering from emotional disorders.)*

For further information about self-help groups:

Garlner, A., & Reissman, F. *Help: A working guide to self-help groups.* New York: New View Point, Vision Books, 1980.

McCormack, N. *Plain talk about mutual help group.* Rockville, Md.: DHHS Publication No. (Adm) 81-113.

National Self Help Clearing House, 33 West 42nd Street, New York, NY 10036, (212) 840-7606.

REFERENCES

Adebimpe, V. R. Overview: White norms and psychiatric diagnosis of black patients. *American Journal of Psychiatry,* 1981, *138*(3) 279–285.

American Psychiatric Association. *Diagnostic and statistical manual of mental disorders* (3rd ed.). Washington, D.C.: APA, 1980.

Antonovsky, A. *Health, stress and coping.* San Francisco: Jossey Bass, 1979.

Beck, A. T., Laude, R., & Bohnert, M. Ideational components of anxiety. *Archives of General Psychiatry,* 1974, *31,* 319–326.

Beck, A. T. *Cognitive therapy and the emotional disorders.* New York: New American Library, 1976.

Bellantuno, C., Reggie, V., Tognoni, G., & Garattini, S. Benzodiazepines: Clinical pharmacology and therapeutic use. *Drug,* 1980, *19,* 195.

Bellock, L., & Small, L. *Emergency psychotherapy and brief psychotherapy*. New York: Grunne & Stratton, 1978.

Benson, H. *The relaxation response*. New York: Morrow, 1975.

Benson, H., Beary, J. F., & Carol, M. P. The relaxation response. *Psychiatry*, 1974, *37*, 37–46.

Benson, H., Greenwood, M. M., & Klenchuk, H. The relaxation response: Psychophysiologic aspects and clinical applications. *International Journal of Psychiatry in Medicine*, 1975, *61*(1–2), 87–98.

Broverman, I. K., Broverman, D. M., Clarkson, F. E., Rosenkrantz, P. S., & Vogel, S. R. Sex role stereotypes and clinical judgment of mental health. *Journal of Counseling and Clinical Psychology*, 1970, *34*, 1–7.

Brown, H. Medical illness and anxiety. In W. Fann, I. Karcon, A. Porkorny, & R. Williams (Eds.), *Phenomenology and treatment of anxiety*. New York: Spectrum, 1979, pp. 205–210.

Burgess, A., & Baldwin, B. *Crisis intervention and practice*. Englewood Cliffs, N.J.: Prentice Hall, 1981, pp. 40–50.

Caplan, G., & Killilea, M. (Eds.). *Support systems and mutual help*. New York: Grune & Stratton, 1976.

Cohen, M. E. The high familial prevalence of neurocirculatory anesthesia, anxiety, neurosis, and effort syndrome. *American Journal of Human Genetics*, 1951, *3*, 126–158.

Cooperstock, R. Sex differences in psychotropic drug use. *Social Science and Medicine*, 1978, *23*, 179–186.

Cooperstock R., & Parnell, P. Research on psychotropic drug use: A review of findings and methods. *Social Science and Medicine*, 1982, *16*, 1179–1196.

Coursey, R. D. Electromyographic feedback as a relaxation technique. *Journal of Consulting and Clinical Psychology*, 1975, *43*, 825–843.

Crowe, R. R., Pauls, D. L., Slymen, D. J., & Noyes, R. A. A family study of anxiety neuroses. *Archives of General Psychiatry*, 1980, *37*, 77–91.

Dennis, J. L., & Hendrie, H. C. Treatment of anxiety states: Some theoretical and practical aspects. *Journal of Indiana State Medical Association*, 1980, *73*(5), 300–305.

Dohrenwend, B. P., Neugebauer, R., & Dohrenwend, B. S. Formulation of hypotheses about the true prevalance of functional psychiatric disorders among adults in the United States. In B. P. Dohrenwend & B. S. Dohrenwend (Eds.), *Mental illness in the United States*. New York: Praeger, 1980.

Elliott, B. R., & Eisdorfer, C. (Eds.). *Stress and human health*. New York: Springer, 1982.

Ellis, A., & Harper, R. A. *A new guide to rational living*. North Hollywood, Calif.: Wilshire, 1977.

Epstein, S. Natural healing processes of the mind. In D. Meichenbaum & M. Jaremko (Eds.), *Stress reduction and management*. New York: Plenum, 1983, pp. 39–65.

Erman, M., & Guggenheim, F. Psychiatric side effects of commonly used drugs. *Drug Therapy*, 1981, *11*, 117–126.

Fiore, N. Fighting cancer: One patient's perspective. *New England Journal of Medicine*, 1979, *300*, 284–289.

Frank, J. D. *Psychotherapy and the human predicament: A psychosocial approach*. New York: Schocken Books, 1978.

Gove, W. R., & Tudor, J. Adult sex roles and mental illness. *American Journal of Sociology*, 1973, *78*, 812–825.

Greenly, J. R., & Mechanic, D. Social selection in seeking help for psychological problems. *Journal of Health and Social Behavior*, 1976, *17*, 249–262.

Guttmacher, L. B., Murphy, D. L., & Insel, T. R. Pharmacologic models of anxiety. *Comprehensive Psychiatry*, 1983, *24*, 312–326.

Hamburg, D. A., Elliott, G., & Parron, D. L. (Eds.). *Health and behavior: Frontiers of biobehavioral science*. Washington, D. C.: National Academy Press, 1982.

Hollister, L. E. *Clinical pharmacology of psychotherapeutic drugs*. New York: Churchill Livingstone, 1978.

Holroyd, K. A. Stress, coping, and the treatment of stress related illness. In J. R. McNamara (Ed.), *Behavioral approaches in medicine: Application and analysis*. New York: Plenum, 1979.

Holroyd, K. A., & Lazarus, R. A. Stress, coping, and somatic adaptation. In I. Golberger & S. Bergmitz (Eds.), *Handbook of stress*. New York: Free Press, 1982.

Howell, E. The influence of gender on diagnoses and treatment. In E. Howell & H. Bayes (Eds.), *Women and mental health*. New York: Basic Books, 1981.

Institute of Medicine. *Report of a study: Sleeping pills, insomnia, and medical practice*. Washington, D.C.: National Academy of Science, 1979.

Jacobson, S. E. *Progressive relaxation* (2nd ed.). Chicago, Ill.: University Press, 1938.

Janis, I. L. Stress inoculation in health care. In D. Meichbaum & M. E. Jaremko (Eds.), *Stress reduction and prevention*. New York: Plenum Press, 1983, pp. 78–84.

Janis, I. L. *Stress and frustration*. New York: Harcourt, Brace & Jovanovich, 1971.

Janis, I. L. *Psychological stress*. New York: Wiley & Sons, 1958.

Karasus, T. B., & Steinmuller, R. I. (Eds.). *Psychotherapeutics in medicine*. New York: Grune & Stratton, 1978.

Lader, M. Behavior and anxiety: Psychological mechanisms. *Journal of Clinical Psychiatry*, 1983, *44*(2), 5–10.

Lazarus, R. S. *Patterns for adjustment*. New York: McGraw-Hill, 1976.

Lazarus, R. S. *Psychological stress and the coping process*. New York: McGraw-Hill, 1966.

Lewis, C. E., & Lewis, M. A. The potential impact of sexual equality on health. *New England Journal of Medicine*, 1977, *297*, 863–869.

Marecek, J. Psychological disorders in women: Indices of role strain. In I. Freise, J. Parsons, P. Johnson, & G. Zellman (Eds.), *Women and sex roles: A social psychological perspective*. New York: W. W. Norton, 1978.

Mechanic, D. (Ed.). *Symptoms, illness behavior, and help seeking*. New York: Prodist, 1982, pp. 1–29.

Meichenbaum, D. Stress prevention and management: A cognitive and behavioral approach. In D. Meichenbaum & M. E. Jaremko (Eds.), *Stress reduction and prevention*. New York: Plenum, 1983.

Mellinger, G. D., & Butler, M. B. Psychotheraputic drugs. In J. P. Morgan & D. V. Kagan (Eds.), *Society and medication: Conflicting signals for prescribers and patients*. Lexington, Mass.: Lexington Books, 1983.

Moulton, R. Some effects of the new feminism. *American Journal of Psychiatry*, 1977, *134*(1), 1–7.

Mulrey, R. *Tension management and relaxation*. St. Louis, Mo.: C. V. Mosby, 1981.

Nemiah, J. C. The psychoanalytic view of anxiety. In D. F. Klein & J. Rabkin (Eds.), *Anxiety: New research and changing concepts*. New York: Raven Press, 1981, 1291–1300.

Noyes, R., Jr. Beta-blocking drugs and anxiety. *Psychosomatics*, 1982, *23*(2), 155–173.

Oakley, A. *Women's work*. New York: Pantheon, 1974.

Paul, S. M., Marangos, P. S., Skolmick, P., & Goodwin, F. K. Biologic substandards of anxiety: Benzodiazepine receptors and endogenous ligands. *L'Encephale*, 1982, *8*, 131–144.

Rapoport, R., and Rapoport, R. N. *Dual career families re-examined*. New York: Harper & Row, 1976.

Raskin, M., Peeke, H. V., Dickman, W., & Pinsker, H. Panic and generalized anxiety disorders. *Archives of General Psychiatry*, 1982, *39*, 687–689.

Rickles, K. Neurobenzodiazepine anxiolytics: Clinical usefulness. *Journal of Clinical Psychiatry*, 1983, *44*(2), 11.

Rickles, K. Clinical comparisons. *Psychosomatics*, 1980, *21* (suppl), 15–20.

Rickles, K. Benzodiazepine in the treatment of anxiety. American Journal of Psychotherapy, 1982, *36*, 358–370.

Raskin, M., Peeke, J. V. S., Dickmen, W., & Pinsker, H. Panic and generalized anxiety disorders: Developmental antecedents and precipitants. *Archives of General Psychiatry*, 1982, *39*(6), 687–689.

Rosenbaum, J. F. Anxiety. In A. Lazare (Ed.), *Outpatient psychiatry, diagnosis and treatment*. Baltimore, Md.: Williams & Wilkins, 1979, pp. 252–256.

Schuckit, M. Anxiety related to medical disease. *Journal of Clinical Psychiatry*, 1983, *44*(2), 11, 31–37.

Schweitzer, L. A., & Adams, G. The diagnosis and management of anxiety for primary care physicians. In W. Fann, I. Karacon, A. Pokorny, & R. Williams (Eds.), *Phenomenology and treatment of anxiety*. New York: Spectrum, 1979, pp. 19–42.

Sexton, M. M. Behavioral epidemiology. In O. F. Pomerleau & J. P. Brady (Eds.), *Behavioral medicine: Theory and practice*. Baltimore: Williams & Wilkins, 1979.

Shader, R. I., & Greenblatt, D. J. Some current treatment options for symptoms of anxiety. *Journal of Clinical Psychiatry*, 1983, *44*(2), 11, 21–30.

Sheehan, B. V., & Sheenan, K. H. The classification of anxiety and hysterical states. *Journal of Clinical Psychopharmacology*, 1982, 2, 225–244.

Skolnick, P., & Paul, S. M. New concepts in the neurobiology of anxiety. *Journal of Clinical Psychiatry*, 1983, *44*(2), 11, 12–18.

Steinmuller, R. I. Psychotherapeutic treatment planning. In B. Karasus & R. I. Steinmuller (Eds.), *Psychotherapeutics in medicine*. New York: Grune & Stratton, 1978, pp. 39–50.

Suinn, R. M., & Deffendacher, J. L. Behavior therapy. In L. A. Schlesinger, *Handbook on stress and anxiety*. San Francisco: Jossey-Bass, 1980.

Strayhorn, J. M. *Foundations of clinical psychiatry*. Chicago, Il.: Year Book Medical, 1982.

Srole, L. Langner, T. S. Michaul, S. T., Otler, M. K., & Rennie, T. A. *Mental health in metropolis. The Midtown Manhattan Study* (Vol. 1). New York: McGraw-Hill, 1962.

Tallman, J. F., Paul, S. M., Skolnick, P., & Gallager, D. W. Receptor sites for the age of anxiety: Pharmacology of the benzodiazepines. *Science*, 1980, *207*, 227–281.

United States Bureau of Labor Statistics. *Perspectives on working women: A data book*. Washington, D.C.: The U.S. Government Printing Office, 1980.

Walker, K., & Wood, M. *Time use: A measure of household production of family goods and services*. Washington, D.C.: American Home Economics Association, 1976.

White, R. B., & Gilland R. M. *Elements of psychopathology; the mechanisms of defense*. New York: Grune & Stratton, 1975, pp. 3–5.

Wilson, T. B., & Lazarus, R. S. Behavior modification and therapy. In T. B. Karsus & R. I. Steinmuller (Eds.), *Psychotherapeutics in medicine*. New York: Grunne & Stratton, 1978, p. 123.

Wolberg, L. *Psychotherapy and the behavioral sciences*. New York: Grune & Stratton, 1966.

Wolfe, J. A cognitive and behavioral approach to working with women alcoholics. In W. Bartel (Ed.), *Women who drink*. Springfield, Ill.: C. C. Thomas, 1979, pp. 197–215.

Zung, W. *How normal is anxiety*. N. Kupash, Michigan: Upjohn, 1980, pp. 5–19.

Zung, W. Assessment of anxiety disorders: Qualitative and quantitative approaches. In W. Fonn, I. Karccon, A. Porkoiny, & R. Williams (Eds.), *Phenomenology and treatment of anxiety*. New York: Spectrum, 1979.

Women As Victims: Education for Prevention

26

Carole A. Anderson

Because women occupy an inferior social position to men, they must, as children, be taught the ways to cope with that position and adapt to their expected role in society. The primary method of adaptation, which women are taught, is that of submission. Submissiveness then becomes the way in which women accommodate to their subordinate position; the net effect of learning and acting submissive is for women to feel powerless and helpless. Inevitably, these feelings prime women to be maltreated, to be victims.

Much has been written during the past several years about the various forms of victimization of women, such as physical abuse of wives by husbands, rape, and medical maltreatment. The mistreatment of women and the lack of ability and societal support to adequately stop or prevent it functions as a self-fulfilling prophecy in reinforcing a woman's sense of powerlessness and helplessness. A further destructive aspect of socialization to an inferior position is that women learn society's definition of them and, in addition to being devalued by the society as a whole, they devalue themselves. This sense of devalued self further accentuates a woman's sense of powerlessness to deal with the exigencies of her daily life.

Indeed, many women seek care in the mental health system for problems of daily living with which they are unable to cope. The typical woman who presents herself for mental health counseling, however, does not suffer from psychopathology of the kind that requires medical intervention. Rather, women who seek therapy are most often anxious and depressed, and are experiencing pain, frustration, confusion, despair, loss, and a pervasive sense of powerlessness (Collier, 1982). Of particular importance is the felt sense of powerlessness.

Power is usually expressed in terms of relationships with others and is the ability to do, to act, and to control one's self or other people (Collier, 1982). Women lack power because society either takes it away or places limits upon it in the course of the normal socialization process. In contrast to men, women possess less financial and political power, are taught not to exercise any power that they might have and to approach men in devious ways to act out their submission (Collier, 1982). This lack of power and concomitant feelings of helplessness preclude many women from taking charge of their lives, and perceiving mistreatment *as* mistreatment and extricating themselves from it. Rather, they are victimized and feel helpless to stop the mistreatment. The more women are victimized the more helpless they feel, a reaction that brings on further maltreatment—a vicious cycle. Central to understanding the place of women in society and the maltreatment imposed on them is the socialization process. Health care providers must not only understand the problems and the forms of victimization that occur to women but must also understand the socialization process that brings women to the point that makes them vulnerable to various kinds of maltreatment.

SOCIALIZATION OF WOMEN

Socialization refers to a life-long process whereby individuals learn the rules of the general society, the norms and values of the social environment, and the occupational skills and the professional roles. The primary agents of socialization are families, social groups, schools, and churches. In recent years, the literature on the socialization of women has pointed to the institutions of our society and the ways in which little girls are taught the traits that will enable them to assume their feminine, albeit subordinate, position as an adult in this society. Of particular importance to women is the socialization that occurs during late childhood and adolescence. These are the years in which a woman learns what it is to be a "woman" and develops traits that will allow her to assume the female role in the culture (see Table 4–3).

In essence, the socialization process teaches men and women what behavioral expectations are held for them. As individuals learn the expectations of their culture, they act in accordance with them. The more people adhere to the normative, gender-specific expectations, the more those actions and traits become firmly gender-linked and are subsequently labeled feminine or masculine; the behavior becomes the gender-specific norm for that society. Behavioral traits that are labeled feminine or the idealized stereotype of normal femininity in our culture are being dependent, passive, fragile, sensitive, noncompetitive, nurturant, intuitive, yielding, receptive, unable to risk, emotionally labile, supportive, and inner-oriented. On the other hand, the traits associated with the idealized masculine role are such things as being independent, aggressive, competitive, task-oriented, assertive, objective, analytical, brave, rational, unsentimental, confident, and in emotional control (Bardwick & Dauran, 1971). These idealized traits then become the adjectives that are used to define the behavior that is desired in a man or a woman. The socialization process teaches little boys and little girls ways to act that conform to the norm. The dilemma for women, of course, is that if a woman incorporates the idealized feminine traits, she will be at odds with what is valued in the society, because society places a higher value on and rewards "masculine" behaviors. In essence, a woman is socialized into an ambivalent role wherein she learns what behaviors are valued in women and what is considered feminine, but she also learns that it is the masculine traits that are rewarded and valued in the culture (Gornick, 1971).

When one looks closely at the traditional traits and behaviors taught to women, it is clear that those qualities do not combine in any woman to make her powerful, independent, self-assertive, or achievement-oriented. Rather, they combine to make women feel inept and unable to control their own fate, and to ward off maltreatment.

One of the most outstanding differences in how boys and girls are socialized is that aggression in men is valued whereas it is not valued in women. Obviously, the ability to act in aggressive ways is essential to being able to control mistreatment. When girls, socialized not to be aggressive, find themselves as adults in a situation of being mistreated, they do not have the repertoire of skills and abilities to fend off mistreatment.

In a study of children's books (Dick and Jane as Victims, 1980), it was found that at the rate of four to one the books portrayed boys in so-called active mastery scenes, those scenes related to creativity, bravery, perseverance, achievement, adventurousness, and ingenuity. Girls, on the other hand, were portrayed as expecting to be helped, being without skills other than domestic, working without monetary compensation, and being led by boys. In addition, scenes of passivity, docility, and dependency featured girls at the ratio of six to one. Also, girls were depicted as rehearsing the traditional female role that involved activities such as cooking and cleaning and being in the kitchen continuously. Of particular note was the fact that contained in these 2760 stories were a hundred stories dealing with meanness in which males were the aggressors against females.

Dowling (1981) offers the thesis that women are trained for dependency and live their lives in an attempt to be kept safe and be taken care of, whereas men are trained for self-sufficiency. She views this dependency, that she has labeled the Cinderella Complex, as the chief force that keeps women oppressed. Women, then, according to Dowling, spend much of their lives looking for people who will "save" them rather than developing or acting out those competencies that will allow them to be self-sufficient, powerful, and in control of their own lives.

In summary, women are rewarded for developing a set of psychological characteristics to accommodate and please men, such as submissiveness, compliance, and passivity. These characteristics are quite costly to women and are antithetical to the use of active mechanisms for coping, resolving conflicts (Carmen, Russo, & Miller 1981), and dealing with aggressive situations.

Women of all ages are particularly vulnerable to victimization. It takes many forms and includes stereotyping, labeling and excluding, sexual harassment, pornography, poverty, incest, physical abuse, rape, and medical maltreatment. This chapter focuses on the latter three forms as examples of the ways in which women are primed to be victimized and how the social structure perpetuates it.

Wife Abuse

Marital violence is a serious and common problem that has come only recently to the attention of the public. This, like other problems of women, has been hidden from public view, and existing statistics grossly underestimate the severity of it. Although wife abuse is not a new problem, it has now been openly acknowledged and discussed due, in large measure, to the efforts of the women's movement that has brought to light the problems of women, illustrating their subordinate social position. At present little is known about wife abuse, but the information is growing and becoming disseminated. The research to date shows that wife abuse is common, widespread, and potentially fatal for women.

Wife abuse is underreported for reasons having to do with such things as societal norms, an unresponsive judicial system, police indifference, and marital laws (Roy, 1977). In 1976 a sample of American households were questioned regarding the occurrence of violence in their families (Straus, 1978). This study empirically validated the belief that physical violence between family members is a common and serious problem.

In spite of what some individuals might think, the severity of violence between family members is quite real. Many women endure years of severe verbal and physical abuse often resulting in a homicide. In fact, due to the unreliable statistics of assaults between husbands and wives, homicide statistics are used instead and reveal a significant number of homicides occurring between family members. Indeed, relatives constitute the single largest category of homicide victims (Boudouris, 1971; Martin, 1976; Straus, 1977; Voss & Hepburn, 1968).

Another indicator of the extent of wife abuse is the frequency of police calls related to domestic disturbances. In many communities domestic disturbance calls are the most frequent call received by police officers. Estimates of interfamily violence can also be obtained by studying couples who are seeking divorce. In one such study, O'Brien (1974) found that 17 percent of the spouses interviewed spontaneously mentioned overt violence in their relationship. In another study, Lebinger (1974) found 36 percent of female divorce applicants complained of being physically abused by their spouses. All of the studies to date leave little doubt that physical abuse of women by men is a very real and serious problem. The statistics are made even more alarming by the knowledge that children growing up in these violent families learn violent ways of relating to one another and are at increased risk for being physically abused themselves as adults or physically abusing their spouses.

Although we know that this is a serious and widespread problem, little evidence exists to identify exact causality. What evidence there is points to a set of individual, cultural, and social organizational factors that combine in a variety of ways to produce family violence (Straus, 1977). Some of these are: cultural norms that legitimate wife abuse as revealed in such things as everyday jokes, cartoons, and sayings about husband and wife interactions; laws that do little to protect a woman from assaults by her husband and often essentially condone the behavior; a reflection of our societal violence; socialization within violent families; the sexist structure of the society; and economic frustrations. Alcohol use and abuse also surfaces as a factor in domestic violence. However, the exact nature of the relationship of alcohol use to domestic violence is unknown. It is thought that alcohol might serve to lower inhibitions and thereby increase the expression of aggressive impulses or that alcohol is used to excuse violent behavior. Very little empirical evidence exists related to alcohol use and domestic violence (Gelles, 1974; Gelles & Straus, 1975).

Women who are beaten are found among all educational, racial, and socioeconomic groups (Steinmetz & Straus, 1974; Straus, 1977). They live in every community and relay personal horror stories that they had kept to themselves. Women who are beaten regularly number more than 200,000, and their shocking stories bring cries of denial and disbelief from those who hear them. Often the question is asked, "Why do women stay in violent relationships?" The answer or the explanation for a woman's frequent immobility rests in the knowledge of the role of women in our society. These women are victims and are immobilized for such reasons as: the societal tendency to "blame the victim"; their own childhood experiences, i.e., socialization into violence; a lack of resources; an unresponsive legal system; a traditional ideology about marriage and the duty of women to stay married "for better or for worse"; and the economic dependency of women on men. Also, the concept of "learned helplessness" put forth by Lenore Walker (1977) is speculated to be another reason why women become immobilized in their situation. Basically, the concept of learned helplessness as it refers to battered women is derived from the theory of Seligman (1972). Seligman's theory was based on his work with animals wherein he was able to interfere with a wide range of adaptive behaviors by subjecting the animals to uncontrollable shocks. The animals in the experiment essentially gave up and became passive when they found that they were unable to control their trauma and mistreatment. He was able to condition them *not* to act out behavior designed to help them survive. Walker (1977) draws an analogy to battered women. Battered women, according to Walker, are also subject to uncontrolled physical trauma. She hypothesizes that the result of this uncontrolled trauma and a woman's inability to control it interferes with her ability to cope, and she becomes helpless; she has learned helplessness.

Many factors function to keep women in violent situations, and to perpetuate their victim status. Their inability to leave is intimately tied to the plight of women in our culture. An understanding of all these forces is vital to assist women in increasing their power to extricate themselves from their victim status. In part, this can be done through the counseling and teaching relationship that a health care provider can and should establish with her women clients. Women who are being beaten must be helped to identify their alternatives and to make difficult choices and changes, otherwise the results are tragic. There is significant physical harm inflicted on women and their children, but more important, violence within that family is perpetuated through the generations. If we are to assist women in identifying their alternatives, making their choices, and provide them with information needed to do so, it is imperative that we understand all the forces that legitimate the use of physical violence by men against women, as well as the social institutions that contribute to the perpetuation of that violence.

Rape

Rape is a crime against women that inflicts pain, terror, humiliation, and physical and psychological harm. Feminists regard rape as the epitome of sexism and a symbol of the oppression of women by men (Brownmiller, 1975; Csida & Csida, 1974; Russel, 1975). Rape is a crime of violence and a woman is the usual victim. However, laws of evidence, an adversarial judicial system, and the fear of convicting an innocent man interact to produce a situation wherein the victim often feels that she, rather than the assailant, is on trial.

The incidence of rape is increasing dramatically, yet many people believe that the official statistics showing this increase still represent only 50 percent of the actual incidence. Although there has been a concomitant increase in other violent crimes over the past several years, increased incidence of rape has surpassed those other increases and is noteworthy (Brownmiller, 1975).

In Brownmiller's (1975) opinion, rape is the natural outcome of the legal subjugation of women to men whereby women become men's property and are utilized by men to express aggression toward other men. Brownmiller cites the pervasive carnage of women that accompanies war as an example of this and illustrates men's expression of the ultimate humiliation perpetrated by the victors against the vanquished.

Contrary to common belief, rape is often planned and involves people who know each other. Rapes occur within conventional social contexts, such as dating, courtships, and friendships, which means that any woman is a potential victim. Victims have reported being raped by fathers, husbands, lovers, and friends (Russel, 1975). Although many would like to focus on the behavior of women to explain "why" rapes occur (e.g., a woman who goes out alone at night, a woman who picks up a strange man in a bar), the feminist perspective views rape as a transgression against a woman by a man that is motivated by *him* rather than provoked by her (Brownmiller, 1975; Csida & Csida, 1974; Russell, 1975; Thompson & Michael, 1974). Rape statistics include victims who are sick, poor, black, white, young, elderly, lonesome, intoxicated, promiscuous, hitchhikers, models, and people with physical disabilities. These groups include virtually all women and therefore cast serious doubt on the notion that rape can be provoked by a certain "kind" of woman. Rather, rape is an aggressive, violent act that brings degradation and humiliation to its victims. No woman enjoys being raped and no woman gives her consent to be raped. However, many women do become submissive in response to physical aggression, verbal coercion, and intimidation (Amir, 1971).

Women who are raped all report feeling degraded (Burgess & Holstrom, 1974). In addition, rape victims experience fear of such things as physical injury, mutilation, and death (Burgess & Holstrom, 1974). The victims of rape experience a clinical syndrome that is akin to any acute stress reaction. This syndrome has been labeled by Burgess and Holstrom (1974) as the "rape trauma syndrome," which is amenable to short-term treatment that focuses on assisting the victim through the immediate stressful situation.

A rape victim's circumstance is compounded by the fact that women often perceive that no one (friends, family, police) really wants to hear details of the rape (Russell, 1975). In response to this perceived reluctance, women often do not discuss what has happened to them beyond the official report (if a report is filed). Their felt shame can be traced to a commonly held belief that a strong, healthy woman cannot be raped by an unarmed man. This belief, to which many women also subscribe, many times provokes the woman's friends and family (including husband) to see her as being responsible for what happened. This loss of support from family and friends compounds the existing shame and degradation felt by the victim.

Rape victims encounter further difficulties when they attempt to bring charges against the rapist. Our judicial–legal system is designed to protect the innocent from false accusation and subsequent prosecution. As a result, often a rape victim is vigorously, and at times aggressively, questioned by the police to determine whether or not a crime (the rape) has actually been committed. This is done in spite of the fact that there are no data to support the contention that false accusations by women are commonplace. This treatment by the legal system has been well publicized by the lay press and many women do not report being raped or do not follow through with their charges to trial. Rapists often go unapprehended and unpunished.

Even under the best of circumstances, rape victims will encounter considerable difficulties with the legal system. Such things as the necessity to recall the exact words and phrases from her original report, the diverse meanings and definitions of consent that exist among and between police, lawyers, jurors, and the victims, and the difficulty in obtaining corroborating evidence to support the charge, are examples of the difficulties that women often encounter. Furthermore, a woman's "role" in the trial of an assailant is that of major witness for the prosecution. As such, she is without legal representation and the assailant's defense attorney, who is acting in the interest of his client, is required to attempt to discredit her (the victim's) testimony. All of these factors combine to make many women reluctant to press charges and to carry the charge to trial. The fact that many women do not prosecute their assailant is often cited as reason to believe that the woman *has not* been raped; she is making a false accusation. Believing this trivializes and minimizes the problem. A more accurate and realistic explanation is that women do not pursue their legal rights because of the enormous difficulty and further shame and humiliation that they will encounter as they attempt to prosecute their assailant.

Closely coordinated services aimed at treating the physical and emotional trauma* experienced by rape victims are crucial in determining the outcome for the woman. As key people in the delivery of the physical and psychological care to victims, health care providers should consider such things as the care of physical injuries, prevention of venereal disease and pregnancy, a complete medicolegal examination, crisis intervention,

---

*See Burgess, A. W., & Holstrom, L. L. *Rape victims of crisis*. Bowie, Md.: Robert Brady, 1974; and Burgess, A. W., & Holstrom, L. L. *Rape crisis and recovery*. Bowie, Md.: Robert Brady, 1979, for a comprehensive understanding of sexual assault, the resultant crisis and trauma, treatment, and factors associated with positive outcomes.

and referral. Because of the complex nature of the rape incident, the victim is in need of comprehensive, sensitive, and humane treatment. Nurses are a major force in the emergency and follow-up treatment of these victims and are able to facilitate the acquisition of services that will help the victim reestablish as soon as possible a normal life pattern.

In summary, rape is an aggressive act that is thought by many to be reflective of social attitudes and beliefs pertaining to definitions of maleness and femaleness, normative sexual role behaviors, and power and privileges. Rape has occurred in every society throughout history and all women are potential victims. The rape victim has numerous needs that must be attended, both in the immediate situation and in the long-term if she is to regain and attain a normal life following the incident. Furthermore, victims also need assistance and support in their efforts to take the legal action that can, in the long run, help them to feel powerful and potent in terms of their ability to obtain vengence for the humiliating transgression against them.

Medical Maltreatment

Even a cursory glance at the statistics from the health care system reveals that today in the United States the health care industry is dependent on women. Not only are women in the majority of the patient population, but they also constitute the largest group of workers. Women, in contrast to men, report more morbidity, are hospitalized more often, receive 63 percent of all surgical operations, consume more drugs, are institutionalized more, and, in the 15 to 44 year age group, experience two and one half times more surgery. The dependence of the system is mutual insofar as women continue to use the system as a principle source of meeting their physiological and emotional needs (Marieskind, 1980). At first glance, it might seem as if this consumption of health and medical services contributes positively to the longevity of women. However, a closer look at the utilization patterns and the statistics reveals that women in the health care system are more often maltreated and sometimes victimized (Corea, 1977; Illich, 1976; Mendelsohn 1981).

The physician's role is to evaluate the complaints of the patient, assess the effect of any objective sounds, signs, and symptoms on the patient and to prescribe and manage care for them (Mechanic, 1976). The doctor–patient relationship can be conceived as an interaction wherein the axis of that interaction becomes the physician's knowledge and the patient's concerns. This interaction obviously rests within a particular social and economic context. A key element within the interaction is the fact that the patient concedes all authority to the physician and assumes an attitude of helplessness and submission to the dominant, superior physician. Literally, patients put themselves in the "hands of the doctor" (Mackenzie, 1979). Because most physicians are men and most patients are women, it becomes readily understandable how it is that this dyad can act out and mutually reinforce traditional and stereotyped images. In essence, both parties, women and physicians, act as they have been trained to act in the patient–physician encounter (Corea, 1977).

In the female world emotional expressiveness is encouraged; women are allowed to be and are more emotionally expressive than men. As part of their medical training, physicians are taught ways to repress their own emotions. Thus we have a situation in which the male physician whose emotional expression has been discouraged through the socialization process and repressed through his training, interacts with a woman who has been socialized quite differently (Notman & Nadelson, 1978). Hence, it is not surprising that physicians can easily misinterpret a woman's symptoms or complaints because not only do they not understand them, but the expression of emotion is also discomforting to them (Corea, 1977; Notman & Nadelson, 1978).

The health care system is a paternalistic one in which sexism abounds. Women are viewed and treated as being less valuable and important than men and are at a disadvantage when compared to men (Bermosk & Porter, 1979; Corea, 1977; Mendelsohn, 1981). In the system, women's problems are often not taken seriously, women are denied authority, power, and control, and often possess unrealistic, sometimes false, expectations of their omnipotent care giver (Bermosk & Porter, 1979).

Furthermore, women are often viewed as a problem by male physicians. In medical school physicians are taught to and do view women primarily through their reproductive function. And, a woman's expression of emotionalism is often labeled as hypochondriacal and the training and texts used perpetuate the myth of the traditional feminine role (Bermosk & Porter, 1979). Mendelsohn, in a recent work, provides an overview of medical practice as one that is characterized by medical and surgical overkill that is routinely inflicted on all Americans but whose "primary victims are women" (Mendelsohn, 1981, p. 10). According to Mendelsohn, male chauvinism pervades American medicine and sexist behavior of male physicians is at the heart of the abuse perpetuated on women. He maintains that women are victims of such things as dangerous and unnecessary surgery, overprescribing of mood altering drugs, and the prescribing of inadequately tested drugs and devices (Mendelsohn, 1981).

According to Marieskind (1980) much of what occurs today can be traced to the growth of the medical profession at the turn of the century and its growing respectability that encouraged increasing numbers of women to seek services. As part of this development, women, particularly the upper classes, came to be viewed as invalids or fragile and delicate. This view was supported by the medical profession, either through sexual surgery or prescribed therapies of inactivity and bedrest. Women became increasingly established as a patient class with promised cures from physicians. Furthermore, the shift of childbirth from home to hospitals, the development of physician-managed contraception, government programs providing prenatal care, third party insurance, and the growth of the medical industrial complex with its promotion of female symptoms and positive cures are all factors that have contributed to defining female morbidity. In the ensuing years, medical education has continued to perpetuate the view of women as being helpless and frail. This has been augmented by such things as medical text books that perpetuate the myths of the traditional female role, sexuality, and maternity care (Bermosk & Porter, 1979; Sculley & Bart, 1972).

Health Care Utilization. Women of all ages visit physicians 22 percent more than men and this figure doubles when visits to accompany children are counted (Marieskind, 1980). Women use the health care system to obtain relief from their distress. Three explanatory models exist to account for the differences in illness episodes and utilization rates: (1) women report illness more than men because it is culturally more acceptable for them to be ill, (2) the sick role is more compatible with women's other role responsibilities, and (3) women have more illness than men because their assigned social roles are more stressful (Mechanic, 1976; Nathanson, 1975, 1977). Yet, the exact interplay of all the possible factors and processes operant in this paradox have yet to be carefully analyzed. Marieskind (1979) believes that physicians have stimulated the need for treatment for conditions that they have constructed as being morbid. One example is menopause. Menopause, a natural physiological event in the reproductive cycle of women and one that is experienced by all women, has been transformed into a disease. Menopause as a disease has been so successfully marketed that American women believe that they must be "treated" for it by physicians and the treatment most often prescribed has been estrogens, which are now known to be carcinogenic (MacPherson, 1981).

The 1977 National Ambulatory Medical Care Survey, documenting office visits by women, is an interesting and provocative report that documents the need for further research on women's health. Some of the highlights of this report are the following:

- Approximately 79 percent of all women in the United States saw a physician at least once during 1977.
- During 1977 an estimated 295 million visits to office-based physicians were made by women 15 years and older, an average of 3.5 visits per woman per year. This rate increased with age. Men visited at the rate of 2.3 per visits per year.
- Approximately 18 percent of women's visits to physicians were for preventive services that included such things as pre- and postnatal care, gynecological examinations, Pap smears, family planning, and contraceptive advice.
- Approximately 40 percent of women's visits were to general and family practitioners and 17 percent to obstetrician/gynecologists.
- Women experienced a higher rate of surgery, 120.2 operations per 1000 women versus 77.8 per 1000 men. Thus, they visited physicians more often for medical and surgical aftercare than men.
- The data revealed that women with arthritis, rheumatism, obesity, and hypertension sought health care more often (67 percent higher rate) than men with the same conditions.
- Women sought health care for symptoms that were referable to psychological and mental disorders more often than men. These include anxiety, nervousness, depression, anger, marital problems, family problems, and social adjustment problems.
- In every age group the problems of men were, on the average, evaluated as serious or very serious proportionately more often than those of women.
- Women were more likely than men to receive specified instructions for a return visit.

What is presented is the picture of an enormous health care complex, dominated by male physicians and wherein women, trained to be submissive toward men, put themselves at increased risk for aggressive medical intervention which, it turns out, is not in their best interests and clearly causes them undue harm.

Unnecessary Surgery. Surgery is performed on women at a much higher rate than it is on men; 120.2 operations per 1000 women versus 77.8 operations per 1000 men (National Ambulatory Medical Care Survey, 1977) and hysterectomies account for much of the surgery on women. During the period from 1966 to 1975 the number of hysterectomies increased by 50 percent or 482,000 hysterectomies in 1966 versus 725,000 in 1977. These figures make hysterectomies the second leading surgical procedure in the United States, second only to dilatation and curettage (*Roundtable Report*, 1980). If the current trend continues, approximately 62 percent of all American women will have had a hysterectomy by the age of 70. Given the number of people involved and the expense of the procedure (considering average length of hospital stay, physician fees, and recovery period), the issue of hysterectomies has become a national one, although very little is known about it. However, one of the striking features of the hysterectomy issue is that 90 percent of them are considered elective (*Roundtable Report*, 1980). Despite strong criticism, government hearings, much lower rates in other countries, and popular press reports on unnecessary hysterectomies, the procedure continues to prevail at the same rate (Marieskind, 1980).

The rate of cesarean sections has increased by 198 percent between the years 1968 and 1978 according the National Hospital Discharge Survey. This astonishing rate persists in spite of the fact that the birth rate has declined in that same period by 17 percent. Marieskind (1979) indicates that the reasons for the rise in cesarean section are complex and that not one factor can be pinpointed to account for it, but, in her view, the increase can be accounted for by a complex interplay of the following factors:

1. Physicians' fear of a malpractice suit.
2. The unwillingness of physicians to go against standard obstetrical practice by allowing a trial of labor in women who have had a previous cesarean section. In other words, physicians are practicing by the early twentieth century norm of once a cesarean, always a cesarean.
3. Physician training, i.e., residents are not trained in normal obstetrics and therefore have little experience with such things as external version, vaginal breech deliveries, etc.
4. The shift in focus from mother to infant to obtain a perfect product and a heavy reliance on technology.
5. Changing indications insofar as more births are classified as complicated and therefore technological intervention is presumed warranted. This factor is also coupled with the reality that there are no uniform criteria for the indications of a cesarean.
6. Shifts in age, parity, and fertility of the child-bearing population. For example, older primiparous women have a higher risk of cesarean and are increasingly in the childbearing population.
7. Economic incentives related to the decreasing number of births and an increasing number of obstetricians.
8. The rising rate of available technology. Marieskind has extensively analyzed the issues concerned with the rise in cesarean section and the reader is referred to her work in this area (Marieskind, 1979) (see also Chapter 17).

Cosmetic Surgery. The majority of cosmetic surgery is done on women and is probably related to the so-called youth cult in our society. There are an estimated one million plastic surgeries performed annually to tuck tummies, augment breasts, and tighten sagging eyelids, chins, cheeks and almost any other part of the anatomy (Marieskind, 1980). Most of this cosmetic surgery is done on women and the cost can be high in both financial and physiological terms. Often, women who have this surgery are unaware of or do not seriously consider the possible complications that range from hemotomas, hair loss, sensory loss, hemorrhage, to facial nerve damage (Marieskind, 1979). Breast augmentation is a popular procedure performed on women and in the past has consisted of injecting liquid silicone enclosed in plastic between the breast tissue and the chest muscle. Up until recently, silicone was injected directly into the breast tissue but this has been found to be extremely dangerous and is now banned by the Food and Drug Administration. In spite of the ban on this practice, however, the practice continues, particularly in offices and clinics not subject to quality control (Marieskind, 1980).

Breast Cancer. Breast cancer is a leading killer of women in the United States. For example, in 1975 there were 40,000 deaths from breast cancer recorded and 90,000 new cases (*Roundtable Report*, 1979). Breast surgery accounts for some of the surgical procedures done on women. However, a controversy is raging about the appropriate treatment. The treatment available today ranges from no surgery to radical surgery with or without radiation and chemotherapy. This controversy and a lack of consensus among physicians puts a woman in a very vulnerable position vis-a-vis the protection of her rights. A part of the controversy has to do with the common practice of asking a woman to give permission preoperatively both for the biopsy and any procedure that the surgeon deems necessary depending on the biopsy results. Women have felt coerced into signing such a consent form and, therefore, are denied the opportunity of having the breast biopsy done, the knowledge of the results, and then the time to thoroughly discuss with their physicians the treatment alternatives, one of which may be surgery. Women with breast cancer have a right to make an informed decision about treatment, whether or not to have surgery, degree of "radicalness" of that surgery, and postoperative drug radiation or chemotherapy (see Chapter 23 for additional information and controversies).

The major issue surrounding the question of whether or not all surgery performed on women is necessary relates directly to the concept of informed consent and whether or not women are given free choice in the matter of surgery, after having been fully informed of all the alternatives and the implications of all those alternatives. The evidence that has accumulated to date leads to the conclusion that women are not given free choice in these matters. Rather, they surrender the decision making about their bodies and their ultimate welfare to the physician whom they view as omnipotent and, thereby, relinquish the opportunity to exert control over themselves, their bodies, and their future well-being.

Contraception. Historically, the burden for preventing unwanted births has rested with women. It is important to note that contraceptive devices and information about contraception has been impeded by numerous social, medical, and legal events that are tied to the traditional role of women as mothers and the traditional childbearing function of women. In the United States the contraceptive information became fully available after the opening of Margaret Sanger's clinic in 1916. In addition, there were laws that prevented the distribution of contraceptive devices, the majority of which were struck down in 1936, except in Connecticut and Massachusetts whose law remained on the books until 1965 and 1966 (Marieskind, 1980).

Many cite the advances in contraceptive technology as one of the primary factors contributing to women's gaining power over their reproductive functioning and the movement of women outside the home. Nonetheless, the contraceptive technology that freed women from unwanted pregnancies has been the source of serious and sometimes lethal side effects.

Only recently have women been afforded contraception that begins to meet the ideal criteria: a low or nonexistent pregnancy rate, easy to use, apart from the act of intercourse, safe, cheap, and reversible. The advent of the Pill and intrauterine device (IUD) are two developments that have brought contraception closest to meeting the ideal. However, both of these methods carry with them numerous side effects resulting in serious problems for women.

The Pill, although coming close to meeting all the criteria for a perfect contraceptive, carries with it significant risks. The reported side effects of the Pill to date involve conditions ranging from minor to major in all of the major physiological systems, including the cardiovascular, gastrointestinal, and neurological. In addition, the risks of the Pill seem to be magnified when taken in combination with other medications or in women who smoke or are over 30 (Marieskind, 1980).

The IUD, a low cost, relatively effective, and convenient contraceptive, has enjoyed widespread usage. Like the Pill, however, the IUD carries with it a certain amount of risk. One brand of the IUD, the Dalkon Shield, introduced in January 1971, was the subject of a class action suit and has been withdrawn from the market by the Food and Drug Administration. The Dalkon Shield was not tested adequately before it was released to the market and has been responsible for serious side effects, such as pelvic inflammatory disease that has affected some 1,100,000 women, 17 of whom have died. To date, $55 million has been paid by the manufacturer's insurance company to victims of side effects of the Dalkon Shield (Mendelsohn, 1981).

For whatever reasons, it has become obvious that some contraceptives have been inadequately tested and the effect of that inadequate testing has caused harm to women. Whether the reasons are centered about the tremendous desire of women to have control over their fertility combined with increasing technological advances, or whether it is more related to a somewhat cavalier attitude on the part of physicians, manufacturers, and drug companies toward women is unknown.

Mental Health. The fact that women have not fared well in the mental health system has become increasingly clear since the landmark study by Broverman and associates (1970) of clinicians' attitudes. Clinicians in this study believed that healthy women differed from men and viewed them as being more submissive, less independent, less adventurous, more suggestable, less competitive, more excitable in minor crisis, more likely to have their feelings easily hurt, more emotional, more conceited about personal appearance, less objective, and less logical than healthy men. The conclusion reached by Broverman was that for a woman to be declared healthy, she must adjust to and accept the behavioral norms for women in our culture, although those norms are less socially desirable and considered to be less healthy than those for the competent, mature adult, which are also the norms associated with maleness. This, then, places a woman in a conflictual situation of whether to exhibit socially desirable mentally healthy, albeit male, attitudes and have her femininity questioned, or to conform to the expectations for women and be viewed as not fulfilling the most desired personal qualities (Broverman, Broverman, & Clarkson, 1970).

Since this landmark study, the subject of sexual stereotyping and therapists' attitudes has been the subject of considerable discussion and research. Sherman (1980) reviewed this empirical work and concluded that, in spite of the many studies flawed by such factors as design problems, variables questionably related to the concept of sexual sterotyping, and biased samples, a therapist's sex role values do operate during therapy and the counseling process and, furthermore, that behavior that does not conform to sexual norms are maladjusted. In addition, Sherman (1980) found evidence in her analysis to support the idea that therapists have inadequate knowledge related to issues that most affect the lives of women.

The opportunity for women to be mistreated in the mental health system emerges from the therapists' lack of understanding, the devalued social position of women in relation to men, negative sanctions imposed on women who do not conform to the traditional female role, the inability to accept a woman's expression of anger at her situation, and the relative disadvantages of women who are married and have children (Carmen, Russo, & Miller, 1981).

Sex bias and sex role stereotyping affect the mental health services delivery system in paradoxical ways insofar as women can be considered to be both underserved and overserved by the system. For disorders considered congruent with sex role sterotypes such as depression, hysteria, conversion, and phobias, women show higher rates of service utilization than do men. However, services that deal with problems that are incongruent with the ideological views of women (and men), such as the aftereffects of rape, incest, and wife abuse, are being ignored. Furthermore, alcohol and drug addiction services also show women to be underserved (Carmen, Russo, & Miller, 1981).

Evidence gathered since the landmark Broverman study in 1970 clearly points to the reality that women are not optimally treated in our mental health care system. Therapists operate from their own perspective shaped by having been socialized in a culture that has definite and different sex role expectations for men and women. This socialization has also been reinforced by their training and they are often employed in mental health care settings that are structured to respond to traditional, societal views of men and women. In addition, theories of human development that form the theoretical foundations upon which therapists base their interventions either lack information or contain misinformation about women.

Women are best served when they actively seek out services and therapists that are dedicated to a nonsexist or feminist ideology. These terms are sometimes used interchangeably. There is a clear distinction between them, however, insofar as feminist therapy incorporates the political and philosophical values of the women's movement whereas nonsexist therapy does not. Nonsexist therapy recognizes the social structure as having produced problems for women but is more dedicated to treating women (and men) from a humanistic perspective (Collier, 1982). Women who feel the need for psychological services need to take an active role in the selection of a therapist who will provide them with optimal, nonsexist services.

Iatrogenic Drug Abuse. Women are using, and often becoming addicted to, drugs at an alarming rate. And, in contrast to men who more often obtain their drugs illegally, women become addicted to drugs that are obtained through prescriptions written by their physicians. Some believe that, as drugs proliferate and health care becomes more fragmented, overprescribing becomes commonplace and that an insidious epidemic is raging among women who are addicted to all kinds of mood altering drugs prescribed by their general physician (as compared to a psychiatrist who is trained to treat altered mood states) to relieve the stresses of daily living such as transition times, loneliness, social isolation, and situations that diminish self-confidence (Nellis, 1980).

A study done in a family practice clinic in Canada (Cooperstock, 1978) compared the treatment given to men and women who came to the clinic with the same emotional symptoms such as crying, nervousness, and depression. The study found that men were *more likely* than women to be sent for laboratory tests or to be given physical therapy and men and women were equally likely to be referred for counseling or social services. However, the major difference in the prescribed therapeutic regimen was that women received significantly more minor tranquilizer prescriptions than did men. Over time, this difference between the groups increased.

Few published works contain information about female drug use/misuse (Bowker, 1977). Related information is available through the review of the literature on alcohol abuse in women because many women are "cross addicted" to alcohol and drugs (Dowling & MacLennan, 1977; Schuckit & Morrissey, 1979). Research into the etiology of female alcoholism falls into the following major categories: early childhood deprivations, the empty nest syndrome, maladaptive sex role performance, and female physiology (Beckman, 1978, 1976, 1975; Belfer, 1971; Bell, 1978; Curlee, 1970; Gomberg, 1974; Kiel, 1978; Lindbeck, 1972; Parker, 1972; Pattison & Sobell, 1977; Podolsky, 1963; Rathod & Thompson, 1971; Schuckit, 1972; Schuckit & Morrissey, 1979, 1976; Schuckit et al., 1969; Wanberg & Horn, 1970; Wanberg & Knapp, 1970). The drug abuse literature on women contains recurring themes relating to mood states, sex roles, sexist views of care providers, and social circumstances.

Schuckit and Morrissey (1979) studied 329 women who were admitted to an alcoholic treatment center and found that two-thirds of them had received prescription drugs, usually hypnotic and antianxiety, from their physicians (one-third had been abusing the prescription drugs). Eighty percent of these women received prescriptions for potentially dangerous drugs while they were actively abusing alcohol.

Jhindmarch (1972) concludes that middle-aged women are at special risk with regard to drug abuse. He maintains that a woman's difficulties in adjusting to middle age produce depression, anxiety, and sleeplessness for which physicians tend to prescribe psychoactive drugs. Furthermore, these complaints are not transient situations, because 50 percent of the patients who had prescriptions for amphetamines or barbiturates had had refills for 4 years or longer (Jhindmarch, 1972).

In one study 87 percent of physicians believed that prescribing Librium to housewives for nervousness was legitimate but not legitimate for "stressed" physicians or anxious college students (Linn, 1971).

Basically, the interaction between a woman and her physician and the resultant prescribing of mood altering drugs begins with the readiness of a woman to seek medical care for her complaints. As previously mentioned, women are socialized to view physicians (mostly men) as being all-powerful and wise. They go to them with their physical complaints and also express emotion. Physicians, in turn, treat their somatic and emotional complaints with mood altering drugs. There is little evidence that physicians take a woman's expression of, for example, loneliness or unhappiness, seriously or that they recommend appropriate counseling. Rather, the expression of emotion reaffirms the physician's view of women as hysterical, dependent, inept, and unable to cope, and is sufficient justification for prescribing mood altering drugs or advising patients to "have a few drinks and relax."

Drug advertisements appearing in medical journals reinforce sexist assumptions in the minds of the readers. Corea (1977) analyzed advertisements in medical journals over a 5-year period and found that the ads tended to associate psychoactive drugs with female patients and nonpsychoactive drugs with male patients.

Housewives are depicted in drug advertisements in medical journals as being oppressed, unfulfilled, and imprisoned. The recommended solution given to the physician reader is to prescribe psychoactive drugs for her rather than to suggest psychological help, social action, or liberation (Seidenberg, 1976).

The 1978 Congressional Hearings on drug abuse in women also supported this contention. At these hearings, several expert witnesses provided vivid, detailed descriptions and examples of the advertising material obtained from medical journals that reinforced sexual stereotypes, thereby encouraging physicians to prescribe mood altering drugs for women. The major point made by those giving testimony was that the Madison Avenue hype advertising encourages physicians to prescribe drugs rather than listen to women and treat their symptoms and life circumstances seriously. The 1978 Congressional Hearings on drug abuse reviewed the federal effort in the treatment of drug abuse and heard expert testimony related to federal treatment programs, public opinion, the media, and high-risk populations. The following statistics related to women were part of that testimony.

- Each year more than 200 million prescriptions are written for tranquilizers, analgesics, barbiturates, and amphetamines. Women receive twice as many of these prescriptions as men.
- Among young people the use of psychotherapeutic drugs among women is increasing at the same rate as the use among men.
- In three major cities in Texas in 1977, the largest percentage of overdose cases were of women and the drug most involved was Valium.
- 5 million women are estimated to have alcohol or substance abuse problems.
- 43 percent of drug-related deaths are female.
- 11 million women took tranquilizers or amphetamines for the first time in 1977.
- In 1974 there were 27.9 million new and 50 million refill prescriptions for Valium and Librium. Over two-thirds of these prescriptions were for women.
- More than 60 percent of all nonpsychoactive drugs and 67 percent of psychoactive drugs are prescribed for women.
- 61 percent of Valium and Librium prescriptions were prescribed by physicians for women (this excludes psychiatric prescriptions).

A 10-year survey of advertisements in medical journals showed that advertisements "push" psychotrophic drugs as the treatment of choice, and they resonate with male anti-female prejudices (Seidenberg, 1976).

From a societal point of view, the consequences of women being a high-risk group for legal drug abuse are monumental. Obviously, there are long-range consequences for the individual woman, but, because women are the primary care providers of young children, the consequences for children who are parented by women in various stages of sedation are also serious. The long-range effects of this level of drug consumption on family life and future generations are unknown, but obviously significant.

Yet, in spite of what appears to be growing evidence of a problem of epidemic proportions, little is known of specific personal or situational factors leading to the prescribing of mood altering drugs, which is too often the first step to the more serious problem of addiciton for women.

WHAT CAN BE DONE?

It should be clear to the reader that women are highly vulnerable to victimization in our culture. Their socialization into a subordinate position results in a diminished self-esteem whereby women feel disenfranchised. Then women, like other members of disenfranchised groups, have difficulty knowing and exercising their rights, and thereby decreasing the probability of becoming a victim. The rights that women need to know and exercise are those human rights that belong to all people in our society, some specific legal rights of women and the legal rights of patients.

Women's Rights. Historically, a great deal of the discrimination against women has been supported by the legal system (Ross & Barcher, 1983). In 1848 the subject of the first women's conference was the low, separate, and unequal status that existed for women at that time, especially married women. Since that first women's conference there have been efforts on the part of feminists to change the laws so that women would enjoy the same constitutional protection that men do. The past 10 years have seen many changes brought about by pressure from feminists. The 1970s were marked by changes in the interpretation of the constitution, the striking down of sex discriminatory laws and practices, and the establishment of new laws outlawing discrimination (Ross & Barcher, 1983). Much progress has been made in spite of the fact that efforts to amend the constitution to provide an equal rights amendment (ERA) have failed. The constitutional doctrine that has been used to create the new laws and strike down existing sexual discrimination laws and practices is the fourteenth amendment. This amendment declares that no state may deny to any person equal protection under the laws (Ross & Barcher, 1983). The equal protection clause, as it is known, has been used to combat discriminatory practices directed against minority groups. It is illegal to segregate jobs by sex, pay men more than women, deny women access to the same educational opportunities as men, arbitrarily deny women credit, or force a woman to use her husband's name. The changes have been the result of individual women filing official complaints of unfair discriminatory practices and receiving judgments in their favor.

Of particular relevance to this chapter is the interpretation of the rights of a woman to control her own body, especially related to birth control, abortion, and sterilization. Two landmark legal decisions were rendered in 1973 and declared that a woman had the right to choose whether or not she will have children. Basically, those legal decisions interpreted the Constitution's statement about rights to privacy to mean that the decision to have or to not have children was a private decision that could be made by a woman alone or in consultation with her physician. These decisions struck down the restrictive abortion laws that existed in most states. Since 1973, however, laws have been enacted in various states in an attempt to regulate abortion clinics, and thus make abortion less available. To date the previous restrictive abortion laws remain outlawed but various, so called "right-to-life" groups have modified the law insofar as they have been successful in getting Congress to vote that federal medicaid funds could not be used for abortions (Ross & Barcher, 1983).

A very important aspect of a woman's right to abortion is that her husband's consent to have one is not necessary. In addition, women have the right to be sterilized, which can also be obtained without a husband's approval.

It is important that women fully understand their rights so that they can exercise them and avoid occurrences over which they feel they have little control.

In addition to legal rights, it is important for women to realize that they have a right to: be treated with respect, i.e., not be degraded, shamed, or humiliated; refuse something without making excuses or feeling guilty; receive information they need to make an informed decision; and to be human and able to express human emotions without becoming labeled or degraded in any way (Chenevert, 1978).

Patients' Rights. Being given complete and accurate information is a key element in understanding the rights of patients vis-a-vis their physicians. The rights of patients derive not only from various legal statutes but, also, from the American Hospital Association's Patient's Bill of Rights, the Joint Commission on Accreditation of Hospitals' (JCAH) Standards, and the American Medical Association principles of medical ethics (Annas, 1975). Patients have a right to be given information related to their diagnosis, treatment, and prognosis. That information is needed to provide their informed consent for treatment. Undergirding all of the specific rights of patients is the concept of self-determination, that is, patients have a right to be self-determined and they, rather than their physician, have the right to determine what happens to them.

That fundamental right is supported by various and specific state legal statutes as well as ethical statements (Annas, 1975).

Not only do patients have certain rights, but those rights *cannot* be defined as subordinate to the physician. Patients have equal rights with physicians, that is, patients have the right to choose their treatment and the right to refuse any treatment. A physician "may not treat a patient until he has explained to the patient the risks and material facts concerning the treatment and its alternatives, including nontreatment, and has secured the patient's competent, voluntary, and understanding consent to proceed" (Annas, 1975, p. 57). In understanding the concept of patients' rights, it must be presumed that all patients are capable of dealing with complete disclosure and, therefore, physicians are obliged to provide a patient with all available relevant information. Furthermore, this information must be provided in understandable, clear, and nontechnical language (Annas, 1975).

A full and complete understanding of women's and patient's rights will go a long way to help women avoid being victimized. However, there are other behavioral characteristics that must be combined with a knowledge of her rights so that a woman can fully exercise her options. Primarily, this refers to the capability of a woman to be assertive.

Strategies for Self-determination. The strategies that are needed to work with women to help them avoid becoming victimized are education, consciousness raising, assertiveness, conflict resolution, and communication skills.

Education. Women need to learn about themselves, their bodies, the sex role socialization process, and the potential problems that they may encounter. The more information a woman has the more able she will be to determine the course most suitable for her, and one that will optimize her own well-being. It is probably critical to begin education aimed at preventing victimization in childhood. Girls need special assistance to express their opinions, to be assertive, and to resist maltreatment. Educating parents and teachers about the potential for victimization of women will facilitate less maltreatment of women in the future.

Teaching can be conducted on a one-to-one basis or in a group setting. Patient education can occur in more or less formal ways, but it is important to be aware of the necessity to include in any educational program for women the psychosocial factors that have had and still do have an effect on women. In general, women are eager to learn, as evidenced by the growth of women's health care collectives and the popularity of publications for women such as *Our Bodies, Ourselves* (Boston Women's Health Book Collective, 1973). Women are an eager audience and health care providers should capitalize on this exciting quality of the learner. The reader will find detailed information about the various educational strategies elsewhere in this book (see Chapters 2 and 3). The use of adult learning strategies may assist women to experience control, gain confidence in their own abilities, and "practice" using their own abilities and knowledge. It is these skills that assist women to resist victimization.

Consciousness Raising. Consciousness raising is a process by which women can be made more aware of the social and cultural forces that have shaped their emotional growth and development. Central to consciousness raising is the analysis and understanding of sex roles in society and, therefore, the common sources of conflict and dissatisfaction for women. It is a process by which conflict and dissatisfaction are identified and understood in terms of a social structure (e.g., legal and educational system, religious groups), rather than in terms of individual intrapersonal or intrapsychic phenomena. In essence, consciousness raising is a form of resocialization (Kirsh, 1974). It is designed to promote personal and social change. Consciousness raising functions to develop an awareness in women of those feminine roles and behaviors into which they have been socialized, their minority group status, the discrimination and prejudice that emerges from that status, and the "personal" problems that emanate from their status and role.

Consciousness raising has traditionally occurred in groups. These groups of women share their individual feelings and needs, focus on the common nature of individual concerns, examine the social order to find the root of their problems, reinforce and support each other to make personal and social changes, and analyze the position of women in our culture and the various ways of changing that status (Kirsh, 1974).

Assertiveness. Assertiveness and assertiveness training for the development of a set of social skills have become very popular topics for women and women's issues. Assertiveness is defined in many ways, but generally includes the ability to stand up for one's own rights, being able to express one's own views, and effective verbal skills (Linehan & Eagan, 1979). Assertion is often contrasted to aggression with the main difference between the two being that aggression contains an element of coercion or denying other people their rights. Assertion or assertiveness is the expression of a person's own wants and preferences without interfering with another person's rights to express individual needs and preferences. Assertiveness and assertiveness training includes various exercises to develop the ability:*

- To express personal needs, wants, preferences, opinions, beliefs, and thoughts
- To express emotions other than anxiety
- To say no
- To ask for favors and make requests
- To express positive *and* negative emotions
- To initiate, continue, and terminate conversations

Assertiveness and assertiveness training also include the development of a certain type of interpersonal style or a presentation of one's self that includes both verbal and nonverbal elements. The verbal elements are those of being direct, open, and comfortable; the nonverbal elements include direct eye contact, a sufficiently audible voice volume, and a facility with words. In addition, assertiveness also involves being brief and unembellished (Linehan & Eagan, 1979).

Assertiveness training has been a popular topic addressed to women because it is believed that women, in deference to men and in response to their subordinate status, have assumed a passive, nonassertive role in their daily lives and activities. This lack of assertiveness is a key element in their vulnerability.

There are a number of assertiveness books for laymen that are available in most bookstores. A sample of these follows:

- Alberte, R. E., & Emmons, M. L. *Your perfect right: A guide to assertive behavior*. San Louis Obispo, Calif.: Impact Publishers, 1970.
- Alberte, R. E., & Emmons, M. L. *Stand up, speak out, talk back!* New York: Pocket Books, 1975.

Source: From Linehan & Egan, 1979.

- Baer, J. *How to be an assertive (not aggressive) woman in life, love and on the job*. New York: New American Library, 1976.
- Fensterheim, H. *Don't say yes when you want to say no*. New York: Dell, 1975.
- Smith, M. J. *When I say no, I feel guilty*. New York: The Dial Press, 1975.
- Taubman, B. *How to become an assertive women*. New York: Pocket Books, 1976.
- *Assert your self, a handbook about assertiveness training for women*. Available from Seattle King County National Organization for Women (N.O.W.), 2252 NE 65th St., Seattle, WA 98115.

Conflict resolution. Conflict is a clash or mutual interference of opposing forces. Interpersonal conflict, the conflict or the clash that occurs between two people, is relevant to this chapter. The ability to resolve conflict is a skill often lacking in violent families and, often, conflict precedes a woman being beaten by her husband. That is not to say that it is always the situation that unresolved conflict causes a beating, but it is a factor in marital relationships and individuals are more or less able to resolve it. The ability to resolve conflict is not totally separate from the ability to be assertive and to express one's needs and wants without denying the other person in the relationship the opportunity to express individual needs and wants. When conflict escalates to the point where a solution to the problem seems impossible, then the opportunity for physical violence becomes greater. Warner (1981) sees physical violence occurring at the end of a five-step process: first, a stressful or conflict situation occurs followed by unsuccessful attempts to deal with the conflict, which then results in increased frustration and anger or depression, and is followed by an act of loss of control and, finally, assault. It is reasonable to assume that if both parties in a situation possessed more effective coping skills or resources their conflict might not escalate to the point of violence. Successful conflict resolution requires that both parties be able to do the following:

- Understand that conflict is normal.
- Succinctly, clearly, and unemotionally express perceptions, points of view, and desires.
- Remain calm, keep voice level audible, and avoid hollering, shouting, or screaming.
- Avoid the use of emotionally charged words.
- Validate that what is being said is being heard.
- Avoid making contradictory statements.
- Understand the other person's point of view.
- Listen carefully to the other person without interrupting.
- Try to leave the situation if the interaction gets "heated."
- Find a compromise to the competing points of view, wishes, or desires.
- Avoid forcing compliance.
- Postpone further discussion if it appears unlikely that a compromise is going to be negotiated at that time.
- Maintain open communication.

Summary

Women are victimized and, in part, that is preventable. The status of women and women's roles in our society is changing rapidly and more and more women are seeking the means to make major personal changes. Health care providers can play a major role in helping women change in ways that will decrease their vulnerability to being victimized. Nurses especially encounter women, most of whom have had some experience in which they were mistreated in all settings. Nurses can help women become aware, not only of their own personal mistreatment, but also of the potential mistreatment that exists for all women. Nurses can educate women about their roles and status and can provide them with information to help them gain the skills necessary to assume greater power in their lives and to help them to become more self-determined. Nurses, as health care providers, can treat women differently; they can develop a cooperative rather than dominant–submissive relationship with them and, thereby, teach women by example, and give them an opportunity to participate fully in their own health care.

Of course, men and men's roles must also change. However, men will not willingly and easily give up their superior status. Why would they? Women, however, can force some changes by behaving differently and taking the opportunity to victimize away from men. Women can also work to change the social structure that perpetuates their subordinate position. Nurses can do this through their work with women and also through their efforts as members of a female-dominated profession.

Women, as a group, must stop being victimized. Victimization functions to diminish a woman's sense of personal worth, self-esteem, and perceived competence. Consequently, these changes prevent women from making optimal contributions to their own lives, the lives of their families, and to society. Nurses by providing appropriate education can help women break old patterns and to become more self-determined. Nurses must also have knowledge of all community resources that can provide services to women victims, to minimize the ill effects of the victimization and to assist women in gaining strength and power with which to resist further mistreatment. Most communities offer counseling and support service for victims. For example, rape crisis, shelters and hotlines for battered women, support groups for single parents, incest victims, welfare mothers, victims assistance, and so on.

Below is a short list of national organizations that serve as resource for women victims and from whom further information may be obtained.*

Center for Women's Policy Studies, 200 P St., N.W., Suite 508, Washington, D. C. 20036. *(Dedicated to increasing public awareness and affecting national policy change on issues involving women.)*
National Coalition Against Domestic Violence, P.O. Box 40132, Portland, OR 97240. *(The coalition has a commitment to address the problem of domestic violence through the support of community-based, direct service programs that involve battered women in the decision-making process.)*
Women's Equity Action League (WEAL), 805 15th St., N. W., Suite 822, Washington, D.C. 20005, (202) 5638-1961. *(Lobbies for pending legislation on battered women.)*
Women's Resource Network, 4025 Chestnut St., Philadelphia, PA 19104. *(Offers training and consultation to law enforcement and criminal justice systems on coping with domestic violence; consultation and education for practitioners and administrative personnel within the mental health and social service fields on counseling victims of abuse; development of workshops, seminars, conferences, and curriculum related to violence in the family; and research and evaluation projects focusing in family violence.)*

BIBLIOGRAPHY

Amir, M. *Patterns in forcible rape*. Chicago: University of Chicago Press, 1971.
Annas, G. J. *The rights of hospital patients*. New York: The American Civil Liberties Union, 1975.
Battered women: Issues of public policy. Proceedings of a consultation sponsored by the U. S. Commission on Civil Rights, Washington, D.C. January 30–31, 1978.

*Source: *Battered women: Issues of public policy*. Proceedings of a consultation sponsored by the U. S. Commission on Civil Rights, Washington, D.C., January 30–31, 1978.

Beckman, L. J. Sex role conflict in alcoholic women: Myth or reality. *Journal of Abnormal Psychology*, 1978, 87, 408–417.

Beckman, L. J. Alcoholism problems and women: An overview. In J. A. Schuckit (Ed.), *Alcoholism problems in women and children*. New York: Grune & Stratton, 1976.

Beckman, L. J. Women alcoholics: A review of social and psychological studies. *Journal of Studies on Alcohol*, 1975, 36(7), 797–823.

Belfer, M. L., Shader, R. I., & Carroll, M., & Harmatz, J. S. Alcoholism in women. *Archives of General Psychiatry*, 1971, 25, 540–544.

Bell, R. G. The chemically dependent woman: An overview of the problem. In J. Dowsling & A. MacLennan (Eds.), *The chemically dependent woman*. Toronto: Addiction Research Foundation, 1978.

Bermosk, L., & Porter, S. *Women's health and human wholeness*. New York: Appleton-Century-Crofts, 1979.

Bernard, J. *The female world*. New York: The Free Press, 1981.

Bardwick, J. M., & Dauvan, E. Ambivalence: The socialization of women. In V. Gornick & B. Maran (Eds.), *Women in sexist society*. New York: Basic Books, 1971.

Boston Women's Health Book Collective. *Our bodies, ourselves: A book by and for women*. New York: Simon & Schuster, 1973.

Boudouris, J. Homicide and the family. *Journal of Marriage and the Family*, 1971, 33, 667–676.

Bowker, L. *Drug use among American women, old and young: Sexual oppression and other themes*. San Francisco: R & E Research Associates, 1977.

Broverman, I. K., Broverman, D. M., Clarkson, F. E., Resenkrantz, P., & Vagel, S. R. Sex role stereotypes and clinical judgment of mental health. *Journal of Consulting Clinical Psychology*, 1970, 34, 1–7.

Brownmiller, S. *Against our will*. New York: Simon & Schuster, 1975.

Burgess, A. W., & Holstrom, L. L. *Rape: Victims of crisis*. Bowie, Md.: Robert J. Brady, 1974.

Carmen, E. H., Russo, N., & Miller, J. B. Inequality of women's mental health. *American Journal of Psychiatry*, 1981, 138(10), 1319–1330.

Chenevert, M. *Special techniques in assertiveness training for women in the health professions*. St. Louis, Mo.: C. V. Mosby, 1978.

Collier, H. C. *Counseling women*. New York: The Free Press, 1982.

Cooperstock, R. Women and psychotropic drug use. In J. Dowsling & A. MacLennan (Eds.), *The chemically dependent woman*. Toronto: Addiction Research Foundation, 1978, 33–39.

Corea, G. *The hidden malpractice*. New York: William Morrow, 1977.

Csida, J. B., & Csida, J. *Rape: How to avoid it and what to do about it if you can't*. Chatsworth, Calif.: Books for Better Living, 1974.

Curlee, J. A comparison of male and female patients at an alcoholism treatment center. *Journal of Psychology*, 1970, 74, 239–247.

Dick and Jane as Victims. Princeton, N.J.: Women on Words and Images, 1980.

Dowling, C. *The cinderella complex*. New York: Summitt Books, 1981.

Dowsling, J., & MacLennan, A. *The chemically dependent woman*. Toronto: Addiction Research Foundation, 1977.

Drug Abuse Treatment, Part I & II. Hearings Before the Select Committee on Narcotics Abuse and Control, House of Representatives, 95th Congress Second Session, June 14, 15, & 22, 1978. Washington, D.C.: U.S. Government Printing Office, 1978.

Gelles, R. J. *The violent home: A study of physical aggression between husbands and wives*. Beverly Hills, Calif.: Sage, 1974.

Gelles, R. J., & Straus, M. Family experience and public support of the death penalty. *American Journal of Orthopsychiatry*, 1975, 45(4), 497–613.

Gomberg, E. S. Women and alcoholism. In V. Franks (Ed.), *Women in therapy*. New York: Brunner/Mazel, 1974.

Gornick, V. Woman as outsider. In V. Gornick & B. K. Maran (Eds.), *Women in sexist society*. New York: Basic Books, 1971.

Illich, I. *Medical nemesis*. New York: Random House/Bantam Books, 1976.

Jhindmarch, J. Drugs and their abuse—Age groups particularly in risk. *British Journal of Addictions*, 1972, 67(3), 209–214.

Kiel, I. J. Sex role variation and women's drinking. *Journal of Studies on Alcohol*, 1978, 39(5), 859–868.

Kirsh, B. Consciousness-raising groups as therapy for women. In V. Franks (Ed.), *Women in therapy*. New York: Brunner/Mazel, 1974, pp. 327–352.

Lebinger, G. Physical abuse among applicants for divorce. In S. K. Steinmetz & M. Straus (Eds.), *Violence in the family*. New York: Harper & Row, 1974, pp. 85–88.

Lindbeck, V. L. The woman alcoholic: A review of the literature. *International Journal of the Addictions*, 1972, 7(3), 567–580.

Linehan, M. M., & Egan, K. J. Assertion training for women. In A. S. Bellack & M. Hersen (Eds.), *Research and practice in social skills training*. New York: Plenum Press, 1979, pp. 237–268.

Linn, L. S. Physician characteristics and attitudes toward legitimate use of psychotherapeutic drugs. *Journal of Health and Human Behavior*, 1971, 12(6), 132–140.

MacPherson, K. Menopause as disease: The social construction of a metaphor. *Advances in Nursing Science*, 1981, 4(2), 95–113.

Mackenzie, W. J. *Power and responsibility in health care*. Oxford, Great Britain: Oxford University Press, 1979.

Marieskind, H. I. *Women in the health care system*. St. Louis, Mo.: C. V. Mosby, 1980.

Marieskind, H. I. *An evaluation of caesarean sections in the U. S*. Washington D.C.: U.S. Dept. of Health Education & Welfare, 1979.

Martin, D. *Battered wives*. San Francisco: Glide, 1976.

Mechanic, D. Sex, illness, illness behavior and the use of health services. *Journal of Human Stress*, 1976, 4, 29–40.

Mendelsohn, R. S. *Malpractice*. Chicago: Contemporary Books, 1981.

Nathanson, C. A. Sex, illness, and medical care: A review of data, theory, and method. *Social Science and Medicine*, 1977, 11, 13–25.

Nathanson, C. A. Illness and the feminine role: A theoretical review. *Social Science and Medicine*, 1975, 9, 57–62.

National Ambulatory Medical Care Survey. *Office visits by women*, 1977.

National Center for Health Statistics. National hospital discharge survey 1968–1977. Washington, D.C.: U. S. Government Printing Office, 1977.

Nellis, M. *The female fix*. Boston: Houghton Mifflin, 1980.

Notman, M. T., & Nadelson, C. The woman patient. In M. T. Notman & C. Nadelson (Eds.), *The woman patient—Medical and psychologic interfaces*. New York: Plenum, 1978.

O'Brien, J. E. Violence in divorce prone families. In S. K. Steinmetz & M. Straus (Eds.), *Violence in the family*. New York: Harper & Row, 1974, pp. 65–75.

Parker, F. B. Sex role adjustment in women alcoholics. *Quarterly Journal of Studies on Alcoholism*, 1972, 33, 647–657.

Pattison, E. M., Sobell, M. B., & Sobell, L. D. *Emerging concepts of alcohol dependence*. New York: Springer, 1977.

Podolsky, E. The woman alcoholic and premenstrual tension. *Journal of the American Medical Woman's Association*, 1963, 18, 816–818.

Rathod, N. H., & Thomson, I. G. Women alcoholics: A clinical study. *Quarterly Journal Studies of Alcoholism*, 1971, 32, 45–52.

Ross, S. D., & Barcher, A. *The rights of women*. New York: Bantam, 1983.

Roy, M. A current survey of 150 cases. In M. Roy (Ed.), *Battered women: A psychosociological study of domestic violence*. New York: Van Nostrand Reinhold, 1977, pp. 25–44.

Russell, D. E. N. *The politics of rape: The victim's perspective*. Briarcliff Manor, N.Y.: Stein & Day, 1975.

Sculley, D., & Bart, P. A funny thing happened on the way to the orifice: Women in gynecology textbooks. *American Journal of Sociology*, 1972, 78(4), 1045–1050.

Schuckit, M. The alcoholic woman: A literature review. *Psychiatry in Medicine*, 1972, 3(1), 37–43.

Schuckit, M., & Morrissey, E. Drug abuse among alcoholic women. *American Journal of Psychiatry*, 1979, *136*(4B), 607–610.

Schuckit, M., & Morrissey, E. Psychiatric problems in women admitted to an alcoholic detoxification center. *American Journal of Psychiatry*, 1979, *136*(4B), 611–616.

Schuckit, M., & Morrissey, E. Alcoholism in women: Some clinical and perspectives with an emphasis on possible subtypes. In M. A. Schuckit (Ed.), *Alcoholism problems in women and children*. New York: Grune & Stratton, 1976, pp. 5–35.

Schuckit, M. A., Pitts, R. N. Jr., Reich, T., King, L. J., & Winokur, G. Alcoholism: Two types of alcoholism in women. *Archives of General Psychiatry*, 1969, *20*, 301–306.

Seidenberg, R. Advertising and drug acculturation. In R. H. Coombs, L. J. Fry & P. G. Lewis (Eds.), *Socialization and drug abuse*. Cambridge, Mass.: 1976.

Seligman, M. Learned helplessness. In A. C. DeGroff & W. P. Cregar (Eds.), *Annual Review of Medicine*, 1972, *23*, 407–411.

Sherman, J. Therapists attitudes and sex role stereotyping. In A. Bradsky & R. H. Mustin (Eds.), *Women and psychiatry*. New York: Guilford Press, 1980, pp. 35–67.

Steinmetz, S. K., & Straus, M. A. *Violence in the family*. New York: Harper & Row, 1974.

Straus, M. A. Wife beating: How common and why? *Victimology*, 1978, *2*, 443–458.

Straus, M. A. A sociological perspective on the prevention and treatment of wife beating. In M. Roy (Ed.), *Battered women: A psychosociological study of domestic violence*. New York: Van Nostrand Reinhold, 1977, pp. 194–238.

Thompson, K., & Michael, A. *Against rape*. New York: Farrar, Strauss & Girous, 1974.

Tyler, S. L., & Woodall, G. M. *Female health and gynecology across the life span*. Bowie, Md.: Robert J. Brady, 1982.

Voss, H. L., & Hepburn, J. R. Patterns in criminal homicide in Chicago. *Journal of Criminal Law, Criminology and Police Science*, 1968, *59*, 488–508.

Walker, L. Battered women and learned helplessness. *Victimology*, 1977, *2*, 525–534.

Wanberg, K. W., & Horn, J. L. Alcoholism symptom patterns of men and women. *Quarterly Journal of Studies on Alcohol*, 1970, *31*(1), 40–61.

Wanberg, K. W., & Knapp, J. Differences in drinking symptoms and behavior of men and women alcoholics. *British Journal of Addictions*, 1970, *64*, 347–355.

Warner, C. G. *Conflict intervention in social and domestic violence*. Bowie, Md.: Robert J. Brady, 1981.

Women and Health Roundtable Report. Federation of Organizations for Professional Women, Washington, D.C., 1979, *4*(4).

Women and Health Roundtable Report. Federation of Organizations for Professional Women, Washington, D.C., 1980, *4*(1).

Women and Health Roundtable Report. Federation of Organizations for Professional Women, Washington, D.C., 1980, *3*(8).

Obstetrical and Perinatal Teaching Needs Form

INSTRUCTIONS

Patient education is an integral part of care provided to the obstetrical and perinatal patient. The Teaching Needs Form provides a method of documentation of patient teaching and assessment of patient learning (Fig. A–1). The following guidelines are provided for the use of this form:

1. Teaching needs are divided according to obstetrical and perinatal categories. Generally, the ambulatory care provider has primary responsibility for antepartum and initial assessment of perinatal teaching needs. The inpatient care provider is usually concerned with the perinatal period. It is expected that these roles will overlap with individual patients; therefore, patient teaching should be documented whenever it is done.

2. The content and objectives for each teaching category are outlined in the attached material (Teaching Needs).

3. Many teaching categories also include written material to augment patient education. When the patient receives written material specified for a given teaching need, indicate this by a $\checkmark$ on the form under the column Written Material Given.

4. Each teaching category must be accompanied by a nursing assessment of patient learning. The care provider writes an assessment of the learner, including learner's abilities and learner's readiness, on the assessment column. Included also should be an overall assessment of the results of the teaching session. If a particular category is problematic and requires extra documentation, a progress note must be written. In the assessment section, refer the reader to the progress note and briefly describe the problem.

5. After completion of the patient assessment, the health care provider must write a plan for follow-up, including a plan for reinforcement of learning. This is to be documented in the column labeled Plan.

6. *Each entry* must be accompanied by the date and the signature of the "teacher," indicating that the teaching has been done according to the content guidelines specific for that teaching category of the "teacher."

These guidelines were prepared by an interdisciplinary team for use in patient education at Strong Memorial Hospital in Rochester, New York. Contributors included Carol Calabrese, Valerie Jones, Colleen Keenan, Beth Knapp, Vivian Littlefield, Joanne Matthews, Anne Marie Pettis, Phyllis Sale, and Mary Lou Wilkins. These guidelines are reproduced here by permission.

OBSTETRIC AND PERINATAL
TEACHING NEEDS

Patient Name

Unit Number

	Date	Signature	Written Mat'l Given	Assessment	Plan
ANTEPARTUM					
Physical/ Emotional Changes					
Fetal Growth/ Development					
Sexuality					
Nutrition/ Weight Gain					
Activity					
Potential Impact: Substance Use					
Danger Signs					
PERINATAL					
Physical/ Emotional Changes					
Labor/ Delivery					
Nutrition/ Exercise					
Sexuality/ Contraception					

10/80

Figure A–1. Obstetrical and perinatal teaching needs form. *(cont.)*

	Date	Signature	Written Mat'l Given	Assessment	Plan
PERINATAL (con't.) Infant Care at Home					
Infant Development/ Sibling Preparation					
Bath Demo					
Infant Feeding Breast Bottle					
Temperature Taking					
Circumcision Care					
Pre- and Post-op Teaching					
Jaundice					
Danger Signs					

Additional Patient Information Given	Date	Signature

Figure A–1. (cont.) Obstetrical and perinatal teaching needs form. *(Source: University of Rochester/Strong Memorial Hospital, Rochester, New York, with permission.)*

7. An additional section is provided to document other pertinent patient information that is not included in the teaching content guidelines. Examples of appropriate information are: how the learner has learned in the past, what facilitates learning for her, what supports the learner has, and if the learner has any special considerations such as a hearing loss or cultural/language barrier.

ANTEPARTUM: PHYSICAL AND EMOTIONAL CHANGES

Behavioral Objectives
The patient will:

1. Identify the major anatomical landmarks of the female reproductive organs on the female pelvic model or illustration.
2. State when pregnancy occurs in relation to the menstrual cycle.
3. Identify physiological discomforts experienced during pregnancy and associated comfort measures.
4. Identify at least one physical and one emotional change that may occur in each trimester.
5. Explore emotional changes experienced and the effect of these changes on relationships with friends and family.
6. Identify and discuss a mood alteration effect on relationship with others.

Teaching Guidelines

1. It is extremely important to assess the patient's past experiences with previous pregnancies, outcomes of those pregnancies, and other problems experienced in prior pregnancies.
2. Discuss basic female pelvic anatomy related to pregnancy.
    A. Utilize models or illustrations to show the major anatomical landmarks.
        (1) External—labia majora, labia minora, urinary meatus, clitoris, vaginal opening, anus
        (2) Internal—vagina, cervix, uterus, fallopian tubes, ovaries
3. Explain the female reproductive system and its function.
    A. Discuss the menstrual cycle emphasizing the fertile period and when pregnancy is most likely to occur.
    B. Discuss the developing fetus, showing changes in fetal size and position, including the resulting differences in the physical appearance of the mother. (See Teaching Needs Form — Fetal Growth and Development.)
    C. Discuss common discomforts associated with the physical changes of pregnancy and common relief measures.
        (1) Backache—pelvic rock exercise
        (2) Constipation—diet changes
        (3) Leg cramps—diet changes and exercise
        (4) Insomnia—changes in sleep positions
    D. Discuss third trimester changes as they relate to the preparation of the body for labor, delivery, and breast-feeding.
        (1) Labor and delivery—change in vaginal secretions, Braxton–Hicks contractions, lower abdominal discomfort, urinary frequency
        (2) Breast-feeding—increasing breast size, colostrum leakage

4. Discuss common emotional changes or mood alterations that may occur during pregnancy, e.g., irritability, increased sensitivity, passivity, introspection, and an increased desire for affection and attention.

Teaching Aids

1. Flip chart—*Birth atlas* (6th ed.). Maternity Center Association, New York, NY.
2. Chart—*Female pelvic organs*. Education Department, Tampax Inc., New York, NY.
3. Flip chart—*Female reproductive organs in health and illness*. Parke, Davis, Detroit, MI.
4. Wall chart—*How a baby grows*. The National Foundation, March of Dimes.

FETAL GROWTH AND DEVELOPMENT

Behavioral Objectives
The patient will:

1. State the length and divisions of a normal pregnancy.
2. State when her baby may be due and how this date was determined.
3. Discuss how the use of certain substances in the first trimester may adversely affect fetal development and growth.
4. Identify the major organs involved in fetal development and the function of each.
5. State when fetal movement is usually felt and the importance of noting this time.
6. Discuss the importance of fetal activity during pregnancy and the need to contact the care provider if there is a decrease in fetal movement.
7. State that the fetus grows at a predictable rate and the importance of keeping prenatal appointments.
8. Discuss second and third trimester maternal and fetal weight gain.
9. Describe at least two measures that may be taken if the fetus is found to be either too large or too small for gestational age.
10. State that during the second trimester and continuing into the third trimester the increasing fetal size will cause changes in body contour and increased pressure on lower body organs and extremities.
11. State that a baby born before 38 weeks is considered premature and, if born at this time, may be at risk of developing problems.
12. State that a baby born after 42 weeks gestational age is considered postdate and if a baby is postdate, tests will be done to determine fetal well-being.

Teaching Guidelines

1. Discuss the length of pregnancy, its divisions, and the calculations of estimated date of confinement.
2. Describe body changes as pregnancy progresses and how the pregnancy stresses other pelvic organs.
3. Discuss the major body organs changes during the first trimester and how substance abuse may affect the fetus.

4. Demonstrate and discuss on an unlabeled diagram the structures involved in fetal development: uterus, placenta, umbilical cord, amniotic sac, cervix, mucous plug, and attachment of uterine ligaments.
5. Demonstrate using pictures or diagrams how the fetus develops during pregnancy.
   A. Emphasize the importance of noting when fetal movement is first felt.
6. Discuss fetal movement and what to do if a decrease in fetal movement is noticed.
7. Describe how fetal growth is monitored, the importance of keeping appointments, and unusual changes to watch for and report.
8. Discuss how the fetus puts on approximately ¾ lb/week in the second and third trimester and the importance of adequate maternal weight gain during this period.
9. Discuss what the care provider may do if fetal size is not consistent with gestational size (ultrasound, check nutritional intake, check continued substance abuse).
10. Discuss prematurity and postmaturity and its meaning to fetal well-being.
11. Discuss what term delivery is and what test may be needed if pregnancy goes postdate (nonstress test, oxytocin challenge test, and weekly to biweekly estriols).

Teaching Aids

1. Flip chart—*How a baby grows*. The National Foundation, March of Dimes.
2. Pamphlet—*Pregnancy series: The reproductive years*. Ortho Reach, Ortho Pharmaceutical Corporation, Raritan, NJ.
3. Flip Chart—*Birth atlas* (6th ed.). Maternity Center Association, New York, NY.

SEXUALITY

Behavioral Objectives
The patient will:

1. Discuss her feelings and concerns regarding sexual activity during her pregnancy.
2. Identify the position of the reproductive organs in relation to the developing fetus and how the fetus is protected within the uterus and amniotic sac.
3. List some contraindications of sexual activity during pregnancy.

Teaching Guidelines

1. Assess the patient's attitudes regarding sexual activity during pregnancy, including advice received from and feeling of the partner, family, and friends.
2. Discuss the position of the developing fetus, uterus, cervix, and vagina in relation to sexual intercourse.
3. Emphasize that sexual activity is not a contraindication during pregnancy, unless given specific instructions by the care provider to refrain from sexual activity.
   A. Review when sexual activity is contraindicated.
      (1) Rupture of membranes
      (2) Bleeding or spotting

      (3) Active herpes infection (self or partner)

      (4) Premature labor

    B. If advised to refrain from sexual activity, review with her (and if possible her partner) the reasons. Encourage patient to discuss with her care provider when sexual relations may be safely resumed.

4. Explain common changes in sexual desire and attitudes during pregnancy.

    A. Change in libido or body image

    B. Breast tenderness or fluid leakage

    C. Fear of harm to fetus

    D. Positional discomforts

    E. Mood swings

    F. Fear of early labor

    G. Effects of nausea and fatigue

5. Suggest alternative methods to alleviate discomforts during sexual activity, such as a change in position.

Teaching Aids

1. Pamphlet—*Sex during pregnancy*. Service to Life series. Lederle: Wayne, N.J., 1980.

NUTRITION AND WEIGHT GAIN

Behavioral Objectives

The patient will:

1. Relate that prenatal nutritional status affects both the energy levels experienced during pregnancy and the outcome of the pregnancy.
2. Name the four basic food groups and the amount of each that is required during pregnancy.
3. Relate the appropriate rate or amount of weight gain needed during pregnancy and the rationale for gaining weight consistently.

Teaching Guidelines

1. Discuss nutrition counseling and evaluation (individually or in a small group setting) as soon as possible after enrollment for prenatal care.
2. Assess prepregnancy and prenatal nutritional status, including attitudes, cultural influences, and knowledge of nutrition.
3. Discuss patient's food preferences and offer suggestions for substitutions, if necessary.
4. Explain *pica* and inquire as to ingestion of clay, starch, and the overuse of foods such as cornstarch and ice.
5. Review the four basic food groups and the required servings of each per day.

    A. Dairy—4 servings

    B. Protein—3 servings

    C. Vegetables and fruit—2 servings of each

    D. Bread—4 servings

6. Explain that the pattern of weight gain during pregnancy is consistent and

steady (i.e., a progressing increase from 3 lb in the 1st trimester, to 14 lb at the end of the 2nd trimester, to approximately 25 lb at term).

7. Explain that the total weight gained includes, in addition to the fetus, maternal stores, fluid, breast tissue, placenta, uterus, and amniotic fluid so that the normal weight gain will not appear excessive to the patient.

8. Explain the direct relationship of maternal nutrition and fetal growth via the placenta and umbilical cord as indicated by increasing fundal height.

9. Assess and encourage patient's use of iron and vitamin supplements. Clarify any medical instructions she may have been given or might have questions about.

10. Review laboratory data and discuss the relationship between anemia, fetal well-being, and proper nutrition at regular intervals throughout the pregnancy.

Teaching Aids

1. Pamphlet—*Be good to your baby before it is born*. The National Foundation, March of Dimes.

2. Chart—*Guide to good eating: A recommended daily pattern* (4th ed.). National Dairy Council, Rosemont, IL.

3. Filmstrip—*Inside my mom*. Cornell University, Ithaca, NY.

ACTIVITY

Behavioral Objectives

The patient will:

1. Continue the normal activities and exercises during the pregnancy with the following exceptions:
   A. Prior to performing any strenuous exercise in which body balance is involved, e.g., diving, horseback riding, surfing, skiing, motorcycle riding, she should discuss it with her care provider.
   B. During long distance traveling requiring sitting for prolonged periods of time, she should periodically stop and walk to improve circulation.

2. Anticiapte that as pregnancy progresses there may be changes in sleep patterns.

Teaching Guidelines

1. Offer reassurance that normal activity can be continued, but body balance changes as pregnancy progresses and body mechanics should be modified.
   A. Explain the change in posture as pregnancy progresses and the stress needed to carry her body in proper alignment. The tilted pelvis will otherwise increase the curvature of the spine.
   B. Teach pelvic tilting (pelvic rock) to increase muscle tone of abdominal muscles and to help transfer the weight of the uterus from the ligaments and muscles to the bodies of vertebra.
   C. Encourage wearing moderate to low heeled shoes to give broad base of support and to lessen inclination of pelvis.
   D. Teach how to pick something up from the floor by using leg muscles (squatting) and not back muscles.
   E. Instruct in tailor sitting and encourage its use for frequent periods during the

day to help promote natural enlargement of the pelvis at the joints and to help with stretching of the perineal and thigh muscles.
   F. Encourage the avoidance of excessive fatigue.
2. Emphasize that travel can be continued throughout pregnancy as long as it does not cause undue fatigue. Stress rest periods on long journey.

Teaching Aids

1. Pamphlet—*Be good to your baby before it is born*. The National Foundation, March of Dimes.
2. *RAMP patient information pamphlet*. University of Rochester, Strong Memorial Hospital, Rochester, NY.

POTENTIAL IMPACT: SUBSTANCE USE

Behavioral Objectives
The patient will:

1. Describe the specific risks involved in smoking, taking drugs, and consuming alcohol during pregnancy.
2. Assess her own use of unprescribed medications, drugs, or smoking during pregnancy and relate this use to fetal development.
3. Discuss not using medications or drugs during pregnancy unless ordered by her care provider.
4. Identify a plan for decreasing her usage of drugs, if she is using an excessive amount.
5. State that douching is not recommended during pregnancy unless ordered by care provider.

Teaching Guidelines

1. Define substance abuse as the use of medications, drugs, alcohol, caffeine, and cigarettes that are not ordered by care provider.
2. Generate a discussion of what substances clients may be taking and the possible consequences of each.
   A. Smoking is associated with low birth weight and smaller head circumference and length of infants. The effect of smoking on the fetus is directly related to how many cigarettes are smoked. The problem is that smaller infants have an increased rate of complications after birth.
   B. Maternal drug addiction causes additional problems, e.g., infection, withdrawal symptoms in the baby, and possible growth retardation. All drugs cross placental barrier and should be minimized. Some have proven tetratogenic effects.
   C. Alcohol in small amounts appears to have limited consequences, but with chronic alcoholics the fetus is usually adversely affected.
3. Discuss that douching is not recommended during pregnancy, especially the use of a hand syringe because of increased risk of air embolism and risk of infection to the uterus. If told to douche by care provider, instruct in how to douche safely.

Teaching Aids

1. Martin, L. *Health care of women*. Philadelphia: J. B. Lippincott, 1978.
2. Reeder, S. R., Mastroianni, L., & Martin, L. L. *Maternity nursing* (14th ed.). Philadelphia: J. B. Lippincott, 1980.
3. Pamphlet—*Deciding about drugs: A woman's choice*. Adapted by Hoffman-La Roche Inc., from original publication by U.S. Dept. of Health Sciences.

DANGER SIGNS OF PREGNANCY

Behavioral Objectives
The patient will:

1. State the major danger signs of pregnancy: bleeding, severe pain, swelling of face and hands, rupture of membranes.
2. Call care provider if a danger sign should occur.
3. Recognize the need to keep a copy of the danger signs of pregnancy and the office and emergency phone numbers of the care provider.

Teaching Guidelines

1. Provide a list of the danger signs of pregnancy.
2. Explain each danger sign and the importance of calling the care provider should a danger sign appear.
   A. Bleeding from the vagina—possible causes are infections, placenta previa, miscarriage, abruption
   B. Severe or continuing nausea and vomiting—danger of dehydration, lack of proper nutrition of mother and newborn
   C. Continuing severe headache — a symptom of preeclampsia
   D. Swelling or puffiness of face or hands or marked swelling of feet or ankles—symptoms of preeclampsia
   E. Blurring of vision or spots before the eyes—symptoms of preeclampsia
   F. Marked decrease in the amounts of urine passed—indicative of kidney complications, preeclampsia
   G. Pain or burning on passing urine—symptom of urinary tract infection
   H. Chills and fever—indicative of maternal infection, danger of premature labor
   I. Sharp or continuous abdominal pain—preeclampsia, abruption
   J. Sudden gush of water from the vagina—indicates rupture of membranes
3. Review all symptoms at 36 week appointment.
4. Review necessary emergency phone numbers and where the patient keeps them.

Teaching Aids

1. List of danger signs.
2. List of emergency phone numbers.

ASSESSMENT OF LABOR

Behavioral Objectives
The patient will:

1. List the signs and symptoms of labor and impending delivery.
2. State the difference between true labor and false labor.
3. State how to time the frequency and duration of a contraction.
4. State what should be done when contractions become regular.

Teaching Guidelines

1. Review the specific signs and symptoms of labor and impending delivery.
2. Discuss false labor and allay any anxieties.
3. Explain what a contraction is, its role in the birth process, and its typical frequency and duration.
4. Explain how to time the duration and frequency of a contraction.
5. Discuss how a friend or relative can help time contractions.
6. Explain when it is required to call the careprovider.
7. Discuss other signs and symptoms that necessitate a call to care provider, e.g., vaginal discharge, bleeding or "show," rupture of membranes.
8. Review the following symptoms that can occur with regular contractions and what can be done to anticipate or relieve them.
   A. Nausea, vomiting—carry or store a paper bag in her hospital suitcase or purse
   B. Diarrhea—commode or bedpan nearby
   C. Pressure on bladder or rectum or both—try to keep bladder empty
   D. Gas pains—daily exercises
   E. Leg cramps—daily exercises, change positions
   F. Light-headedness or dizziness—not get up or be left alone

Teaching Aids

1. Watch or clock with a second hand.

PERINATAL: PHYSICAL CHANGES

Behavioral Objectives
Prior to discharge the patient will:

1. Describe the physiological changes of the uterus, vagina, breasts, bowels, perineum, vascular system, and abdominal wall that occur during the puerperium.
2. Identify 4 to 6 weeks as the expected time frame for completion of puerperal physiological changes.
3. State that vaginal bleeding, which includes larger clots, is abnormal and must be reported to the health care provider.
4. List two signs and symptoms of breast engorgement.
5. Identify three measures that relieve discomfort associated with breast engorgement.
6. Describe three measures to use for relief of constipation.

Teaching Guidelines

1. Review the following physical changes that take place during the postpartum period.
   A. Involution of the uterus
      (1) First pospartum day— fundus is midline and one finger breadth above umbilicus.
      (2) Uterus involves at rate of one finger breadth a day.
      (3) Within 2 weeks—no longer palpable above symphysis.
      (4) With 5–6 weeks—prepregant size.
   B. The abdominal wall
      (1) Soft and relaxed after delivery.
      (2) Return to normal tone and appearance depends upon prepregant muscle control and performance of postpartum exercises.
   C. Afterpains
      (1) Caused by involution of uterus.
      (2) Most intense activity during first 2–3 days.
      (3) Increased activity with multiparity and breast-feeding.
   D. Lochia
      (1) Variable amount of nonfoul uterine discharge.
      (2) First 3 days—bright red.
      (3) Within 3–8 days—brown or pink.
      (4) By the 10th day—yellowish-white in color.
   E. Vascular system
      (1) Blood volume decreases to its prepregnant level.
      (2) Diuresis occurs.
   F. The perineum
      (1) Considerable tenderness and edema if an episiotomy or laceration repair is present.
      (2) Sutures usually dissolve in about 3 weeks.
      (3) Personal hygiene is essential in the care of the perineum.
   G. Menstruation
      (1) In nonlactating mothers, ovulation usually occurs within 4–6 weeks and menstruation within 6–12 weeks after delivery.
      (2) In lactating mothers, ovulation is inhibited for varying amounts of time.
      (3) Discourage lactation as a means of contraception.
   H. The vagina
      (1) The distended vagina becomes relaxed and edematous and gradually diminishes in size.
      (2) The vagina never regains its nulliparious state.
   I. Breasts
      (1) Prior to the onset of lactation, engorgement may occur. It usually peaks between the 3rd and 5th day and lasts about 48 hr.
      (2) Signs and symptoms of breast discomfort ranging from mild swelling and tenderness to very heavy, hot, tender, and painful breasts.
      (3) Relief measures for breast discomfort.
         a. Use of a good supportive bra, heat or ice packs.
         b. Use of a mild analgesic.

      c. If breast-feeding, the breast should be emptied, if not, medication may be needed to suppress lactation.

  J. Bowels

    (1) Constipation may occur due to any of the following factors:

      a. Relaxed abdominal and intestinal muscles

      b. A cleansing enema during labor

      c. Lack of solid food during labor

      d. Postpartum diuresis

      e. The demand of lactating breasts for fluid

      f. Painful episiotomy and/or sore hemorrhoids may prevent bearing down to aid in elimination.

    (2) Early ambulation, sitz baths, stool softeners, mild cathartics, small enemas, or suppositories may relieve perineal discomfort and aid elimination.

Teaching Aids

1. Flip chart—*Female reproductive organs in health and illness*. Parke, Davis, Detroit, MI.
2. Chart—*Female pelvic organs*. Educational Department, Tampax Inc., New York, NY.

PERINATAL: EMOTIONAL CHANGES

Behavioral Objectives

Prior to discharge the patient will:

1. Describe any mood alterations and their effect on the postpartum woman's relationship with others.
2. Describe the phases of emotional change potentially experienced during the postpartum period.
3. Describe some common mood variations postpartum, including transitory states of emotional distress.

Teaching Guidelines

1. Review the following phases of emotional change.

  A. "Taking-in phase" (dependent phase): usually lasts 2–3 days and is characterized by:

    (1) Passivity.

    (2) Concern for own needs, including food, sleep, reviewing labor and delivery experience, being cared for and about, and ego support.

  B. "Taking-hold phase": usually begins on the 3rd postpartum day and lasts about 10 days.

    (1) Characterized by desire to take command and become autonomous.

    (2) A concentration on the present and on getting organized.

    (3) Mothering tasks become a priority with an inner drive to master them. Inability to perform these tasks perfectly may elicit anxiety and frustration.

    (4) Openness to learning about her baby.

    C. "Letting-go phase"
      (1) Acceptance of the infant as an individual and separate from herself.
      (2) A sense of emptiness and grief may be experienced.
  2. Explain postpartum blues.
    A. Transitory states of emotional distress during the postpartum period are common for new mothers including unexplainable sadness and frequent crying.
    B. Emotional lability may be due to a combination of environmental pressures, role changes, hormonal changes, and interpersonal conflict.

Teaching Aids

1. Boston Women's Health Book collective. *Our bodies, ourselves*. New York: Bantam Books, 1977.
2. Rubin, R. Basic maternal behavior. *Nursing Outlook,* 1961, 9(1), 683–686.
3. Rubin, R. Binding-in in the pospartum period. *Maternal–Child Nursing Journal,* 1977, 6, 67–75.

LABOR AND DELIVERY

Behavioral Objectives

The patient will:

1. Identify three symptoms signaling the onset of true labor.
2. Discuss responses to the onset of labor, including emergency telephone number of care provider, when to come to hospital, and plans for transportation.
3. Identify needs regarding her labor and delivery including a support person, classes or groups for childbirth preparation, alternative birthing procedures such as LeBoyer, birthing room, or labor room delivery.
4. Attend the prepared childbirth education classes of choice.
5. Review the normal progression of labor through the states of early labor through delivery.

Teaching Guidelines

1. Identify current knowledge and attitudes about labor and the birth process, including common myths and the influence of family and friends.
2. Explain the difference between false labor and true labor and reinforce the necessity of notifying the care provider when the bag of water ruptures or contractions occur at regular intervals and increase in strength and duration.
3. Discuss the protective qualities of the amniotic sac and that the patient must notify care provider or come to hospital if there is a possibility that her membranes may be ruptured.
4. Teach the patient to time contractions.
5. Document the patient's labor support.
6. Discuss the value of preparation for labor and delivery by attending prenatal classes or groups and the use of psychoprophylactic measures during labor.
7. Refer patient to and encourage attendance in prepared childbirth education classes and document her attendance.

8. Review with the patient her medical history. Discuss the possibility of cesarean birth and when a cesarean may be medically indicated.

Teaching Aids

1. Pamphlets describing local childbirth preparation groups or classes.
2. Watch or clock with second hand.

MATERNAL NUTRITION

Behavior Objectives
The patient will:

1. Name the four basic food groups and the number of required daily servings of each group.
2. State the approximate daily caloric intake.
3. Identify the amount and composition of daily fluid intake.
4. State the rationale for not dieting during lactation.
5. State the importance of daily iron, vitamins, and adequate fluid intake.

Teaching Guidelines

1. All patients will receive nutrition counseling on the postpartum unit.
2. Review the four basic food groups and the required servings of each per day
   A. For the lacating woman:
      (1) Protein—4 servings
      (2) Dairy—5 servings
      (3) Vegetables and fruit—2 servings of each
      (4) Bread—3 servings
   B. For the nonlactating woman:
      (1) Protein—3 servings
      (2) Dairy—3 servings
      (3) Vegetables and fruit—2 servings of each
      (4) Bread—3 servings
3. Discuss patient's food preference and offer suggestions for substitutions, e.g., yogurt or cheese instead of milk, etc.
4. Explain that after delivery she may resume a balanced diet of 1200–1600 calories per day.
5. Identify the increased caloric need of the lactating woman, at least 300–500 calories per day above the normal daily allowance.
6. Explain the increased daily fluid needs of the lactating woman: 2–3 quarts of fluid should be comprised mostly of water, juices, and milk.
   A. Explain the higher sodium and sugar content of soft drinks and powdered mixes and other "empty calories."
7. If breast-feeding, suggest ways the woman can insure her fluid intake.
   A. Drink 2 glasses of liquid with meals.
   B. Drink 1–2 glasses of liquid each time before she breast-feeds.
8. Explain the relationship between maternal nutrition and infant nutrition and

emphasize that dieting should *not* be done during lactation except under *close* observation by her care provider.

9. Inform the patient that her care provider may prescribe iron and vitamins to be taken daily while lactating for additional nutritional support.
10. Refer to community health nursing services, if necessary.

Teaching Aids

1. Pritchard, J. A., & Macdonald, P. C. *Williams obstetrics* (16th ed.). New York: Appleton-Century-Crofts, 1980.
2. Pamphlet—*Guide to good eating: A recommended daily pattern* (4th ed.). National Dairy Council, Rosemont, IL.
3. Pamphlet—*Understanding breastfeeding*. Patient Information Library, 345-G, Serramonte Plaza, Daly City, CA: PAS Publishing.
4. Pamphlet—*Breastfeeding your baby*. Ross Laboratories, Columbus, OH.
5. Pamphlet—*Bottle feeding your baby*. University of Rochester, Strong Memorial Hospital, Rochester, NY.

PERINATAL EXERCISES

Behavioral Objectives
The patient will:

1. State the purpose for exercising.
2. Explain the reason for planning a progressive exercise program—least strenous to strenous.
3. State the "danger signs" of overexertion postpartum and how to amend the exercise program should any occur.
4. Perform the exercises outlined for days 1 to 3.

Teaching Guidelines

1. Refer to exercise sheet entitled "10 Exercises after Pregnancy."
2. Explain the occurrence of diastasis recti postpartum and demonstrate.
3. Explain the need to strengthen and tone the rectus muscles through abdominal tightening exercises and sit-ups.
4. Discuss the possibility of back strain and muscle "pulls" if the exercises are not done properly or in progression.
5. Identify the danger signs of overexertion postpartum—muscle weakness, dizziness, a change in the color or increase in the amount of the lochia or both.
   A. Explain that should any of these occur, the patient should rest for the reminder of that day. Notify care provider of signs and care provider may suggest an exercise plan for the patient.
6. Supervise and demonstrate the exercises for days 1 to 3.
7. Explain and demonstrate the remaining seven exercises.
8. Refer to community health nursing services if needed.

Teaching Aids

1. Pamphlet—*10 exercises after pregnancy*. Lederle reprint from R. C. Benson, *Handbook of obstetrics and gynecology* (5th ed.). Los Altos, Calif.: Lange, 1974.

SEXUALITY AND CONTRACEPTION

Behavioral Objectives
The patient will:
1. Identify and describe the various types of birth control.
2. Discuss contraceptive method or methods as preferred by patient.
3. State the percent-effectiveness of each preferred method and its relationship to method compliance.
4. State instructions for use of each preferred method and how it relates to the act of intercourse.
5. Identify advantages and disadvantages for each preferred method.
6. Identify "maintenance factors" involved with each preferred method, e.g., monthly or yearly renewal, expense, need for medical intervention/supervision, care of the device.

Teaching Guidelines
1. Assess knowledge of and preferences for specific contraceptive methods.
2. Focus teaching and support on patient's contraceptive preferences.
    A. Review the various methods of contraception—barrier, chemical, natural, and surgical.
        (1) Explain the approximate percent-effectiveness of each method and that effectiveness can approach 100%. Pill, nearly 100%; IUD and diaphragm, over 95%; foam/condom, 85%; sterilization, nearly 100%; NFP, percent-effectiveness is directly related to couple's motivation to use it. These figures represent method effectiveness *not* usage effectiveness. Improper use of any method will result in lowered effectiveness.
        (2) Detail the duration of use of each method—long-term or permanent versus interim.
    B. Discuss the use of each method of contraception, detailing provision of the method, daily responsibility (if any), and use in relationship to intercourse.
        (1) *Sterilization*—a (usually) irreversible operative procedure.
        (2) *Pill*—by prescription only. Discuss procedure for using the 21- versus the 29-pill pack.
        (3) *IUD*—inserted into the uterus by the care provider and remains in place for 3–5 years depending on the type. Discuss how and when to check for presence of the string.
        (4) *Diaphragm*—by prescription. Must be used with contraceptive cream or jelly.
            a. Insert vaginally up to 6 hours prior to intercourse and leave in place for 6 hours after intercourse.
            b. Additional cream or jelly must be inserted vaginally without removing the diaphragm if repeated intercourse occurs after initial insertion. The "6-hours after" time period is calculated from the time of the last intercourse.
            c. Wash and dry the diaphragm, may apply cornstarch prior to storage and return it to the container.
        (5) *Condoms/Foam*—over-the-counter. Should be used together and applied immediately prior to intercourse.
        (6) *NFP*—Woman must take her tempature daily upon awakening and before

getting out of bed. This value is charted on a temperature graph, which is started on the first day of the menstrual cycle. The cervical dilatation, position, and mucus are also assessed daily for signs of fertility. These signs are logged in on the temperature graph and together show the couple when they are fertile and need to abstain.

3. Discuss "method maintenance" for each form of contraception.
   A. *Sterilization*—no maintenance, one-time hospitalization and surgery fees.
   B. *Pill*—by perscription, must remember to have it filled, monthly cost, must have regular appointments with care provider at least every 3 months.
   C. *IUD*—one-time cost for 3–5 years for contraception.
   D. *Diaphragm*—by prescription. Yearly cost for diaphragm, maintenance cost of refills of cream or jelly. Must be refitted:
      (1) Yearly
      (2) After every *pregnancy*
      (3) After a weight gain *or* loss of 20 lb or more.
   E. *Condoms*—no maintenance, cost of supply.
   F. *NFP*—cost of basal body temperature thermomenter and temperature graphs. Cost of classes on use of this method varies.
4. Discuss the impact each method may have on sexuality and the couple's relationship.
5. Refer specific questions about the patient's medical ability to use a particular method to her care provider.

Teaching Aids

1. Sample pill packages, IUDs, diaphragms, foam and applicators, condoms, and BBT thermometer.
2. Pelvic model.
3. Pamphlets from Ortho Pharmaceutical Corporation, Raritan, NJ, 08869:
   After your doctor prescribes the Pill
   After your doctor prescribes your Ortho diaphragm
   A guide to the methods of contraception
   A guide to the use of Ortho vaginal contraception
   Lippes loop—Your intrauterine contraceptive
   The Pill
   Understanding conception and contraception
4. Pamphlet—*Choosing a birth control method*. The EMKO Co.
5. Pamphlet—*Important facts about post-partum sterilization*. American College of Obstetricians and Gynecologists, Suite 2700, One East Wacker Drive, Chicago, IL.
6. Pamphlet—*The natural way of planning your family*. Natural Family Planning Education of Rochester, New York, Kearney Building, 89 Genesee Street, Rochester, NY.

INFANT CARE AT HOME

Behavioral Objectives:

Before discharge, the patient will:

1. List the necessary infant supplies needed for safe care after discharge.
2. Have a plan for obtaining supplies not presently at home.

3. Identify a person(s) to be utilized as home support.
4. List the services provided by public assistance and that are appropriate for them.

Teaching Guidelines

1. Review supplies necessary for safe infant care, i.e., car seat, clothes, diapers, breast pump and/or formula, living arrangements, crib.
2. Discuss the New York State child care seat law:
   A. Passengers under the age of five riding in certain passenger motor vehicles registered in New York State must be in a "specially designed detachable or removable seat" that meets the current Federal Motor Vehicle Safety Standards relating to such seats. A safety belt may be substituted for a child care seat for a child over the age of four but under the age of five.
   B. The operator of the vehicle and the vehicle owner who "knowingly permits" operation in noncompliance are both responsible for compliance with the law.
   C. Failure to observe the law is subject to a fine of not more than $25, although the court will waive or excuse the fine on presentation of proof of purchase or rental of the required safety seat.
   D. The child seat law does not apply to buses, commercial vans, taxis, motorcycles, or authorized emergency vehicles.
3. Review measures to ensure child safety in the home.
4. Assess knowledge of child care and offer support.
5. Review a plan for obtaining needed supplies.
6. Discuss support persons during pregnancy and available to help at home after discharge.
7. Discuss services provided and appropriateness of public assistance programs, e.g., Medicaid, WIC, Public Health Nurse.
8. Refer to community health nursing services if necessary.

Teaching Aids

1. Pamphlet—*Your baby's safety: The important first year*. Ross Growth & Development Program, Columbus, OH 43216
2. Pamphlet—*Child care & feeding*. University of Rochester, Strong Memorial Hospital, Rochester, NY.
3. Local "Poison Control Pamphlet"
4. Pamphlets regarding the Women, Infant, and Children's (WIC) program and local community health nursing services.
5. Fact sheet: New York State Child Care Seat Law. State of New York, Governor's Traffic Safety Committee, Rockefeller Empire State Plaza, Albany, NY 12228.

INFANT DEVELOPMENT AND SIBLING PREPARATION

Behavioral Objectives

The patient will:

1. State at least two reasons why siblings need to feel part of the birth experience.
2. Discuss with children at their developmental level the changes a new baby will mean in their lives.
3. Allow children to help prepare for the baby's arrival.

4. Have plans for child care during hospitalization.
5. Discuss feelings regarding sibling visitation.

Teaching Guidelines

1. Review the family's plans for integrating infant into the family unit and suggest ways of minimizing the negative effects on older siblings.
   A. Plan special ways for them to help, e.g., move into new room before time for baby's arrival, plan for daily time to spend with older sibling, allow privileges.
2. Discuss how siblings may take part in the birth process.
   A. Accompany parent to prenatal visits and classes.
   B. Hear the fetal heart.
   C. Hear stories and see pictures of babies.
   D. Help prepare the baby clothes, and baby's sleeping area.
3. Assess patient's plans for assistance at house while hospitalized and following delivery.
4. Discuss sibling visitation policy and encourage the mother to invite her children to the hospital to visit their new brother(s) or sister(s).
5. Review plans for coping with sibling rivalry and jealousy should these become manifest.
6. Discuss household pets, if any—they may also show jealousy and resentment toward the baby.

Teaching Aids

1. Pamphlet—*The phenomena of early development*. Ross Laboratories, Columbus, OH.
2. Fraiberg, S. H. *The magic years: Understanding and handling the problems of early childhood*. New York: Scribner, 1959.
3. Erickson, E. *Childhood and society* (2nd ed.). New York: Norton, 1978.

BATH DEMONSTRATION

Behavioral Objectives
Prior to discharge, the patient will:

1. Describe an ideal time and place to bathe the baby.
2. Describe and/or demonstrate safe handling and sponge bathing of the newborn.
3. Discuss feelings and concerns regarding her ability to hold, bathe, and care for this baby.
4. Discuss and/or role-play various infant responses to the bath and possible reactions to the baby.
5. List the necessary equipment used to bathe a baby.
6. Describe and/or demonstrate the care of the umbilicus.
7. Describe and/or demonstrate the use of the bulb syringe.
8. Discuss the physical characteristics of the normal newborn.
9. Describe and/or demonstrate the care of the newborn genitalia.

Teaching Guidelines

1. Offer support and encouragement to the family.
2. Emphasize that the bath:
   A. Should be relaxed and enjoyable.
   B. Can occur at any time before a feeding or at least one hour after a feeding.
   C. Location should be comfortable for the mother and the baby and be draft-free.
3. Emphasize that daily baths are unnecessary and frequent bathing increases drying of the newborn's already dry skin.
   A. Every other day bathing is adequate.
   B. Use a mild soap.
   C. Use alcohol to keep the cord clean and dry.
   D. Sponge baths and not immersion baths should be used at least until the cord falls off and the umbilicus has healed.
4. Emphasize having all needed bath equipment gathered together prior to starting the baby's bath.
   A. Basin or sink
   B. Washcloth
   C. Soap, e.g., castile, Ivory, J & J baby soap, etc.
   D. Blankets for drying and rewrapping
   E. Bulb syringe
   F. Fresh diaper and fresh set of baby clothes
5. Discuss and demonstrate bathing procedure.
   A. Emphasize bathing baby starting at head and going to feet.
   B. Review bath safety.
6. Discuss use of cornstarch, lotions, and powders and some lotions and powders may trap urine and irritate skin. Discuss use of a vitamin supplemented skin ointment or medicated powder for diaper rashes.
7. Discuss and demonstrate diapering using cloth, plastic, and paper diapers.
8. Review cleansing of ears and genital areas.

Teaching Aids

1. Bath equipment.
2. Samples of mild soaps, lotions, and powders.
3. Samples of vitamin supplemented skin ointment and medicated powder.
4. Samples of cloth and paper diapers.

INFANT FEEDING: BREAST

Behavioral Objectives
The patient will:

1. Decide on a feeding method and state rationale for her choice.
   A. List 2–3 benefits of either breast- or bottle-feeding.
2. Eat a well-balanced diet consisting of the four basic food groups.
3. State amount of fluid intake necessary while lactating and proper fluids to drink.

4. Discuss signs and symptoms of mastitis.
5. Understand the cause of engorged breasts and sore nipples.
6. Demonstrate understanding of breast self-examination.
7. Discuss organizations that provide support.
8. Demonstrate good hand washing and breast care.
9. Demonstrate several different positions of holding the baby while breast-feeding.
10. Demonstrate positioning of baby after feeding.
11. Demonstrate knowledge of baby's readiness to feed, eliciting rooting reflex.
12. Demonstrate breaking suction.

Teaching Guidelines

1. Document feeding choice decision and support.
   A. Evaluate patient's knowledge and experience with both breast and bottle feeding.
   B. Discuss the benefits of breast-feeding and bottle feeding including nutritional information, maternal postpartum activities (e.g., school, work).
2. Discuss feeding behavior of the individual baby. Position baby on either side or abdomen at all times to prevent aspiration.
3. Review importance of comfortable position to breast-feed, for mother and baby, e.g., sitting, lying down, football hold, resting baby on pillow, aligning the baby's head with the breast.
4. Discuss feeding procedure.
   A. Review good handwashing techniques.
      (1) Wash hands before each feeding. Breast cleanliness—wash once a day with soap.
      (2) More frequent cleaning may be needed before each feeding if using masse cream, lanolin, or vitamin supplemented ointment. Some babies do not like the taste.
   B. Review positioning of baby to prevent aspiration.
   C. Discuss inappropriateness of propping bottles.
   D. Promote emptying of breast
      (1) Start feeding with the breast that baby finished last feeding on. Suggest placing a safety pin on the bra to indicate which breast to begin on.
      (2) Encourage the let-down reflex by responding to times infant is hungry, i.e., feeding baby or pumping breast.
   E. Discuss feeding reflexes: let-down, rooting.
   F. Burp the baby between each breast and during feeding—a burp may not be elicited between breasts, but should be after both breasts. Babies take in less air when breast-feeding.
   G. Demonstrate breaking suction.
   H. Wear a clean supportive bra—preferably cotton, or cotton lining to enhance airing of nipple.
5. Review signs and symptoms of mastitis and ways to avoid. Some women are more prone to sore nipples than others.
   A. May start by nursing the baby 5 minutes on each side and progress by increasing to 15 minutes on each side (if baby is alert enough) and decreasing if nipples become very tender.

   B. Prevention and treatment of sore nipples:
      (1) Exposing of breast to air for 15–20 minutes after each feeding; exposing breasts to sunlight at home or bake light in hospital.
      (2) Use of masse cream, vitamin supplemented ointment, or lanolin after each feeding.
      (3) Use of breast shields.
      (4) Offer the less sore nipple first and change nursing position.

Teaching Aids

   1. Pamphlet—*The care and feeding of a newborn baby.* University of Rochester, Strong Memorial Hospital, Department of Obstetrics and Gynecology, Rochester, NY.
   2. Pamphlet—*Helpful information for prospective parents.* University of Rochester, Strong Memorial Hospital, Department of Obstetrics and Gynecology, Rochester, NY.

INFANT FEEDING: BOTTLE

Behavioral Objectives

The patient will:

   1. Decide on a feeding method and state rationale for choice.
      A. List 2–3 benefits of either breast- or bottle-feeding.
   2. Discuss preparation of formula to be used.
   3. Discuss how to increase formula feedings.
   4. Demonstrate positions for burping baby.
   5. Demonstrate positioning of baby on either side or stomach to prevent aspiration after feeding.
   6. Demonstrate how to encourage baby to feed.
      A. Eliciting rooting reflex
      B. Unwrapping baby
      C. Burp frequently, at approximately every one ounce rub the nipple against the roof of the mouth.
   7. Discuss frequency of feeding.
   8. Discuss and demonstrate breast self-examination.
   9. Discuss with baby's pediatrician increasing formula appropriately with weight gain of baby.

Teaching Guidelines

   1. Document feeding choice decision and support.
      A. Evaluate patient's knowledge and experience with both breast and bottle feeding.
      B. Discuss the benefits of breast-feeding and bottle-feeding, including nutritional information, maternal postpartum activities (e.g., school, work).
   2. Review the three different types of formula preparations and refrigeration after preparation, including proper cleaning of bottles and nipples; not to reuse formula from same bottle.
      A. Ready to feed

    B. Concentrate

    C. Powder

  3. Discuss feeding behavior of individual baby.

    A. Review and discuss demand feeding, modified demand, and scheduled feedings (approximately between 2 to 5 hours).

    B. Formula is to be increased by one ounce when baby is wakening more frequently than normal pattern.

  5. Discuss bottle feeding technique.

    A. Review good handwashing technique.

    B. Review positioning of baby to prevent aspiration.

    C. Discuss inappropriateness of propping bottles.

Teaching Aids

  1. Pamphlet—*The care and feeding of a newborn baby*. University of Rochester, Strong Memorial Hospital, Department of Obstetrics and Gynecology, Rochester, NY.

  2. Pamphlet—*Helpful information for prospective parents*. University of Rochester, Strong Memorial Hospital, Department of Obstetrics and Gynecology, Rochester, NY.

TEMPERATURE TAKING

Behavioral Objectives

Before discharge, the postpartum patient will:

  1. Identify two modes of temperature taking for an infant and one mode of temperature-taking for herself.

  2. Demonstrate correct temperature-taking procedures on an infant and on herself.

  3. Locate the mercury line on the thermometer.

  4. Accurately identify the temperature reading indicated by the mercury line on the thermometer.

  5. Contrast the range of normal temperatures for an infant and an adult.

  6. List two or three symptoms of an abnormal temperature in infants and in adults.

  7. State the importance of veryifying the degree of temperature elevation in an infant, and in postpartum women.

  8. State two or three nursing care activities for infants and adults with abnormal temperature readings.

  9. State when and how often to recheck abnormal temperatures.

  10. State when to call the doctor to report abnormal temperatures.

Teaching Guidelines

  1. Explain that an infant's temperature may be taken:

    A. By the axillary route

    B. By the rectal route

  2. A woman's temperature may be taken by the oral route.

  3. Explain and demonstrate how to perform correct temperature taking on an infant:

     A. Axillary temperature—keep the thermometer bulb tucked securely in the axilla for 3–5 minutes

     B. Rectal temperature—lubricating the bulb and ½ inch of the thermometer before insertion into the rectum for 3–5 minutes

5. Explain and demonstrate how to perform an oral adult temperature.
6. Explain and demonstrate how to find the silver mercury line between the calibration lines and the numbers on the thermometer.
7. Explain the calibration of the thermometer and where the range of normal infant temperature is and the range for normal postpartum is.
8. Explain the signs and symptoms of an abnormal temperature in an infant:
   A. Appears unusually fussy or irritable
   B. Feels too warm or too cold
   C. Consistently refuses feedings
9. Explain that an adult need only check own temperature if feeling too warm or does not "feel well."
10. Explain home treatment for an abnormal temperature.
    A. Below normal infant temperatures: the infant should be wrapped with an extra blanket.
    B. Above normal infant temperatures:
       (1) Extra clothing should be removed
       (2) Extra fluids, especially glucose water, may be encouraged.
       (3) Before giving any antipyretics to a newborn the care provider should be consulted.
    C. Above normal adult temperatures:
       (1) Take extra fluids
       (2) Avoid chilling self
11. Explain that all abnormal temperatures should be rechecked in 1 hour.
12. Emphasize that two consecutive abnormal temperatures should be reported to the doctor.

Teaching Aids

1. Sample centigrade or Fahrenheit thermometer.
2. Pamphlet—*Infant temperature taking*. University of Rochester, Strong Memorial Hospital, 601 Elmwood Avenue, Rochester, NY.

CIRCUMCISION CARE

Behavioral Objectives

Before discharge, the infant's mother will:

1. State what a circumcision entails.
2. State the possible complications of a circumcision.
3. Identify the organs involved in the procedure.
4. List the reasons for performing this procedure.
5. List the preparations needed before and during the procedure.
6. List the care needed during the healing process.
7. Demonstrate care of the healing circumcision site.

8. List abnormal signs that may be seen during the healing process.
9. State when to call the pediatrician.

Teaching Guidelines

1. Assess previous experience and cultural or religious background regarding circumcisions.
2. Explain the operative procedure.
3. Identify the location of the foreskin and glands.
   A. Discuss the most common reasons for performing a circumcision, which are
      (1) Social reasons
      (2) Religious reasons
      (3) A slight chance of developing a phimosis (constriction of the glands by the foreskin).
   B. Review possible complications of the procedure.
   C. Explain the preparations involved in the circumcision:
      (1) Infant is NPO for 1 hour prior to the procedure to prevent possible aspiration.
      (2) A consent form should be signed by the parent before the procedure is done.
      (3) Infant is taken to the designated circumcision area, usually in the nursery.
      (4) Parents may watch the procedure with the obstetrician given advanced knowledge of this request.
4. Review possible complications of the procedure.
   A. Ascertain whether or not surgeon has spoken with parents and if not arrange for this prior to operation.
   B. Assess and clarify family's understanding of the procedure.
   C. Discuss the complications of infection and hemorrhage.
5. Explain the normal healing process for the circumcision.
   A. Healing occurs from the inside outward, as the surrounding tissue heals.
   B. The plastic ring will gradually slide off the end of the penis.
   C. The plastic bell (ring) will fall off after the tissue heals completely, in approximately 7 to 10 days.
6. Explain and demonstrate care of the circumcision.
   A. Rinse site with plain water (no soap) at least three times a day
   B. No ointment is necessary
   C. Allow bell to fall off on its own to ensure complete healing
7. Discuss the abnormal signs possibly seen during the healing process:
      (1) Difficulty with urination
      (2) Yellow puslike drainage
      (3) Swelling and readness of the glands
      (4) Coolness of the glands
8. Emphasize that the pediatrician should be notified immediately if any of the abnormal signs appear.

Teaching Aids

1. Pamphlet—*Now that your baby has been circumcised.* Hollister Inc., Chicago, IL.

PRE- AND POSTOPERATIVE TEACHING

Behavioral Objectives
The patient will:

1. Identify the reason for cesarean section.
2. State the preparation required for the cesarean.
3. Verbalize her knowledge and concerns regarding an operative procedure.
4. List available resources, e.g., pediatrics, anesthesia, nursing.

Teaching Guidelines

1. Explain when a cesarean section is necessary.
2. Obtain signature on consent forms for an operative procedure.
3. Explain the need for a Foley catheter.
   A. Explain procedure during insertion.
4. Explain the need for abdominal prep.
   A. Explain procedure during prep.
5. Explain the need for an intravenous line and when it will be started.
6. Assist the patient onto the operating room table and stay with her.
7. Before preparing the abdomen with antiseptic solution take the fetal heart rate.
8. Explain the need for a leg place strap.
9. Explain when the anesthesia will be started.
10. Explain that she will be taken to the recovery room afterwards. Assure her that she will be informed of the outcome of the delivery if she awakens before leaving the operating room.
11. Provide reassurance and allay anxiety of patient, spouse, and/or significant others.
12. If the patient requests the father in the room during the cesarean, refer to the OB/GYN policy manual.

Teaching Aids

1. Pamphlet or handout describing operating room and procedures in regards to cesarean sections.

FETAL MONITORING

Behavioral Objectives
The patient will:

1. State the need for monitoring fetus.
2. Verbalize feelings and reactions to continuous monitoring.
3. Give a brief explanation of the fetal monitor procedure.

Teaching Guidelines

1. Inform the patient and explain the specific need for fetal monitoring.
2. Review with the patient a copy of "Monitoring Your Baby at SMH."
3. Discuss questions or concerns that she may have regarding continuous monitoring; offer reassurance and support.

4. Apply the monitor according to standard OB/GYN nursing fetal monitoring procedure.
5. Explain the use of the monitor by reviewing systematically the tubigrip transducer, toco, and graph paper. Explain the lights and sounds that emanate from the machine.
6. Inform the patient of how long she can anticipate being monitored and rationale.
7. Explain that the external monitor may need to be readjusted from time to time, but that wearing a monitor should not inhibit her activities in the labor room.

Teaching Aids

1. Pamphlet—*Monitoring your baby at SMH*. University of Rochester, Strong Memorial Hospital, Department of Obstetrics and Gynecology, Rochester, NY.

PHYSIOLOGICAL JAUNDICE OF THE NEWBORN

Behavioral Objectives

The parent or parents will:

1. Describe jaundice as a yellow appearance of the whites of eyes and skin of the newborn.
2. Identify the appearance of jaundice in the first 24 hours of life as a serious condition requiring immediate notification of the care provider.
3. Identify the cause of physiological jaundice as normal immaturity of the infant's liver.
4. Demonstrate awareness of the test and treatment the infant with physiological jaundice may undergo, such as:
   A. Heel punctures for bilirubin
   B. Need for increased feedings, fluids
   C. Use of natural light at home
   D. Phototherapy when appropriate
5. Verbalize feelings and reactions to jaundice in the newborn.

Teaching Guidelines

1. Review physiology of jaundice in newborns.
2. Discuss tests for and treatment of newborns who have physiological jaundice.
3. Offer reassurance and support. Allay any anxieties parent(s) may have.

Teaching Aids

1. Pamphlet—*Jaundice in newborn babies*. Ross Laboratories, Columbus, OH.

DANGER SIGNS POSTPARTUM

Behavioral Objectives

Prior to discharge the patient will:

1. State the major postpartum danger signs and symptoms.
2. State the proper response when danger signs appear.

Teaching Guidelines

1. Review and explain each danger sign.
   A. Temperature—100.4°F or 38°C.
   B. Breasts—mass (lump) in breast, reddened, warm, firm area decrease or absence of milk flow discharge from nipple.
   C. Lochia—clots or tissue expelled, foul-smelling lochia, large amount of bright red bleeding during or post cessation of lochial flow.
   D. Episiotomy—continuing or increased soreness extending past 2 weeks, foul-smelling discharge, swelling, separation.
   E. Abdomen—redness or swelling at surgical site, separation of the wound, foul-smelling discharge.
   F. Pain—any site (abdominal, uterine, breast, leg).
   G. Legs—calf pain or tenderness; warm over site; increase in calf circumference; obvious veins that look swollen.
2. Instruct patient that each of the above danger signs requires medical consultation/follow-up. If it occurs after the patient is home, instruct her to contact her care provider.
3. Instruct patient as to proper response should she experience any of the above symptoms.
4. Review with her the written discharge instructions for cesarean section or vaginal delivery.

Teaching Aids

1. Written discharge instructions for vaginal delivery.
2. Written discharge instructions for cesarean section.

APPENDIX B

Diabetic Guidelines and Teaching Tool

INSTRUCTIONS: DIABETIC TEACHING TOOL

Patient education is an integral part of the care provided to the diabetic antepartum and postpartum patient. The diabetic teaching tool provides a method of documenting assessment of patient learning and patient teaching (Fig. B–1). The following guidelines are provided for the use of this tool:

1. Teaching needs are divided according to antepartum, perinatal, and postpartum categories. Generally, the ambulatory care provider has primary responsibility for antepartum and initial assessment of intrapartum and postpartum teaching needs. The inpatient provider is usually concerned with the postpartum period. It is expected that these roles will overlap with individual patients and the provider should document patient teaching whenever it is done.
2. The content and the objectives for each teaching category are outlined in the attached material (Teaching tool).
3. Many teaching categories also include written material to augment patient education. When the patient receives written material specified for a given teaching need, indicate this by a checkmark on the form under the column Written Material Given.
4. Each teaching category must be accompanied by a nursing assessment of patient learning. The care provider writes an assessment of the learner, including learner's abilities and learner's readiness, on the assessment column. Included also should be an overall assessment of the results of the teaching session. If a particular category is problematic and requires extra documentation, a progress note must be written. In the assessment section, refer the reader to the progress note and briefly describe the problem.
5. After completion of the patient assessment, the health care provider must write a plan for follow-up, including a plan for reinforcement of learning. This is to be documented in the column labeled Plan.
6. *Each entry* must be accompanied by the date and the signature of the "teacher,"

These guidelines were prepared by an interdisciplinary team for use in patient education at Strong Memorial Hospital in Rochester, New York. Contributors included Patricia Allen, Terry Callison, Amy Finkle, Vivian Littlefield, Sr. Barbara Lum, Jules Moodley, Nancy Peco, Sophie Pines, Phyllis Sale, Sheryl Silberman, Elaine Trescott, Sr. Mary John Van Atta, Cheryl Wagner, Laurie Walsh, Mary Lou Wilkins, and Sue Zigrossi. These guidelines are reproduced here by permission.

	Date	Signature	Written Material Given	Assessment	Plan
Antepartum					
General information					
Diabetes/Predisposing factors					
Definitions					
Course in pregnancy					
Nutritional management					
Weight gain					
Diet plan					
Concentrated CHO					
Basic four food groups					
Hospital menu completion					
Reviews adequacy of tray					
Sample menu for home use					
Effects on fetus					
Glucose metabolism					
SGA/LGA					
Glucose storage					
Testing for optimal delivery					
Prematurity					
ICN/SCN/Tour					
Hypoglycemia					
Hyperglycemia					
Ketoacidosis					
Maternal infection					
Prevention					
UTI					
Vaginitis					
Activity					
Insulin					
Insulin types					
Injection technique					
Equipment and storage					
Urine tests for fetal well-being					
S/A					
Blood glucose testing					
Testing					
FBS					
2 hr PP					
GTT					
NST/CST					
U/S (see pamphlets)					
Kick count (see pamphlets)					
Amniocentesis					

Figure B–1. Diabetic teaching tool. *(cont.)*

	Date	Signature	Written Material Given	Assessment	Plan
Intrapartum Routine blood/urine assessment Insulin/glucose control Fetal monitoring Time and mode of delivery Delivery team					
Postpartum *Newborn* Glucose metabolism Hypoglycemia Critical time period Screening method Treatment					
Maternal Insulin requirements Diet Projected family size Contraceptive alternatives Community resources Contacting care provider					

Additional Patient Information Given	Date	Signature

Figure B–1. (cont.) Diabetic teaching tool.

indicating that the teaching has been done according to the content guidelines specific for that teaching category.

7. An additional section is provided to document other pertinent patient information that is not included in the teaching content guidelines. Examples of appropriate information are: how the learner has learned in the past, what facilitates learning for her, what supports the learner has, and if the learner has any special considerations such as a hearing loss or cultural/language barrier.

ANTEPARTUM TEACHING OBJECTIVES

The client will:

1. Explain diabetes.
   A. Define
      (1) Diabetes as a disease caused either by increased demand of insulin, an inadequate supply of insulin, or a combination of the two.

        (2) The pancreas as

           a. A large gland located behind and below the stomach and liver

           b. A major producer of insulin

        (3) Insulin as a hormone produced by the pancreas.

    B. List three predisposing factors.

        (1) Pregnancy—aggravates diabetes by increasing the need for insulin production.

        (1) Heredity—diabetes may have been transmitted in the family.

        (2) Obesity—requires more insulin to metabolize food.

    C. Discuss metabolism in diabetes mellitus.

        (1) Three main constituents of food

           a. Carbohydrates

           b. Fats

           c. Protein

        (2) Role of insulin

           a. Explain one major way in which insulin affects the body's use of glucose. Give one effect of the lack of insulin in carbohydrate metabolism.

           b. State one way in which insulin acts on fats. Give one effect of lack of insulin on fat metabolism.

           c. State one way in which insulin affects protein use by the body. Give one effect of the lack of insulin on protein metabolism.

        (3) Gestational or insulin-dependent diabetic

           a. State whether insulin-dependent or noninsulin-dependent.

              i. Pregnancy may cause a change in insulin dependency.

              ii. Discuss the meaning of gestational diabetes, noting increased susceptibility to diabetes later in life.

              iii. List three factors other than pregnancy that can aggravate diabetes.

    D. Discuss the course in pregnancy.

        (1) Review changes in diabetic needs as pregnancy progresses, which may necessitate hospitalization to determine insulin and diet requirements.

        (2) List three complications of diabetes during pregnancy.

        (3) Discuss feelings about being a pregnant diabetic.

2. Hypoglycemia

    A. Define as a less than normal level of glucose in the blood.

    B. Cause

        (1) State two possible causes of hypoglycemia.

        (2) State how pregnancy aggravates hypoglycemia.

    C. Symptoms

        (1) State three symptoms of hypoglycemia.

    D. Prevention

        (1) State four ways to prevent hypoglycemia.

        (2) Describe symptoms of hypoglycemia.

    E. Treatment—State two ways to treat hypoglycemia.

3. Hyperglycemia

    A. Define as a greater than normal level of glucose in the blood.

    B. Cause

        (1) State two possible causes of hyperglycemia.

        (2) State how pregnancy aggravates hyperglycemia.

    C. Symptoms
        (1) Describe three symptoms of hyperglycemia.
    D. Prevention
        (1) Describe four ways to prevent hyperglycemia.
        (2) Describe symptoms of hyperglycemia.
    E. Treatment
        (1) State one way to treat hyperglycemia.
4. Ketoacidosis
    A. Define as an acid condition of the body resulting from overproduction of ketones.
    B. Cause
        (1) State one cause of ketoacidosis.
        (2) Describe two possible precipitating factors of ketoacidosis.
    C. Symptoms
        (1) State two symptoms of depressed central nervous system activity.
    D. Prevention
        (1) State importance of testing urine routinely.
        (2) State when it is necessary to report urine testings to health care provider.
    E. Treatment
        (1) State that hospitalization may be necessary for effective treatment.

ANTEPARTUM TEACHING GUIDELINES

1. Explanation of diabetes: Assess what each client knows about diabetes. It is extremely important to assess the patient's past experiences with previous pregnancies, outcomes of those pregnancies, and other problems experienced in prior pregnancies.
    A. Definitions
        (1) Diabetes—an inability to use and store glucose normally because of a decrease or lack of insulin production or ineffective insulin production by the pancreas.
        (2) Pancreas—a large gland located behind and below the stomach and liver. A major function is the production of insulin.
        (3) Insulin—a highly specialized protein with powerful hormonal actions; secreted by beta cells of the Islets of Langerhans in the pancreas (Burrow & Ferris, 1975).
    B. Predisposing factors
        (1) Pregnancy
            a. "Host–parasite relationship"—Maternal glucose is transferred to the fetus.
            b. Anti-insulin effect.
            c. Human placental lactogen (HPL), a growth hormone produced by the placenta, increases mobilization of free fatty acids and diminishes the effect of maternal insulin. Highest levels are in the third trimester (Burrow & Ferris, 1975).
            d. Steroids
                i. Estrogen increases as gestation advances. Is thought to act as an insulin antagonist.

      ii. Progesterone may decrease peripheral effectiveness of insulin.

      iii. Cortisol is thought to cause maternal hypoglycemia by increasing gluconeogenesis (Schuler, 1979).

   e. White's Classification of Diabetes in Pregnancy (Burrows & Ferris, 1975):

      i. Class A—Gestational diabetes

      ii. Class B—Onset after age 20; duration less than 10 years

      iii. Class C—Onset before age 20; duration 10–20 years

      iv. Class D—Duration more than 20 years, or onset before age 10; benign retinopathy

      v. Class F—Nephropathy

      vi. Class R—Malignant retinopathy

(2) Heredity—Predisposes to diabetes; however, the pattern of inheritance is unclear.

   a. Analyze the family history. Investigate tissues and blood type, and ascertain degree of glucose tolerance (Melunsky, 1979).

(3) Obesity—requires a larger amount of insulin to utilize the food they eat.

C. Metabolism in diabetes mellitus (Epenshade, 1979).

(1) Explain the three main constituents of food.

   a. Carbohydrates—composed mainly of sugars and starches.

   b. Fats—occur in nearly pure form as liquids or solids, such as oils and margarine, may be a component of other foods, and may be of animal or vegetable origin. Fats have a higher energy content than any other food.

   c. Proteins—made up of amino acids with higher concentrations found in milk, eggs, fish, meat, dried beans and peas. Proteins are essential constituents of all living cells and are the nitrogen-containing nutrient.

(2) Explain the role of insulin—"An understanding of how insulin affects the body's use of carbohydrates, fats, and protein and what happens when there is a lack of it is basic to understanding why diabetics develop the signs and symptoms they do" (Epenshade, 1979, p. 26).

   a. Insulin and carbohydrates:

      i. Without insulin, the glucose cannot get into the cells to be burned, the glucose cannot be stored in the liver, and the liver breaks down the glycogen it has stored. This results in hyperglycemia, fatigue, and no glucose reserves.

   b. Insulin affects availability of glucose in three ways:

      i. "Insulin allows movement of glucose from blood into fat and muscle cells. To use an analogy between the body and a car, the ignition key must be turned before gasoline can move through the gas line to the engine. Just as your car cannot get gas to run unless you turn the key, so the body cannot get glucose for energy without insulin. Thus, insulin is like the key, glucose is like the gasoline, the blood is like the gas line, and the cell is like an engine" (Epenshade, 1979, p. 26).

      ii. "Insulin stimulates the storage of glucose as glycogen in the liver."

      iii. "Insulin inhibits the breakdown of glycogen to glucose" (Epenshade, 1979).

      c. Insulin and fat
         i. The lack of insulin results in the breakdown of fat tissue and thus weight loss. One product of the fat breakdown is ketones. When too many ketones build up in the blood, ketonuria and then ketoacidosis occur.
        ii. Insulin acts in two ways in relation to fat (Epenshade, 1979).
           (a) Insulin promotes conversion of foods to fat tissue.
           (b) Insulin inhibits breakdown of fat tissue.
      d. Insulin and protein
         i. When the body lacks insulin, less protein is synthesized. In children, growth does not progress well and in adults, damaged tissue does not heal rapidly. Also, when there is not enough insulin, the body converts protein to glucose and this results in more blood sugar (Epenshade, 1979).
           (a) Insulin stimulates protein synthesis within tissues.
           (b) Insulin inhibits the conversion of protein to glucose (Epenshade, 1979).
  (3) Gestational or insulin-dependent diabetic
      a. Gestational diabetes is a period of abnormal glucose tolerance occurring during pregnancy and controlled by diet and possibly insulin.
      b. The insulin-dependent diabetic requires a combination of diet and insulin therapy to control diabetes.
      c. The advancing pregnancy causes a decrease in glucose tolerance and an increase in insulin requirements (Guthrie & Guthrie, 1977). A gestational diabetic develops diabetes during pregnancy which disappears after delivery (usually within 6 weeks). She is more prone to develop diabetes within 15 years (Schuler, 1979, p. 449).
  (4) Factors other than the diabetogenic effect of pregnancy can aggravate diabetes.
      a. Emotional factors:
         i. Response to pregnancy
        ii. Outside stress placed upon mother, e.g., lack of finances, unstable family situation
      b. Decreased activity levels in pregnancy
      c. Nausea and vomiting
      d. Anorexia
      e. Metabolic problems, e.g., T4 increases, Cushing's syndrome
D. Course of diabetes in pregnancy.
  (1) The insulin dependent diabetic may need her dosage adjusted frequently during her pregnancy (Schuler, 1979). As pregnancy advances and levels of HPL, estrogen, progesterone, and cortisol increase, diabetes intensifies.
      a. First trimester—the drain of maternal glucose for fetal development results in decreased insulin requirements. Because of this, diabetics are more prone to hypoglycemic reactions. As pregnancy advances and levels of HPL, estrogen, progesterone, and cortisol increase, diabetes intensifies.
      b. Second trimester—diabetes intensifies and a tendency toward maternal acidosis increases.
      c. Third trimester—still further increase of diabetogenic state causes con-

stant changes in insulin requirements. Will need frequent evaluation and regulation.

(2) The diabetic is more prone to develop complications and problems during pregnancy (Schuler, 1979).
   a. Vaginal infections and pregnancy-induced hypertension
   b. Pre-eclampsia
   c. Hyperglycemia and ketoacidosis
   d. Increased incidence of still births
   e. Large for gestational age (LGA) babies in Class A, B, and C diabetics and small for gestational age (SGA) babies in Class D, F, and R diabetics
   f. Polyhydramnios

(3) Discuss patient's concerns and feelings about being diabetic and pregnant.

2. Hypoglycemia
  A. Definition—a less than normal level of glucose in the blood (Guthrie & Guthrie, 1977).
  B. Possible causes—too much insulin is taken; insufficient amount of food is ingested; increase in amount of exercise with additional food; and hyperglycemic effects of certain drugs. May be aggravated in pregnancy by fetus syphoning glucose from maternal system and/or from nausea and vomiting that may occur in early pregnancy (Guthrie & Guthrie, 1977).
  C. Symptoms—each diabetic may experience different symptoms and should be aware of how the body reacts to hypoglycemia (Guthrie & Guthrie, 1977).
    (1) Primary level symptoms—nervousness, shakiness, weakness, sweatiness, headache, blurred vision, and hunger.
    (2) Secondary level symptoms—severe headache, blurred vision, disorientation, light-headedness, and finally, unconsciousness.
  D. Prevention
    (1) Do not alter activity states beyond what is normal.
    (2) Do not skip meals, eat less than prescribed at a given time, or change time of meals.
    (3) Promptly report illness and infections.
    (4) Avoid emotional stress.
    (5) Know how your own body reacts (Guthrie & Guthrie, 1977).
  E. Treatment—emphasize knowing and understanding symptoms and treating all reactions immediately.
    (1) Eat a simple, fast-acting sugar, e.g., 4 oz orange juice, 2 lumps sugar, 4 oz of a sweetened beverage, 1–2 hard candies.
    (2) If no improvement after 5 min, repeat same dose of sugar, candy, etc.
    (3) If no improvement in 15 min, have someone bring you to a hospital or call an ambulance.
    (4) If immediate treatment works, then 1 hour afterward take one glass of milk or eat a meal (if it is mealtime). The reason for this is to be sure your blood sugar does not get too low again.
    (5) Overtreatment should be avoided. Usually 10 g of glucose is all that is needed.
    (6) If the diabetic woman is not alert enough to swallow, do not force fluids. An injection of glucagon should be given. Every person on insulin should have glucagon available at home, with a family member instructed in its use.

3. Hyperglycemia
    A. Definition—a greater than normal level of glucose in the blood (Guthrie & Guthrie, 1977).
    B. Possible causes—increased dietary intake of large quanitities of carbohydrates especially when exercise does not increase at the same time; infection and fever; emotional stress; drugs, i.e., thiazides and corticosteroids during pregnancy, the diabetogenic effect increases as gestation increases (Guthrie & Guthrie, 1977).
    C. Symptoms
        (1) "In the earlier stages, symptoms are polyuria, polydipsia, dry mouth and polyphagia" (Guthrie & Guthrie, 1977).
        (2) "As it progresses to ketonuria and acidosis, then feelings of tiredness, abdominal cramps, nausea, decreased appetite and Kussmaul's respirations may develop. With further depression the client may go into ketoacidosis" (Guthrie & Guthrie, 1977).
        (3) Watch for signs of infection and notify your health care provider if it occurs.
    D. Prevention
        (1) Do not omit insulin.
        (2) Eat meals at regularly scheduled times; do not overeat.
        (3) Avoid emotional stress.
        (4) Awareness of body reaction to hyperglycemia.
        (5) If unable to eat solids, take insulin and liquids.
        (6) Test urine daily (Guthrie & Guthrie, 1977).
    E. Treatment
        (1) Call health care provider.
        (2) Take insulin if forgotten.
        (3) Have someone stay with client.
        (4) Go to bed.
        (5) Take one cup of hot liquid, e.g., salty broth, tea, or coffee every hour.
        (6) Test urine for sugar and acetone every time you urinate; keep a written record of the results.
        (7) Hospitalization is usually indicated for severe cases.
4. Ketoacidosis: Maternal ketoacidosis presents the greatest risk to the fetus during pregnancy (Clark & Alfonso, 1979).
    A. Definition—an acid condition of the body resulting from overproduction of ketones.
    B. Caused by a shift from carbohydrates to fat metabolism for energy because of lack of insulin or inability to utilize available insulin; the end effect of hyperglycemia. May be precipitated by emotional or physical stress, infection, surgery, or failure to take insulin. Diabetes may be previously undiagnosed (Guthrie & Guthrie, 1977).
    C. Symptoms—same as hyperglycemia.
        (1) Symptoms of central nervous system depression—headache, stupor, decreased muscle tone and reflexes, coma (Guthrie & Guthrie, 1977).
    D. Prevention—recognize symptoms of hyperglycemia
        (1) Routinely check urine and report any ketonuria to health care provider.
    E. Treatment—"Will be hospitalized in intensive care to restore normal carbohy-

drate, fat and protein metabolism; fluid balance; and to recognize and treat any circulatory complications" (Guthrie & Guthrie, 1977).

BIBLIOGRAPHY

Burrow, G. N., & Ferris, T. F. *Medical complications during pregnancy*. Philadelphia: W. B. Saunders, 1975.

Clark, A. L., & Alfonso, D. *Childbearing: A nursing perspective* (2nd ed.). Philadelphia: F. A. Davis, 1979.

Epenshade, J. *Staff manual for teaching patients about diabetes mellitus*. U.S. Dept. of Health, Education, and Welfare (in cooperation with the American Hospital Association), 1979.

Guthrie, D. W., & Guthrie, R. A. *Nursing management of diabetes mellitus*. St. Louis, Mo.: C. V. Mosby, 1977.

Melunsky, A. *Know your genes*. New York: Avon, 1979.

Miller, B. F., & Keane, C. B. *Encyclopedia and dictionary of medicine and nursing*. Philadelphia: W. B. Saunders, 1972.

Schuler, K. When a pregnant woman is diabetic: Antepartal care. *American Journal of Nursing*, 1979, 79(3), 448–450.

Steinberg, A. G. Heredity and diabetes. *Eugenics Quarterly*, 1955, 2, 26.

Tucker, S. M. *Fetal monitoring and fetal assessment in high risk pregnancy*. St. Louis, Mo.: C. V. Mosby, 1978.

Ziegel, E. E., & Cranley, M. S. *Obstetric nursing*. New York: Macmillan, 1978.

NUTRITIONAL MANAGEMENT TEACHING OBJECTIVES

The client will:

1. Consume adequate calories and nutrients distributed properly to meet needs of pregnancy as evidenced by appropriate weight gain and determined by care provider.
2. Describe diet plan based on diet history, food likes and dislikes.
3. Comply with diet, both in hospital and at home, as evidenced by the following:
   A. Instruction and assessment
      (1) Avoid concentrated carbohydrates.
      (2) Place foods in Basic Four Food Groups.
      (3) Complete hospital menu with accuracy.
      (4) Complete sample menu for home use based on diet prescription.
4. Modify diet for home use with assistance.

NUTRITIONAL TEACHING GUIDELINES

1. Coordinate the client's learning needs—instructing the client, referring appropriately, and reinforcing dietary instructions.
   A. Ensure that client is receiving the appropriate number of calories to meet the energy needs of pregnancy based on height, weight, and other factors.
   B. Methods used to determine the caloric needs of a pregnant woman include the following:
      (1) Allow approximately 40 kcal/kg of body weight during pregnancy. It has

been shown that energy intakes below 36 kcal/kg impair adequate protein utilization in pregnancy (Oldham & Sheft, 1951).

(2) Calorie needs may be calculated by first calculating basal energy expenditure (BEE):

  a. For women: BEE = 665 + (9.6 × present weight) + 1.7 × present height − (4.7 × age)

  b. For weight maintenance: BEE × 1.20 (Blackburn et al., 1977).

(3) Caloric need may also be calculated by determining a patient's ideal body weight (IBW).

  a. IBW: women 100 lb for the first 5 ft of height plus 5 lb for each additional inch.

   i. Small frame subtract 10% × IBW

   ii. Large frame add 10% × IBW

  b. To determine total calories needed:

   i. BEE + IBW × 10

   ii. Add activity Kcals:

    (a) sedentary: IBW × 3

    (b) moderate: IBW × 5

    (c) strenuous: IBW × 10 (American Diabetes Association, 1976).

C. All methods of determining caloric needs are approximations and may need to be adjusted to fit the individual. Frequent weights are the best measurement of whether caloric needs are being met. The average weight gain during the first trimester is 2 to 4 lb, and approximately 1 lb each week thereafter. Adjustments may be needed for teens, underweight, or highly active individuals.

D. Caloric needs will be recalculated postpartum for weight maintenance, weight loss, or lactation prior to discharge.

2. Interview patient and establish rapport as you obtain diet history. Ask open-ended questions.

A. Assess adequacy of diet patterns and life-style as it relates to nutrition.

  (1) Gather data regarding the family meals, food preparation, shopping, occupations, weight patterns, etc.

  (2) Record typical food, snack, or beverage items ingested at meals.

B. Assess patient's understanding of diabetes.

C. Assess patient's motivation and ability to comply with prescribed diet.

D. Assess pateint's eating habits, likes, dislikes. Record typical food, snack, or beverage items ingested at meals.

3. Calculation of diet

A. Nutrient balance

  (1) Once the proper caloric level is determined, the next step is to ensure proper nutrient balance.

  (2) Carbohydrate intake should not be disproportionately reduced for the diabetic. However, carbohydrates should be provided in complex forms such as breads, cereals, and vegetables whenever possible. Concentrated carbohydrates are quickly absorbed, resulting in greater increments in blood glucose. Adequate carbohydrates are important for diabetic control as well as fetal demands for glucose. This need translates to approximately 45 percent of total Kilocalories as carbohydrates (Worthington & Roberts, 1977).

  (3) Optimum protein is also important in diabetic control, because protein

needs are increased during pregnancy. Ther diet should contain approximately 2 g protein/kg body weight. This translates to approximately 20 percent of total calories from protein (Worthington & Roberts, 1977).

(4) Thus the remainder of total calories (30–35 percent) should come from fat. This is adequate to meet the requirements of the pregnant diabetic.

B. Distributive balance

(1) Provide ³⁄₁₀ at breakfast, ³⁄₁₀ at lunch, ³⁄₁₀ at dinner, and ¹⁄₁₀ at snack. This serves to provide total Kilocalories in much the same distribution. It is necessary for the distribution of food throughout the day to balance with insulin activity to avoid insulin or diabetic reactions and provide for sustained release of glucose (Worthington & Roberts, 1977).

(2) Once the patient is discharged, the Kilocalories may be dispersed in three meals and three snacks, if desired. While in the hospital, however, three meals plus an evening snack is the standard for glucose monitoring unless otherwise ordered.

(3) A sheet can be developed for calculating the diet. Exchange lists and explanations of how to calculate a diabetic diet can be provided by the Hospital Dietician.

(4) For convenience, standard patterns for various Kilocalorie levels can be developed by the dietetics department. These can be used temporarily for the newly admitted patient who has not yet been seen by the dietician, who will individualize the pattern to conform to the patient's needs and preferences.

4. Monitoring tolerance and compliance to diet

Once the diet plan has been established, the patient is visited regularly by the dietician or nurse for further assessmment of tolerance and compliance with diet. The dietician or nurse emphasizes the importance of eating all items on trays for consistency of intake during this period of insulin adjustment. The patient may have suggestions or complaints that can be attended to by modifications in the diet. The dietician documents and monitors the patient's intake and feelings of hunger or satiety. Persistent problems may indicate that a change in caloric level is necessary. The patient's menu is checked daily by a dietician to ensure accuracy in meeting the diet prescription.

A. Instruction and assessment

Diet instruction is an ongoing process throughout the hospital stay. Formal instruction takes place during a session in which the dietician gives the patient a dietary instruction booklet and explains the diet. Based on the dietician's or nurse's assessment of the patient's level of understanding, a decision is made as to whether to use the yellow, more basic copy, or the white standard copy. Both follow the commonly used American Diabetic Association exchange system and contain the patient's individualized diet as planned by the dietician.

(1) Instructions incorporate the following principles:

 a. Uses the American Diabetic Association exchange system.

 b. Rationale for diet in relation to blood glucose and insulin.

 c. Avoidance of concentrated carbohydrates.

 d. Regulation of eating pattern.

(2) Instruction will vary greatly from patient to patient based on needs, interest, and intelligence level. The dietician asks questions to assess the pa-

tient's understanding of aforementioned principles. The patient may make daily menu selections that are checked for accuracy by the dietician. The patient may be asked to complete a sample home menu following her plan. This allows the dietician to assess both subjectively and objectively the progress, understanding, and expected compliance of the patient.

B. Diet modifications for home use
  (1) Prior to discharge, a few changes in the patient's diet plan may be made to adjust for the home environment. These changes usually involve redistribution of foods to allow for snacks and smaller meals.
  (2) The patient is given the dietician's name and business phone number on an instruction sheet, should further questions arise.
  (3) Available glucose diets.
      From time to time the pregnant diebetic may require four 6-hour glucose feedings. This diet is inflexible in terms of amounts and kinds of foods; however, these are only temporary conditions. The rationale and guidelines for solid and liquid glucose diets can be developed at each hospital.

BIBLIOGRAPHY

American Diabetes Association, Inc. *Exchange lists for meal planning*. New York: The American Dietetic Association, 1976.

Blackburn, L., Vermeersch, J., & Rodwell Williams, S. Nutritional and metabolic assessment of the hospitalized patient. *Journal of Parenteral and Enteral Nutrition*, 1977, *1*, 1–11.

Committee on Maternal Nutrition, Food and Nutrition Board, National Research Council, National Academy of Sciences. *Maternal nutrition and course of pregnancy*. Washington, D.C.: U.S. Government Printing Office, 1970.

Oldham, H., & Sheft, B. B. Effect of caloric intake on nitrogen utilization during pregnancy. *Journal of American Dietetic Association*, 1951, 27(10), 847–854.

Recommended Dietary Allowances (rev. ed.). Washington, D.C.: Food and Nutrition Board, National Academy of Sciences, National Research Council, 1979.

Worthington, B., & Roberts, S. *Nutrition in pregnancy and lactation*. St. Louis, Mo.: C. V. Mosby, 1977.

EFFECTS ON FETUS: TEACHING OBJECTIVES

The client will:

1. Describe briefly the process of glucose metabolism during fetal life.
2. State how growth of the fetus is affected, depending on the classification of diabetes.
3. Explain how the fetus stores glycogen to prepare for birth.
4. Explain why it may be necessary to deliver the infant before 40 weeks' gestation.
5. Explain the various tests used to help the medical staff decide the optimal time for delivery of the infant.
6. Discuss the meaning of prematurity, and what this could mean in terms of the infant.
7. Discuss and tour special care units.
   A. Discuss why the infant would be admitted to Intensive Care Nursery or Special Care Newborn Nursery.

B. Tour Intensive Care Nursery and Special Care Newborn units prior to delivery.

EFFECTS ON FETUS: TEACHING GUIDELINES

1. Process of glucose metabolism during fetal life.
   A. During fetal life, energy consumption is high. The fetus must meet the needs of growth, energy storage, and metabolic maintenance.
   B. During gestational development, glucose is transferred continuously across the placenta from mother to fetus. Glucose is the fetus' primary energy source. Other sources do not appear to be significant *in utero*.
   C. Concentration of glucose in the plasma of the fetus is about 70–80 percent of the maternal level. As maternal glucose levels fluctuate from high and low, the fetus is subjected to these changes.
   D. Maternal insulin does not cross the placenta; therefore, the fetus is dependent on his or her own supply of insulin for development. This production is stimulated by increased glucose available from the maternal circulation.
2. Growth of the fetus in relation to the mother's classification of diabetes.
   A. Class A, B and C usually deliver large for gestational age (LGA) babies.
      (1) Fetal hyperglycemia, which results from high maternal levels of blood sugar, provides a continuous stimulus to the islets for insulin production, as evidenced by their hyperplasia. Fetal hyperinsulinism and hypoglycemia ultimately lead to excessive growth and deposition of fat (Korones, 1976, p. 207).
   B. Class D, F, and R are more likely to deliver small for gestational age (SGA) babies.
      (1) This is due to vascular and kidney involvement and the compromised placental function associated with these classes of diabetes.
3. The fetus stores glycogen to prepare for birth.
   A. As the pregnancy proceeds, the liver glycogen increases and placenta glycogen slowly declines. At about 20–24 weeks of gestation the fetal liver becomes the primary storage site for glycogen, while placental deposits gradually diminish. Glycogen stored in the fetal heart and skeletal muscle simultaneously increases as pregnancy proceeds to term. These glycogen supplies, particularly those of the liver and heart, are indispensable sources of energy (Korones, 1976, p. 204). Before this time the placenta has a high glycogen content, and has enzymes for glucose release and therefore is able to regulate the fetal blood glucose level until the liver is ready to assume this function. Energy appears to be stored rapidly near term. Glycogen reaches about 5 percent by weight in the liver and up to 4 percent in heart muscle. These energy stores are decreased by prematurity and intrauterine malnutrition. It is felt that these stores are utilized during the process of birth, and the fetus may rely on the stores of energy during this time. If the birth is complicated by malnutrition or prematurity, storage may be inadequate, and the birth process may be very stressful for the fetus.
4. Delivery before 40 weeks gestation.
   A. It might be necessary to deliver the fetus before term. The medical goal is to achieve all possible advantages to the fetus from its intrauterine environment,

and to detect and deliver the fetus when the intrauterine environment becomes disadvantageous or dangerous. This may occur when the placenta malfunctions, and needs to be assessed on an individual basis through the various tests available to the medical team:

(1) Ultrasonic measurement of the biparietal diameter
(2) Estriol assays
(3) NST/CST
(4) L/S ratio
(5) PG assay

5. Prematurity—38 to 42 weeks is the average length of gestation.
   A. The baby born before 37 weeks is called premature, immature, or preterm.
   B. A baby born before the mother's delivery date sometimes needs surroundings that provide some of the same things the mother provided, e.g., warmth, nourishment. The body will be completely formed when the infant is born prematurely; however, some body systems may be immature. This means (s)he will probably not be as mature as a full-term baby until at least the mother's expected delivery date.

6. The infant of a diabetic is at risk for a number of problems.
   A. Macrosomia—excessive fetal size for gestational age. These infants characteristically have a round, cherubic face and an increase in length proprotionate to their weight. Most commonly seen in Class A and B, but may be seen in Class C (Felig, 1975, p. 183).
   B. Hypoglycemia—due primarily to a temporary state of hyperinsulism in response to the high glucose load imposed by the mother. The neonate's larger glycogen stores thus are rapidly depleted (Jensen, Benson, & Bobak, 1977, p. 500).
   C. Prematurity—resulting in respiratory distress syndrome (RDS) and other immaturity of various body systems.
   D. Hyperbilirubinemia—more frequently seen among infants of diabetic mothers than in babies of like gestational age who are born of nondiabetic mothers. Characteristics and treatment of this disorder are identical in all premature infants (Korones, 1976, p. 208).
   E. Hypocalcemia—occurs in 30 percent of infants of diabetic mothers and infants of mothers of gestational diabetes. This condition is related to the associated high incidence of preterm delivery and perinatal asphyxia.
   F. Birth trauma and perinatal asphyxia occur in 20–35 percent of infants of diabetic mothers. Examples include the following: cephal hematoma, paralysis of facial nerve, fracture of the clavicle, bronchial plexus palsy, phrenic nerve palsy (Jensen, Benson, & Bobak, 1977, p. 599).

7. Congenital anomalies—occur two or three times more frequently than in the general population. The incidence is greatest among infants of the diabetic mother at Classes C–F. The more frequently occurring anomalies include:
   A. CNS—anencephaly, encephalocele, meningomyelocele, hydrocephalus.
   B. Caudal regression syndrome—sacral agenesis with weakness or deformities or both at the lower extremities, malformation and fixation of the hip joints, and shortening or deformity of the femurs.
   C. Tracheoesophageal fistula.
   D. Congenital heart malformations—increased threefold compared to infants of

nondiabetic mothers (Jensen, Benson, & Bobak, 1977, p. 264, 600; Korones, 1976, p. 209).

8. Admission to Neonatal Intensive Care unit and Special Care Nursery. Infants of Class A diabetes will be admitted to normal Newborn Nursery if they have had an uneventful delivery. All other diabetic newborns will go to a Special Care Nursery for the first 24 hours, or as needed.

   A. Tour—Parents and grandparents are encouraged to visit in the nursery often after delivery. Parents should tour the Intensive and Special Care nurseries before delivery, whenever possible. Explain equipment and various aspects of the nursery to lessen their anxiety. Siblings may "window visit."

BIBLIOGRAPHY

Burrow, G., & Ferris, T. F. (Eds.). *Medical complications during pregnancy*. Philadelphia: W. B. Saunders, 1975.

Felig, P. Diabetes mellitus. In G. Burrow & T. F. Ferris (Eds.), *Medical complications during pregnancy*. Philadelphia: W. B. Saunders, 1975.

Jensen, M., Benson, R. C., & Bobak, I. *Maternity care: The nurse and the family*. St. Louis, Mo.: C. V. Mosby, 1977, pp. 263–269, 599–601.

Korones, S. B. *High-risk newborn infants*. St. Louis, Mo.: C. V. Mosby, 1976, pp. 204–209.

MATERNAL INFECTION TEACHING OBJECTIVES

The client will:

1. Discuss predisposition of diabetics to infection.
   A. State that diabetics are more susceptible to all types of infection and more highly during pregnancy.
2. Discuss prevention of infection.
   A. Describe routine perineal care during pregnancy.
   B. Describe four skin care practices to be maintained.
   C. Describe seven foot care practices to be maintained.
   D. Describe mouth care during pregnancy.
      (1) State one reason why dental care is important during pregnancy.
      (2) State two dental care practices to prevent caries.
   E. State one symptom of viral disturbance that must be reported to the care provider.
3. Discuss urinary tract infections.
   A. List two reasons pregnancy predisposes diabetics to urinary tract infections.
   B. List two possible effects of urinary tract infections that may affect pregnancy.
   C. List five symptoms of a urianry tract infection.
   D. List three ways of preventing urinary tract infections.
4. Discuss vaginitis.
   A. Cause
      (1) List two organisms that commonly cause vaginitis.
      (2) List one reason the diabetic is prone to vaginal infections.
   B. Distinguish between characteristics and origin of normal vaginal discharge during pregnancy and those of vaginitis.

    C. List two symptoms of monilial vaginitis.
    D. List three ways of preventing vaginitis.
    E. Reporting of symptoms
      (1) State the importance of early reporting of symptoms to the care provider.
5. Discuss skin care.
    A. List the elements of good skin care.
6. Discuss foot care.
    A. List the elements of good foot care.
7. Discuss mouth care.
    A. List the elements of good dental care.
8. Discuss eye care.
    A. List the elements of good eye care
9. Discuss the reporting of symptoms.

MATERNAL INFECTION: TEACHING GUIDELINES

Assess each client's knowledge about diabetes. Patient education needs are dependent upon current knowledge and level of comprehension.

1. Predisposition
    A. Diabetics are highly susceptible to all types of infection. Some factors responsible for increased susceptibility include peripheral vascular insufficiency and high levels of glucose in soft tissues. Pregnancy may additionally predispose the diabetic to urinary tract infection.
2. Prevention of infection and personal care practices.
    A. Perineal care
      (1) Bathe or shower daily.
      (2) Eliminate douching unless prescribed by health care provider.
      (3) Note and report changes from normal vaginal discharge.
      (4) Cleanse from front to back after voiding or a bowel movement.
3. Urinary tract infections
    A. Predisposing causes
      (1) Pregnant women are apt to develop urinary tract infection due to stasis of urine, caused by
        a. Mechanical pressure of gravid uterus on ureters.
        b. Physiological effects of progesterone on smooth muscle (which decreases contractility).
      (2) In pregnancy complicated by diabetes, these problems are compounded by glycosuria, which is a favorable environment for bacteriuria.
    B. Complications
      (1) Urinary tract infection is a predisposing factor in prematurity.
      (2) Urinary tract infection increases the incidence of pyelonephritis, a serious complication of pregnancy.
      (3) Diabetes becomes temporarily more severe with infection and requires reestablishment of control.
    C. Symptoms—In addition to screening for infection with a clean catch midstream urine during prenatal visits, some common symptoms that may be experienced with a urinary infection include:

          (1) Dysuria 38°C/100.4°F.
          (2) Fever.
          (3) Urgency of need to urinate.
          (4) Frequency of urination.
          (5) Lower abdominal pain.
          (6) Back pain (tenderness in region of kidney, just below waistline).
    D. Prevention of urinary tract infection
          (1) Screen for infection on prenatal visits with midstream clean catch urine collections.
          (2) Ingest adequate fluid intake to flush out bacteria in urine.
          (3) Comply with described diabetic treatment.
          (4) Report any symptoms to care provider.
          (5) Cleanse from front to back after stool or void; one wipe and dispose of tissue.
4. Vaginitis
    A. Cause
          (1) Simple vaginitis is caused by *E. coli*, staphylococcus, streptococcus.
          (2) Monilial vaginitis is caused by *Candida albicans*, which thrives in an environment rich in sugar. Therefore, monilial vaginitis is common in patients with poorly controlled diabetes.
    B. Normal vaginal discharge of pregnancy
          (1) Vaginal discharge increases during pregnancy. It arises from the cervical glands and often appears thick, white, and stringy.
          (2) Vaginal discharge has strong acid reaction due to lactic acid content, which is believed to help keep vagina relatively free of pathogenic bacteria.
    C. Symptoms
          (1) Thick, white, cheese-like vaginal discharge.
          (2) Vaginal and vulvar region may appear either normal or have acute inflammation, which may involve urethra and cause dysuria.
          (3) Pruritis.
    D. Prevention
          (1) Maintain hygiene with daily bathing or showering.
          (2) Maintain diabetic control.
          (3) Report symptoms of increased vaginal discharge to health care provider.
          (4) Eliminate douching.
5. Skin care
    A. Elements of care
          (1) Bathe or shower daily.
          (2) Use lotion to avoid cracking and drying.
          (3) Maintain exercise and activity levels in moderation to promote good circulation.
          (4) Check skin for bruises, abrasions, lacerations.
          (5) Promptly report and seek care provider's treatment for injury.
6. Foot care
    A. Elements of care
          (1) Keep feet clean and dry thoroughly between toes; trim toenails straight across.
          (2) Wear shoes to avoid injuries to bare feet.

        (3) Wear properly fitted shoes.
- a. Avoid stockings that restrict circulation, including knee highs or round garters.

        (4) Avoid extremes of heat, cold, and exposure to strong chemicals.

        (5) Maintain exercise and activity in moderation to promote good circulation.
- a. Avoid crossing knees; elevate legs whenever possible when sitting.
- b. Avoid pressure at back of knees when sitting.
- c. When traveling, stop hourly and walk for 10 minutes.

        (6) Inspect feet carefully and routinely for calluses, corns, blisters, abrasions, and ingrown toenails, with early treatment of foot problems by podiatrist. Client should avoid treating own foot problems.

7. Mouth care
  A. Elements of care
     (1) The diabetic is susceptible to periodontal disease, commonly called pyorrhea. Periodontal disease does not always appear as an obvious swelling and bleeding of the gums, and it sometimes goes undetected until dental examination.
     (2) Poor oral hygiene resulting in accumulation of dental plaque invites periodontal disease. Therefore, good dental care includes:
- a. Daily brushing and flossing to remove dental plaque
- b. Dental checkups every 6 months.
- c. Reporting of oral complaints to dentist, particularly the swelling or bleeding of gums.

8. Eye care
  A. Retinopathy is by far the most common eye problem for the diabetic, and this may occur without visual impairment. Therefore, good eye care involves:
     (1) Periodic checks of retina by physician or ophthalmologist.
     (2) Maintenance of annual eye and visual checkups.
     (3) Reporting of visual changes, including blurred vision, to care provider.

9. Reporting of symptoms
  A. Early detection and successful treatment of infection and complications are enhanced when the patient reports any symptoms of urinary tract infection, vaginitis, injuries to skin or feet, or visual changes. If in doubt, it is better to check with the appropriate care provider than wait and jeopardize pregnancy and diabetes control.

ACTIVITY TEACHING OBJECTIVES

The client will:

1. Discuss maintaining normal activity levels during pregnancy.
  A. Discuss the effect of exercise in diabetic control.
  B. Discuss activity levels during hospitalization.
     (1) List ways of maintaining activity levels that closely resemble home.
     (2) Name at least one beneficial effect of this activity level during hospitalization.

ACTIVITY TEACHING GUIDELINES

1. Maintenance
   A. Effect of exercise in diabetic control.
      (1) Is beneficial, and pregnant women are encouraged to continue usual activities as long as they do not become fatigued.
      (2) May necessitate need for rest periods, as pregnancy progresses.
      (3) Is highly individualized and needs to be discussed with your care provider.
      (4) In diabetes, the balance of physical activity with rest becomes even more crucial in adjusting insulin dosages.
      (5) Exercise promotes metabolism and utilization of carbohydrates, decreasing insulin requirements; therefore, exercise enhances the effect of insulin.
      (6) It is important to maintain reasonable consistency in the length of exercise and rest periods.
   B. Activity level during hospitalization for control.
      (1) Encourage maintaining activity levels similar to those in their home situation. Activities may include showering, dressing in street clothes, walking, reading, and doing crafts.
      (2) Activity levels resembling "at home" situations help the care provider to institute adjustments in the American Dietetic Association diet and insulin requirements, which will be appropriate when the patient is discharged.

INSULIN: TEACHING OBJECTIVES

The client will:

1. Discuss the types and administration of insulin.
   A. State the type(s) of insulin they are using, including duration and peak time for the insulin(s).
   B. State appropriate techniques to follow for administering insulin.
   C. Administer own insulin, following appropriate techniques.
   D. Mix two kinds of insulin appropriately (if needed).
2. Discuss need for an injection schedule.
   A. State time for these injections.
   B. State schedule for obtaining insulin base line and reason for its use.
   C. State importance of eating regular meals when taking insulin.
3. Discuss choice and care of injection sites.
   A. State three injection sites.
   B. State one reason for rotation of injection sites (include diagram).
4. Discuss insulin and syringe maintenance.
   A. State where and at what temperature insulin should be stored.
   B. Describe appropriate care of syringes.

INSULIN: TEACHING GUIDELINES

1. Preface to teaching insulin injection.
   A. Expect some anxiety when a patient is learning to give insulin. Incorporate principles of learning when teaching self-administration of insulin.

(1) Proceed from simple to complex tasks.
(2) Reinforce learning.
(3) Break down learning into manageable segments of information.
B. Assess special needs of patients, including:
(1) Illiteracy
(2) Minimal level of literacy or comprehension
(3) Visual impairment
(4) Handicap(s) that interfere with insulin administration
2. Insulin
A. Types
(1) *Regular insulin*—duration 5–8 hours; peaks in 2–3 hours
(2) *Lente insulin*—duration 24 hours; peaks 8–10 hours
(3) *NPH insulin*—duration 24 hours; peaks 8–10 hours
(4) *Ultra Lente*—duration 36 hours; peaks 12–16 hours
B. Injection technique for administering insulin.
(1) Collect equipment (syringe, needle, alcohol and cotton, or alcohol swabs).
(2) Wash hands
(3) If NPH or Lente insulin, roll between hands to mix (also warms insulin if it has been stored in refrigerator).
(4) Wipe top of bottle with alcohol.
(5) Measure number of units of air; push into bottle.
(6) Turn bottle upside down; withdraw number of units of insulin needed.
(7) Get rid of all air bubbles in syringe.
(8) Check dose; remove needle from bottle; cap needle.
(9) Wipe skin with alcohol.
(10) Pinch skin up with thumb and forefinger.
(11) Uncap needle; hold like a pencil.
(12) Push needle straight into the skin at a 90-degree angle.
(13) Release pinched skin; inject insulin into skin.
(14) Remove needle from skin.
(15) Wipe skin with alcohol.
C. Instruct patient in administering own insulin using the proper technique
D. Mix two kinds of insulin
(1) Roll NPH or Lente between hands.
(2) Wipe bottle tops with alcohol.
(3) Measure number of units of air; inject into bottle of NPH or Lente; withdraw needle.
(4) Draw up number of units of air; inject into regular insulin
(5) Turn bottle upside down; withdraw number of units of insulin; check for bubbles in syringe.
(6) Reinsert needle into NPH or Lente; withdraw number of units needed.
3. Injection schedule
A. Time of injections
(1) During pregnancy the most common times for injections are before breakfast and before dinner.
(2) Combining regular and NPH or Lente offers the best coverage.
B. When hospitalized for regulation, to obtain a base line for daily insulin needs,

regular insulin is given every 6 hours prior to meals (6 AM, 12 noon, 6 PM, 12 midnight).
C. Consistency in technique and adherence to schedule.
4. Injection sites
   A. Appropriate sites include:
      (1) Upper arm
      (2) Upper thigh
      (3) Buttocks
      (4) Abdomen
   B. Rotation of sites is important to prevent skin breakdown. Once a site is used, it should not be used again for at least 14 days; however, a spot 1 inch away from previous site can be used.
      (1) May be helpful to keep a record of injection sites on a diagram (Fig. B–2).
5. Insulin and syringe maintenance
   A. Insulin must be kept at room temperature (68°–78°F). Extra insulin can be kept in the refrigerator (avoid freezing).
   B. Syringes
      (1) If using disposable syringes, they must be broken after use and disposed of properly.
      (2) If using glass syringes, they must be taken apart and sterilized by boiling for 10–15 minutes.
      (3) Alcohol and cotton balls can be used for cleaning injection sites.
      (4) Alcohol balls and alcohol swabs are available at the local drug store.

URINE TESTING: TEACHING OBJECTIVES

The client will:

1. Accurately test urine
   A. Accurately perform at least one method of urine testing.
   B. State one reason that daily fractional urine testing of sugar and acetone (ketones) and strict accurate record keeping are an important part of the medical management of diabetes.
2. Accurately record and report sugar and acetone levels.
   A. Accurately accomplish at least one method of recording and reporting sugar and acetone levels.
3. Accurately test, record, and report blood glucose.
   A. Test blood glucose levels using a reagent strip impregnated with glucose oxidase and a lancet.
   B. Record appropriately.
   C. Report results to care provider.

URINE TESTING: TEACHING GUIDELINES

1. Relevancy of urine testing. Urine testing: a diabetic has an adequate supply of carbohydrates that cannot be properly utilized because of an inadequate supply of insulin. Because the diabetic has a tendency to disordered carbohydrate metabo-

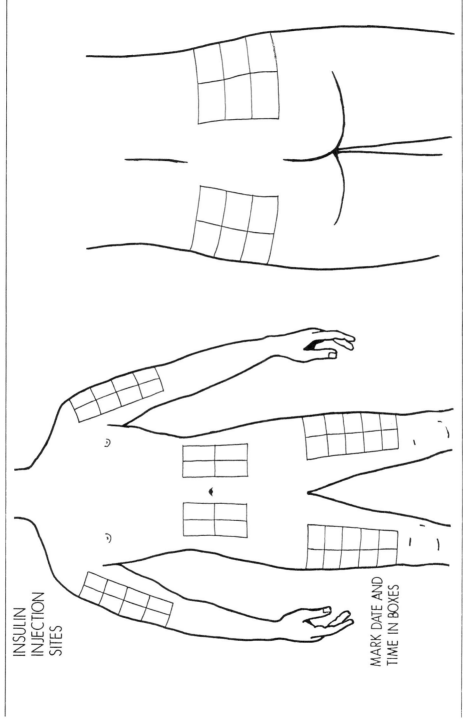

INSULIN
INJECTION
SITES

MARK DATE AND
TIME IN BOXES

Figure B–2. Form for recording insulin injection sites. (Source: University of Rochester/Strong Memorial Hospital, Rochester, New York, with permission.)

lism and the further difficulty of control in pregnancy, the glucose tolerance must be continually monitored. This provides a *rough* guide as to control.

A. Instruction for the use, care, and interpretations of the reagent strips are part of the packaging of the reagents. Encourage the patient to be totally familiar with all aspects.

    (1) Testing described is with the use of keto-diastiks. If the patient uses another testing material, e.g., Clinitest tabs, Test-tape, or Acetest tabs, then the patient needs instruction in the use of those materials.

B. Stress strict adherence to procedure and technique to insure accuracy.

    (1) Method:

        a. Use the double-voided specimen technique.

        b. Empties bladder, waits 15–30 minutes and voids again into a container.

        c. Test this urine sample with a keto-diastix in the urine and tap lightly on the container to remove excess urine.

        d. Compare the ketone test area (originally buff-colored) to the ketone color chart on the bottle *exactly* 15 seconds after wetting.

        e. Note the results printed above the color blocks on the bottle that most closely match the test areas at the specified reading times. Ignore color changes that occur after these times.

C. Instruct the patient to follow the instructions of the care provider as to the frequency of urine testing and notification of results.

2. Stress importance of strict, accurate record keeping. Record sheets should include date, time of last meal, time of testing glucose and ketone columns.

A. Ketones or acetone:

    (1) Check color of the reagent area at 15 seconds after wetting and compare to the ketone color chart on the bottle label.

    (2) State that the color blocks indicate the relative amounts (small, medium, large) of ketones present.

B. Glucose:

    (1) Check color of the reagent area at 30 seconds after wetting and compare to the glucose color chart on the bottle label.

    (2) State that the color blocks indicate the amounts of glucose present in units per percent, and also in milligrams per deciliter (mg/d) for metric system results.

3. Blood glucose testing. Because diabetic pregnancy outcome is directly related to the degree of control maintained throughout gestation, it is essential to closely monitor blood glucose levels. With the advent of available materials for home monitoring of these levels, it is now possible to achieve this control without repeated hospital admissions.

A. At this institution* the procedure followed for blood glucose testing is the one developed by Bio-Dynamics, Inc. for use with Chemstrip B.G.

B. Technique for proper use of B.G. Chemstrips.

    (1) Be sure that the expiration date on the B.G. Chemstrip bottle has not been reached.

    (2) Use only B.G. Chemstrip bottles that are properly capped, *and recap*

---

*Strong Memorial Hospital, Rochester, New York.

after use. B.G. Chemstrip bottles without caps may be exposed to excessive moisture, decreasing the accuracy of the strips.

(3) Use a time piece with an accurate second hand; exposure of blood on a reagent pad should be for 60 seconds exactly.

(4) Interpret the reagent strip *under bright lighting only*, not in the dark recesses of a patient's room.

(5) Use only the bottle from which you obtained the B.G. Chemstrip to interpret the glucose concentration. *Each bottle has an individual color code* that must be used to interpret the glucose value.

TESTS FOR FETAL WELL-BEING: TEACHING OBJECTIVES

The client will describe purpose and technique for:

1. Fasting blood sugar
2. 2-hour postprandial (PP) blood sugar
3. Glucose tolerance test (GTT)
4. Nonstress test (NST)
5. Oxytocin challenge test/contraction stress test (OCT/CST)
6. Ultrasound (Fig. B–3)
7. Amniocentesis (Fig. B–4)
8. Kick count (Figs. B–5 and B–6)

TESTS FOR FETAL WELL-BEING: TEACHING GUIDELINES

Assess motivation and ability of patient to follow instructions for testing procedure(s). The nurse and pregnant diabetic should have thorough knowledge of normal and diabetic alterations of carbohydrate metabolism in pregnancy.

1. Fasting blood sugar
   A. Measures glucose in the blood when fasting.
   B. Method
      (1) No food is taken 12 hours prior to testing; water is the only fluid allowed.
      (2) Blood is drawn by venipuncture.
   C. Interpretations
      (1) Normal range 80/100 mg.
      (2) Therapeutic goal is to maintain the fasting level at 100 mg.
2. Postprandial blood sugar (2-hour PP)
   A. Measures blood sugar following a meal.
   B. Method
      (1) Patient eats a meal containing 100 g of carbohydrates.
      (2) Blood is usually drawn by venipuncture 2 hours after meal.
   C. Interpretation
      (1) Normal range 80/100 mg.
      (2) Therapeutic goal is to maintain the postprandial level below 150 mg.
3. Glucose tolerance test (GTT): Explain necessity for using blood glucose rather than urine tests for management, regulation, and control.

What's an Ultrasound Exam?

Your doctor has scheduled you to have a <u>painless</u>, non-invasive procedure which takes about 30 minutes to perform. <u>No x-rays are involved.</u> Sound waves at frequencies above the range of human hearing are transmitted by a scanner held against your abdomen by a technologist. Echoes from various structures in your abdomen are displayed on a TV screen and photographed. You will be asked to lie on your back and mineral oil will be spread on your abdomen to assure good contact of the scanner with your skin. (See picture on opposite page.)

Measurements and appropriate pictures of the pelvic structures will be obtained. This information will be interpreted by the physician in the OB/GYN Ultrasound Laboratory at Strong Memorial Hospital and the results will be sent to your doctor, usually within three days. Please do not ask the technologists in the laboratory to comment on the results of your examination. It is the lab's policy that the results of your exam be given only to your physician.

The examination takes place in Room   on the second floor of Strong Memorial Hospital. It is essential that you have a <u>full urinary</u> bladder for the exam. <u>Drink one quart of water or juice one hour before your scheduled examination time. Do not empty your bladder.</u>

There is a charge for the ultrasound exams. One part of this is a hospital charge to cover the use of the equipment, the films, supplies, and technical personnel. There is also a physician's fee for the interpretation of the films as well as the written and/or oral consultation with your physician. For your convenience our billing department (   ) is located near the Ultrasound Laboratory. Please bring any appropriate claim forms with you at the time of your visit. You will be expected to pay that portion of the physician's fee not covered by your insurance.

Most women find that the examination is actually fun. It is painless, quick, and safe for you and your developing baby. Each year approximately 7,000 women have such examinations done in our Laboratory.

If you still have questions or need to change your appointment time, please call us at   . Patients who are late for their appointment will be rescheduled.

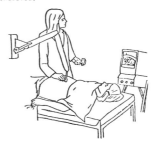

Your appointment is with the Department of OB-GYN Ultrasound Laboratory, Room   Strong Memorial Hospital.

NAME _____

DATE _____ TIME _____

Please report to Out-Patient Registration (near main lobby) 1/2 hour prior to each ultrasound examination.

A <u>full bladder is necessary</u> for this examination. <u>Drink 1 quart of water or juice 1 hour before your appointment. Do not empty your bladder.</u> If unable to keep this appointment, please call

Figure B–3. Patient education pamphlet on ultrasound. (*Source: University of Rochester/Strong Memorial Hospital, Rochester, New York, with permission.*)

A. Purpose
  (1) Measures response to a measured dose of glucose.
B. Method
  (1) Patient is prepared for test by ingesting a high carbohydrate diet (minimum 200 g carbohydrate per day) for 3 days preceding test. No food is taken 12 hours prior to or during test. No smoking, tea, or coffee are allowed during the test (alters body's response to carbohydrates). Minimal activity (alters glucose metabolism), and no stress (epinephrine and cortisone raise glucose levels) are the regimen.
  (2) See Tests and Procedures Protocol (Fig. B–7).
  (3) The test is begun with a fasting blood and urine specimen obtained from the patient.
    a. One hundred (100) mg of glucose are administered orally, over a 5-minute period.
    b. Blood samples are then drawn at 1-, 2-, and 3-hour intervals.
    c. Watch for signs and symptoms of dizziness, sweating, weariness, nausea, vomiting, or diarrhea during the test.

AMNIOCENTESIS

Your doctor has asked that an amniocentesis be performed for you. This means that some of the fluid which surrounds your unborn baby will be removed with a thin needle. The fluid is then sent for testing.

The amniocentesis will be done by an obstetrician. Since an ultrasound scan is always performed prior to the actual amniocentesis to help the physician determine where to place the needle, you will need to have a full urinary bladder. You will be asked to sign a consent form before we begin.

How?

Your abdomen will be cleaned with an antiseptic solution and a sterile towel will be draped over your abdomen. The doctor will then insert the needle through the abdomen into the uterus where the amniotic fluid surrounds the baby. You will feel the sting of the needle when it first penetrates your skin. However, there are relatively few nerves beneath the skin; you should only feel pressure as the fluid--about one ounce-- is removed. Most patients find that amniocentesis is no more uncomfortable than having a blood sample drawn.

When the test has been completed, the fluid will be sent to the laboratory. The doctor will let you know when the test results will be available.

After the amniocentesis

Occasional cramping pain is common after an amniocentesis. You should inform your obstetrician if any of the following happen: a) cramping which becomes more frequent in the hours following the procedure; b) vaginal bleeding; c) clear fluid being passed vaginally; d) decrease in fetal movement.

In the 24 hours following the procedure you should avoid strenuous exercise or lifting of heavy objects.

Why?

Some of the common reasons for having an amniocentesis are:

1. Genetic studies to detect an inherited disorder or to determine if Down's Syndrome (Mongolism) is present. A blood sample may be drawn before a genetic amniocentesis.

2. For detection of bilirubin levels if Rh sensitization is present. In this way the doctor can make a better judgment about when to deliver the baby.

3. To test for the maturity of the baby, especially the lungs, if the doctor is planning to deliver the baby early because of a maternal condition such as diabetes, high blood pressure, or bleeding.

4. To check for signs of infection after premature rupture of membranes.

Where?

The amniocentesis is done in the Obstetrics-Gynecology Ultrasound Laboratory on the second floor in the new hospital (Room #   ). If you should need to change the time of your appointment, please phone

YOUR APPOINTMENT IS:

DAY _____

DATE _____

TIME _____

[Please report to **Out-Patient Registration** in the Main Lobby ½ **hour** prior to your appointment time. Thank you!]

Figure B–4. Patient education pamphlet on amniocentesis. (*Source: University of Rochester/ Strong Memorial Hospital, Rochester, New York, with permission.*)

C. Interpretation
   (1) Plasma glucose level:
      a. Normal fasting   105 mg
      b. One-hour   190 mg
      c. Two-hour   165 mg
      d. Three-hour   145 mg
   (2) Abnormal GTT is two or more values outside the normal range.
   (3) Special considerations
      a. Every effort must be made to give careful instructions about the procedure, its importance, and the necessity of completeness of collection for accuracy.
      b. Provide supportive care!! The 24-hour urinary collection is often one of the more annoying and stressful aspects of the patient's medical regimen.
      c. When possible, provide a collection container that fits under the toilet seat, along with a leakproof container for storing urine.
      d. Label with identifying data (patient name, date, times of start and finish of collection).

Your doctor has requested that you keep a KICK COUNT on your baby. This is simply a record of your baby's movement in utero (womb). Some movements may feel like the baby's rolling around while other movements feel like the baby is kicking.

Recording the KICK COUNT is a simple procedure which is to be done twice each day, once in the morning and once in the early evening. While doing this you should focus your attention on your baby's movements. This means you should not watch T.V., read, or be involved in any other activity.

It is often possible to THINK your baby is moving less, when in reality it is not. Record only the movement(s) you are certain of at the time you feel it. If the baby seems to move half as much as the previous day, you should call the doctor IMMEDIATELY.

An active baby is a healthy baby and this information will be helpful to your doctor in assessing your baby's condition.

INSTRUCTIONS

1. You should not be without food for more than 4 hours.

2. Lie on left side.

3. Count each movement occuring during a one hour period.

4. Do this twice each day, once in the morning, once in the early evening at approximately the same time each day.

5. Record the date, time and number of movements on the sheet provided.

6. Notify your doctor IMMEDIATELY if the baby moves one-half as many times as the previous day.

7. Call 275-2401 between 8:30 a.m.- 4:30 p.m. Monday through Friday. 275-3131 after 4:30 p.m. and on weekends.

8. Bring the record sheet with you to your next visit to the clinic.

Figure B–5. Patient education pamphlet on fetal movement recording (kick count). *(Source: University of Rochester/Strong Memorial Hospital, Rochester, New York, with permission.)*

```
                              FETAL MOVEMENT RECORD
                                   KICK COUNT

        Patient Name:_____

        Unit #:_____
```

| | | MORNING | | | EVENING | |
DATE	TIME BEGUN	TIME ENDED	NUMBER OF MOVEMENTS	TIME BEGUN	TIME ENDED	NUMBER OF MOVEMENTS

Figure B–6. Fetal movement record sheet. *(Source: University of Rochester/Strong Memorial Hospital, Rochester, New York, with permission.)*

(4) Urinary creatinine is done to assure that the 24-hour urine collection is complete. The output of creatinine in a 24-hour urine is relatively constant. The average daily creatinine excretion in the last month of pregnancy is 1.35 g to 0.14 g (SD). Creatinine levels below 1.0 g indicate an unreliable urine collection.

4. Nonstress test (NST):
   A. Purpose
      (1) The placenta is vital to fetal life. It serves as lungs, intestinal tract, and kidneys for the fetus throughout intrauterine life. The placenta transports oxygen and metabolites from mother to fetus, eliminates waste products from the fetus to maternal circulation, and assists in production of protein and steroid hormones to accommodate needs of the fetus and pregnancy. The health—and sometimes survival—of the fetus is dependent on placental function. Uteroplacental insufficiency can affect the fetus in varying

degrees. Gradually developing insufficiency can affect fetal nutritional status; rapidly developing insufficiency can produce hypoxemia, acidosis, and subsequent fetal death. When hypoxia, acidosis, or drugs depress the fetal central nervous system, there may be a reduction in baseline variability of fetal heart rate and absence of accelerations with fetal movement. This can be assessed by nonstress testing (NST) (Figs. B–8 and B–9).

(2) The mechanical force of a uterine contraction (spontaneous or induced) impedes placental blood flow. When the fetus is under stress from the contraction and is unable to compensate due to decreased reserves, which may result from maternal diabetes, fetal distress develops. The oxytocin challenge test and contraction stress test provide a means for assessing uteroplacental reserve.

(3) The normal, healthy fetus demonstrates a characteristic fetal heart rate

---

Tests and Procedures Protocol: High Carbohydrate Diet for Preparation for Glucose Tolerance Test (Approximately 300 gm CHO)

Instructions

For your glucose tolerance test to give accurate results, it is important for you to eat a high carbohydrate diet for 3 days before the test. A pattern for the diet is given below. Be sure to eat both the right *kinds* and the right *amounts* of food. Especially, be sure to eat the carbohydrate foods (bread, potatoes, fruits, milk, sweet desserts). Sweetened beverages (pop or koolaid) and candy may be included as well. If there is something on the diet you cannot eat, please check with the care provider or clinic dietitian.

Breakfast

    1 cup (8 oz) orange or grapefruit juice or a large serving of other fruit.
    1 egg
    2 slices toast, or toast and cereal
    Butter or margarine, as desired
    1 Tablespoon or more, jam, jelly or honey for toast, or sugar for cereal
    1 cup (8 oz) milk
    Coffee or tea, as desired

Lunch

    Sandwich: 2 slices bread
               2 slices meat or cheese, or 2 tablespoons peanut butter (jelly may be added)
               Butter, margarine, or mayonnaise as desired
    Saltines or 2 graham crackers, or another slice of bread
    Vegetables, as desired
    Large serving of fruit or a sweet dessert such as cake, cookies, jello, etc.
    Coffee or tea, as desired

Dinner

    Medium-sized serving (3 oz or more) meat
    1 cup potatoes, rice, macaroni, or noodles
    1 slice bread or 1 roll, muffin, or biscuit
    Vegetables, as desired
    Butter, margarine, salad dressing, as desired
    Large serving of fruit or a sweet dessert such as jello, cake, cookies, etc.
    1 cup (8 oz) milk
    Coffee or tea, as desired

Snack

    Large serving fruit or juice or 1 cup (8 oz) milk
    4 graham crackers or 2 slices bread, or toast, cereal, cookies, etc.

Figure B–7. Test and procedures protocol: High carbohydrate diet.

NON STRESS TEST

Your doctor has requested that you have a Non-Stress Test (N.S.T.). The purpose of this test is to provide information about how well your baby is doing.

The test is performed with you lying in a bed or lounge chair. A light elastic band is used to hold small sensors from a fetal monitor on your abdomen. The fetal monitor is used to record your baby's heart rate and any contractions. The reaction of the baby's heart rate to its movements within the uterus is recorded.

The results will be given to your doctor to help him plan the care that is best for you and your baby.

The test should take about 40 minutes.

Your appointment is scheduled for _____ at _____ .

If you have any questions, please call _____ .

Instructions

1. You may eat your regular meal before the test. You should not be without food for more than 6 hours.

2. Wear comfortable, loose-fitting clothing.

3. Please stop at the Outpatient Registration Office located to the left of the Information Desk located on the first floor to register.

4. Before your appointment, empty your bladder to insure comfort during the test.

5. Then, please come to the FETAL MONITORING LAB WAITING ROOM # and give your name to the receptionist.

DIRECTIONS TO FETAL MONITORING LAB WAITING ROOM

After registering:

1. Left at Cashier

2. To elevators at green carpet

3. Up to 2nd Floor SOUTH CORRIDOR

4. Follow sign: FETAL MONITORING LAB WAITING ROOM # .

Figure B–8. Patient education pamphlet on the nonstress test (NST). (*Source: University of Rochester/Strong Memorial Hospital, Rochester, New York, with permission.*)

pattern. This can be assessed by external monitoring (fetal monitor) techniques without stress or stimulus to the fetus. Observation of average baseline variability and acceleration of fetal heart rate (FHR) in response to fetal movement is a reassuring sign that the fetus has good uteroplacental reserve. Decreased variability and absence of accelerations with fetal activity suggest the need for further evaluation of fetal well-being.

B. Procedure
(1) Have patient empty bladder to ensure comfort.
(2) Patient is placed in semi-Fowler's position (30 degree elevation of head) to avoid supine hypotension.
(3) Apply external monitor (transducer and tocodynamometer). Record FHR, contraction pattern, if any, and fetal activity. Fetal movements (FM) include visible, palpable, audible, or other perceivable fetal activity.
(4) Record baseline blood pressure and pulse; repeat every 15 minutes. Record on tracing.

C. Interpretation
(1) Reactive: Two or more accelerations in response to FM, amplitude of 15 bpm lasting 15 seconds in a 10-minute period, *or* five accelerations in a 20-minute period with same amplitude and duration.
    a. Management: Reassuring fetal well-being. Should labor occur within 1 week, fetus would be born in good condition.
(2) Nonreactive: Less than two accelerations with amplitude below 15 bpm or

lasting less than 15 seconds, *or* less than five accelerations in a 20-minute period with diminished amplitude and duration.

    a. Management: Proceed to oxytocin challenge test and contraction stress test.

5. Contraction stress test (CST)/Oxytocin challenge test (OCT):

   A. Purpose

      (1) The CST and OCT constitute a means of determining fetal well-being by assessing the degree of uteroplacental reserve. Uteroplacental circulation serves to provide the fetus with both nutritive and respiratory life support systems. The ability of the fetus to withstand a decreased oxygen supply can be assessed by providing a physiological stress, i.e., uterine contraction. Fetal response can be evaluated by simultaneous recording (fetal monitor) of spontaneous or induced contractions and FHR. The healthy fetus will exhibit reassuring FHR patterns (average baseline variability and accelerations of FHR with fetal movement). The compromised fetus will exhibit a nonreassuring FHR pattern (consistent late decelerations, decreased FHR variability, absence of acceleration with fetal movement, decreased or absent fetal activity).

   B. Procedure

      (1) Have patient empty bladder to insure comfort.

      (2) To avoid supine hypotension place patient in semi-Fowler's position.

      (3) Apply external monitor (transducer and tocodynomometer) and record baseline FHR and contraction pattern for 10 minutes, noting rate and reactivity.

CONTRACTION STRESS TEST

Your doctor has requested that you have a Contraction Stress Test (C.S.T.). The purpose of the test is to provide your doctor with information about how your baby is doing.

The test is performed with you lying in a bed. A light elastic band is used to hold small sensors from a fetal monitor on your abdomen. The fetal monitor is used to record your baby's heart rate and any contractions. The reaction of the baby's heart rate to its movements within the uterus is recorded. Your doctor also wants to see how a contraction affects the heart activity of your unborn baby. You will be given a small amount of a hormone--pitocin--by an intravenous (IV), which will cause you to have a few mild contractions.

The results will be given to your doctor to help him plan the care that is best for you and your baby.

The test should take about 40 minutes.

Your appointment is scheduled for _____ _____ at _____ .

If you have any questions, please call _____ .

INSTRUCTIONS

1. You may eat your regular meal before the test. You should not be without food for more than 6 hours.

2. Wear comfortable, loose-fitting clothing.

3. Please stop at the Outpatient Registration Office located to the left of the Information Desk located on the first floor to register.

4. Before your appointment, empty your bladder to insure comfort during the test.

5. Then, please come to the FETAL MONITORING LAB WAITING ROOM # and give your name to the receptionist.

DIRECTIONS TO FETAL MONITORING LAB WAITING ROOM

After registering:

1. Left at Cashier

2. To elevators at green carpet

3. Up to 2nd Floor SOUTH CORRIDOR

4. Follow Sign: FETAL MONITORING LAB WAITING ROOM # .

Figure B–9. Patient education pamphlet on the contraction stress test (CST). *(Source: University of Rochester/Strong Memorial Hospital, Rochester, New York, with permission.)*

      a. Note on tracing any periodic FHR changes, especially accelerations associated with fetal movements, which include visible, palpable, audible, or other perceivable fetal activity.

      b. If spontaneous uterine activity is such that there are three contractions within 10 minutes (3/10), obtain 30 minutes of contractions. If you obtain 3/10 and good quality contractions with interpretable FHR, it is not necessary to give oxytocin.

(4) Baseline blood pressure and pulse: Take initial BP and pulse; repeat every 15 minutes and *record* on tracing.

(5) Oxytocin administration:

      a. Oxytocin is piggybacked into intravenous set-up.

      b. Oxytocin: 1 ampule (10 units/1000 cc solution of Dextrose 5 in water) ½ ampule (5 units/500 cc solution of Dextrose 5 in water)

      c. Use lactated Ringers for diabetics.

      d. Using an intravenous infusion pump, start oxytocin at 0.5 mu/min or 3 cc/hr. Every 15 minutes increase oxytocin until contractions are established, moderately palpable (40–60 sec), and three contractions occur within a 10-minute period.

         i. Rate   3 cc/hr   0.5 mu/min

                     6 cc/hr   1.0 mu/min

                 15 cc/hr   2.5 mu/min

                 30 cc/hr   5.0 mu/min

                 60 cc/hr   10.0 mu/min

               120 cc/hr   20.0 mu/min

(6) Three contractions within 10 minutes, with good quality contractions and interpretable FHR, constitute a test period.

(7) When rate has been established, discontinue oxytocin. Continue monitoring until uterine activity returns to preoxytocin stimulation levels and heart rate is showing no signs of uteroplacental insufficiency.

C. Interpretation

(1) Negative: Three contractions within 10-minute period, moderately palpable, average baseline variability, acceleration of FHR with fetal movement; *no* late decelerations.

      a. Management: Assurance that fetus is likely to survive labor, should it occur in 1 week.

(2) Positive: Consistent late decelerations, even with less than three contractions within 10 minutes; variability may be decreased; FHR may not accelerate with fetal movement.

      a. Management: Further fetal assessment studies.

(3) Suspicious: Inconsistent but definite late decelerations that do not persist with continued uterine activity; baseline variability may be average or decreased; acceleration may be present.

      a. Management: Repeat in 24 hours.

(4) Hyperstimulation: Contractions more often than every 2 minutes or longer than 90 seconds; stress is considered enough to exceed normal uteroplacental reserve.

      a. Management: Repeat in 24 hours.

(5) Unsatisfactory: Quality of recording is not sufficient to interpret, e.g., artifact or unestablished contraction pattern.

      a. Management: Repeat in 24 hours.

AMNIOCENTESIS: TEACHING OBJECTIVES

The client will:

1. Define amniocentesis as the removal of amniotic fluid from the amniotic cavity by needle puncture.
2. Describe and state the reason for the procedure.
3. State that there is less than 1 percent risk to mother and fetus.
4. Describe amniotic fluid as consisting of fetal cells and secretions.
5. State that the lecithin to sphingomyelin (L/S) ratio is an indicator of fetal lung maturity.
6. State that in diabetic gestations, a mature L/S does not indicate that the neonate will not suffer from respiratory distress syndrome (RDS).
7. State that phosphatidyl glycerol (PG) present with a mature L/S is indicative that the neonate will not have RDS.

AMNIOCENTESIS: TEACHING GUIDELINES

1. Definition: Removal of fluid from the amniotic cavity by needle puncture.
2. Procedure
   A. See amniocentesis protocol (Fig. B–10).
   B. Variations in method may be employed, e.g., local anesthesia may be used to anesthetize the puncture site. Ultrasound may not be used to determine fetal position, dress of physician, etc.
   C. Consent forms.

Amniocentesis Protocol

Amniocentesis is a procedure in which a needle is inserted into the uterine cavity through the abdominal wall and a portion of the amniotic fluid is withdrawn.

Prior to the amniocentesis, an ultrasound examination will usually be performed to provide important information related to the amniocentesis. The ultrasound will determine gestational age, position of the fetus, location of the placenta, fetal heart activity and, most importantly, whether there is sufficient amniotic fluid to perform the amniocentesis safely. It will determine both depth and angle of needle insertion needed to reach the fluid.

Either the physician or ultrasound technologist will mark the patient's abdomen with a special dye where the needle is to be inserted. The site will be cleansed with betadine, and a sterile drape with hole will be placed over the area. The patient is not usually given lidocaine, because we have found that this does not make a difference. The physician will insert a 20 G spinal needle (3-½) to the proper depth, and up to 25 cc of amniotic fluid will be withdrawn.

After fluid is obtained, the needle will be withdrawn and a small Band-Aid will be placed over the puncture site. The ultrasound technologist will measure and record the distance between the symphysis and the puncture site. (S)he will also observe fetal activity.

The patient will be instructed to watch for signs of vaginal bleeding, leakage of amniotic fluid, or severe cramping. Although it is unlikely that any problems would occur, she must contact her care provider if they should. She is advised to refrain from strenous activity for 24 hours; no other precautions are given.

Women who are Rh negative and unsensitized will receive Rh immune globulin within 72 hours of the amniocentesis to prevent possible sensitization that could occur as a result of this procedure.

Figure B–10. Procedures protocol: Amniocentesis.

3. Risks
   A. Overall complications are less than 1 percent for both mother and fetus.
      (1) Maternal—hemorrhage, fetomaternal hemorrhage with possible isoimmunization, infection, labor, abruption, damage to intestine or bladder, amniotic fluid embolism.
      (2) Fetal—death, hemorrhage, infection (amnionitis), direct injury from the needle, abortion or premature labor, leakage of amniotic fluid.
4. Amniotic fluid analysis
   A. Amniotic fluid consists primarily of fetal urine and secretions and contains fetal cells. The sample is centrifuged to separate cells from the fluid.
   B. Lecithin to sphingomyelin (L/S) ratio
      (1) Primarily contains phospholipids
      (2) Surfactant acts as a surface detergent at the air–liquid interface of the alveoli, preventing their collapse at the end of expiration.
      (3) Without surfactant a neonate develops RDS, a condition associated with immaturity in which the lung collapses with each expiration.
   C. Color
      (1) Bloody tap—changes the level of other amniotic fluid constituents in the direction of predicting a less mature fetus.
      (2) Greenish-tinged or thick dark green sample—indicates the presence of meconium, associated with fetal hypoxia. Presence of meconium interferes with reliability of tests in L/S ratio and bilirubin delta OD.
5. Lecithin and sphingomyelin (L/S)
   A. Two phospholipids assessed by L/S ratio
   B. Comprise largest part of surfactant complex
   C. During gestation, sphingomyelin concentrations are less than lecithin until about 26 weeks. At 26–34 weeks, the concentration of the lecithin to sphingomyelin is fairly equal. From 34–36 weeks, there is a sudden increase in lecithin and the ratio rapidly rises.
   D. Ratio of 2.0 or greater indicates pulmonary maturity, and RDS will rarely occur in the neonate.
      Note: At SMH, 2.5 or greater is the accepted ratio.
   E. In a macrosomic fetus, as occurs in diabetic gestation, L/S is unreliable as an indicator of fetal lung maturity; RDS has been reported in neonates with mature L/S ratios.
6. Lung profile
   A. Measures interrelationships among surfactant phospholipids
      (1) L/S ratio
      (2) Disaturated (acetone precipitated) lecithin
7. Phosphatidyl inositol (PI) and phosphatidyl glycerol (PG)
   A. Acts as a lung stabilizer
   B. When present in diabetic gestations with a mature L/S, is a good predictor that RDS will not occur.

INTRAPARTUM: TEACHING OBJECTIVES

The client will:

1. Discuss the reason for monitoring glucose levels in blood and urine specimens obtained at periodic intervals during labor.

2. State that during labor insulin will be provided either subcutaneously or intravenously.
3. Describe the purpose and procedure for internal and external fetal monitoring during labor.
4. Discuss some reasons why diabetics are delivered prior to their anticipated due date by either labor induction or cesarean section.
5. State that a pediatrician will be in attendance at delivery and will assess the newborn's physiological needs.

INTRAPARTUM: TEACHING GUIDELINES

1. Energy needs during labor increase the amount of insulin due to:
   A. Increased uptake of glucose by the cells.
   B. Increased efficiency of glucose utilization.
   C. Mobilization of maternal glycogen stores.
   D. Patients are watched closely for hypoglycemia; the goal is to keep glucose levels constant and normal throughout labor, and to be aware of any sharp drop in insulin requirements postlabor and delivery.
2. Insulin needs are determined by closely monitoring blood glucose levels. During labor the route of choice for insulin is IV, because the patient will already be receiving IVs; however, some physicians may prefer the subcutaneous route (Fig. B–11).
3. Mechanical Fetal Monitoring Procedure
   A. Explain purpose of fetal monitoring.
      (1) The woman's physician will determine the need for fetal monitoring and type to be used, e.g., external or internal.
      (2) To have available a continuous and clear recording of the fetal heart and/or uterine activity for diagnostic purposes of the antepartal and intrapartal woman.
         a. Intended to assist the physician and nurse to render better care.
         b. Reassure that this procedure is not necessarily indicative of a problem.
         c. Reassure that the procedure will not hurt the mother and there are minimal risks to the fetus.
            i. With internal leads there is a small chance of scalp abcess or infection.
         d. Machine is sensitive and may show interference.
         e. Alarms indicate fetal heart rate changes, interference, or movement.
   B. Discuss external monitoring procedure if this procedure was requested (refer to procedure manual).
      (1) Directions accompany each machine and will vary with the machine.
      (2) Explain that leads may need readjusting when patient changes position.
      (3) Label all tracings appropriately.
   C. Discuss internal monitoring procedure if this procedure was requested. (Refer to facility procedure manual.)
      (1) Refer to directions accompanying machine.
      (2) Disconnect external cable to obtain recordings. Allow 15–30 seconds for adequate readout to begin.
      (3) Label all tracings appropriately.
4. It is the care provider's responsibility to explain the risk to benefit ratio for

IV Insulin Protocol

1. Purpose
   A. To achieve optimal glucose control for 48 hours prior to delivery of insulin dependent diabetics.
   B. To provide continuous insulin, pulsed to meals.
2. Method
   A. Enabling facts: Addition of albumin to insulin solution eliminates glass or plastic binding of insulin.
   B. Solution preparation:
       500 ml of normal saline
       50 units of regular insulin
   C. Infusion rates:
        5 cc/hr   0.5 unit insulin/hr
       10 cc/hr   1.0 unit insulin/hr
       15 cc/hr   1.5 unit insulin/hr
       20 cc/hr   2.0 unit insulin/hr
       25 cc/hr   2.5 unit insulin/hr
       30 cc/hr   3.0 unit insulin/hr
       Always piggyback insulin to D_5LR at 30 cc/hr.
   D. Control: Heparin lock for blood glucoses. First 6 hours sample every hours. Then 2 hr pc and fasting.
   E. Patients able to eat while on intravenous fluids:
       (1) Meals: Approximately every 6 hours: Equally divided calories and glucose load.
       (2) Infusions: Approximately 1–3 hours at 1.5 times calculated hourly requirement, then hours 1–6, 0.5 the hourly requirement.
           a. Calculation of hourly insulin requirement:
               i. Total calories ÷ total insulin = cal/unit
               ii. Total calories ÷ 24 hours = cal/hour
               iii. Cal/hour ÷ cal/unit = unit/hour
           b. Patients on IV glucose (uniform infusion): Infuse at constant rate.
               i. 50 g glucose/6 hours = 8.3 g/hr or $D_{10}W$ at 83 cc/hr (33 cal/hr)
               ii. 33 cal/hr ÷ cal/unit = units/hour (4 cal/g glucose)
       (3) *Example:* 19-year-old Class C diabetic on 2200 cal diet and 44 units of insulin per 24 hours period: Diet order (1) 2200 cal every 5 hours; feedings equally divided.
           a. Diet: Calculation of hourly rate of insulin requirement:
               i. Total cal ÷ total insulin = cal/unit
                  2200 cal ÷ 44 units = 50 cal/unit
               ii. Total cal ÷ 24 hours = cal/hour
                  2200 cal ÷ 24 = 91.6 cal/hour
               iii. Cal/hour ÷ cal/unit = units/hour
                  91.6 cal/hour ÷ 50 cal/unit = 1.8 units hour
               Mean insulin requirement is therefore 1.8 units/hour.

Figure B–11. Procedures protocol: IV insulin.

delivery to the patient. The patient should understand that the aim is to deliver when the fetus is healthiest.

A. Class D, F, and R diabetics often have small for gestational age babies (SGA). These babies may be delivered by low forceps or cesarean section to prevent CNS pressure during delivery.

B. The large for gestational age (LGA) baby could encounter problems during delivery because of excessive size, thus resulting in a "tight fit" in the maternal pelvis and birth canal. To facilitate delivery of the LGA baby, the mother usually has to push longer and often must have a low forceps delivery, vacuum extraction, or cesarean section. (Macrosomia is not encountered as often as in previous years due to better control of pregnant diabetic women.)

5. The obstetrician will decide whether or not a pediatrician will be in attendance at the delivery. The client should be encouraged to discuss with the obstetrician plans regarding pediatrician involvement.

IV INSULIN PROTOCOL

1. Purpose
   A. To achieve optimal glucose control for 48 hours prior to delivery of insulin-dependent diabetics.
   B. To provide continuous insulin infusion, pulsed to meals.
2. Method
   A. Enabling facts: Addition of albumin to insulin solution eliminates glass or plastic binding of insulin.
   B. Solution preparation:
      500 ml of normal saline
      50 units of regular insulin
   C. Infusion rates:
      5 cc/hour = 0.5 unit insulin/hour
      10 cc/hour = 1.0 unit insulin/hour
      15 cc/hour = 1.5 unit insulin/hour
      20 cc/hour = 2.0 unit insulin/hour
      25 cc/hour = 2.5 unit insulin/hour
      30 cc/hour = 3.0 unit insulin/hour
      Always piggyback insulin to D_5LR at 30 cc/hour.
   D. Control: Heparin lock for blood glucoses. First 6 hours sample every hour. Then 2 hour p.c. and fasting.
   E. Patients able to eat while on intravenous fluids:
      (1) Meals: Approximately every 6 hours: Equally divided calories and glucose load.
      (2) Infusions: Approximately 1–3 hours at 1.5 times calculated hourly requirement, then hours 1–6, .5 the hourly requirement.
         a. Calculation of hourly insulin requirement:
            i. Total calories ÷ total insulin = *cal/unit*
            ii. Total calories ÷ 24 hours = *cal/hour*
            iii. Cal/hour ÷ cal/unit = *units/hour*
         b. Patients on IV glucose (uniform infusion): Infuse at constant rate.
            i. 50 gm glucose/6 hours = 8.3 gm/hour or $D_{10}W$ at 83 cc/hour (33 cal/hour)
            ii. 33 cal/hour ÷ cal/unit = *units/hour* (4 cal/gm glucose)
      (3) Example: 19 year old Class C diabetic on 2200 cal diet and 44 units of insulin per 24 hours period: Diet order (1) 2200 cal every 5 hours; feedings equally divided.
         a. Diet: Calculation of hourly rate of insulin requirement:
            i. Total cal ÷ total insulin = cal/unit
               2200 cal ÷ 44 units = 50 cal/unit
            ii. Total cal ÷ 24 hours = cal/hour
               2200 cal ÷ 24 = *91.6 cal/hour*
            iii. Cal/hour ÷ cal/unit = units/hour
               91.6 cal/hour ÷ 50 cal/unit = 1.8 units/hour
      Mean insulin requirement is therefore 1.8 units/hour.

b. *Infusion Protocol:*

0–3 hours
1.5 × hourly requirement
1.5 × 1.8 units/hour = 2.7 units/hour

3–6 hours
0.5 × hourly requirement
0.5 × 1.8 units/hour = 0.9 units/hour

For q6 hr diet, then infusion rates of:
0–3 hours
2.7 units/hour = *27 cc/hour*
(10 cc/hour = 1 unit/hour) 2.7 × 10 = 27 cc/hour

3–6 hours
0.9 units/hour = 9 cc/hour
(10 cc/hour = 1 unit/hour) = 0.9 units/hour = (0.9) × (10) or 9 cc/hour

F. IV Glucose only—no oral fluids or food.
    (1) Per protocol 83 cc/hour $D_{10}W$ = 33 cal/hour
        33 cal/hour ÷ cal/unit = units/hour
        33 cal/hour ÷ 50 cal/unit = 0.66 units/hour
    (2) Infusion rate: 0.6 units/hour at 10 cc/hour = 1 unit/hour = 6.6 or 7 cc/hour

Note: One may need to adjust insulin rates slightly based on blood glucose values. Two intravenous infusion systems are required for intravenous glucose/insulin administration.

POSTPARTUM NEWBORN: TEACHING OBJECTIVES

The client will:

1. Discuss glucose metabolism in the newborn.
    A. Describe briefly the process of glucose metabolism in the newborn, during the immediate neonatal period, prior to adequate oral intake.
    B. Identify the time, postdelivery, when the newborn's blood glucose is normally lowest.
2. Define hypoglycemia in the newborn period as a temporary problem that will be resolved by the time of discharge.
3. Discuss screening methods for hypoglycemia in the newborn.
4. Describe treatment of hypoglycemia in the newborn.

POSTPARTUM NEWBORN: TEACHING GUIDELINES

1. Glucose metabolism
    A. It is extremely important for the nurse to obtain a history related to pregnancy experiences. The fetus has had all nutrients delivered via the placenta, but after birth the newborn is entirely dependent upon the external environment. Energy is required for muscular activity, respiration, and maintenance of body temperature. This energy must be derived from the infant's own body

store, or from an oral or intravenous intake source. As energy demands increase, the maternal glucose supply is no longer available and the neonate responds by glucogenesis, which is the formation of glucose from noncarbohydrate sources such as protein and possible fats. Glucogenesis occurs in the liver under such conditions as low carbohydrate intake or starvation; therefore, immediate attention to blood dextrostixs and feeding are essential.

  B. Blood glucose. The blood glucose of a newborn usually reaches its lowest level at 1 or 2 hours of age. A spontaneous rise in glucose usually follows, attaining acceptable levels by about age 4 to 6 hours. However, there are infants who will not have a spontaneous rise and will become hypoglycemic.

2. Hypoglycemia in the newborn period
  A. Hypoglycemia occurs when blood glucose in the newborn should be maintained above 40 mg/100 ml. Hypoglycemia is a temporary condition that will be resolved before discharge of the baby.

3. Screening methods
  A. Dextrostix are checked on admission and every 30 minutes until the dextrostix is over 45 mg% × 3, then before each feeding for 24 hours. If the dextrostix is below the normal range, a blood glucose level will be drawn to determine if the newborn is hypoglycemic. If the blood glucose is below the normal range, treatment will be instituted.

4. Treatment of hypoglycemia in the newborn
  A. Prophylactic care should be initiated as soon as an infant is identified to be "at risk." Early oral or tube feedings should be started, if appropriate. If not, as in the case of respiratory distress, an intravenous solution of Dextrose 10 in water would be started. This is accomplished with an infusion pump, and continues until the baby can take adequate oral feeding to maintain blood glucose levels within a normal range. During this period, frequent assessments by dextrostix will be continued. As the infant is able to maintain appropriate blood glucose levels, the intravenous infusion must be gradually decreased.

POSTPARTUM MATERNAL: TEACHING OBJECTIVES

The client will:

1. Describe insulin requirements of a postpartum mother within the first 24–48 hours, 48 hours to 6 weeks, and 6 weeks thereafter.
2. Describe a postpartum diet.
3. Discuss future projected family size.
4. Verbalize concerns during the postpartum period to the care provider.
5. Describe appropriate contraceptive alternatives for use by the diabetic.
6. Identify local community resources available to the diabetic.
7. State when it is necessary to contact the care provider.

POSTPARTUM MATERNAL: TEACHING GUIDELINES

1. Insulin requirements
  A. "Within the first 24 to 48 hours after delivery, the diabetic mother's insulin requirement will rapidly fluctuate" (Rancilio, 1979).

(1) Frequently, the mother will need less insulin than she required prior to becoming pregnant; individual needs will vary. "As soon as the baby is born, the mother's endocrine system will reverse gestation-induced requirements. Therefore, you may see a decrease in serum blood sugars, human growth hormone (HGH), and human placental lactogen (HPL)" (Rancilio, 1979). During this time, little or no insulin may be needed.

B. From 48 hours to 6 weeks after delivery, the mother's insulin needs will be evaluated by the care provider. The increase in the mother's physical activity after delivery tends to reduce insulin needs for a time. A combination of long-acting and regular insulin may be used.

C. At approximately 6 weeks, when all body systems have returned to homeostasis, the mother's insulin requirements will probably return to that of the prepregnant state.

D. If the mother is breast-feeding or medical complications occur, the insulin dosage may need to be adjusted accordingly.

2. Diet
   A. For nonlactating mothers, diet would not be altered to any great extent. The diet would simply be a calorie-regulated ADA diet, per care provider's decision.
   B. For lactating mothers, diet needs to be increased within the range of 400–800 calories a day to compensate for loss by milk production. Some of these extra calories could easily be absorbed in increased fluids, such as fruit juices or milk, which would also help in milk production.
   C. When complications, e.g., hemorrhage or infection, occur during the involution period, diet will need to be altered. Also, if breast-feeding is interrupted or stopped, the patient will need to contact her care provider to regulate diet and insulin needs.

3. Considerations for future family size
   A. Medical complications
      (1) The obstetrical risk factor for future pregnancies is determined by the patient's diabetic condition, based on White's classification (Burrow & Ferris, 1975).
      (2) Parity: because of residual complications from each pregnancy, subsequent pregnancies place the patient at increased risk.
      (3) Age: the age of the mother is an important consideration. When planning future children, there is a 5–10 percent risk of birth defects with diabetic mothers, and the risk increases with age (Burrow & Ferris, 1975, p. 180).

4. The client should contact the care provider for any alteration in diet, method of infant feeding, contraception, or physical and emotional status, because control of diabetes may be directly related to these factors.
   A. Stress factors
      Because pregnancy is a stressful time (Caplan, 1961) and diabetics experience an even higher degree of stress (Galloway, 1976), it is imperative to consider the following issues when discussing family planning: frequent antepartum hospitalizations, increased financial demands, home care for family, interruption of family life, and previous obstetrical and neonatal outcomes.
   B. Location (distance from home to high risk unit)
      Because of the need for an experienced and skilled medical team in managing pregnancy and diabetes, it is important to consider such issues as location of

perinatal center and distance from home, accessibility, and cost of frequent travel.

C. Desire for more children

The desire of both the woman and her partner should be considered when discussing family planning, method of birth control, and problems childbirth can present to the diabetic woman.

5. Contraception

A. Birth control pills have been shown to have a diabetogenic effect. Alterations may occur in carbohydrate metabolism; therefore, insulin requirements may change. Vascular problems associated with diabetes may be potentiated with the use of oral contraceptives (Pritchard, MacDonald, & Gant, 1985, p. 604); therefore, oral contraceptives are not usually recommended for diabetic women.

B. Intrauterine device (IUD)

"The risk of pelvic infection from an intrauterine device is a very likely increased in the diabetic woman" (Pritchard, MacDonald, & Gant, 1985, p. 604).

C. Barrier method and foam

Barrier methods and foam are good methods for a well-motivated woman. There are no increased risks for the diabetic woman who chooses to use these methods.

D. Sterilization: Bilateral tubal ligation (BTL), vasectomy

These methods are appropriate for patients who have either completed their families or have a medical reason for limiting family size.

E. Natural Family Planning

This method uses neither artificial nor mechanical contraceptives and, therefore, is not contraindicated for use by the diabetic patient.

6. Communication

The care provider must create an atmosphere in which the client will feel comfortable in expressing concerns.

7. Community resources: In addition to the patient's primary health care provider, there are several support agencies that may offer a variety of services.

A. *American Diabetic Association*—2 Park Avenue, New York, NY 10016. (Membership includes a bimonthly magazine, *Diabetic Forecast*, and quarterly national and chapter newsletters. The magazine and newsletters provide useful information on diabetes care, as well as recipes for the diabetic.) Check with your local chapter.

B. *March of Dimes*—1275 Marmaroneck Avenue, White Plains, NY 10605. Check with your local chapter.

C. Women Infants and Children (W.I.C.) Program—check with your local department of health or social services.

D. County Department of Health—check with your local health department.

GLOSSARY

Acceleration. Periodic increases in fetal heart rate.

Acidosis. A condition resulting from accumulation of acid or depletion of alkaline reserves in the blood and body tissues.

Adrenal. Near the kidney; produced by the adrenal gland.

Adrenalin. *See* epinephrine.

Amniocentesis. Needle aspiration of fluid surrounding fetus.

Amniotic sac. Membranous sac enveloping the fetus and the fluid surrounding the fetus.

Amplitude. Wideness of range.

Analgesia. Absence of normal sense of pain.

Anorexia. Lack or loss of appetite.

ARM. Artifical rupture of membranes by means of an amnihood (resembles a crochet hook) done during a vaginal examination and does not hurt any more than the examination. The color, consistency, and amount of the fluid is noted.

Bacteriuria. Presence of bacteria in the urine.

Biosynthesis. Formation of a chemical compound by enzymes.

Candida albicans. (Monilia) A genus of yeast-like fungus. May flare up during pregnancy because of the increased glycogen content of the vaginal epithelium.

Carbohydrate. Sugars and starches in the diet.

Cervix. The narrow, lower end of the uterus extending into the vagina and serving as a passageway between the two organs.

Chronic. Persisting for a long time.

Cortisone. A carbohydrate-regulating hormone from the adrenal cortex.

CPD. Cephalopelvic disproportion. This cannot always be foreseen. There may be forewarnings during measurement of mother's pelvis of a "border line" pelvis, but more factors come into play.

Creatinine clearance. A laboratory test for measuring kidney function.

Deceleration. Periodic decreases in fetal heart rate.

Demerol. A white, odorless, crystalline compound, soluble in water, and has an analgesic effect similar to morphine.

Diabetes mellitus. A disease of metabolism characterized by high blood sugar and a deficiency of insulin.

Diabetogenic. Produces diabetes.

Dysuria. Painful urination.

Eclampsia. A major toxemia of pregnancy accompanied by hypertension, albuminuria, oliguria (scant urine), edema, convulsions, and coma. The kidneys, brain, heart, liver, and placenta can be involved.

Effacement. The thinning-out of the normally thick cervix in the early stage of labor to facilate dilatation.

Embryo. The product of conception during the first 3 months of gestation.

Epidural (continuous). A type of anesthesia given by means of a plastic catheter into the epidural space of the spinal canal. An intervenous line must always be in place, FH and P monitoring. The nurse helps the patient maintain the "arched cat" position for the insertion of the catheter after the proper cleansing of the area. Under sterile conditions, the catheter is taped in place and a syringe attached to the top end by the shoulder, and taped safely, usually to the gown.

Epinephrine (adrenalin). Chief hormone secreted at nerve synapses.

Estriols. Predominant estrogenic metabolite found in urine.

Estrogen. A female sex hormone.

Fats. Compounds consisting of carbon, hydrogen, and oxygen in various chemical combinations.

Fetal. Pertaining to developing fetus in the uterus.

Fetus. The product of conception after the third month of gestation.

Forceps. A pair of tongs for holding or extracting the fetus. There are many different types.

Genetic. Hereditary.

Gestation. Period of intrauterine fetal development. Synonyms: pregnancy, gravidity.

Gestational age. Developmental age of fetus.

Glucose. A simple sugar.

Glycosuria. Abnormally high sugar content in the urine.

Hormone. A chemical substance secreted by a gland that circulates in the bloodstream and produces effects elsewhere in the body.

HPL. Human placental lactogen. A hormone produced by the placenta that increases the mobilization of free fatty acids and diminishes the effect of maternal insulin.

Hyperglycemia. High blood sugar.

Hypoglycemia. Low blood sugar.

Hypoxemia. Deficient oxygen in the blood.

Insulin. A hormone produced by the pancreas that facilitates the passage of glucose from the blood into the body cells, resulting in lowering of the level of the blood sugar.

Intrauterine. Within the uterus.

Ketoacidosis. A severe, life-threatening illness in diabetes caused by the accumulation of ketones in the blood in which the body fluids become acid.

Ketonuria. Ketones in the urine.

Kidneys. Two bean-shaped, glandular organs that secrete urine and are located in the lumbar region. Their function is to regulate the content of water and other substances in the blood and to remove various wastes from the blood.

Lethargy. Stupor or coma resulting from disease.

LGA. Large for gestational age.

Liver. A large gland located in the upper right portion of the abdomen.

MBE. Micro blood examination. A minute specimen of blood is obtained from the baby's scalp with the aid of a special scope and probe during a vaginal examination and examined rapidly for pH of baby's blood denoting degree of acidosis present, to safely continue labor or quickly deliver via forceps, vacuum or C-section.

Meconium. The first feces of a newborn infant, greenish black or light brown, tarry consistency, almost odorless. When present before or during birth is usually an indication of some degree of fetal distress, especially if the fetus is less than 36 weeks.

Metabolic. Concerns metabolism.

Metabolism. Sum total of physical and chemical processes and reactions of the body.

Metabolites. Compounds produced during metabolism.

Nausea. The distressing feeling that vomiting may occur.

Obesity. Excessive accumulation of fat in the body.

Oxytocin. Hormone produced by the pituitary gland that acts as a stimulant to pregnant uterus, resulting in contractions.

Pancreas. A gland in the abdomen located just behind the stomach that manufactures insulin and secretes it into the bloodstream when the blood sugar level of the body is increased.

Perceivable. To become aware of through the senses.

Perfusion. Passing of a fluid through spaces.

Peridontal. A disease process affecting the tissues about a tooth.

Physiological. Normal.

Placenta. The organ that transfers glucose, oxygen, and other components in the blood from the mother to the fetus.

Polyhydramnios. An excess of amniotic fluid in the amniotic sac. Can be associated with other problems, e.g., congenital anomalies.

Prandial. Pertaining to a meal.

Preeclampsia. A toxemia (poisoning) of pregnancy of unknown etiology (cause) characterized by hypertension, which increases headaches, protein in the urine, and edema of lower extremities. If untreated, can progress to a more serious disease, eclampsia.

Prenatal. Period before birth.

Presenting part. Term applied to the manner in which the fetus presents itself to the examining finger, at the mouth (cervix) of the uterus.

Progesterone. A progestational hormone, which induces changes in the endometrium to prepare the uterus for implantation of the fertilized ovum and maintenance of pregnancy.

Protein. Compounds containing carbon, hydrogen, oxygen, sulphur, phosphorus, especially nitrogen. Necessary for building and repair of body tissues.

Pyorrhea. A discharge of pus.

Retinopathy. Disease of the retina. Occurs with prolonged, poorly controlled diabetes and involves abnormal growth of and bleeding from the capillary blood vessels in the eye.

SGA. Small for gestational age.

Supine. Lying flat, face upward.

Tachycardia. Abnormally rapid heart rate.

Tetanic contraction. A constant muscular contraction of the uterus.

Tocodynamometer. Monitors uterine activity.

Transducer. Monitors fetal heart rate.

Ureter. A narrow, muscular, foot-long tube that conducts urine from the kidney to the urinary bladder.

Urinary bladder. A hollow sac with muscular walls into which the urine drains.

Urinary tract. The system composed of the kidneys, urinary bladder, ureters, and the urethra.

Uteroplacental. Relating to the uterus and the placenta.

Vacuum extraction. A type of delivery accomplished by the means of a lubricated metal cap, applied to the fetus' caput, and increasing amounts of air forced through a tube to help pull the fetus down and out. The obstetrician pulls down as the mother pushes to facilitate delivery. The gauge is monitored to maintain and increase the vacuum pressure. The resultant swelling in the baby's head is harmless and disappears within a few days.

Vagina. Musculomembranous canal that extends from the lower part of the vulva to the cervix, connecting the external and internal reproductive organs.

Variability. Normal irregularity of cardiac rhythm.

Venipuncture. Puncture of vein for collection of blood specimens.

Vulva. The external parts of the female reproductive system that surround the opening of the vagina.

BIBLIOGRAPHY

Burrow, G. N., & Ferris, T. A. (Eds.). *Medical complications during pregnancy*. Philadelphia: W. B. Saunders, 1975.

Caplan, G. *An approach to community mental health*. New York: Grune & Stratton, 1961.

Galloway, K. The uncertainty and stress of high-risk pregnancy. *Maternal–Child Nursing*, 1976, *1*(5), 294–299.

Lilly Research Laboratories. *Diabetes mellitus*. Indianapolis, Ind.: Eli Lilly, 1973.

Merkatz, I. R., & Adams, P. A. J. (Eds.). *The diabetic pregnancy: A perinatal perspective*. New York: Grune & Stratton, 1979.

Pritchard, J. A., MacDonald, P. C., & Gant, F. G. *Williams obstetrics* (17th ed.). Norwalk, Conn.: Appleton-Century-Crofts, 1985.

Rancilio, N. When a pregnant women is diabetic: Postpartal care. *American Journal of Nursing*, 1979, 79(3), 453–456.

Gynecological Care Plans

University of Rochester
Strong Memorial Hospital

SMH# 626

7/81

OB/GYN NURSING

PATIENT CARE PLAN

VAGINAL PROCEDURE

DATE	INT.	Prob. #	NURSING DIAGNOSIS/ PATIENT PROBLEM	EXPECTED OUTCOMES/ GOALS	NURSING INTERVENTION	PROBLEM STATUS REVISED/RESOLVED/RESPONSE
		1	Knowledge deficit related to pre/postoperative routine.	1. Prior to surgery, the patient will: a. state what sens- ations/procedures to expect. b. state that all ques- tions have been answered.	Based on assessment: ā surgery conduct discussion with patient in- cluding expected: pre/post-op routine; fluids/diet/activity limit- ations and resumption; incision and drainage, discomfort and medications; pulmonary toilet; catheter use and voiding; review normal pelvic anatomy as it relates to procedure. allow for expression of feelings; clarify misconceptions.	
		2	Altered patterns of urinary elimination r/t prox. of bldr/ureters to operative field; catheter.	1. Pt. maintains urine output of > 30 cc/hr. 2. Within 24 hrs. post- op pt. voids spontan- eously, and continues without discomfort there- after, OR pt. will void with <100 cc residuals after catheter removal.	Maintain hydration; check catheter patency/connections, spgr, BUN. Perineal care b.i.d. and prn. Assess and record freq./quan. of voids, bladder distention/abd. discomfort; dysuria. Attempt to stimulate voiding, if HNV in 8° notify HO. See OB/GYN Nursing Procedure entitled Nursing Care of the Patient With Suprapubic Drainage.	

Primary Nurse _____ Associate Nurse _____

Adm. Date	Trans. Date	OR Date	Emergency Phone #	Diagnosis
Room #	Name	Age	Doctor	

Figure C–1. Gynecological care plan: Vaginal procedure. (cont.)

717

OB/GYN Nursing VAGINAL PROCEDURE

DATE	INT.	Prob #	NURSING DIAGNOSIS/ PATIENT PROBLEM	EXPECTED OUTCOMES/ GOALS	NURSING INTERVENTION	PROBLEM STATUS	
						REVISED	RESOLVED RESPONSE
		3	Ineffective breathing patterns r/t anesthesia discomfort; narcotics used.	1. Within 48 hours post-operatively, the patient will have normal breath sounds c̄ prod. cough.	Immed. post-op initiate pulmonary regimen at least q2°. Assess breath sounds, VS prn. Ambulate ASAP post-op, as ordered.		
		4	Alteration in bowel elimination: nausea r/t anesthesia.	1. Pt. does not have emesis postoperatively.	Assess and record; abdomen, bowel sounds, flatus, intake, prn. Evaluate effectiveness of antiemetic.		
			Constipation r/t anesthesia and operative manipulations.	2. Patient will evacuate bowel before discharge.	Enc. amb; avoid gaseous foods once on liquids; give prune j., coffee. Apply heating pad prn. Assess and record effectiveness of measures to stimulate bowel evacuation.		
		5	Alteration in comfort: Pain r/t incision and/ or surgical manipulation.	1. Within 48 hours post-op, patient's pain is at level allowing amb. and nml. self-care activities.	Assess patient discomfort at least q3° x 24° then prn. Institute comfort measures. Reinforce body mech. to pain. Assess and record effectiveness of pain medication.		
		6	Potential for injury: hemorrhage.	During hospital stay pt. does not experience hypovolemia as noted by: VS within pt.'s baseline; drainage <200 cc. per site per shift.	Assess and record: VS, LOC, quan/qual of drainage prn. Assist c̄ position q2° x 24°.		

INT	FULL SIGNATURE	TITLE	INT	FULL SIGNATURE	TITLE	INT	FULL SIGNATURE	TITLE

Figure C–1. (cont.) Gynecological care plan: Vaginal procedure. (cont.)

University of Rochester
Strong Memorial Hospital

SMH# 626
7/81

OB/GYN NURSING
PATIENT CARE PLAN

Page 3 of 3

VAGINAL PROCEDURE

DATE	INT.	Prob #	NURSING DIAGNOSIS/ PATIENT PROBLEM	EXPECTED OUTCOMES/ GOALS	NURSING INTERVENTION	PROBLEM STATUS REVISED/RESOLVED/RESPONSE
			thromboembolism.	Remains free of thrombo-embolism.	Remove antiems, bid. Assess LE for heat/redness/Homan's sign. Have patient ambulate; do leg exercises. Do not allow crossed legs or sitting c̄ knees bent for >20 min. Record pt. activity and tolerance.	
		7	Potential for ineffective indiv. coping r/t impact on fertility/sexuality.	1. The patient will communicate fears/concerns.	Supply accurate info pre/post-op re: common fears/myths. Review normal anatomy. Record pt. response/questions. Determine sexual interests/practices, any post-op limitations. Involve partner as needed.	
		8	Potential for infection related to surgical procedure.	1. Throughout hospitalization, the patient remains infection-free.	Assess and record q shift and prn; VS; urine/wound/vaginal drainage (color/odor/quan.) Check CBC and culture results.	
		9	Potential for impaired home maintenance management r/t post-op limitations and recuperation after discharge.	Patient returns home with assistance as needed and as arranged prior to discharge.	On day of admission and throughout hospitalization, assess pt/family for actual/potential postdischarge problems. If problem suspected, verify with pt/family. Confer with them, other providers and community resources to develop and implement plan.	
			Approved 9/83 Revised 11/83			

Primary Nurse

Associate Nurse

Adm. Date	Trans. Date		OR Date		Emergency Phone #	Diagnosis
Room #	Name		Age		Doctor	

Figure C–1. (cont.) Gynecological care plan: Vaginal procedure. *(Source: University of Rochester/Strong Memorial Hospital, Rochester, New York, with permission.)*

University of Rochester
Strong Memorial Hospital

SMH# 626

7/81 LAPAROTOMY

OB/GYN NURSING
PATIENT CARE PLAN

Page 1 of 3

DATE	Prob. #	INT.	NURSING DIAGNOSIS/ PATIENT PROBLEM	EXPECTED OUTCOMES/ GOALS	NURSING INTERVENTION	PROBLEM STATUS REVISED/RESOLVED/RESPONSE
	1		Knowledge deficit related to pre/postoperative routine.	1. Prior to surgery, the patient will: a. state what sensations/ procedures to expect. b. state that all questions have been answered.	Based on assessment; a surgery conduct discussion with patient including expected: pre/post-op routine, fluids/ diet/activity limitations and resumption; incision and drainage; discomfort and medications, pulmonary toilet; catheter use and voiding; review normal pelvic anatomy as it relates to procedure. Allow for expression of feelings; clarify misconceptions.	
	2		Altered patterns of urinary elimination r/t prox. of bldr/ureters to operative field; catheter.	1. Pt. maintains urine output of ≥ 30 cc/hr. 2. Within 24 hrs. post-op pt. voids spontaneously, and continues as without discomfort thereafter.	Maintain hydration; check catheter patency/connections, spgr, BUN. Perineal care b.i.d. and prn. Assess and record freq./quan. of voids, bladder distention/abd. discomfort; dysuria. Attempt to stimulate voiding, if HNV in 8° notify HO.	
	3		Ineffective breathing patterns r/t anesthesia, discomfort, narcotics used.	1. Within 48 hours postoperatively, the patient will have normal breath sounds & prod. cough.	Immed. post-op initiate pulmonary regimen at least q2°. Assess breath sounds, VS prn. Ambulate ASAP post-op, as ordered	

Primary Nurse

Adm. Date	Trans. Date	OR Date	Emergency Phone #	Diagnosis
Room #	Name	Age	Doctor	

Associate Nurse

Figure C–2. Gynecological care plan: Laparotomy. (cont.)

OB/GYN Nursing LAPAROTOMY

DATE	INT	Prob #	NURSING DIAGNOSIS/ PATIENT PROBLEM	EXPECTED OUTCOMES/ GOALS	NURSING INTERVENTION	PROBLEM STATUS REVISED / RESOLVED / RESPONSE
		4	Alteration in bowel elimination: nausea, r/t anesthesia.	1. Pt. does not have emesis post-operatively	Assess and record: abdomen, bowel sounds, flatus, intake, prn. Evaluate effectiveness of antiemetic. Enc amb; avoid gaseous	
			Constipation r/t anesthesia and operative manipulations.	2. Patient will evacuate bowel before discharge.	foods once on liquids; give prune j., coffee. Apply heating pad prn. Assess and record effectiveness of measures to stimulate bowel evacuation.	
		5	Alteration in comfort: pain r/t incision and/or surgical manipulation.	1. Within 48 hrs. post-op, patient's pain is at level allowing amb. and nml self-care activities.	Assess patient discomfort at least q3° x 24° then prn. Institute comfort measures. Reinforce body mech. to ↓ pain. Assess and record effectiveness of pain medication.	
		6	Potential for injury: hemorrhage.	During hospital stay pt. does not experience hypovolemia as noted by VS within pt.'s baseline; drainage <200 cc. per site per shift.	Assess and record: VS, I0C, quan/qual of drainage prn. Assist c̄ position q2° x 24°	
			thromboembolism.	Remains free of thromboembolism.	Remove antiems. b.i.d. Assess LE for heat/ redness/Homan's sign. Have patient ambulate; do leg exercises. Do not allow crossed legs or sitting c̄ knees bent for >20 min. Record pt. activity and tolerance.	

INT	FULL SIGNATURE	TITLE	INT	FULL SIGNATURE	TITLE	INT	FULL SIGNATURE	TITLE

Figure C–2. (cont.) Gynecological care plan: Laparotomy. (cont.)

APPLETON/Littlefield 141-F
Final Page No. 721

University of Rochester
Strong Memorial Hospital

SMH# 626
7/81   LAPAROTOMY

OB/GYN NURSING

PATIENT CARE PLAN

DATE	INT	Prob #	NURSING DIAGNOSIS/ PATIENT PROBLEM	EXPECTED OUTCOMES/ GOALS	NURSING INTERVENTION	PROBLEM STATUS REVISED/RESOLVED/RESPONSE
		7	Potential for ineffective indiv. coping r/t impact on fertility/sexuality.	1. The patient will communicate fears/concerns.	Supply accurate info pre/post-op, re: common fears/myths. Review normal anatomy. Record pt. response/questions. Determine sexual interests/ practices, any post-op limitations. Involve partner as needed.	
		8	Potential for infection related to surgical procedure.	1. Throughout hospitalization, the patient remains infection free.	Assess and record q shift and prn: VS; urine/wound/vaginal drainage (color/ odor/quan.) Check CBC and culture results.	
		9	Potential for impaired home maintenance management r/t post-op limitations and re-cuperation after discharge.	Patient returns home with assistance as needed and arranged prior to discharge.	On day of admission and throughout hospitalization, assess pt/family for actual/potential postdischarge problems. If problem suspected, verify with pt/family. Confer with them, other providers and community resources to develop and implement plan.	

Approved 9/23
Rev'sed 11/83

Primary Nurse				Associate Nurse	
Adm. Date	Trans. Date	OR Date	Emergency Phone #	Diagnosis	
Room #	Name	Age	Doctor		

Figure C–2. (cont.) Gynecological care plan: Laparotomy. (Source: University of Rochester/ Strong Memorial Hospital, Rochester, New York, with permission.)

722

Index

Italicized page numbers refer to figures and tables.